Advances in Geriatric Diseases

Advances in Geriatric Diseases

Editor

Francesco Mattace-Raso

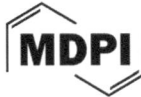

Basel • Beijing • Wuhan • Barcelona • Belgrade • Novi Sad • Cluj • Manchester

Editor
Francesco Mattace-Raso
Erasmus MC University
Medical Center
Rotterdam
The Netherlands

Editorial Office
MDPI AG
Grosspeteranlage 5
4052 Basel, Switzerland

This is a reprint of articles from the Special Issue published online in the open access journal *Journal of Clinical Medicine* (ISSN 2077-0383) (available at: https://www.mdpi.com/journal/jcm/special_issues/Geriatric_Diseases).

For citation purposes, cite each article independently as indicated on the article page online and as indicated below:

Lastname, A.A.; Lastname, B.B. Article Title. *Journal Name* **Year**, *Volume Number*, Page Range.

ISBN 978-3-7258-2567-7 (Hbk)
ISBN 978-3-7258-2568-4 (PDF)
doi.org/10.3390/books978-3-7258-2568-4

© 2024 by the authors. Articles in this book are Open Access and distributed under the Creative Commons Attribution (CC BY) license. The book as a whole is distributed by MDPI under the terms and conditions of the Creative Commons Attribution-NonCommercial-NoDerivs (CC BY-NC-ND) license.

Contents

About the Editor ix

Francesco Mattace-Raso
It Is Time for Senescience
Reprinted from: *J. Clin. Med.* **2022**, *11*, 4542, doi:10.3390/jcm11154542 1

Cristina Lirio-Romero, Rocío Palomo-Carrión, Helena Romay-Barrero, Asunción Ferri-Morales, Virginia Prieto-Gómez and María Torres-Lacomba
Age Differences in Motor Recruitment Patterns of the Shoulder in Dynamic and Isometric Contractions. A Cross-Sectional Study
Reprinted from: *J. Clin. Med.* **2021**, *10*, 525, doi:10.3390/jcm10030525 4

Sławomir Kujawski, Agnieszka Kujawska, Radosław Perkowski, Joanna Androsiuk-Perkowska, Weronika Hajec, Małgorzata Kwiatkowska, et al.
Interaction between Subjective Memory Decline and Depression Symptom Intensity in Older People. Results of the Second Wave of Cognition of Older People, Education, Recreational Activities, Nutrition, Comorbidities, and Functional Capacity Studies (COPERNICUS)
Reprinted from: *J. Clin. Med.* **2021**, *10*, 1334, doi:10.3390/jcm10071334 16

Chan-Young Kwon and Boram Lee
Acupuncture for Behavioral and Psychological Symptoms of Dementia: A Systematic Review and Meta-Analysis
Reprinted from: *J. Clin. Med.* **2021**, *10*, 3087, doi:10.3390/jcm10143087 28

Jeannette A. Goudzwaard, Sadhna Chotkan, Marjo J. A. G. De Ronde-Tillmans, Mattie J. Lenzen, Maarten P. H. van Wiechen, Joris F. W. Ooms, et al.
Multidimensional Prognostic Index and Outcomes in Older Patients Undergoing Transcatheter Aortic Valve Implantation: Survival of the Fittest
Reprinted from: *J. Clin. Med.* **2021**, *10*, 3529, doi:10.3390/jcm10163529 44

Encarnación Blanco-Reina, Lorena Aguilar-Cano, María Rosa García-Merino, Ricardo Ocaña-Riola, Jenifer Valdellós, Inmaculada Bellido-Estévez and Gabriel Ariza-Zafra
Assessing Prevalence and Factors Related to Frailty in Community-Dwelling Older Adults: A Multinomial Logistic Analysis
Reprinted from: *J. Clin. Med.* **2021**, *10*, 3576, doi:10.3390/jcm10163576 54

Salman Hussain, Ambrish Singh, Benny Antony, Rolando Claure-Del Granado, Jitka Klugarová, Radim Líčeník and Miloslav Klugar
Association of Acute Kidney Injury with the Risk of Dementia: A Meta-Analysis
Reprinted from: *J. Clin. Med.* **2021**, *10*, 4390, doi:10.3390/jcm10194390 65

Chi-Di Hung, Chen-Cheng Yang, Chun-Ying Lee, Stephen Chu-Sung Hu, Szu-Chia Chen, Chih-Hsing Hung, et al.
Polypharmacy Is Significantly and Positively Associated with the Frailty Status Assessed Using the 5-Item FRAIL Scale, Cardiovascular Health Phenotypic Classification of Frailty Index, and Study of Osteoporotic Fractures Scale
Reprinted from: *J. Clin. Med.* **2021**, *10*, 4413, doi:10.3390/jcm10194413 77

Sang-Wook Lee, Jae-Sik Nam, Ye-Jee Kim, Min-Ju Kim, Jeong-Hyun Choi, Eun-Ho Lee, et al.
Predictive Model for the Assessment of Preoperative Frailty Risk in the Elderly
Reprinted from: *J. Clin. Med.* **2021**, *10*, 4612, doi:10.3390/jcm10194612 87

Andrea Corsonello, Luca Soraci, Francesco Corica, Valeria Lago, Clementina Misuraca, Graziano Onder, et al.
The Interplay between Anticholinergic Burden and Anemia in Relation to 1-Year Mortality among Older Patients Discharged from Acute Care Hospitals
Reprinted from: *J. Clin. Med.* **2021**, *10*, 4650, doi:10.3390/jcm10204650 98

Chenglei Fan, Carmelo Pirri, Caterina Fede, Diego Guidolin, Carlo Biz, Lucia Petrelli, et al.
Age-Related Alterations of Hyaluronan and Collagen in Extracellular Matrix of the Muscle Spindles
Reprinted from: *J. Clin. Med.* **2022**, *11*, 86, doi:10.3390/jcm11010086 110

Øystein Bruserud, Anh Khoi Vo and Håkon Rekvam
Hematopoiesis, Inflammation and Aging—The Biological Background and Clinical Impact of Anemia and Increased C-Reactive Protein Levels on Elderly Individuals
Reprinted from: *J. Clin. Med.* **2022**, *11*, 706, doi:10.3390/jcm11030706 123

Mohammed S. Salahudeen, Adel Alfahmi, Anam Farooq, Mehnaz Akhtar, Sana Ajaz, Saud Alotaibi, et al.
Effectiveness of Interventions to Improve the Anticholinergic Prescribing Practice in Older Adults: A Systematic Review
Reprinted from: *J. Clin. Med.* **2022**, *11*, 714, doi:10.3390/jcm11030714 158

Iwona Bonikowska, Katarzyna Szwamel and Izabella Uchmanowicz
Adherence to Medication in Older Adults with Type 2 Diabetes Living in Lubuskie Voivodeship in Poland: Association with Frailty Syndrome
Reprinted from: *J. Clin. Med.* **2022**, *11*, 1707, doi:10.3390/jcm11061707 176

Femke C. M. S. Overbeek, Jeannette A. Goudzwaard, Judy van Hemmen, Rozemarijn L. van Bruchem-Visser, Janne M. Papma, Harmke A. Polinder-Bos and Francesco U. S. Mattace-Raso
The Multidimensional Prognostic Index Predicts Mortality in Older Outpatients with Cognitive Decline
Reprinted from: *J. Clin. Med.* **2022**, *11*, 2369, doi:10.3390/jcm11092369 194

Víctor Mayoral Rojals, Ángeles Canós Verdecho, Begoña Soler López and the Team DUO
Assessment of the Management of Patients with Chronic Pain Referred to a Specialized Pain Unit: A Cross-Sectional Multicenter Study (the DUO Project)
Reprinted from: *J. Clin. Med.* **2022**, *11*, 3586, doi:10.3390/jcm11133586 203

Encarnación Blanco-Reina, Ricardo Ocaña-Riola, Gabriel Ariza-Zafra, María Rosa García-Merino, Lorena Aguilar-Cano, Jenifer Valdellós, et al.
Prevalence and Clinical Conditions Related to Sarcopaenia among Older Persons Living in the Community
Reprinted from: *J. Clin. Med.* **2022**, *11*, 3814, doi:10.3390/jcm11133814 216

Lisanne Tap, Andrea Corsonello, Mirko Di Rosa, Paolo Fabbietti, Francesc Formiga, Rafael Moreno-González, et al.
Inflammaging and Blood Pressure Profiles in Late Life: The Screening for CKD among Older People across Europe (SCOPE) Study
Reprinted from: *J. Clin. Med.* **2022**, *11*, 7311, doi:10.3390/jcm11247311 229

Else-Marie van de Vreede, Floor van den Berg, Parsa Jahangiri, Kadir Caliskan and Francesco Mattace-Raso
The Effect of Age on Non-Invasive Hemodynamics in Chronic Heart Failure Patients on Left-Ventricular Assist Device Support: A Pilot Study
Reprinted from: *J. Clin. Med.* **2023**, *12*, 29, doi:10.3390/jcm12010029 239

Natalia Sosowska, Agnieszka Guligowska, Bartłomiej Sołtysik, Ewa Borowiak, Tomasz Kostka and Joanna Kostka
Better Handgrip Strength Is Related to the Lower Prevalence of Pain and Anxiety in Community-Dwelling Older Adults
Reprinted from: *J. Clin. Med.* **2023**, *12*, 3846, doi:10.3390/jcm12113846 249

Rada Artzi-Medvedik, Robert Kob, Mirko Di Rosa, Fabrizia Lattanzio, Andrea Corsonello, Ilan Yehoshua, et al.
Quality of Life and Kidney Function in Older Adults: Prospective Data of the SCOPE Study
Reprinted from: *J. Clin. Med.* **2023**, *12*, 3959, doi:10.3390/jcm12123959 260

Magdalena Szklarek, Tomasz Kostka and Joanna Kostka
Correlates of Restless Legs Syndrome in Older People
Reprinted from: *J. Clin. Med.* **2024**, *13*, 1364, doi:10.3390/jcm13051364 273

Eryk Wacka, Jan Nicikowski, Pawel Jarmuzek and Agnieszka Zembron-Lacny
Anemia and Its Connections to Inflammation in Older Adults: A Review
Reprinted from: *J. Clin. Med.* **2024**, *13*, 2049, doi:10.3390/jcm13072049 285

Neng Pan, Zbigniew Ossowski, Jun Tong, Dan Li and Shan Gao
Effects of Exercise on Frailty in Older People Based on ACSM Recommendations: A Systematic Review and Meta-Analysis of Randomized Controlled Trials
Reprinted from: *J. Clin. Med.* **2024**, *13*, 3037, doi:10.3390/jcm13113037 307

Jie Sui, Pia Rotshtein, Zhuoen Lu and Magdalena Chechlacz
Causal Roles of Ventral and Dorsal Neural Systems for Automatic and Control Self-Reference Processing: A Function Lesion Mapping Study
Reprinted from: *J. Clin. Med.* **2024**, *13*, 4170, doi:10.3390/jcm13144170 331

About the Editor

Francesco Mattace-Raso

Francesco Mattace-Raso is a Professor of Geriatrics at the Erasmus MC University Medical Center of Rotterdam, The Netherlands. He chairs the Division of Geriatric Medicine and is the Principal Investigator of the Vascular Aging Science Center, Erasmus MC. From 2010 to 2021, he served as the Head of the Postgraduate School of Geriatrics at the Erasmus MC University Medical Center of Rotterdam.

His main research interest includes investigating the causes and consequences of age-related cardiometabolic changes and understanding the complex biological process of senescence and the possible consequences on individual vitality. An author of many milestone studies and co-author of guidelines and expert papers, in this field, Francesco Mattace-Raso has played a leading role internationally.

He has been involved in 6 significant EU projects and has acted as the principal and/or co-investigator of several clinical trials and scientific networks.

Up to date, Francesco has supervised 15 PhD candidates and more than 50 master's thesis at the Erasmus University of Rotterdam, has written several book chapters and guidelines and is the author of >300 peer-reviewed publications (h 62).

Francesco is an Associate Editor of Age and Ageing and a member of the Editorial Board of Hypertension, the American Journal of Hypertension, Clinical Interventions in Aging, Artery Research, and Panminerva Medica.

Within the European Society of Geriatric Medicine, Francesco is a member of the Full Board, and he is a member of the SIG Cardiovascular Diseases and the SIG Comprehensive Geriatric Assessment, where he has served as member of the Academic Board. He is Co-Chair of the International Course on Cognitive Disorders.

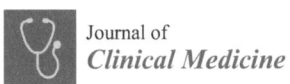

Editorial

It Is Time for Senescience

Francesco Mattace-Raso

Section of Geriatrics, Department of Internal Medicine, Erasmus MC University Medical Center, 3015 GD Rotterdam, The Netherlands; f.mattaceraso@erasmusmc.nl; Tel.: +31-10-7035979

Citation: Mattace-Raso, F. It Is Time for Senescience. *J. Clin. Med.* **2022**, *11*, 4542. https://doi.org/10.3390/jcm11154542

Received: 18 July 2022
Accepted: 1 August 2022
Published: 4 August 2022

Publisher's Note: MDPI stays neutral with regard to jurisdictional claims in published maps and institutional affiliations.

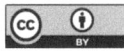

Copyright: © 2022 by the author. Licensee MDPI, Basel, Switzerland. This article is an open access article distributed under the terms and conditions of the Creative Commons Attribution (CC BY) license (https://creativecommons.org/licenses/by/4.0/).

Aging is the most impressive demographic phenomenon in human history. Due to fast medical developments, in addition to developments in the fields of transport, communication and economics, the world's population is aging progressively and globally.

Humans have always reached extreme ages; it is not uncommon for historical individuals to have reached one hundred years of age. However, the pace of population aging today is much faster than in the past, and as a consequence of this, the percentage of persons reaching extreme longevity has increased beyond expectation. The number of persons aged 80 years or older is expected to triple worldwide in the next thirty years, with a projected 426 million octogenarians in 2050 [1].

As physicians, we will see a substantial increase in patients with chronic conditions, multimorbidity, and polypharmacy. Moreover, more and more patients will be faced with progressive functional and cognitive decline. Physicians have begun to encounter this novel category of patients: patients who were not included in our textbooks, and have only recently come to be described. The significant improvements in medicine in recent decades means that young adult patients have been able to survive diseases which were considered fatal in the past. Additionally, we have been able to prolong the prognosis of diseases which are still, unfortunately, fatal. In this way, we have 'created' a new category of patients who will undergo sophisticated mini-invasive and complex interventions, will use more and more medicines and, possibly, will have advantages with the support of technology.

Therefore, the study of age-related disorders is of paramount importance, and we must embrace a new concept: **SENESCIENCE**. This is a novel term to indicate the scientific approach of age-related physiology and disease.

This novel vision requires a novel approach from bench to bedside, and beyond. Only with a translational approach we will be able to understand and classify age-related disorders, unravel underlying mechanisms, discover new treatments and develop technology to adequately treat older patients and, when necessary, give adequate support in order to maintain independency and quality of life. Some of these topics have been treated in the Topical Collection "New Frontiers in Geriatric Diseases" of the *Journal of Clinical Medicine*.

Evidence-Based Medicine and Not Eminence-Based Medicine

There is a major need to expand and standardize medical guidelines for older patients. One of the pitfalls of geriatric medicine is that we miss, almost completely, the inclusion of older participants in clinical randomized control trials. This means that almost every medical treatment applied in older patients is an extrapolation of a treatment which has been shown to be effective and possibly harmless in young adults. Only recently have several large randomized control trials (RCT) included systematically older patients. The treatment of hypertension in older adults, for example, has been a matter of debate in recent decades. Is the treatment harmless and effective? What levels of blood pressure are recommended in persons aged >80 years? Recent RCTs have given answers to these questions. The HYVET trial showed, for the first time and conclusively, the benefits of blood pressure-lowering drug treatment in people aged 80 years or older [2]. Thereafter, other trials have investigated whether intensive blood-pressure-lowering intervention is safe and effective in older hypertensive patients. The SPRINT trial showed that an intensive blood pressure treatment results in significant cardiovascular benefit in high-risk patients with hypertension compared with routine blood pressure control [3]. Moreover, this study was the first trial on the treatment of hypertension stratifying for frailty. These studies, along with other RCTs, have provided high-quality knowledge which has been extremely useful to update (inter)national guidelines. Additionally, of course, we have to remember that treating old, frail patients will always require a tailored approach [4]. Finally, we cannot forget relevant topics when dealing with medications in frail patients: polypharmacy, drug–drugs interactions, and the balance between efficacy and safety [5–7].

Stratification and Advanced Care Planning

Information on prognosis is a necessity to optimize tailored treatments in older patients. It can be very challenging to establish an exact prognosis in persons with multimorbidities. Competing risk, drug interactions, reduced homeostasis and the risk of multiorgan failure, for example, are insidious enemies. Several attempts have been made to develop prediction tools. One of the most effective tools that has been produced in recent years is the multidimensional prognostic index (MPI) [8]. International and multicentric studies performed in different settings have shown that the MPI is useful to predict mortality and risk of hospitalization in community-dwelling and hospitalized older individuals. A multidimensional assessment of older people admitted to hospital may facilitate appropriate clinical and post-discharge management.

Evidence from these studies has prompted MPI_AGE Investigators to formulate recommendations for healthcare providers, policy makers and the general population, which may help to improve the cost-effectiveness of appropriate healthcare interventions for older patients [9]. The application of this tool in specific categories of patients has shown that the MPI can be a useful tool to assess frailty and predict which patient will have a higher chance of benefiting from a TAVI procedure [10]. Moreover, also in heterogeneous populations, such as patients suffering from cognitive decline, the MPI has been able to predict mortality. These findings need to be confirmed in larger and even more heterogeneous populations of patients with cognitive decline. If confirmed, the MPI could be used as a novel tool for risk stratification and medical decisions in this specific category of patients with a high need for tailored support [11].

From Bench to Bedside

Finally, to better understand age-related disease, it is necessary to understand age-related cellular mechanisms, DNA repair, and the degradation of tissue. In vitro investigations are strongly needed. A recent experimental study found that alterations in the extracellular matrix where the muscle spindles are embedded could help to partly explain the peripheral mechanisms underlying age-related decline in functional changes [12]. The knowledge acquired by these approaches will determine future developments.

The last concept with must consider is domotics: a technology which can be used by older individuals experiencing functional and/or cognitive decline to assist in controlling devices or events in their environment. The recent developments in this field are promising, and have given much inspiration to gerotechnology.

In conclusion, aging is here to stay, and we must grasp the opportunities offered by this unknown phenomenon in order to grapple with the future of older patients.

Funding: This research received no external funding.

Conflicts of Interest: The author declares no conflict of interest.

References

1. World Health Organization. Ageing and health. Available online: www.who.int/news-room/fact-sheets/detail/ageing-and-health (accessed on 15 July 2022).
2. Beckett, N.S.; Peters, R.; Fletcher, A.E.; Staessen, J.A.; Liu, L.; Dumitrascu, D.; Stoyanovsky, V.; Antikainen, R.L.; Nikitin, Y.; Anderson, C.; et al. Treatment of hypertension in patients 80 years of age or older. *N. Engl. J. Med.* **2008**, *358*, 1887–1898. [CrossRef] [PubMed]
3. Williamson, J.D.; Supiano, M.A.; Applegate, W.B.; Berlowitz, D.R.; Campbell, R.C.; Chertow, G.M.; Fine, L.J.; Haley, W.E.; Hawfield, A.T.; Ix, J.H.; et al. Intensive vs Standard Blood Pressure Control and Cardiovascular Disease Outcomes in Adults Aged ≥ 75 Years: A Randomized Clinical Trial. *JAMA* **2016**, *315*, 2673–2682. [CrossRef] [PubMed]

4. Mattace-Raso, F.; Rajkumar, C. Medicine is a science of uncertainty and an art of probability. Blood pressure management in older people. *Age Ageing* **2021**, *50*, 59–61. [CrossRef] [PubMed]
5. Hung, C.D.; Yang, C.C.; Lee, C.Y.; Hu, S.C.; Chen, S.C.; Hung, C.H.; Chuang, H.Y.; Chen, C.Y.; Kuo, C.H. Polypharmacy Is Significantly and Positively Associated with the Frailty Status Assessed Using the 5-Item FRAIL Scale, Cardiovascular Health Phenotypic Classification of Frailty Index, and Study of Osteoporotic Fractures Scale. *J. Clin. Med.* **2021**, *10*, 4413. [CrossRef] [PubMed]
6. Corsonello, A.; Soraci, L.; Corica, F.; Lago, V.; Misuraca, C.; Onder, G.; Volpato, S.; Ruggiero, C.; Cherubini, A.; Lattanzio, F. The Interplay between Anticholinergic Burden and Anemia in Relation to 1-Year Mortality among Older Patients Discharged from Acute Care Hospitals. *J. Clin. Med.* **2021**, *10*, 4650. [CrossRef] [PubMed]
7. Salahudeen, M.S.; Alfahmi, A.; Farooq, A.; Akhtar, M.; Ajaz, S.; Alotaibi, S.; Faiz, M.; Ali, S. Effectiveness of Interventions to Improve the Anticholinergic Prescribing Practice in Older Adults: A Systematic Review. *J. Clin. Med.* **2022**, *11*, 714. [CrossRef] [PubMed]
8. Pilotto, A.; Veronese, N.; Daragjati, J.; Cruz-Jentoft, A.J.; Polidori, M.C.; Mattace-Raso, F.; Paccalin, M.; Topinkova, E.; Siri, G.; Greco, A.; et al. Using the Multidimensional Prognostic Index to Predict Clinical Outcomes of Hospitalized Older Persons: A Prospective, Multicenter, International Study. *J. Gerontol. A Biol. Sci. Med. Sci.* **2019**, *74*, 1643–1649. [CrossRef]
9. Cruz-Jentoft, A.J.; Daragjati, J.; Fratiglioni, L.; Maggi, S.; Mangoni, A.A.; Mattace-Raso, F.; Paccalin, M.; Polidori, M.C.; Topinkova, E.; Ferrucci, L.; et al. Using the Multidimensional Prognostic Index (MPI) to improve cost-effectiveness of interventions in multimorbid frail older persons: Results and final recommendations from the MPI_AGE European Project. *Aging Clin. Exp. Res.* **2020**, *32*, 861–868. [CrossRef] [PubMed]
10. Goudzwaard, J.A.; Chotkan, S.; De Ronde-Tillmans, M.J.A.G.; Lenzen, M.J.; van Wiechen, M.P.H.; Ooms, J.F.W.; Polinder-Bos, H.A.; de Beer-Leentfaar, M.; Van Mieghem, N.M.; Daemen, J.; et al. Multidimensional Prognostic Index and Outcomes in Older Patients Undergoing Transcatheter Aortic Valve Implantation: Survival of the Fittest. *J. Clin. Med.* **2021**, *10*, 3529. [CrossRef] [PubMed]
11. Overbeek, F.C.M.S.; Goudzwaard, J.A.; van Hemmen, J.; van Bruchem-Visser, R.L.; Papma, J.M.; Polinder-Bos, H.A.; Mattace-Raso, F.U.S. The Multidimensional Prognostic Index Predicts Mortality in Older Outpatients with Cognitive Decline. *J. Clin. Med.* **2022**, *11*, 2369. [CrossRef]
12. Fan, C.; Pirri, C.; Fede, C.; Guidolin, D.; Biz, C.; Petrelli, L.; Porzionato, A.; Macchi, V.; De Caro, R.; Stecco, C. Age-Related Alterations of Hyaluronan and Collagen in Extracellular Matrix of the Muscle Spindles. *J. Clin. Med.* **2021**, *11*, 86. [CrossRef]

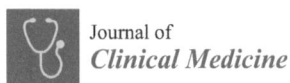

Article

Age Differences in Motor Recruitment Patterns of the Shoulder in Dynamic and Isometric Contractions. A Cross-Sectional Study

Cristina Lirio-Romero [1,2], Rocío Palomo-Carrión [1,2,*], Helena Romay-Barrero [1,*], Asunción Ferri-Morales [1], Virginia Prieto-Gómez [3] and María Torres-Lacomba [3]

[1] Faculty of Physiotherapy and Nursing, Physiotherapy and Occupational Therapy Department, University of Castilla-La Mancha, Avda. Carlos III s/n, 45004 Toledo, Spain; Cristina.Lirio@uclm.es (C.L.-R.); Asuncion.Ferri@uclm.es (A.F.-M.)
[2] GIFTO Research Group, Avda. Carlos III s/n, 45004 Toledo, Spain
[3] Physiotherapy in Women's Health (FPSM) Research Group, Physiotherapy Department, Faculty of Medicine and Health Sciences, University of Alcalá, Alcalá de Henares, 28805 Madrid, Spain; v.prieto@uah.es (V.P.-G.); maria.torres@uah.es (M.T.-L.)
* Correspondence: Rocio.Palomo@uclm.es (R.P.-C.); Helena.Romay@uclm.es (H.R.-B.)

Citation: Lirio-Romero, C.; Palomo-Carrión, R.; Romay-Barrero, H.; Ferri-Morales, A.; Prieto-Gómez, V.; Torres-Lacomba, M. Age Differences in Motor Recruitment Patterns of the Shoulder in Dynamic and Isometric Contractions. A Cross-Sectional Study. *J. Clin. Med.* **2021**, *10*, 525. https://doi.org/10.3390/jcm10030525

Academic Editor: Francesco Mattace-Raso
Received: 30 December 2020
Accepted: 25 January 2021
Published: 2 February 2021

Publisher's Note: MDPI stays neutral with regard to jurisdictional claims in published maps and institutional affiliations.

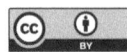

Copyright: © 2021 by the authors. Licensee MDPI, Basel, Switzerland. This article is an open access article distributed under the terms and conditions of the Creative Commons Attribution (CC BY) license (https://creativecommons.org/licenses/by/4.0/).

Abstract: Aging processes in the musculoskeletal system lead to functional impairments that restrict participation. Purpose: To assess differences in the force and motor recruitment patterns of shoulder muscles between age groups to understand functional disorders. A cross-sectional study comparing 30 adults (20–64) and 30 older adults (>65). Surface electromyography (sEMG) of the middle deltoid, upper and lower trapezius, infraspinatus, and serratus anterior muscles was recorded. Maximum isometric voluntary contraction (MIVC) was determined at 45° glenohumeral abduction. For the sEMG signal registration, concentric and eccentric contraction with and without 1 kg and isometric contraction were requested. Participants abducted the arm from 0° up to an abduction angle of 135° for concentric and eccentric contraction, and from 0° to 45°, and remained there at 80% of the MIVC level while isometrically pushing against a handheld dynamometer. Differences in sEMG amplitudes (root mean square, RMS) of all contractions, but also onset latencies during concentric contraction of each muscle between age groups, were analyzed. Statistical differences in strength (Adults > Older adults; 0.05) existed between groups. No significant differences in RMS values of dynamic contractions were detected, except for the serratus anterior, but there were for isometric contractions of all muscles analyzed (Adults > Older adults; 0.05). The recruitment order varied between age groups, showing a general tendency towards delayed onset times in older adults, except for the upper trapezius muscle. Age differences in muscle recruitment patterns were found, which underscores the importance of developing musculoskeletal data to prevent and guide geriatric shoulder pathologies.

Keywords: shoulder; musculoskeletal disorders; surface electromyography; age groups; aging

1. Introduction

Aging leads to a regression of physical capacities and a decrease in functionality in older people [1,2]. Around 35% of people over 65 years of age suffer from neuromuscular disorders [3,4]. The proportion of older people will increase in the coming decades [5], so establishing normative data in order to improve diagnosis, prevention, and treatment is a necessity to reduce costs due to absence of information.

In mid-adulthood, age-related changes appear that progressively decrease muscle function [1,6]. These natural aging changes are clinically defined as geriatric sarcopenia [7,8]. With age, the muscle mass in skeletal muscle decreases, especially for type II fibers, which lead to a decrease in strength, with a consequent increase in muscle weakness [9]. In addition, neuronal factors are also altered and are responsible for the loss of muscle function [10].

Regarding upper limbs, shoulder muscle function decreases with less use of arms and hands in daily activities. Furthermore, it appears to impair balance, which increases the risk of falls mainly in older adults [11]. The typical recruitment pattern of shoulder muscles has already been studied in healthy adults [12], as well as their differences between the sexes [13]. Furthermore, as previously mentioned, the literature shows physiological changes with age [7,9,14]. However, no evidence has been found linking these changes with possible differences in motor recruitment patterns. Therefore, it is essential to understand age-related physiological alterations from different activities of the upper limb, such as dynamic and isometric movements involved in daily tasks—previous subjects of study in the lower limb [15,16].

Abduction is the shoulder movement commonly used for function evaluation because it gives useful information on the control and quality of the movement of the upper limb [17]. The scapula is in a favorable position during abduction since metabolic energy has not been required by passive scapulothoracic forces [18]. Analysis of muscle recruitment patterns has been used through surface electromyography (sEMG) to understand functional differences in muscles recruitment [19,20]. sEMG is also used by physical therapists to better understand the function and dysfunction of the neuromusculoskeletal system [20].

The present study aims to describe muscle recruitment patterns during dynamic and isometric contractions of abduction movement to identify age-related muscle function. The objective was to provide electromyography data on motor recruitment during shoulder abduction in adults and older adults, both healthy, to facilitate a preventive or therapeutic approach to loss of upper limb function.

Additionally, the implication of possible motor disorders of the shoulder complex muscles in older people on the loss of force, mobility, and functionality of the upper limb is intended to be observed.

2. Materials and Methods

2.1. Design

A descriptive cross-sectional study in two age groups was carried out (Registry: NCT04706169) [21], in which the sEMG activity (amplitude and onset) of the middle deltoid (MD), upper trapezius (UT), infraspinatus (IS), lower trapezius (LT), and serratus anterior (SA) was compared in adults and older adults.

All study participants were informed about the purpose of the study, signed the informed consent, and participated voluntarily. The Ethics Committee "Clinical Research of the University of Alcalá (Madrid, Spain)" approved the study (2012/038/01/20,120,924).

2.2. Participants

Participants attended, from December 2015 to March 2019, the laboratory of the Research Group "Physiotherapy in Women's Health Research Group", at Teaching and Research Unit in Physiotherapy of the University of Alcalá (Madrid, Spain) and Ocaña Senior Center (Toledo, Spain) voluntarily after reading an advertisement about the need to recruit healthy people for a research study. A physical therapist (C.L.-R.), experienced and trained in sEMG recordings, performed the assessment.

Participants, without symptoms in the shoulder and/or cervical area during the last year, were assigned to the respective age groups: over 65 years (Older adults) and 20 to 64 years (Adults). Participants with rheumatological diseases, moderate or severe cognitive impairment, tumors, massive osteoarthritis, circulatory disorders, dermatological problems, sedentary people, or those who had received physiotherapy within the 12 months prior to sEMG assessment were excluded from the study as well as those who took medication that could have repercussions in motion processing.

2.3. Assessments/Interventions

sEMG was used to measure the amplitude and onset of five shoulder muscle activities performing glenohumeral abduction. In this movement, the middle deltoid muscle was selected because it is a main motor. The infraspinatus muscle represented the rotator cuff muscle group. The middle deltoid muscle was selected as the representative of shoulder abduction because it is a main motor in this movement [22]. The trapezius muscle and especially the serratus anterior muscle were chosen as representative, established of the ascending scapular rotator muscles [18].

For determination of the force values by means of the maximum isometric voluntary contraction (MIVC), necessary to normalize the signal and maintain the isometric contraction, the participants held a dynamometer (MicroFET®2, Hoggan Health Industries, West Jordan, UT, USA) [23]. To detect MIVC, the participants raised their arm to 45° of glenohumeral abduction. The handheld dynamometer was placed on the forearm at a medium distance between the wrist and the elbow. This position was marked to ensure the reliability of the dynamometer measurement during submaximal force tests. Next, the participant isometrically abducted his arm with maximum effort while the dynamometer was firmly fixed by the physical therapist (C.L.-R.). The participants repeated this three times, and the average value was used to determine the MIVC value.

The submaximal level of isometric contraction was determined at 80% of the MIVC. Prior to electromyographic evaluation, submaximal tests were performed. The physical therapist instructed the participants to perform an isometric glenohumeral abduction at 45° for 5 s using the hand dynamometer to mark the respective submaximal force level. To record the electrical activity during the submaximal isometric contraction, elevation of the arm was requested for 2 s in the abduction movement from 0° to 45° [24], and maintained for 5 s once they reached the value of 80% of their MIVC. The abduction displacement was recorded/registered by the electronic goniometer (MLTS700, ADInstruments, Oxford, UK).

In addition, a physiotherapist (C.L.-R.) trained with participants how to perform abduction movements up to 135° for 7 s and return to the starting position of 0° (without weight and with a 1 kg weight in hand). Subjects chose weight they thought they would lift in their normal daily activities (range = 1–3 kg) [25–27]. As for the older adults, they lifted the weight that allowed them to complete the range of movement (1 kg).

Once proofs had been performed and MIVC values were taken, electrodes were placed to record the activity of the five muscles, as well as the electric goniometer to record movement. The surface electromyograph used was a PowerLab 15T (ADInstruments, Oxford, UK). The experienced physical therapist placed sEMG electrodes for precise positioning. Conductive adhesive hydrogel surface electrodes (27 mm diameter) (Kendall™ 100 series Foam Electrodes, Covidien, MA, USA) were used, using a 30 mm electrode gap. The skin was wiped with alcohol and two electrodes were placed on the midline of the respective muscle bellies, aligned along the muscle fibers. In addition, ground electrodes were placed on bone sites (processus spinosus C6, C7, and the posterior part of the acromion). The electric goniometer was positioned so that one sensor was fixed on the upper part of the scapula and the other on the back of the arm at a 90° angle between both sensors and preset in the 0° position (i.e., neutral position) in the sEMG registration software. Adhesive tape was used to fix the electrodes and cables. sEMG (gain: 1000) and goniometric signals were sampled at a rate of 1000 samples per second, using a 16-bit AD converter.

The sEMG signals were band-pass filtered (10–500 Hz, eighth Bessel filter) to improve the signal-to-noise ratio. LabChart® Software (ADInstruments, Oxford, UK) was used to simultaneously capture sEMG data on a PC. Root mean square (RMS) values were obtained automatically, within the time interval of 2 to 4 s after the start of the contraction and were normalized according to the respective MIVC. Muscle onset values were obtained from analysis graphs that included the arm displacement recorded simultaneously with sEMG (Figure 1). The onset was obtained as the time distance of the interception between the level of pre-activation relative to the onset of arm displacement during dynamic contraction and the linearly interpolated RMS slope [12,19].

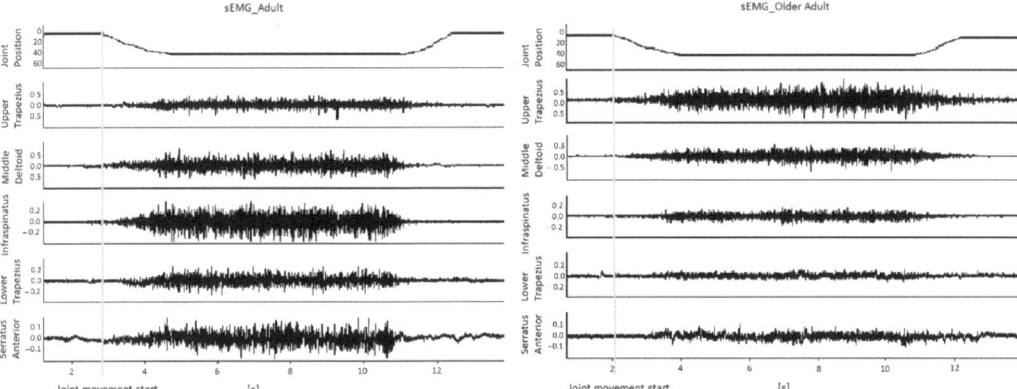

Figure 1. Raw surface electromyography (sEMG) recordings of the five muscles (indicated on the **left**) simultaneously displaying the abduction movement (from 0° to 45°). These have been obtained from one representative participant from the Older Adults group and one from the Adults groups, displaying the abduction movement.

To obtain reliable electromyographic signal data, we have tried to reduce crosstalk, motion artifacts, skin contact impedance, and power supply noise by correct electrode placement and filters [19].

sEMG data of all the investigated muscles were simultaneously recorded (Figure 1). They were requested to perform (a) 3 repetitions of glenohumeral abduction up to 135° and return to position 0, (b) 3 equal repetitions, but with a 1 kg weight in their hand, and (c) 3 repetitions of isometric abduction (intervals between tests of 2 min). The mean sEMG values of the 3 repetitions were used for further analysis.

Demographic variables were collected: age, sex, dominant body side, height and weight (body mass index), and physiotherapy treatments within the 12-months prior to sEMG assessment. This last issue was registered to understand any possible variation despite the healthy condition of all subjects during the last year. The MIVC, glenohumeral range of motion (ROM), and the Shoulder Disability Questionnaire were analyzed as clinical variables. As was previously reported, we determined the MIVC at 45° of abduction [28] by a hand dynamometer. These data served as reference values to normalize the sEMG signal and to determine the levels of submaximal isometric contraction previously reported.

Glenohumeral ROM was measured with a universal goniometer (Enraf Nonius Ibérica®, Madrid. Spain): flexion, internal and external rotation, and abduction. To assess possible shoulder dysfunction, although with no complaints, the Shoulder Disability Questionnaire was used. The Shoulder Disability Questionnaire is widely used in research and clinical practice in several countries. It consists of 16 items about shoulder complaints during tasks performed in the last 24 h (yes, no, or not applicable). The ratio of the number of items with an affirmative answer over the number of applicable items was multiplied by 100. Scores range from 0 (no functional limitation) to 100 (affirmative to all items); higher scores mean higher disability [29].

A sEMG variable result was the amplitude of muscle activity quantified through the normalized RMS. Additionally, the onset(s) of muscle contraction was registered/recorded during dynamic contraction. Therefore, the time between the start of the abduction movement and the start of the contraction of each muscle was calculated [19,30].

2.4. Sample Size

We determined the sample size considering differences in the levels of MIVC between the two groups of 30 participants each. Assuming within the group a standard deviation of 20.9 N, a standard deviation of 30.1 N could be detected in the ANOVA between groups with type I error of 0.05 and 80% power. Furthermore, to detect group differences, a difference of 21 N was reported assuming identical power and variations within the group [13].

2.5. Statistical Analysis

Data were analyzed using IBM SPSS Statistics 20 for Windows (SPSS Inc., 2011, IBM Corp, Armonk, NY, USA). The Shapiro–Wilks test was used to test normal or non-normal distribution of variables. The mean and standard deviations, as central tendency measures, were estimated in the normal distributed variables, and the median and interquartile range in the not normally distributed variables. Student's t-test and Mann–Whitney U test were used to calculated significant differences between adults and older adults. A 95% confidence interval for each estimator was used.

3. Results

The flow chart shows the process for selecting participants (Figure 2).

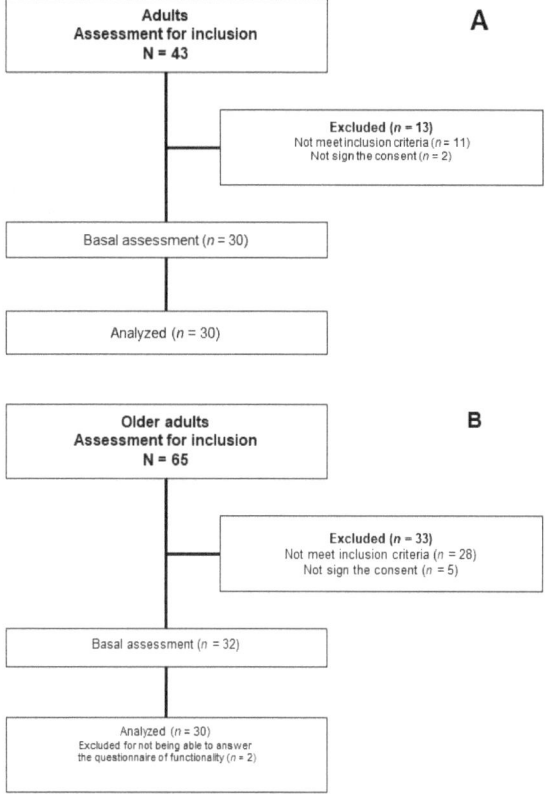

Figure 2. Flow of participants. (**A**) Adults; (**B**) Older adults.

3.1. Age-Related Differences in Demographic and Clinical Data

Statistically significant differences were observed between age groups in functionality and body mass index ($p < 0.01$, Adults < Older adults) as well as in MIVC ($p < 0.01$, Adults

> Older adults), active ROM $p < 0.05$, Adults > Older adults), and previous physiotherapy treatments ($p < 0.05$, Adults < Older adults). Respective values are shown in Table 1 for each group.

Table 1. Demographic and clinical characteristics.

Variables	Adults n = 30	Older Adults n = 30	p-Value [†]
Age Median (IR *)	45.5(27.5)	70.5(8.3)	<0.01
Gender n women (%)	15(50)	16(53.3)	0.80
Dominant limb n right (%)	30(100)	28(93.3)	0.16
Previous physiotherapy treatments n yes (%)	2(6.7)	11(36.7)	<0.05
Body mass index Mean (SD **)	24.4(3)	29.2(3.6)	<0.01
MVIC [Newton] Mean (SD **)	122.9(44)	75.7(26)	<0.01
SDQ Median (IR *)	0(0)	0(12.5)	<0.01
Glenohumeral Flexion Mean (SD **)	160.5(9.5)	151.2(9.3)	<0.01
Glenohumeral Internal Rotation Mean (SD **)	73.8(10.6)	70.7(22.7)	0.49
Glenohumeral External Rotation Mean (SD **)	85.5(8.4)	71.8(15.1)	<0.01
Glenohumeral Abduction Mean (SD **)	160.8(11.8)	147.5(9.5)	<0.01

SDQ—Shoulder Disability Questionnaire; * IR—Interquartile Range; ** SD Standard Deviation; [†] p-value obtained by Mann–Whitney U test, χ^2 test and Student t-test.

3.2. Age-Related Differences in sEMG Signal

In general, the RMS values showed a decrease in older subjects (Older adults) with respect to adults in all muscles analyzed in terms of the three types of contraction (concentric, eccentric, and isometric) with and without added weight. However, no statistically significant differences were found in dynamic contractions regardless of load (Figure 3). Statistically significant differences were only found for isometric contraction ($p < 0.05$). In addition, the SA muscle showed statistically significant differences in terms of eccentric contractions with or without weight and concentric with weight ($p < 0.05$, Adults > Older adults).

The rest of the analysis referring to concentric and eccentric contractions with or without weight did not show statistically significant differences ($p > 0.05$), although a decrease in the amplitude of the sEMG signal of all contractions was observed in the Older adults group (Figure 3).

Regarding onset times, the tests performed showed in all muscles analyzed during glenohumeral abduction that they progressively delayed with age with the exception of the UT muscle, which showed an advance for Older adult group (Figure 4). The delay observed between age groups was significantly different for the scapula stabilizers, LT and SA ($p < 0.01$, adults < Older adults) and for DM and IS ($p < 0.05$, Adults < Older adults). In general, a different order of recruitment between age groups was observed. Not observed in adults, the UT muscle was the first one to be recruited in older adults. UT muscle was recruited before the beginning of the abduction movement compared with the adults group that showed later UT contraction ($p > 0.05$)

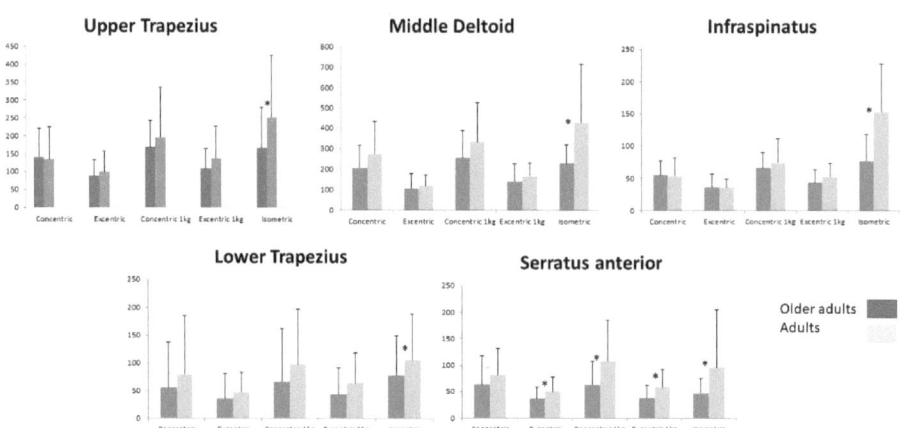

Figure 3. Means (standard deviation) of RMS for each muscle are shown for every muscle contraction: dynamics (concentric and eccentric; with and without 1 kg resistance) and isometric. * $p < 0.05$ between age groups.

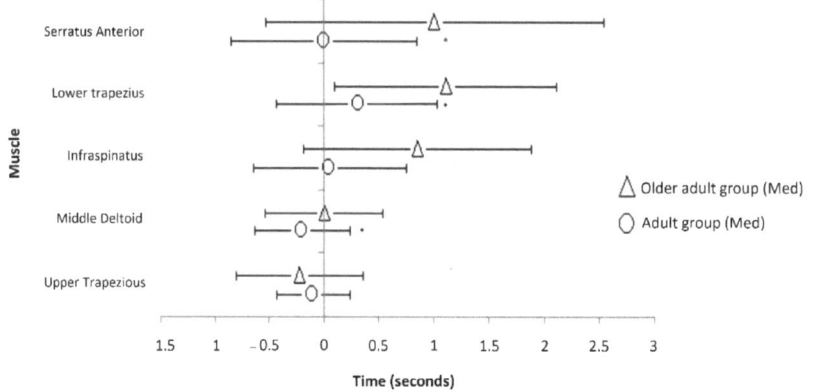

Figure 4. Onset time of muscles contraction. The onset of concentric contraction was averaged for each muscle during shoulder joint abduction for all subjects in Adults and Older adults. Median (±RI) values for each muscle are shown. The vertical line at zero seconds represents the start of the abduction movement. The anticipated contraction is showed to the left (negative) of the zero line. * $p < 0.05$ between age groups.

4. Discussion

The present study compared the motor recruitment patterns of shoulder muscles between the adults and older adults groups during dynamic and isometric glenohumeral abduction, observing differences in isometric (against high resistance) and especially SA muscle in both types of contractions. The sEMG amplitude and onset time of contractions were the primary outcome measures. Older people showed lower sEMG amplitudes during abduction compared to the adults group. With increasing age, the onset of glenohumeral abduction contraction in most of the times analyzed was found to be delayed in older people. Differences between age groups were found in shoulder ROM, body mass index, shoulder function, and previous physiotherapy treatments. The decrease in shoulder functionality has previously been related to age [31], and to loss of muscle mass and range of motion [17].

To understand the age-related changes found in MIVC levels, it is not possible to contrast these data with sEMG amplitude [32], but it is necessary to consider degenerative alterations in the composition, size, and number of muscle fibers [33], and the replacement of the contractile structure by connective tissue or fat [34]. The loss of fibers is related to the decrease in the number of motor neurons with age [14]. Plow et al. tried to explain the loss of motor neurons and the alteration in the number of fibers because of changes in the motor cortex with age but did not obtain such findings [35].

4.1. sEMG Signal

As with previous studies [12,13,36], differences in sEMG amplitude with age are indicative of differences in the patterns of recruitment and its consequent tendency towards functional alteration. In opposition to the results found in the isometric contraction, the dynamic contractions (concentric and eccentric) did not show statistically significant differences between age groups. This variation in EMG signal between types of contraction has previously been reported [15,37].

Starting from the planning of the contractions, it is necessary to clarify that it was intended to imitate the muscular action that the muscles analyzed perform in daily activities. Everyday tasks require dynamic actions that use more easily achievable static forces [38]. Dynamic contractions are commonly performed over wide ranges of motion and with no or light load (especially in older people), and isometric contractions are frequently performed against resistance. In addition, posture, together with impaired coordination of the scapular musculature, are factors that influence the strength of dynamic contractions and reduce the range of motion [39]. Knowing the functioning of contractions is key to understanding the greater significance in the results of submaximal isometric contraction, where higher motor units are recruited. In fact, during isometric contractions, motor units generally show higher recruitment thresholds than in dynamic contractions [40]. However, we can deduce that when evaluating a healthy population with symptoms, we can see that age is not a relevant factor in dynamic contractions, but rather in requests for isometric contractions against submaximal resistance. However, the disadvantages previously reported in the normalization of the sEMG signal in different age groups [41] prevent us from affirming that the submaximal isometric contraction changes more with age than the dynamic contractions.

Focusing on submaximal isometric glenohumeral abduction at 45°, the UT, LT, and SA muscles function as stabilizers of the scapula [18]. It is worth highlighting the results regarding the differences between age groups found in SA that show a tendency to lose scapular stability with age, which in turn explains the loss in the last degrees of glenohumeral abduction, although without clinical symptoms, and loss of shoulder function in the healthy older population. Shoulder pathologies also have reported similar motor patterns of decreasing SA muscle activity [42,43]. Since the activity of the SA depends not only on force production but also on neuromuscular control and recruitment, a precise coordinated activity may occur at the right moment. This proper firing pattern and recruitment requires coupling of the serratus anterior muscle with the trapezius that results in "force couples", necessary for normal scapular orientation [44]. Non-appropriate activity of these muscles in older adults could depend on lower proprioception, more effort and heaviness associated with the muscular activity, and worse perceived timing of muscle contraction with aging [45]. SA muscle recruitment deficits in older adults have been manifested by its altered pattern of recruitment or its altered timing (delayed muscle onset), which can reduce shoulder movement. Given that, only significant differences were evidenced in dynamic contractions in the SA muscle. It can be assumed to be the most altered muscle found in older adults under healthy conditions, which is of interest to understand the functional deterioration of the upper limb with age. However, as a low correlation between the SA muscle signals has been found using surface and intramuscular electrodes, sEMG to assess muscle activation levels in the SA muscle is not the best option [46], also considering the possible influence that higher body mass index may exert, thereby disturbing data recordings in older adults [47].

The onset was significantly different between adults and older adults in all muscles analyzed as shown by previous studies [48], except for UT muscle. The delay in the start of contraction with the normal aging process has been explained by neuromuscular impairments in transmission or by muscle weakness. Kwon et al. relate this delay with an alteration in the co-activation of the antagonist musculature with age [49]. As suggested by Kibler [50,51], the co-activation of the upper trapezius and serratus anterior hold the activation of the rotator cuff muscles. The balance between the glenohumeral internal and external rotators may be compromised by the alteration in upper trapezius and serratus anterior recruitment patterns, which also could be related to less shoulder function in older adults. However, it is not possible to understand why there was more significant differences in all glenohumeral ROM, except for internal rotation. Differences with age in movement are not the result of a decrease in force or speed, but rather central factors that affect movement coordination [52,53].

The present study was able to demonstrate that the main stabilizing muscle of the scapula showed the most notable decrease in the amount of recruitment in addition to a delay tendency in the onset of contraction in older people. Its known tendency towards reduction in scapular stability is pointed out as the basis of certain shoulder disorders. As has been shown in previous evidence [13,43], UT muscle anticipation could compensate the delay of SA and LT muscles. Moreover, possible latent trigger points in the muscle analyzed could be present in subjects of both groups. In an asymptomatic population, latent trigger points could alter the muscle activity signal. Regarding muscle contraction onset, a large variability in the onset times displayed has previously been observed for muscles with latent trigger points [27].

The present arguments hope to provide a tool for prevention and treatment of geriatric disorders, paying special attention to the prevention of loss of activity of the scapular stabilizer muscles.

4.2. Limitations and Clinical Implications

The study design considered the inherent problems in measuring sEMG. The greater difficulty in normalizing the signal in older people should be noted, as well as the non-normalization of the sEMG signal muscle by muscle, but in general for the five muscles according to the MIVC. This was performed in this way to avoid loss of interest mainly of the participants of the older adults group.

Furthermore, the great variability in sEMG results between subjects limits their analysis. This may be due to individual factors in degree of physical activity and hormonal or pharmacological factors, which could have been recorded. We found a high variability when referring to the sEMG values in the reviewed studies and latent trigger points must be considered in following studies about muscle activity differences. This made the discussion and interpretation of the data presented more difficult.

Important age-dependent differences have been identified in the motor recruitment patterns of the shoulder muscles, especially for high resisted isometric contractions, showing that they undergo alterations with age, especially in relation to scapula stabilization and coordination between SA and UT muscle. Healthcare professionals can use the present findings for prevention or treatment; given the great difficulty that exists to carry out activities against high resistance as one common musculoskeletal complain in geriatric diseases. It is a wake-up call to attention to the tending deterioration of the SA muscle.

5. Conclusions

The results showed age differences in muscle recruitment patterns in static maintenance of shoulder lift, but not in its dynamic contraction, which can influence loss of force, range of movement, and functionality even in a healthy population, emphasizing the serratus anterior as the more challenging muscle and its tendency to reduce its activity. This underscores the importance of developing an early treatment approach from adulthood to prevent and guide geriatric shoulder pathologies. This is intended to awaken interest in launching new studies that evaluate possible therapeutic approaches that address the desynchronization found in older shoulder muscles.

Author Contributions: Conception and design, C.L.-R., R.P.-C., H.R.-B. and M.T.-L.; provision of participants, M.T.-L.; provision of interventions, C.L.-R., data analysis and interpretation. C.L.-R., R.P.-C., H.R.-B., A.F.-M., V.P.-G. and M.T.-L. collection and assembly of data, C.L.-R., manuscript writing and editing, C.L.-R., R.P.-C., H.R.-B. and M.T.-L., supervision, M.T.-L., V.P.-G. and A.F.-M. All authors have read and agreed to the published version of the manuscript.

Funding: This research received no external funding.

Institutional Review Board Statement: The study was conducted according to the guidelines of the Declaration of Helsinki and approved by the Ethics Committee for Clinical Research of the University of Alcalá (Madrid, Spain) (2012038/01/20,120,924).

Informed Consent Statement: Informed consent was obtained from all subjects involved in the study.

Acknowledgments: The authors are grateful to the laboratory of the "Physiotherapy in Women's Health Research Group", at the Teaching and Research Unit in Physiotherapy of the University of Alcalá (Madrid, Spain) and Ocaña Senior Center (Toledo, Spain) Research Group for the loan of their facilities.

Conflicts of Interest: The authors declare no conflict of interest.

References

1. Dziechciaż, M.; Filip, R. Biological Psychological and Social Determinants of Old Age: Bio-Psycho-Social Aspects of Human Aging. *Ann. Agric. Environ. Med.* **2014**, *21*, 835–838. [CrossRef] [PubMed]
2. Tuna, H.D.; Edeer, A.O.; Malkoc, M.; Aksakoglu, G. Effect of Age and Physical Activity Level on Functional Fitness in Older Adults. *Eur. Rev. Aging Phys. Act.* **2009**, *6*, 99–106. [CrossRef]
3. Carneiro, J.A.; Ramos, G.C.F.; Barbosa, A.T.F.; de Mendonça, J.M.G.; de Costa, F.M.; Caldeira, A.P. Prevalência e Fatores Associados à Fragilidade Em Idosos Não Institucionalizados. *Rev. Bras. Enferm.* **2016**, *69*, 435–442. [CrossRef] [PubMed]
4. Faurot, K. Epidemiology of Aging. In Proceedings of the APHA's 2019 Annual Meeting and Expo, Philadelphia, PA, USA, 2–6 November 2019; American Public Health Association: Philadelphia, PA, USA, 2019.
5. WHO. Ageing and Health. 2018. Available online: https://www.who.int/ageing/about/facts/es/ (accessed on 11 December 2020).
6. Farr, J.N.; Almeida, M. The Spectrum of Fundamental Basic Science Discoveries Contributing to Organismal Aging. *J. Bone Miner. Res.* **2018**, *33*, 1568–1584. [CrossRef] [PubMed]
7. Dhillon, R.J.S.; Hasni, S. Pathogenesis and Management of Sarcopenia. *Clin. Geriatr. Med.* **2017**, *33*, 17–26. [CrossRef] [PubMed]
8. Larsson, L.; Degens, H.; Li, M.; Salviati, L.; Lee, Y.I.; Thompson, W.; Kirkland, J.L.; Sandri, M. Sarcopenia: Aging-Related Loss of Muscle Mass and Function. *Physiol. Rev.* **2019**, *99*, 427–511. [CrossRef]
9. Ohlendiec, K. Proteomic Profiling of Fast-to-Slow Muscle Transitions during Aging. *Front. Physiol.* **2011**, *2*, 105. [CrossRef]
10. Khosa, S.; Trikamji, B.; Khosa, G.S.; Khanli, H.M.; Mishra, S.K. An Overview of Neuromuscular Junction Aging Findings in Human and Animal Studies. *Curr. Aging Sci.* **2019**, *12*, 28–34. [CrossRef]
11. Sanders, O.; Hsiao, H.Y.; Savin, D.N.; Creath, R.A.; Rogers, M.W. Aging Changes in Protective Balance and Startle Responses to Sudden Drop Perturbations. *J. Neurophysiol.* **2019**, *122*, 39–50. [CrossRef]
12. Wickham, J.; Pizzari, T.; Stansfeld, K.; Burnside, A.; Watson, L. Quantifying 'Normal' Shoulder Muscle Activity during Abduction. *J. Electromyogr. Kinesiol.* **2010**, *20*, 212–222. [CrossRef]
13. Lirio-Romero, C.; Anders, C.; de La Villa-Polo, P.; Torres-Lacomba, M. Implications on Older Women of Age- and Sex-Related Differences in Activation Patterns of Shoulder Muscles: A Cross-Sectional Study. *J. Women Aging* **2019**, *31*, 492–512. [CrossRef] [PubMed]
14. Faulkner, J.A.; Larkin, L.M.; Claflin, D.R.; Brooks, S.V. Age-related changes in the structure and function of skeletal muscles. *Clin. Exp. Pharmacol. Physiol.* **2007**, *34*, 1091–1096. [CrossRef] [PubMed]
15. Smith, C.M.; Housh, T.J.; Hill, E.C.; Keller, J.L.; Johnson, G.O.; Schmidt, R.J. Are There Mode-Specific and Fatigue-Related Electromechanical Delay Responses for Maximal Isokinetic and Isometric Muscle Actions? *J. Electromyogr. Kinesiol.* **2017**, *37*, 9–14. [CrossRef] [PubMed]
16. Smith, C.M.; Housh, T.J.; Hill, E.C.; Johnson, G.O.; Schmidt, R.J. Dynamic versus Isometric Electromechanical Delay in Non-Fatigued and Fatigued Muscle: A Combined Electromyographic, Mechanomyographic, and Force Approach. *J. Electromyogr. Kinesiol.* **2017**, *33*, 34–38. [CrossRef] [PubMed]

17. Namdari, S.; Yagnik, G.; Ebaugh, D.D.; Nagda, S.; Ramsey, M.L.; Williams, G.R.; Mehta, S. Defining Functional Shoulder Range of Motion for Activities of Daily Living. *J. Shoulder Elb. Surg.* **2012**, *21*, 1177–1183. [CrossRef]
18. Veeger, H.E.J.; van der Helm, F.C.T. Shoulder Function: The Perfect Compromise between Mobility and Stability. *J. Biomech.* **2007**, *40*, 711–714. [CrossRef]
19. McManus, L.; de Vito, G.; Lowery, M.M. Analysis and Biophysics of Surface EMG for Physiotherapists and Kinesiologists: Toward a Common Language with Rehabilitation Engineers. *Front. Neurol.* **2020**, *11*, 576729. [CrossRef]
20. Medved, V.; Medved, S.; Kovač, I. Critical Appraisal of Surface Electromyography (SEMG) as a Taught Subject and Clinical Tool in Medicine and Kinesiology. *Front. Neurol.* **2020**, *11*, 560363. [CrossRef]
21. Clinical Trials.gov. U.S. National Library of Medicine. 2021. Available online: https://clinicaltrials.gov (accessed on 12 January 2021).
22. Kapanji, A. *The Physiology of the Joints, Vol. 1, the Upper Limb*; Churchill Livingstone: Edinburgh, UK, 2007.
23. Celik, D.; Dirican, A.; Baltaci, G. Intrarater Reliability of Assessing Strength of the Shoulder and Scapular Muscles. *J. Sport Rehabil.* **2012**, *21*, 1–5. [CrossRef]
24. Ashour, A.A. Relationship between Isometric Muscle Force and Surface EMG of Wrist Muscles at Different Shoulder and Elbow Angles. *J. Am. Sci.* **2014**, *10*, 26–34.
25. Rolf, O.; Ochs, K.; Bohm, T.D.; Baumann, B.; Kirschner, S.; Gohlke, F. Rotator cuff tear—An occupational disease? An epidemiological analysis. *Z. Orthop. Ihre Grenzgeb.* **2006**, *144*, 519–523. [CrossRef] [PubMed]
26. Magermans, D.J.; Chadwick, E.K.J.; Veeger, H.E.J.; Van Der Helm, F.C.T. Requirements for upper extremity motions during activities of daily living. *Clin. Biomech.* **2005**, *20*, 591–599. [CrossRef] [PubMed]
27. Lucas, K.R.; Rich, P.A.; Polus, B.I. Muscle activation patterns in the scapular positioning muscles during loaded scapular plane elevation: The effects of latent myofascial trigger points. *Clin. Biomech.* **2010**, *25*, 765–770. [CrossRef] [PubMed]
28. Andersen, K.S.; Christensen, B.H.; Samani, A.; Madeleine, P. Between-Day Reliability of a Hand-Held Dynamometer and Surface Electromyography Recordings during Isometric Submaximal Contractions in Different Shoulder Positions. *J. Electromyogr. Kinesiol.* **2014**, *24*, 579–587. [CrossRef] [PubMed]
29. van der Heijden, G.J.M.G.; Leffers, P.; Bouter, L.M. Shoulder Disability Questionnaire Design and Responsiveness of a Functional Status Measure. *J. Clin. Epidemiol.* **2000**, *53*, 29–38. [CrossRef]
30. Villarroya Aparicio, M.A. Electromiografía Cinesiológica. *Rehabilitación* **2005**, *39*, 255–264. [CrossRef]
31. Raz, Y.; Henseler, J.F.; Kolk, A.; Tatum, Z.; Groosjohan, N.K.; Verwey, N.E.; Arindrarto, W.; Kielbasa, S.M.; Nagels, J.; 't Hoen, P.A.C.; et al. Molecular Signatures of Age-Associated Chronic Degeneration of Shoulder Muscles. *Oncotarget* **2016**, *7*, 8513–8523. [CrossRef]
32. Farina, D.; Merletti, R.; Enoka, R.M. The Extraction of Neural Strategies from the Surface EMG: An Update. *J. Appl. Physiol.* **2014**, *117*, 1215–1230. [CrossRef]
33. Doherty, T.J. Invited Review: Aging and Sarcopenia. *J. Appl. Physiol.* **2003**, *95*, 1717–1727. [CrossRef]
34. Merletti, R.; Farina, D.; Gazzoni, M.; Schieroni, M.P. Effect of Age on Muscle Functions Investigated with Surface Electromyography. *Muscle Nerve* **2002**, *25*, 65–76. [CrossRef]
35. Plow, E.B.; Varnerin, N.; Cunningham, D.A.; Janini, D.; Bonnett, C.; Wyant, A.; Hou, J.; Siemionow, V.; Wang, X.-F.; Machado, A.G.; et al. Age-Related Weakness of Proximal Muscle Studied with Motor Cortical Mapping: A TMS Study. *PLoS ONE* **2014**, *9*, e89371. [CrossRef]
36. Raz, Y.; Henseler, J.F.; Kolk, A.; Riaz, M.; van der Zwaal, P.; Nagels, J.; Nelissen, R.G.H.H.; Raz, V. Patterns of Age-Associated Degeneration Differ in Shoulder Muscles. *Front. Aging Neurosci.* **2015**, *7*, 236. [CrossRef] [PubMed]
37. Tsai, A.-C.; Hsieh, T.-H.; Luh, J.-J.; Lin, T.-T. A Comparison of Upper-Limb Motion Pattern Recognition Using EMG Signals during Dynamic and Isometric Muscle Contractions. *Biomed. Signal Process. Control* **2014**, *11*, 17–26. [CrossRef]
38. McDonald, A.C.; Savoie, S.M.; Mulla, D.M.; Keir, P.J. Dynamic and Static Shoulder Strength Relationship and Predictive Model. *Appl. Ergon.* **2018**, *67*, 162–169. [CrossRef]
39. Radaelli, R.; Bottaro, M.; Weber, F.; Brown, L.E.; Pinto, R.S. Influence of Body Position on Shoulder Rotator Muscle Strength during Isokinetic Assessment. *Isokinet. Exerc. Sci.* **2010**, *18*, 119–124. [CrossRef]
40. Linnamo, V. Motor Unit Activation and Force Production during Eccentric, Concentric and Isometric Actions. *Stud. Sport Phys. Educ. Health* **2002**, *82*.
41. Baggen, R.J.; van Dieën, J.H.; Verschueren, S.M.; van Roie, E.; Delecluse, C. Differences in Maximum Voluntary Excitation Between Isometric and Dynamic Contractions Are Age-Dependent. *J. Appl. Biomech.* **2019**, *35*, 196–201. [CrossRef] [PubMed]
42. Lirio-Romero, C.; Torres-Lacomba, M.; Gómez-Blanco, A.; Acero-Cortés, A.; Retana-Garrido, A.; de la Villa-Polo, P.; Sánchez-Sánchez, B. Electromyographic Biofeedback Improves Upper Extremity Function: A Randomized, Single-Blinded, Controlled Trial. *Physiotherapy* **2020**, *15*, S0031-9406(20)30016-X. [CrossRef] [PubMed]
43. Phadke, V.; Camargo, P.; Ludewig, P. Scapular and Rotator Cuff Muscle Activity during Arm Elevation: A Review of Normal Function and Alterations with Shoulder Impingement. *Braz. J. Phys. Ther.* **2009**, *13*, 1–9. [CrossRef] [PubMed]
44. Kibler, B.W.; McMullen, J. Scapular dyskinesis and its relation to shoulder pain. *J. Am. Acad. Orthop. Surg.* **2003**, *11*, 142–151. [CrossRef]
45. Comerford, M.J.; Mottram, S. *Diagnosis of Uncontrolled Movement, Subgroup Classification and Motor Control Retraining of the Shoulder Girdle*; KC International: Ludlow, UK, 2010.

46. Hackett, L.; Reed, D.; Halaki, M.; Ginn, K.A. Assessing the validity of surface electromyography for recording muscle activation patterns from serratus anterior. *J. Electromyogr. Kinesiol.* **2014**, *24*, 221–227. [CrossRef] [PubMed]
47. Nordander, C.; Willner, J.; Hansson, G.; Larsson, B.; Unge, J.; Granquist, L.; Skerfving, S. Influence of the Subcutaneous Fat Layer, as Measured by Ultrasound, Skinfold Calipers and BMI, on the EMG Amplitude. *Eur. J. Appl. Physiol.* **2003**, *89*, 514–519. [CrossRef] [PubMed]
48. Hong, J.-S.; Kim, J.-H.; Hong, J.-H.; Chun, K.-J. Electromyograph Analysis during Isokinetic Testing of Shoulder Joint in Elderly People. *J. Biomech. Sci. Eng.* **2012**, *7*, 379–387. [CrossRef]
49. Kwon, M.; Chen, Y.-T.; Fox, E.J.; Christou, E.A. Aging and Limb Alter the Neuromuscular Control of Goal-Directed Movements. *Exp. Brain Res.* **2014**, *232*, 1759–1771. [CrossRef] [PubMed]
50. Kibler, W.B.; Chandler, T.J.; Shapiro, R.; Conuel, M. Muscle activation in coupled scapulohumeral motions in the high performance tennis serve. *Br. J. Sports Med.* **2007**, *41*, 745–749. [CrossRef] [PubMed]
51. Kibler, W.B.; Ellenbecker, T.; Sciascia, A. Neuromuscular adaptations in shoulder function and dysfunction. *Handb. Clin. Neurol.* **2018**, *158*, 385–400. [CrossRef]
52. Chadnova, E.; St-Onge, N.; Courtemanche, R.; Kilgour, R.D. Kinematics and Muscle Activation Patterns during a Maximal Voluntary Rate Activity in Healthy Elderly and Young Adults. *Aging Clin. Exp. Res.* **2017**, *29*, 1001–1011. [CrossRef]
53. Škarabot, J.; Ansdell, P.; Brownstein, C.G.; Hicks, K.M.; Howatson, G.; Goodall, S.; Durbaba, R. Reduced Corticospinal Responses in Older Compared with Younger Adults during Submaximal Isometric, Shortening, and Lengthening Contractions. *J. Appl. Physiol.* **2019**, *126*, 1015–1031. [CrossRef]

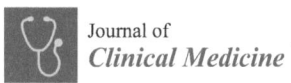

Article

Interaction between Subjective Memory Decline and Depression Symptom Intensity in Older People. Results of the Second Wave of Cognition of Older People, Education, Recreational Activities, Nutrition, Comorbidities, and Functional Capacity Studies (COPERNICUS)

Sławomir Kujawski [1,*], Agnieszka Kujawska [2,3], Radosław Perkowski [2], Joanna Androsiuk-Perkowska [2], Weronika Hajec [2], Małgorzata Kwiatkowska [2], Natalia Skierkowska [2], Jakub Husejko [2], Daria Bieniek [4], Julia L. Newton [5], Paweł Zalewski [1] and Kornelia Kędziora-Kornatowska [2]

Citation: Kujawski, S.; Kujawska, A.; Perkowski, R.; Androsiuk-Perkowska, J.; Hajec, W.; Kwiatkowska, M.; Skierkowska, N.; Husejko, J.; Bieniek, D.; Newton, J.L.; et al. Interaction between Subjective Memory Decline and Depression Symptom Intensity in Older People. Results of the Second Wave of Cognition of Older People, Education, Recreational Activities, Nutrition, Comorbidities, and Functional Capacity Studies (COPERNICUS). *J. Clin. Med.* **2021**, *10*, 1334. https://doi.org/10.3390/jcm10071334

Academic Editors: Jaakko Tuomilehto and Francesco Mattace-Raso

Received: 14 January 2021
Accepted: 17 March 2021
Published: 24 March 2021

Publisher's Note: MDPI stays neutral with regard to jurisdictional claims in published maps and institutional affiliations.

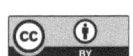

Copyright: © 2021 by the authors. Licensee MDPI, Basel, Switzerland. This article is an open access article distributed under the terms and conditions of the Creative Commons Attribution (CC BY) license (https://creativecommons.org/licenses/by/4.0/).

1 Department of Hygiene, Epidemiology, Ergonomics and Postgraduate Education, Division of Ergonomics and Exercise Physiology, Collegium Medicum in Bydgoszcz, Nicolaus Copernicus University in Toruń, 85-094 Bydgoszcz, Poland; p.zalewski@cm.umk.pl
2 Department of Geriatrics, Collegium Medicum in Bydgoszcz, Nicolaus Copernicus University in Toruń, 85-094 Bydgoszcz, Poland; agajos11@gmail.com (A.K.); perkowski.radoslaw@gmail.com (R.P.); joannaandrosiuk@gmail.com (J.A.-P.); weronika.topka.bydg@gmail.com (W.H.); malgorzata.gajos0904@gmail.com (M.K.); nataliaskierkowska1@gmail.com (N.S.); kubahusejko@gmail.com (J.H.); kasiakor@interia.pl (K.K.-K.)
3 Department of Physiology, Collegium Medicum in Bydgoszcz, Nicolaus Copernicus University in Toruń, 85-092 Bydgoszcz, Poland
4 Department of Gastroenterology and Nutrition Disorders, Collegium Medicum in Bydgoszcz, Nicolaus Copernicus University in Toruń, 85-168 Bydgoszcz, Poland; daria.bieniek2@wp.pl
5 Population Health Sciences Institute, The Medical School, Newcastle University, Newcastle-upon-Tyne NE2 4AX, UK; julia.newton@ncl.ac.uk
* Correspondence: skujawski@cm.umk.pl; Tel.: +48-52-585-3615

Abstract: Background: Prevalence of subjective memory impairment (SMC), with or without objective memory impairment, and the mediating role of depression symptom intensity was examined in older people. Methods: n = 205 subjects (60 years old and older) were examined and followed up at two years. Cognitive function was examined using the Montreal Cognitive Assessment (MoCA) Delayed Recall (DR) subtest. Geriatric Depression Scale (GDS) was used as a screening tool for depression. Statistical analysis was performed using linear mixed models. Results: A total of 144 subjects (70.24%) had SMC. MoCA Delayed Recall scores were not significantly changed in relation to time and SMC. Dynamics of SMC significantly influenced changes in GDS score (p = 0.008). Conclusions: SMC and objective memory impairment do not fully overlap each other. Subjects without SMC for longer than two years noted less intensity of depression symptoms in comparison to subgroup with SMC. However, occurrence of SMC in subjects who were previously free of SMC, was not related to increase in depression symptom intensity.

Keywords: cognitive function; older people; gerontology

1. Introduction

Subjective memory complaints (SMC) form a core component of the criteria for Mild Cognitive Impairment (MCI) [1,2]. However, results of a meta-analysis on objective vs. subjective memory performance noted minimal correlation between objective performance and subjective assessments, with regards to memory function in general. This highlights the need for caution when only relying on the latter [3].

SMC could be related to depression in late life [4]. However, changes over time in this relationship needs further investigation. Results showed that SMC at baseline increased the risk of increased depressive symptom intensity after four [5] and ten years [6,7]. A recent analysis concludes that SMC in cognitively normal older people might contribute to the development of depressive symptoms in the future [4]. A subgroup with SMC were shown to be at a higher risk for developing depressive symptoms [4–6]. Findings from the English Longitudinal Study of Ageing show that in patients with objective cognitive impairment, depressive symptoms might show increased SMC, but this did not affect objective impairment [8]. In contrast, Lehrner et al. noted that depression is related to increase in SMC, regardless of objective cognitive function [9]. In summary, based on the results from previous studies, the relationship exacted between SMC, objective memory impairment, and depression severity, seemed to be unclear. A systematic review suggested that further studies examining relationship between those factors should be performed in a longitudinal manner [10].

Cognition of Older People, Education, Recreational activities, NutritIon, Comorbidities, fUnctional capacity Studies (COPERNICUS) is the first longitudinal study on aging in Poland [11]. A multidisciplinary approach is needed to examine the potential factors influencing cognitive function because of the well-described relationship between cognitive function and physical exercise [12], level of physical activity [13], and cognitive activity [14], in addition to traditional indicators of cognitive reserve, such as education level and occupational attainment [15]. In this study, we examined the prevalence of SMC, with or without objective memory impairment, and explored the mediating role of depression symptom intensity in older people.

2. Materials and Methods

2.1. Enrolment

Figure 1 presents the process of study enrolment. In total, from $n = 407$ examined in the baseline cohort, $n = 202$ participants were lost to follow-up in the second wave of the study.

Participants were enrolled into studies based on advertisement, using regional TV and radio, during health-promoting lectures, in Day Care Centers for the Elderly, and at various meeting-groups for older people. Messages included information regarding an opportunity to a take part in a free-of-charge physical, physiotherapeutic, dietary, social, and cognitive assessment for people 60 years old and over. Age under 60 years old was the only excluding factor from participation in study. The lack of other factors excluding participation was underlined to collect the most representative sample of an older, Polish cohort, as much as possible. The study was approved by the Ethics Committee, Ludwik Rydygier Memorial Collegium Medicum in Bydgoszcz, Nicolaus Copernicus University, Torun (KB 340/2015, date of approval: 21 April 2015); and written informed consent was obtained from all participants.

2.2. Measurement

2.2.1. Subjective Questionnaire

Subjective problems with memory were assessed twice—at the baseline and after 2-years follow-up. Data from both time-points was included in the statistical analysis. Participants were divided into subjective memory complainers (SMC) and non-subjective memory complainers (NSMC), depending on their answers to the question "Have You observed memory decline?" "Yes" was coded as "1", "no" as "0". At the 2-year follow-up, the time frame of this question was over the last 2 years. Then, the following answers on dynamics of memory decline could be chosen—"once it was better once worse", "slow rate of memory decline", "rapid", and "it is hard to describe". One of three answers on the presence of memory performance fluctuation during the day could be chosen—"yes", "no", or "it is hard to describe". The time of day when the memory impairment could be described using one of the following options "worsen during the day", "at the evening", "at the morning", "it is hard to describe", and "none".

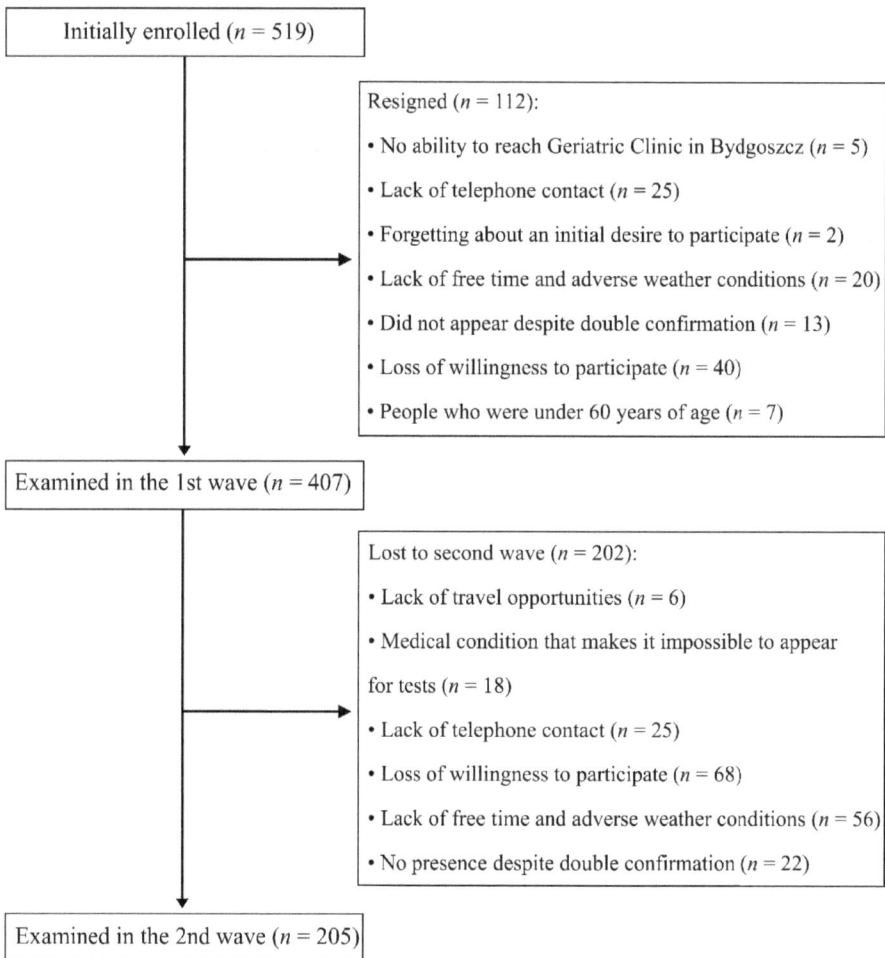

Figure 1. Flow chart of the study.

2.2.2. Cognitive Tests

Neuropsychological tests were conducted by two staff, who underwent common training in the procedures. Almost all (97.1%) neuropsychological tests were conducted by the same person. First, a questionnaire on subjective memory complaints was conducted. Cognitive functioning was assessed with the Mini-Mental State Examination (MMSE), Montreal Cognitive Assessment (MoCA), and Trail Making Test Part B (TMT B). MMSE is a well-known 30-points questionnaire used in neuropsychological assessment, it measures orientation to time and place, immediate recall, and short-term verbal memory, calculation, language, and construct ability. A higher score indicates better cognitive performance [16]. MMSE accuracy and efficiency seems to be worse than other screening tests aiming to measure cognitive function in older people [17]. However, it was widely used in previous research on older patients in Poland [18–20].

The MoCA assesses several cognitive domains [21,22]. It measures all main cognitive domains; namely visuospatial skills, short-term memory recall, executive functioning (examined by a mini-form of Trail Making Test part B, phonemic fluency task, and a two-item verbal abstraction task). Attention, concentration, and working memory, as well as naming and other language skills were evaluated. In MoCA, test results of two subtests (Verbal Fluency subtest and Delayed Recall of five nouns) were taken into account separately during analysis. The Verbal Fluency subtest result is the number of words in Polish starting with the letter "S", which are not own nouns (conjugation prohibited). In the case of Delayed Recall, two score was taken into analysis—first was the number of words recalled without the help of person carrying out the test (MoCA Delayed Recall subtest). The second score was the overall number of words recalled without help, and number of words recalled after the category of the word recalled and the number of words were correctly chosen from a list of three words (MoCA Delayed Recall subtest overall score). Results from the Delayed Recall subtest served as an indicator of verbal short-memory performance. Result of this subtest was used to address the primary outcome of the study, namely the relationship between subjective and objective memory impairment with depression severity. The Polish version of MoCA was shown to be accurate in assessing the cognitive function level in previous research [23].

Trail Making Test part B is a fast-to-assess neuropsychological tool, which measures various skill from the executive functioning domain—visuospatial skills, task switching, and working memory, to mention a few [24].

2.2.3. Emotional State Assessment

The 15-item Geriatric Depression Scale (GDS) is a self-report measure of depression dedicated to older patients' assessment [25]. This shorter version was proven to be useful among very old people, with and without cognitive impairment [26]. Questions concerning assessment of retrospection, the quality of life, current state, activities, mental state, life attitude, and other questions were asked. Answers were presented in dichotomized (yes/no) format. The higher the score, the higher the severity of depression. GDS sensitivity and specificity was calculated as 84% and 95%, respectively [25,27].

2.2.4. Functional Performance Assessment

A six-minute walk test (6MWT) was performed [28]. Eight feet up-and-go result is an indicator of functional performance, gait speed, and balance, in a dynamic manner. Subject was asked to get up from the chair and walk a distance of 8 feet, to and around a marker placed on floor, get back and sit on the chair again, as fast as possible [29].

2.2.5. Activity Level Assessment

Answers on questions about the frequency of current physical, cognitive and social activities, and diet, were coded in the following way—"never" was coded as 0, "once a year" as 1, "several times a year" as 2, "1–2 times a month" as 3, "once a week" as 4, "few times a week" as 5, and "daily" as 6. The result of the questionnaire was the overall score from all questions. The following questions on cognitive and social activities were asked—reading press, reading books, watching TV, listening to the radio, going to the café, restaurant, going to the cinema, going to the theater or concert, going to church, going to visit friends or family, taking part in social group meetings, computer use, card game, chess/checkers, and solving crosswords. In addition, questions on the following physical activities—short walks around the house place, long walks, gymnastics, cycling, running/jogging, swimming, skiing, team games, sailing, horse riding, Nordic walking, tennis/table tennis, dance, and work on the plot or in the garden/mushroom collection. The following questions on frequency of travel activities in the last 3 years were asked: 1-day trips without accommodation, multi-day sightseeing trips, pilgrimages, wandering (with accommodation in hostels, campsites), stays at campsites, with accommodation, holiday/holiday stays, trips stationary, leisure trips to friends, stays on plot (outside your home), spa stays (prophylactically without referrals to the sanatorium), and stays in sanatoria on the basis of a referral. Frequency of consumption of beer, wine, vodka, and other strong alcohols was assessed. Overall frequency was the score of ethanol consumption. Financial status was calculated indirectly, based on particular items in an activity questionnaire (such as frequency of going to restaurants, traveling abroad etc.).

2.3. Statistical Analysis

All statistical analyses were performed using the statistical package R [30]. Mean and standard deviation (SD) values are presented. To assess the relationship of SMC with changes in objective short-term verbal memory decline (before vs. after two years) and GDS score, a linear mixed model with a restricted maximum likelihood approach, and *t*-tests (using the Satterthwaite method) was used. Analysis was carried out in R statistical packages (Lme4 and LmerTest packages was used [31]). The subject and time factors were determined as random effects. Plots were created to show the interaction between SMC and time (before vs. after 2 years). The vertical lines denote the 95% confidence interval. Post-hoc tests results were adjusted using the Holm method to counteract the problem of multiple comparisons using lsmeans and multcomp packages [32].

3. Results

3.1. Baseline Data from Those Participating in the Follow-Up Compared to Those Not Participating

Table 1 shows the comparison between baseline data from those participants lost to follow up in the second wave compared to those who were re-examined. The age of participants lost to follow-up were not significantly different as compared to those re-examined. Scores of MMSE, MoCA, and TMT B were significantly worse in subjects lost to follow-up. Moreover, the group of re-examined subjects who spent significantly more years in education, were characterized by higher cognitive, social, and overall activity level, as well as better financial status.

Table 1. Comparison of lost to follow-up vs. re-examined subjects.

Variable	Not Examined in the Second Wave (*n* = 202) Mean ± SD	Re-Examined (*n* = 205) Mean ± SD	z or t	*p*-Value
Age (years)	69.84 ± 6.3	69.66 ± 6.0	0.01	0.99
Age of memory impairment (years)	64.75 ± 7.3	65.12 ± 7.7	−0.96	0.34
MMSE (points)	27.33 ± 2.4	27.80 ± 2.1	−2.24	0.03
MoCA (points)	22.74 ± 3.7	23.63 ± 3.5	−2.46	**0.01**
MoCA Delayed Recall (words)	2.26 ± 1.7	2.25 ± 1.6	0.10	0.92
MoCA DR in overall (words)	4.62 ± 0.8	4.76 ± 0.5	−1.31	0.19
MoCA Verbal Fluency (words)	12.02 ± 4.4	12.73 ± 4.5	−1.59	0.11
TMT B (seconds)	162.74 ± 99.4	136.90 ± 88.5	3.33	**<0.01**
GDS (points)	3.37 ± 2.8	3.23 ± 2.8	0.71	0.48
Health self-assessment-currently (points)	6.73 ± 1.6	7.05 ± 1.5	−1.75	0.08
Health self-assessment-10 years ago (points)	8.09 ± 1.7	8.00 ± 2.0	0.03	0.97
Years of education (years)	13.55 ± 3.1	14.37 ± 3.4	−2.24	**0.02**
Mental and social activity lvl (points)	40.06 ± 8.5	42.72 ± 8.2	−3.05	**<0.01**
Physical activity lvl (points)	19.48 ± 7.9	20.06 ± 7.2	−0.74	0.46
Touristic activity lvl (points)	6.42 ± 3.6	6.44 ± 3.4	−0.21	0.83
Sum of rich in antioxidants food intake (points)	22.91 ± 6.2	24.11 ± 5.7	−1.23	0.22
Ethanol intake (points)	4.27 ± 3.6	4.76 ± 3.5	−1.41	0.16
Total cognitive + physical + touristic activity lvl (points)	65.95 ± 14.9	69.22 ± 14.2	−2.24	**0.02**
Financial status (points)	10.95 ± 5.3	13.12 ± 5.3	−3.96	**<0.01**

MMSE—Mini–Mental State Examination; MoCA—Montreal Cognitive Assessment; MoCA Delayed Recall—number of word correctly recalled without examiner help in the short-term verbal memory test; MoCA DR in overall—number of words correctly recalled after category and list cues in Delayed Recall subtest of MoCA, TMT B -Trail Making Test Part B, GDS—Geriatric Depression Scale; *p*-values lower than 0.05 are bolded.

At baseline, subjective memory impairment was noticed by 73.8% of the subgroup lost to follow-up and by 79% of the re-examined participants. One hundred twenty-five subjects reported SMC at baseline and after 2 years. Thirty-seven subjects reported SMC at the baseline, however, were free of SMC after 2 years (Table 2).

Table 2. Comparison of SMC prevalence at the baseline and after 2 years.

SMC Baseline	SMC after 2 Years	Count (n)	Frequency (%)
yes	yes	125	61
no	yes	20	9.8
yes	no	37	18
no	no	23	11.2

SMC—Subjective memory complaints presence.

3.2. Comparison of Measures in the Cohort with Baseline and Follow-Up Data

In the cohort of 205 re-examined subjects, 144 (70.24%) had SMC. Twenty subjects (13.99%) with SMC noted memory impairment fluctuation during the day. At the baseline, ninety-five participants had a history of arterial hypertension, of which 58 received antihypertensive treatment.

Interaction between time and SMC factors in the results of MoCA Delayed Recall subtest score (which is the number of word recalled without the examiners help) was not statistically significant (-0.09 (-0.6; 0.4), $t = -0.34$, $p = 0.73$) (Figure 2).

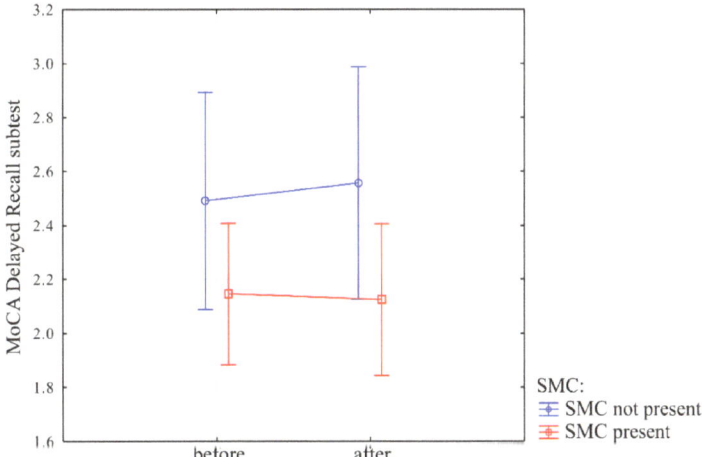

Figure 2. Interaction between time and subjective memory complaint (SMC) presence and results of MoCA Delayed Recall subtest. Y-axis (MoCA Delayed Recall subtest) represents the number of words recalled correctly in short-term verbal memory test in MoCA without the help of staff conducting the examination. X-axis ("before" and "after") denotes the initial time-point and after two years, respectively. Blue line indicates subgroup without subjective memory complaints, while red line indicates scores of participants with subjective memory complaint.

Interaction between time and SMC and the overall results of the MoCA Delayed Recall subtest was not statistically significant (-0.14 (-0.39; 0.11), $t = -1.01$, $p = 0.31$) (Figure 3).

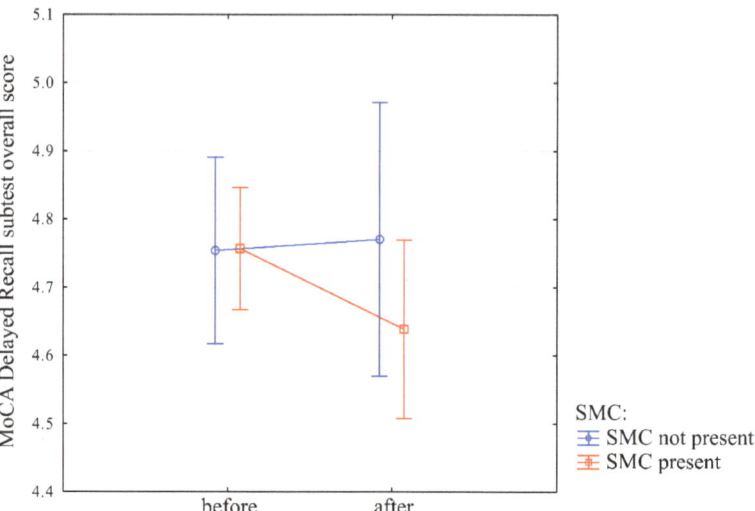

Figure 3. Interaction between time and subjective memory complaint (SMC) presence and results of the overall MoCA Delayed Recall subtest. Y-axis represents the number of words overall recalled correctly in the short-term verbal memory test in MoCA, after category, and the list cues. First, a category of word was recalled, then the participant was asked to choose the correct word from a list of three words from the same category. Sum of the overall number of words recalled by the participant themselves, with the category and list cue. X-axis ("before" and "after") denotes the initial time-point and after two years, respectively. Blue line indicates a subgroup without subjective memory complaints, while the red line indicates scores of participants with subjective memory complaint.

The interaction between time and SMC and the other tests (MMSE, MoCA, TMT B) were also non-significant. Participants with SMC in the second wave (follow up) were significantly older, had worse TMT B, showed higher depression severity, a slower gait, and a worse aerobic capacity compared to subgroup without SMC in the baseline (Table 3).

Table 3. Difference in variables measured in the baseline between subgroups with subjective memory complaint (SMC) present vs. non-present after two years.

Variable	Subjective Memory Complaint Present				z	p-Value
	Present (n = 162)		Not Present (n = 43)			
	Mean	Std. Dev.	Mean	Std. Dev.		
Age (years)	70.25	6.1	67.44	5.2	2.67	**0.01**
Years of education (years)	14.23	3.5	14.91	3.2	−1.56	0.12
MMSE (points)	27.69	2.2	28.21	1.7	−1.35	0.18
MoCA (points)	23.67	3.6	23.51	3.1	0.63	0.53
MoCA Verbal Fluency (words)	12.67	4.5	12.95	4.7	t = −0.36	0.72
MoCA Delayed Recall (words)	2.28	1.6	2.12	1.5	0.63	0.53
TMT B (seconds)	142.66	89.3	115.33	82.7	2.33	**0.02**
GDS (points)	3.46	2.8	2.35	2.7	2.69	**0.01**
8 ft test (seconds)	6.14	2	5.58	2	2.19	**0.03**
6MWT (meters)	496.95	97.9	535.33	105.8	−2.54	**0.01**

MMSE—Mini-Mental State Examination; MoCA—Montreal Cognitive Assessment; MoCA Delayed Recall—number of word correctly recalled without examiner help in the short-term verbal memory test; TMT B—Trail Making Test Part B; GDS—Geriatric Depression Scale, 8 ft test—8 ft up-and-go—8 ft test; and 6MWT—Six-minute walk test; p-values lower than 0.05 are bolded.

Subjects with SMC and objective verbal memory decline in the second wave had significantly lower years of education, better MoCA, Delayed Recall subtest scores, and worse TMT B performance, as compared to subgroup without subjective and objective memory impairment in the baseline (Table 4).

Table 4. Difference in variables measured in the baseline between subgroups with SMC present vs. non-present after two years.

Variable	Subjective and Objective Memory Impairment				z	p-Value
	Present (n = 60)		Not Present (n = 145)			
	Mean	Std. Dev.	Mean	Std. Dev.		
Age (years)	70.38	6	69.37	6	−1.20	0.23
Years of education (years)	13.55	3.3	14.71	3.4	2.54	**0.01**
MMSE (points)	27.78	2.2	27.81	2.1	−0.28	0.78
MoCA (points)	24.68	3.2	23.20	3.6	−2.74	**0.01**
MoCA Verbal Fluency (words)	12.53	4.4	12.81	4.6	t = 0.4	0.69
MoCA Delayed Recall (words)	3.22	1.2	1.85	1.6	−5.55	**<0.0001**
TMT B (seconds)	158.78	101.1	127.78	81.3	−2.02	**0.04**
GDS (points)	3.72	2.9	3.03	2.8	−1.71	0.09
8 ft test (seconds)	6.15	2.1	5.97	2	−0.74	0.46
6MWT (meters)	495.68	93.8	508.42	103.2	0.53	0.59

MMSE—Mini-Mental State Examination; MoCA—Montreal Cognitive Assessment; MoCA Delayed Recall—number of word correctly recalled without examiner help in the short-term verbal memory test; TMT B—Trail Making Test Part B; GDS—Geriatric Depression Scale, 8 ft test—8 ft up-and-go—8 ft test; and 6MWT—Six-minute walk test. p-values lower than 0.05 are bolded.

GDS was included as a dependent variable with SMC, before and after 2 years as a fixed effect, while subject and time factors were set as random effects. Dynamics of SMC was significantly related to changes in GDS scores (F = 4.9, p = 0.008). Participants who did not report SMC at both time-points of the GDS score was significantly lower (2.39 ± 2.2 before vs. 2 ± 1.8 after two years) in comparison to subjects who reported SMC at both time-points (3.62 ± 2.8 before vs. 3.62 ± 2.7 after two years) (p = 0.04). Moreover, among participants who did not report SMC before and reported SMC after two years, the GDS score was significantly lower (2.3 ± 3.3 before vs. 1.95 ± 2.4 after two years) in comparison to subjects who reported SMC at both time-points (3.62 ± 2.8 before vs. 3.62 ± 2.7 after two years) (p = 0.04) (Figure 4).

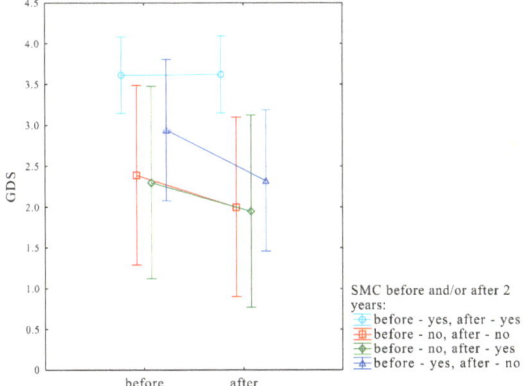

Figure 4. Results of linear mixed model predicting GDS score change over two years in relation to the presence of subjective and objective verbal memory decline. Y-axis represents the score on the Geriatric Depression Scale (GDS). X-axis ("before" and "after") denotes the initial time-point and after two years, respectively. Light blue line indicates the subgroup of subjective memory complaint (SMC) at both time-points, red line indicates subgroup without SMC at both time-points. Green line indicates participants who were free of SMC at the initial time-point, but it changed after two years (after). Dark blue line denotes subgroup with SMC at the initial time-point and who was free of SMC after two years (after).

4. Discussion

In the above study, higher depression symptom severity at baseline assessment was associated with a higher risk of both SMC and objective decline of short-term verbal memory. This finding was consistent with a recent analysis, where depression was shown to be related to an increase in SMC [9]. In addition, in a similar study, the authors concluded that perception of decline of memory functioning rather than current memory functioning might be a significant predictor of increase in depressive symptoms in older adults [4]. In addition, previous studies revealed the same association, i.e., that SMC at baseline increases the risk of increased depressive symptom intensity [5,7].

Subjective memory complaints might occur more frequently in people experiencing negative mood [33,34]. In contrast, deficits in memory and attention are often associated with depression [35,36]. Balash et al. noted that SMC could be related to sub-syndromal depression and anxiety in cognitively intact older subjects [37]. Recent findings also indicate that depression severity might occur both before and after objective cognitive decline is noted [38].

Schmand et al. reported that SMC indicates "realistic" self-observation of cognitive decline. However, our results indicate that SMC was not significantly related to changes in short-term verbal memory test [39]. On the other hand, our results support those of a study conducted on a population from Germany, which confirmed that SMC is more strongly related to depression than objective memory decline [40].

In our study, 37 subjects (18%) reported SMC at baseline, however, were free of SMC after 2 years. Therefore, one can speculate that SMC could be transient in some older patients. In line with the above results, in a longitudinal study on 543 subjects from a rural Chinese population, 265 (49%) answered "yes" to the question "Do you have trouble with your memory?" at the baseline and 209 (39%) answered the same after 3 years [41]. It seems important to conduct further studies to explore the relationship between SMC with objective memory decline and depression severity. SMC is one of the components of a Mild Cognitive Impairment (MCI) diagnosis proposed by Petersen et al. [42]. However, some authors suggest that SMC might be more related to emotional disturbance rather than objective cognitive impairment [43], while some even strongly suggest that SMC should be excluded from the MCI criteria [44]. Therefore, further studies on mechanisms underlying SMC are needed. Moreover, understanding the underlying background of SMC might improve treatment of comorbidities of older patients with SMC.

One of the potential limitations of our study was that it used a questionnaire to capture the subjective memory complaints at only two time-points, without specifying the exact time-frame. Moreover, complaints in other cognitive domains and associated worries were not examined. One factor that could affect both the frequency and usability of an SMC is how it is measured [45]. Questions could be focused on current memory performance assessment, comparison of performance with peers, or reflect on whether the memory deteriorated over time [46]. Research examining how older adults interpret memory performance questions shows that these different types of questions do actually assess different aspects of perception of issues with memory [47,48]. Moreover, further studies should incorporate more time-points to fully reveal the relationship between the dynamics of SMC and depression intensity. In addition, further longitudinal studies on the relationship between SMC, objective memory decline and depression severity, should incorporate bigger sample sizes and examine the effects of comorbidities and treatment on this relationship. It seems that side-effects from certain groups of pharmacological agents could be associated with episodic memory decline [49]. On the other hand, deep brain stimulation in patients with Parkinson Disease presumably could lead to short-term improvement in depression [50] On the other hand, the above study is the first in Polish population to examine the relationship between depression, subjective, and objective memory decline in a longitudinal manner.

5. Conclusions

Our results suggest that groups of older people with SMC and objective short-term verbal memory decline do not fully overlap each other. Participants with SMC after two years were older, had a worse executive function, showed higher depression severity, a slower gait, and worse aerobic capacity.

Older people without SMC for longer than two years showed less intensity of depression symptoms in comparison to a subgroup with SMC for longer than two years. However, the occurrence of SMC in older people who were previously free of SMC, was not related to an increase in depression symptoms intensity.

Author Contributions: Conceptualization, S.K., P.Z., K.K.-K., and A.K.; methodology, S.K., P.Z., K.K.-K., and A.K.; software, S.K.; validation, R.P., J.A.-P., M.K., N.S., J.H., and D.B.; formal analysis, S.K.; investigation, S.K., A.K., R.P., J.A.-P., M.K., N.S., J.H., and D.B.; resources, S.K.; data curation, R.P., J.A.-P., M.K., N.S., J.H., and D.B.; writing—original draft preparation, S.K. and A.K.; writing—review and editing, S.K., A.K., R.P., J.A.-P., W.H., M.K., N.S., J.H., D.B., J.L.N., P.Z., and K.K.-K.; visualization, S.K.; supervision, P.Z. and K.K.-K.; project administration, P.Z. and K.K.-K.; funding acquisition, S.K. All authors have read and agreed to the published version of the manuscript.

Funding: This research received no external funding.

Institutional Review Board Statement: The study was conducted according to the guidelines of the Declaration of Helsinki, and approved by the Ethics Committee, Ludwik Rydygier Memorial Collegium Medicum in Bydgoszcz, Nicolaus Copernicus University, Torun (KB 340/2015, date of approval: 21 April 2015).

Informed Consent Statement: Informed consent was obtained from all subjects involved in the study.

Data Availability Statement: Individual data are available from the corresponding author S.K. on request.

Conflicts of Interest: The authors declare no conflict of interest.

References

1. Winblad, B.; Palmer, K.; Kivipelto, M.; Jelic, V.; Fratiglioni, L.; Wahlund, L.O.; Nordberg, A.; Bäckman, L.; Albert, M.; Almkvist, O.; et al. Mild cognitive impairment–beyond controversies, towards a consensus: Report of the International Working Group on Mild Cognitive Impairment. *J. Intern. Med.* **2004**, *256*, 240–246. [CrossRef] [PubMed]
2. Portet, F.; Ousset, P.J.; Visser, P.J.; Frisoni, G.B.; Nobili, F.; Scheltens, P.; Vellas, B.; Touchon, J. MCI Working Group of the European Consortium on Alzheimer's Disease (EADC). Mild cognitive impairment (MCI) in medical practice: A critical review of the concept and new diagnostic procedure. Report of the MCI Working Group of the European Consortium on Alzheimer's Disease. *J. Neurol. Neurosurg. Psychiatry* **2006**, *77*, 714–718. [CrossRef] [PubMed]
3. Crumley, J.J.; Stetler, C.A.; Horhota, M. Examining the relationship between subjective and objective memory performance in older adults: A meta-analysis. *Psychol. Aging* **2014**, *29*, 250. [CrossRef] [PubMed]
4. Mogle, J.; Hill, N.L.; Bhargava, S.; Bell, T.R.; Bhang, I. Memory complaints and depressive symptoms over time: A construct-level replication analysis. *BMC Geriatr.* **2020**, *20*, 1–10. [CrossRef] [PubMed]
5. Heun, R.; Hein, S. Risk factors of major depression in the elderly. *Eur. Psychiatry* **2005**, *20*, 199–204. [CrossRef]
6. Potvin, O.; Bergua, V.; Swendsen, J.; Meillon, C.; Tzourio, C.; Ritchie, K.; Dartigues, J.F.; Amieva, H. Anxiety and 10-year risk of incident and recurrent depressive symptomatology in older adults. *Depress. Anxiety* **2013**, *30*, 554–563. [CrossRef] [PubMed]
7. Singh-Manoux, A.; Dugravot, A.; Ankri, J.; Nabi, H.; Berr, C.; Goldberg, M.; Zins, M.; Kivimaki, M.; Elbaz, A. Subjective cognitive complaints and mortality: Does the type of complaint matter? *J. Psychiatr. Res.* **2014**, *48*, 73–78. [CrossRef]
8. Brailean, A.; Steptoe, A.; Batty, G.D.; Zaninotto, P.; Llewellyn, D.J. Are subjective memory complaints indicative of objective cognitive decline or depressive symptoms? Findings from the English Longitudinal Study of Ageing. *J. Psychiatr. Res.* **2019**, *110*, 143–151. [CrossRef]
9. Lehrner, J.; Moser, D.; Klug, S.; Gleiß, A.; Auff, E.; Dal-Bianco, P.; Pusswald, G. Subjective memory complaints, depressive symptoms and cognition in patients attending a memory outpatient clinic. *Int. Psychogeriatr.* **2014**, *26*, 463–473. [CrossRef]
10. Brigola, A.G.; Manzini, C.S.S.; Oliveira, G.B.S.; Ottaviani, A.C.; Sako, M.P.; Vale, F.A.C. Subjective memory complaints associated with depression and cognitive impairment in the elderly: A systematic review. *Dement. Neuropsychol.* **2015**, *9*, 51–57. [CrossRef]
11. Kujawski, S.; Kujawska, A.; Gajos, M.; Topka, W.; Perkowski, R.; Androsiuk-Perkowska, J.; Newton, J.L.; Zalewski, P.; Kędziora-Kornatowska, K. Cognitive functioning in older people. Results of the first wave of cognition of older people, education, recreational activities, nutrition, comorbidities, functional capacity studies (COPERNICUS). *Front. Aging Neurosci.* **2018**, *10*, 421. [CrossRef]

12. Kramer, A.F.; Colcombe, S. Fitness effects on the cognitive function of older adults: A meta-analytic study—Revisited. *Perspect. Psychol. Sci.* **2018**, *13*, 213–217. [CrossRef] [PubMed]
13. Weuve, J.; Kang, J.H.; Manson, J.E.; Breteler, M.M.; Ware, J.H.; Grodstein, F. Physical activity, including walking, and cognitive function in older women. *JAMA* **2004**, *292*, 1454–1461. [CrossRef] [PubMed]
14. Marquine, M.J.; Segawa, E.; Wilson, R.S.; Bennett, D.A.; Barnes, L.L. Association between cognitive activity and cognitive function in older Hispanics. *J. Int. Neuropsychol. Soc.* **2012**, *18*, 1041. [CrossRef] [PubMed]
15. Stern, Y.; Barnes, C.A.; Grady, C.; Jones, R.N.; Raz, N. Brain reserve, cognitive reserve, compensation, and maintenance: Operationalization, validity, and mechanisms of cognitive resilience. *Neurobiol. Aging* **2019**, *83*, 124–129. [CrossRef]
16. Folstein, M.F.; Folstein, S.E.; McHugh, P.R. "Mini-mental state". A practical method for grading the cognitive state of patients for the clinician. *J. Psychiatr. Res.* **1983**, *12*, 189–198. [CrossRef]
17. Mitchell, A.J. The Mini-Mental State Examination (MMSE): Update on its diagnostic accuracy and clinical utility for cognitive disorders. In *Cognitive Screening Instruments*; Springer: Cham, Switzerland, 2017; pp. 37–48.
18. Uchmanowicz, I.; Jankowska-Polańska, B.; Mazur, G.; Froelicher, E.S. Cognitive deficits and self-care behaviors in elderly adults with heart failure. *Clin. Interv. Aging* **2017**, *12*, 1565–1572. [CrossRef] [PubMed]
19. McFarlane, O.; Kozakiewicz, M.; Kędziora-Kornatowska, K.; Gębka, D.; Szybalska, A.; Szwed, M.; Klich-Rączka, A. Blood Lipids and Cognitive Performance of Aging Polish Adults: A Case-Control Study Based on the PolSenior Project. *Front. Aging Neurosci.* **2020**, *12*, 590546. [CrossRef]
20. Kapusta, J.; Kidawa, T.M.; Rynkowska-Kidawa, M.; Irzmański, T.R.; Kowalski, T.J. Evaluation of frequency of occurrence of cognitive impairment in the course of arterial hypertension in an elderly population. *Psychogeriatrics* **2020**, *20*, 406–411. [CrossRef]
21. Freitas, S.; Simoes, M.R.; Marôco, J.; Alves, L.; Santana, I. Construct validity of the montreal cognitive assessment (MoCA). *J. Int. Neuropsychol. Soc.* **2012**, *18*, 242–250. [CrossRef]
22. Nasreddine, Z.S.; Phillips, N.A.; Bédirian, V.; Charbonneau, S.; Whitehead, V.; Collin, I.; Cummings, J.L.; Chertkow, H. The Montreal Cognitive Assessment, MoCA: A brief screening tool for mild cognitive impairment. *J. Am. Geriatr. Soc.* **2005**, *53*, 695–699. [CrossRef]
23. Magierska, J.; Magierski, R.; Fendler, W.; Kłoszewska, I.; Sobów, T.M. Clinical application of the Polish adaptation of the Montreal Cognitive Assessment (MoCA) test in screening for cognitive impairment. *Neurol. Neurochir. Pol.* **2012**, *46*, 130–139. [CrossRef]
24. Reitan, R.M. Validity of the Trail Making Test as an indicator of organic brain damage. *Percept. Mot. Skills* **1958**, *8*, 271–276. [CrossRef]
25. Almeida, O.P.; Almeida, S.A. Short versions of the geriatric depression scale: A study of their validity for the diagnosis of a major depressive episode according to ICD-10 and DSM-IV. *Int. J. Geriatr. Psychiatry* **1999**, *14*, 858–865. [CrossRef]
26. Conradsson, M.; Rosendahl, E.; Littbrand, H.; Gustafson, Y.; Olofsson, B.; Lövheim, H. Usefulness of the Geriatric Depression Scale 15-item version among very old people with and without cognitive impairment. *Aging Ment. Health* **2013**, *17*, 638–645. [CrossRef]
27. Albiński, R.; Kleszczewska-Albińska, A.; Bedyńska, S. Geriatryczna Skala Depresji (GDS). Trafność i rzetelność różnych wersji tego narzędzia–przegląd badań. *Psychiatry Pol.* **2011**, *45*, 555–562.
28. Roomi, J.; Johnson, M.M.; Waters, K.; Yohannes, A.; Helm, A.C.M.J.; Connolly, M.J. Respiratory rehabilitation, exercise capacity and quality of life in chronic airways disease in old age. *Age Ageing* **1996**, *25*, 12–16. [CrossRef]
29. Rikli, R.E.; Jones, C.J. Development and validation of a functional fitness test for community-residing older adults. *Aging Phys. Act.* **1999**, *7*, 129–161. [CrossRef]
30. R Core Team. *R: A Language and Environment for Statistical Computing*; R Foundation for Statistical Computing: Vienna, Austria, 2013.
31. Bates, D.; Mächler, M.; Bolker, B.; Walker, S. Fitting linear mixed-effects models using lme4. *arXiv* **2014**, arXiv:1406.5823.
32. Hothorn, T.; Bretz, F.; Westfall, P. Simultaneous inference in general parametric models. *Biom. J.* **2008**, *50*, 346–363. [CrossRef] [PubMed]
33. Cargin, W.J.; Collie, A.; Masters, C.; Maruff, P. The nature of cognitive complaints in healthy older adults with and without objective memory decline. *J. Clin. Exp. Neuropsychol.* **2008**, *30*, 245–257. [CrossRef]
34. Farrin, L.; Hull, L.; Unwin, C.; Wykes, T.; David, A. Effects of depressed mood on objective and subjective measures of attention. *J. Neuropsychiatry Clin. Neurosci.* **2003**, *15*, 98–104. [CrossRef]
35. Donaldson, C.; Lam, D.; Mathews, A. Rumination and attention in major depression. *Behav. Res.* **2007**, *45*, 2664–2678. [CrossRef] [PubMed]
36. Rock, P.L.; Roiser, J.P.; Riedel, W.J.; Blackwell, A.D. Cognitive impairment in depression: A systematic review and meta-analysis. *Psychol. Med.* **2014**, *44*, 2029. [CrossRef] [PubMed]
37. Balash, Y.; Mordechovich, M.; Shabtai, H.; Giladi, N.; Gurevich, T.; Korczyn, A.D. Subjective memory complaints in elders: Depression, anxiety, or cognitive decline? *Acta Neurol. Scand.* **2013**, *127*, 344–350. [CrossRef] [PubMed]
38. Desai, R.; Charlesworth, G.M.; Brooker, H.J.; Potts, H.W.; Corbett, A.; Aarsland, D.; Ballard, C.G. Temporal Relationship Between Depressive Symptoms and Cognition in Mid and Late Life: A Longitudinal Cohort Study. *Am. Med. Dir. Assoc.* **2020**, *21*, 1108–1113. [CrossRef] [PubMed]
39. Schmand, B.E.N.; Jonker, C.; Geerlings, M.I.; Lindeboom, J. Subjective memory complaints in the elderly: Depressive symptoms and future dementia. *Br. J. Psychiatry* **1997**, *171*, 373. [CrossRef] [PubMed]

40. Schütz, H.; Caspers, S.; Moebus, S.; Lux, S. Prevalence and psychosocial correlates of subjectively perceived decline in five cognitive domains. Results from a population-based cohort study in Germany. *Int. J. Geriatr. Psychiatry* **2020**, *35*, 1219–1227. [CrossRef] [PubMed]
41. Wang, P.N.; Wang, S.J.; Fuh, J.L.; Teng, E.L.; Liu, C.Y.; Lin, C.H.; Shyu, H.Y.; Lu, S.R.; Chen, C.C.; Liu, H.C. Subjective memory complaint in relation to cognitive performance and depression: A longitudinal study of a rural Chinese population. *J. Am. Geriatr. Soc.* **2000**, *48*, 295–299. [CrossRef]
42. Petersen, R.C.; Doody, R.; Kurz, A.; Mohs, R.C.; Morris, J.C.; Rabins, P.V.; Ritchie, K.; Rossor, M.; Thal, L.; Winblad, B. Current concepts in mild cognitive impairment. *Arch. Neurol.* **2001**, *58*, 1985–1992. [CrossRef]
43. Yates, J.A.; Clare, L.; Woods, R.T.; MRC CFAS. Subjective memory complaints, mood and MCI: A follow-up study. *Aging Ment. Health* **2017**, *21*, 313–321. [CrossRef] [PubMed]
44. Lenehan, M.E.; Klekociuk, S.Z.; Summers, M.J. Absence of a relationship between subjective memory complaint and objective memory impairment in mild cognitive impairment (MCI): Is it time to abandon subjective memory complaint as an MCI diagnostic criterion? *Int. Psychogeriatr.* **2012**, *24*, 1505–1514. [CrossRef]
45. Molinuevo, J.L.; Rabin, L.A.; Amariglio, R.; Buckley, R.; Dubois, B.; Ellis, K.A.; Subjective Cognitive Decline Initiative (SCD-I) Working Group. Implementation of subjective cognitive decline criteria in research studies. *Alzheimers Dement.* **2017**, *13*, 296–311. [CrossRef] [PubMed]
46. Hertzog, C.; Hülür, G.; Gerstorf, D.; Pearman, A.M. Is subjective memory change in old age based on accurate monitoring of age-related memory change? Evidence from two longitudinal studies. *Psychol. Aging* **2018**, *33*, 273. [CrossRef]
47. Hill, N.L.; Mogle, J.; Whitaker, E.B.; Gilmore-Bykovskyi, A.; Bhargava, S.; Bhang, I.Y.; Sweeder, L.; Tiwari, P.A.; Van Haitsma, K. Sources of response bias in cognitive self-report items: "Which memory are you talking about?". *Gerontologist* **2019**, *59*, 912–924. [CrossRef] [PubMed]
48. Mogle, J.; Hill, N.; Bhang, I.; Bhargava, S.; Whitaker, E.; Kitt-Lewis, E. Time frame, problem specificity, and framing: The implicit structures of questions about memory in older adults. *Aging Ment. Health* **2020**, *24*, 56–62. [CrossRef] [PubMed]
49. Papenberg, G.; Bäckman, L.; Fratiglioni, L.; Laukka, E.J.; Fastbom, J.; Johnell, K. Anticholinergic drug use is associated with episodic memory decline in older adults without dementia. *Neurobiol. Aging* **2017**, *55*, 27–32. [CrossRef] [PubMed]
50. Couto, M.I.; Monteiro, A.; Oliveira, A.; Lunet, N.; Massano, J. Depression and anxiety following deep brain stimulation in Parkinson's disease: Systematic review and meta-analysis. *Acta Med. Port.* **2014**, *27*, 372–382. [CrossRef] [PubMed]

Review

Acupuncture for Behavioral and Psychological Symptoms of Dementia: A Systematic Review and Meta-Analysis

Chan-Young Kwon [1,*,†] and Boram Lee [2,†]

[1] Department of Oriental Neuropsychiatry, Dong-eui University College of Korean Medicine, 52-57 Yangjeong-ro, Busanjin-gu, Busan 47227, Korea
[2] Department of Clinical Korean Medicine, Graduate School, Kyung Hee University, 26 Kyunghee-daero, Dongdaemun-gu, Seoul 02447, Korea; qhfka9357@naver.com
* Correspondence: beanalogue@deu.ac.kr; Tel.: +82-51-850-8808
† Chan-Young Kwon and Boram Lee are co-first authors.

Abstract: Dementia is an important health issue worldwide, and non-pharmacological strategies for the management of behavioral and psychological symptoms of dementia (BPSD) are considered to be important. This review analyzes the effectiveness and safety of acupuncture for BPSD. Thirteen electronic databases were comprehensively searched to find clinical studies using acupuncture on BPSD, published up to December 2020. Five randomized controlled clinical trials and two before-after studies, mainly on Alzheimer's disease (AD), were included. Meta-analysis suggested that the total effective rate based on BPSD symptoms in the acupuncture combined with psychotropic drugs group was significantly higher than that in the psychotropic drugs group (risk ratio, 1.27; 95% confidence interval, 1.11 to 1.45; $I^2 = 51\%$). In terms of other outcomes related to BPSD, acupuncture as an adjunctive therapy, but not as monotherapy, was associated with significant benefits in most included studies. However, the included studies did not have optimal methodological quality. Our review highlights the limited evidence proving the effectiveness and safety of acupuncture for BPSD in patients with AD. Although some clinical studies have reported the potential benefits of adjuvant acupuncture in managing BPSD, the evidence is not robust and is based on small studies. Therefore, high-quality research in this field is needed.

Keywords: dementia; BPSD; acupuncture therapy; acupuncture; systematic review

1. Introduction

Dementia refers to a clinical syndrome that significantly impairs an individual's activities of daily living (ADL) with gradual cognitive decline, and it is an important health issue worldwide [1]. Along with strategies to prevent the occurrence of dementia based on an understanding of its multifactor pathology, strategies to reduce the burden of dementia patients and their caregivers as well as the socioeconomic burden is becoming increasingly important [1]. According to estimates, the number of patients with Alzheimer's disease (AD), a representative type of dementia, is expected to be 13.8 million in the United States and 115.4 million globally as of 2050 [2,3].

Behavioral and psychological symptoms of dementia (BPSD), which most patients with dementia experience, are thought to be the main cause of the dementia-related burden [4,5]. Therefore, the management of BPSD is a promising strategy to reduce the burden of dementia, and a non-pharmacological approach is particularly preferred in terms of benefit-risk ratio [6,7]. However, psychosocial interventions for BPSD are still not implemented systematically, and pharmacological interventions that can be associated with a number of negative health outcomes are being used [8–10]. As many non-pharmacological interventions are difficult to implement in actual clinical settings due to barriers related to resident unavailability and external barriers [11], it is necessary to explore non-pharmacological interventions that are individualized, can be easily implemented, are accessible, and are effective and safe for patients with dementia, in terms of evidence-based medicine (EBM).

Acupuncture, a promising non-pharmacological intervention, is recommended worldwide for some conditions such as pain [12] although it is not evaluated to have robust evidence to be officially recommended for the management of BPSD [13]. Acupuncture has been studied not only for pain conditions, but also for a wide range of health conditions such as neoplasms/cancer, pregnancy or labor, mood disorders, stroke, nausea/vomiting, sleep, and paralysis/palsy [14], and has the potential to improve overall health [15]. In addition, this modality appears to be generally safe [16]. In this context, acupuncture can be considered a promising treatment for the elderly population. Psychiatric manifestations in patients with dementia have been well documented in neuroimaging and neuropathology studies [17]. The effects of acupuncture on the nervous system of human subjects and animal models with neurological diseases including AD have also been reported [18]. It has been stated that acupuncture can influence AD pathology through the inhibition of accumulation of toxic proteins, regulation of glucose metabolism, reduction of neuronal apoptosis, and neuroprotective effects [18]. Therefore, this treatment may have a therapeutic effect on BPSD, which accompanies AD pathology [19,20].

However, there have been insufficient studies to examine the applicability of acupuncture for BPSD by comprehensively and systematically collecting previously published literature. Examining the applicability of acupuncture from the perspective of EBM potentially improves the management of dementia, thereby contributing to the reduction of the burden caused by dementia. Therefore, this systematic review aimed to analyze the effectiveness, safety, and research status of acupuncture in BPSD management.

2. Materials and Methods

The protocol of this systematic review was registered in the OSF registries (URL: https://osf.io/hu5ac) (Accessed on 30 November 2020) and the International Prospective Register of Systematic Reviews (registration number: CRD42020211005) before the start of the study. The protocol for this study was published in an international academic journal [21]. This systematic review complied with the Preferred Reporting Items for Systematic Reviews and Meta-Analyses (PRISMA) statement (Supplement 1) [22].

2.1. Information Sources and Search Strategy

A comprehensive study search was conducted in 13 electronic databases, including Medline via PubMed, EMBASE via Elsevier, the Cochrane Central Register of Controlled Trials, Allied and Complementary Medicine Database via EBSCO, Cumulative Index to Nursing and Allied Health Literature via EBSCO, PsycARTICLES via ProQuest, Oriental Medicine Advanced Searching Integrated System, Koreanstudies Information Service System, Research Information Service System, Korean Medical Database, Korea Citation Index, China National Knowledge Infrastructure, and Wanfang Data on December 28, 2020. All studies published from their inception to the search date were considered. To find additional gray literature such as theses or conference abstracts, relevant literature reference lists and trial registries, including clinicaltrials.gov, were reviewed. In addition, consultations with experts in this area were conducted. The study search process was conducted by a single researcher (BL). The search strategies and results in each database are described in Supplement 2.

2.2. Eligibility Criteria

The inclusion criteria for this review were as follows: (1) *Population*: Patients with dementia regardless of the type in long-term care facilities, community, or specialized geriatric assessment and psychiatric units was allowed. Only patients with dementia, with standard diagnostic criteria or validated tools, were included. The standard diagnostic criteria for dementia included the Diagnostic and Statistical Manual of Mental Disorders, the International Classification of Diseases, the National Institute of Neurological and Communicative Disorders and Stroke and the Alzheimer's Disease and Related Disorders Association, and other recommended diagnostic criteria. There were no restrictions on sex, age, or race/ethnicity of the patients. (2) *Intervention*: Acupuncture regardless of the type as monotherapy or adjunctive therapy to psychotropic drugs such as anxiolytics, antidepressants, and antipsychotics, with or without routine care for dementia as treatment interventions were included. Studies that did not list details such as the treatment period and treatment points (i.e., acupoints) were excluded. In addition, studies involving psychotherapy as treatment or control interventions were excluded. (3) *Comparator*: Wait-list, placebo (sham-acupuncture), or psychotropic drugs such as anxiolytics, antidepressants, and antipsychotics, with or without routine care for dementia, as control interventions were allowed. (4) *Outcome*: The severity of BPSD symptoms, such as Behavior Pathology in Alzheimer Disease Rating Scale (BEHAVE-AD) [23], Neuropsychiatric Inventory (NPI) [24], and Brief Psychiatric Rating Scale (BPRS) [25] were considered as the primary outcomes. The secondary outcome measures included the total effective rate (TER) for BPSD symptoms; ADL of patients such as Barthel Index [26]; instrumental ADL such as ADL Prevention Instrument [27]; quality of life (QOL) of patients with dementia such as Alzheimer Disease Related Quality of QOL [28]; caregiver burden of caregivers such as Caregiver Burden Inventory [29]; QOL of caregivers such as the Short Form 36 Health Survey (SF-36) [30]; placement in long-term care facility from home; and safety data such as incidence of adverse events (AEs). (5) *Study design*: clinical studies, regardless of the type, such as randomized controlled clinical trials (RCTs), non-randomized controlled clinical trials, and before-after studies. There were no restrictions on the publication language or publication status.

2.3. Study Selection

All documents retrieved from the study search process were imported into EndNote X8 (Clarivate Analytics, Philadelphia, PA, USA). After removing duplicates, the titles and abstracts of the documents were screened for inclusion. After the initial screening, the full texts of the remaining documents were carefully reviewed to evaluate the final inclusion. The study search process was conducted by two independent researchers (C.Y.K. and B.L.). Any disagreements between the two researchers were resolved through a consensus.

2.4. Data Extraction

In the data extraction process, a pre-defined form in Excel 2016 (Microsoft, Redmond, WA, USA) was used by two independent researchers (C.Y.K. and B.L.). The following items were extracted from the included studies: first author's name, publication year, country of publication, sample size and withdrawals, details of participants, treatment and control intervention, duration of intervention, outcome measures and results, AEs, and information for assessing the risk of bias (RoB). In particular, details of acupuncture procedures, such as acupoints, stimulation method, and needle retention time, were extracted. The authors contacted the corresponding authors of the original studies via e-mail, when the data in each included study were insufficient or ambiguous. Any disagreements between the two researchers were resolved through a consensus.

2.5. Risk of Bias Assessment

The RoB evaluation tools of the included studies were applied differently according to the study type. The inclusion criteria of the systematic review allowed all original clinical studies regardless of the study type, but the types included were limited to RCTs and before-after studies. In the case of RCTs, the Cochrane Collaboration's Rob tool was used to evaluate RoB. Using this tool, the RoB of RCTs can be evaluated by categorizing it into random sequence generation, allocation concealment, blinding of participants, personnel, and outcome assessors, completeness of outcome data, selective reporting, and other biases. For other biases, a statistical baseline imbalance of participants' mean age, sex, disease period, or disease severity between the treatment and control groups was considered. Each domain was evaluated as "low risk," "unclear risk," or "high risk," and the evaluation method of the Cochrane Handbook was followed [31]. The results of the RoB assessment were presented as figures using Review Manager software (version 5.4; Cochrane, London, UK). In case of before-after studies, the Quality Assessment Tool for Before-After (Pre-Post) Studies With No Control Group produced by the US National Heart Lung and Blood Institute was used [32]. The RoB assessment process was conducted by two independent researchers (C.Y.K. and B.L.), and any disagreements between the two researchers were resolved through consensus.

2.6. Data Synthesis and Analysis

A qualitative analysis of all included studies, including demographic characteristics of participants, details of interventions, and outcomes, was conducted. Quantitative synthesis was performed with the outcome measures if there were two or more studies using the same type of treatment and control interventions. The meta-analysis was conducted and presented as forest plots using Review Manager software (version 5.4; Cochrane, London, UK). For continuous outcomes, the mean differences with 95% confidence intervals (CIs) were calculated. For binary outcomes, the risk ratios (RRs) with 95% CIs were calculated. Heterogeneity between the studies in terms of effect measures was assessed using both the χ^2 test and the I^2 statistic, and I^2 values greater than 50% and 75% were interpreted as substantial and considerable heterogeneity, respectively. In the meta-analysis, a random-effects model was used if included studies had significant heterogeneity (an $I^2 > 50\%$), while a fixed-effect model was used if the heterogeneity was not significant or if the number of studies included in the meta-analysis was less than 5 [33,34]. According to the protocol [21], subgroup analyses based on severity of dementia, type of dementia, severity of BPSD, and treatment duration were planned; however, these were not conducted because the number of studies included and the relevant data were insufficient. Sensitivity analysis in meta-analyses was planned to remove studies with high RoB and outliers that are numerically distant from the rest of the data, but this was not conducted for the same reason.

2.7. Publication Bias

Assessment of publication bias using a funnel plot was planned in the protocol [21]; however, the assessment was not conducted, as there were no more than 10 studies included in each meta-analysis.

3. Results

3.1. Study Selection

A total of 8715 documents were identified through initial database searches, and 1600 duplicates were excluded. After reviewing the titles and abstracts of the remaining 7115 documents, 44 potentially relevant articles were selected. The full texts of the 44 articles were assessed for the final inclusion. Among them, the following numbers of studies were excluded: not clinical studies ($n = 3$), not report the standard diagnostic criteria or validated tools for participants ($n = 3$), not on acupuncture ($n = 1$), comparing two different kinds of acupuncture ($n = 2$), not reporting outcomes related to BPSD ($n = 18$), without details about the study ($n = 5$), using same data (thesis or conference abstract) ($n = 3$), using the same data (published in another journal) ($n = 1$), and not available full-text ($n = 1$) (Supplement 3). Finally, a total of seven studies (five RCTs [35–39] and two before-after studies [40,41]) were included in this review (Figure 1).

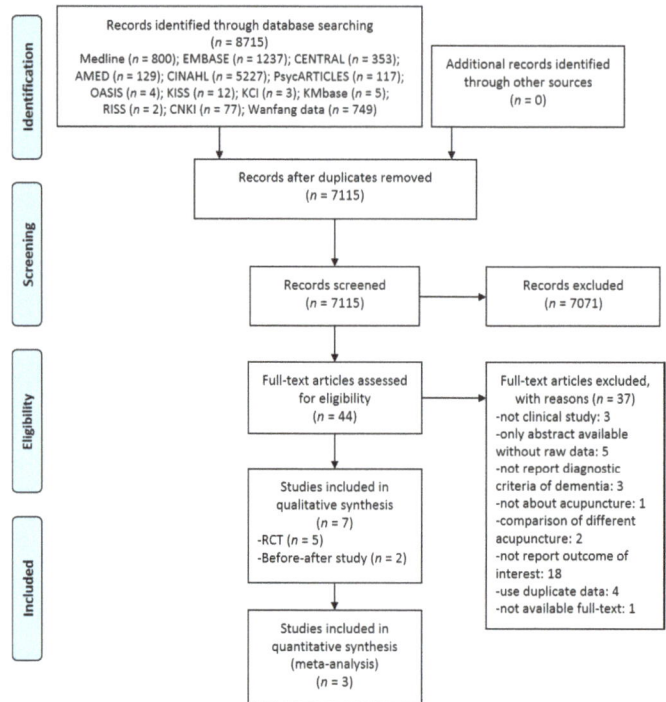

Figure 1. A PRISMA flow diagram of the literature screening and selection processes. AMED, Allied and Complementary Medicine Database; CENTRAL, Cochrane Central Register of Controlled Trials; CINAHL, Cumulative Index to Nursing and Allied Health Literature; CNKI, China National Knowledge Infrastructure; KCI, Korea Citation Index; KISS, Korean Studies Information Service System; KMbase, Korean Medical Database; OASIS, Oriental Medicine Advanced Searching Integrated System; RCT, randomized controlled trial; RISS, Research Information Service System.

3.2. Study Characteristics

Among the seven included studies, six [35–39,41] were conducted in China, and the remaining study [40] was conducted in America. As for the type of publication, there was one thesis [41], and the remainder [35–40] were journal articles. As for the type of dementia, except for one study [40] involving patients with AD or vascular dementia (VD), all studies [35–39,41] were in patients with AD. As for the type of acupuncture, three [37,40,41] used manual acupuncture, three [35,38,39] used electroacupuncture, and one [36] used scalp acupuncture.

Among the five RCTs [35–39], there were three [35,36,38] comparing acupuncture combined with psychotropic drugs and psychotropic drugs alone, one [37] comparing acupuncture and anti-dementia drugs, and one [39] comparing acupuncture combined with routine care and routine care alone. No study recruited participants according to pattern identification. The treatment period ranged from 4 weeks to 12 years, of which 8 weeks was the most common in the two RCTs [35,36]. Only one RCT [37] conducted a follow-up assessment after completion of treatment. Two RCTs [37,39] were approved by the institutional review board for the study, and three RCTs [37–39] received consent forms from the participants. The two before-after studies used manual acupuncture for 9–12 weeks [40] and 8 weeks [41], respectively. In addition, the two studies [40,41] also did not use pattern identification in recruiting participants. The two studies [40,41] did not describe approval by the institutional review board for the study; however, they reported that they received consent forms from participants (Tables 1 and 2).

Table 1. Characteristics of included studies.

Study, Year, [Reference]	Sample Size(Included→Analyzed)	Mean Age (yr)	Sex (M:F)	Population	Intervention	Treatment Duration/F/U	Outcome
Ou, 2000, [35]	30(16:14) →30(16:14)	TG: 65.5 ± 6.8 CG: 64.7 ± 7.6	TG: 16(10:6) CG: 14(9:4)	-AD (mild, moderate) -baseline BPRS TG: 42.85 ± 5.25 CG: 41.91 ± 4.88	TG: EA + perphenazine (4–30 mg/d) CG: perphenazine (8–40 mg/d)	8 wk/none	1. TER (BPRS) 2. BPRS 3. CGI
Huang 2014, [36]	100(50:50) →100(50:50)	TG: 70.9 ± 8.6 CG: 71.5 ± 7.9	TG: 50(24:26) CG: 50(23:27)	-AD (mild, moderate, severe) -baseline HAMD TG: 22.30 ± 6.93 CG: 21.45 ± 7.01	TG: SA + fluoxetine (20 mg/d) CG: fluoxetine (20 mg/d)	8 wk/none	1. TER (HAMD) 2. HAMD 3. ADL
Jia 2017, [37]	87(43:44) →80(41:39)	TG: 75.11 ± 6.53 CG: 74.50 ± 6.83	TG: 43(13:30) CG: 44(16:28)	-AD (mild, moderate) -baseline NPTTG: 9.28 ± 2.49 CG: 8.97 ± 2.69	TG: MA CG: donepezil (first 4 weeks: 5 mg/d; thereafter: 10 mg/d)	12 wk/12 wk	1. ADAS-cog 2. CIBIC + 3. ADCS-ADL23 4. NPI
Zhang 2017, [38]	82(41:41) →82(41:41)	TG: 66.12 ± 11.33 CG: 65.25 ± 10.62	TG: 41(23:18) CG: 41(22:19)	-AD -baseline PSQI TG: 14.12 ± 2.12 CG: 14.91 ± 3.32	TG: EA + midazolam (7.5 mg/d) CG: midazolam (7.5 mg/d)	30 d/none	1. TER (PSQI) 2. PSQI
Zhao 2020, [39]	120(60:60) →120(60:60)	TG: 72.0 ± 10.9 CG: 70.9 ± 11.2	TG: 60(30:30) CG: 60(28:32)	-AD -baseline MMSE TG: 14.34 ± 2.87 CG: 14.62 ± 3.01	TG: EA + passive music therapy + routine care (routine nursing, psychological comfort, daily cognitive training, diet modification) CG: routine care	4 wk/none	1. TER (MMSE, MoCA, SF-36) 2. MMSE 3. MoCA 4. ADL 5. BEHAVE-AD 6. SF-36 7. Levels of acetylcholine, choline acetylase, acetylcholinesterase, norepinephrine, 5-HT, and dopamine

Table 1. Cont.

Study, Year, [Reference]	Sample Size(Included→Analyzed)	Mean Age (yr)	Sex (M:F)	Population	Intervention	Treatment Duration/F/U	Outcome
Lombardo 2001, [40]	11→11	76	11(3:8)	-AD or VD -baseline MMSE 21.9 ± 5.2	MA	9–12 wk/none	1. POMS-anxiety 2. STAI-state anxiety 3. CSDD 4. GDS 5. MMSE 6. Boston naming test 7. Controlled oral word association test 8. Caregiver: SF-36-vitality, anxiety, depression 9. Patient: SF-36-vitality, anxiety, depression
Ying 2006, [41]	33→30	74.96 ± 5.41	30(12:18)	-AD -baseline MMSE 12.47 ± 2.62 -baseline BEHAVE-AD 18.90 ± 6.67	MA	8 wk/none	1. BEHAVE-AD 2. MMSE 3. ADL 4. TCM symptom score

Abbreviations. AD, Alzheimer's disease; ADCS-ADL23, Alzheimer's disease cooperative study—activities of daily living, 23-item scale; ADL, activities of daily living; BEHAVE-AD, the behavior pathology in Alzheimer's disease rating scale; BPRS, the brief psychiatric rating scale; CG, control group; CGI, clinical global impression; CSDD, Cornell scale for depression in dementia; EA, electro-acupuncture; GDS, geriatric depression scale; HAMD, the Hamilton depression rating scale; MA, manual acupuncture; MMSE, mini-mental state examination; MoCA, Montreal cognitive assessment; NPI, the Neuropsychiatric inventory; POMS, profile of mood states; PSQI, the Pittsburgh sleep quality index; SF-36, short form 36 health survey; STAI, state-trait anxiety inventory; TCM, traditional Chinese medicine; TER, total effective rate; TG, treatment group; VD, vascular dementia. Note. Among outcomes, those that have been bolded fall within the scope of this systematic review.

Table 2. Methods of acupuncture performed.

Study, Year, [Reference]	Type of Acupuncture	Acupoints	Stimulation Method	Needle Retention Time	Treatment Frequency
Ou, 2000, [35]	EA	GV20, Yintang, GV14	De qi GV20 to Yintang or GV20 to GV14 Wave: continuous wave; Frequency: 2–4 Hz; Intensity: visible twitching of the local muscles, but comfortable and tolerable.	30 min	6 session/wk
Huang 2014, [36]	SA	anterior vertex zone, frontal zone	Manual stimulation	NR	6 session/wk

Table 2. Cont.

Study, Year, [Reference]	Type of Acupuncture	Acupoints	Stimulation Method	Needle Retention Time	Treatment Frequency
Jia 2017, [37]	MA	-Basic acupoints: CV17, CV12, CV6, ST36, TW5, SP10-Additional acupoints: LV3, GB39, ST40, BL17, ST44, ST25, CV4	De qi	30 min	3 session/wk
Zhang 2017, [38]	EA	GV20, GV24, EX-HN1, Anmian, Taiyang, P6, HT7, SP6, KI1	De qi Taiyang to EX-HN1 Wave: dilatational wave; Frequency: 2–100 Hz; Intensity: 2–4 V	25 min	1 session/d for 10d and rest for 3d
Zhao 2020, [39]	EA	GV20, BL23	Not reporting on De qi Around GV20 to GV20, around BL23 to BL23 Wave: continuous wave; Frequency: 50 Hz; Intensity: 2 V, 1 mA	20 min	1 session/d for 7d and rest for 1d
Lombardo 2001, [40]	MA	-Basic acupoints: GB3, GV16, GV20, GV23, GV24, PC6, HT7, SP6, EX-HN1, Yintang -Additional acupoints: ST36, LI4, GB20, GV17, SP4, KI3, SI3, BL62, BL23, GV26, EX-B2	NR	30 min	3 session/wk (1–2 wk), 2–3 session/wk (additional 7–10 wk)
Ying 2006, [41]	MA	-Basic acupoints: GV24, HT7, GV20, GV16, GV14, EX-B2 -Additional acupoints: BL23, GB39, LV3, SP6, HT5, HT7, ST36, SP10, BL17	De qi Manual stimulation every 10 min during needle retention	30 min	1 session/d for 6d and rest for 1d

Abbreviations. EA, electro-acupuncture; MA, manual acupuncture; NR, not recorded; SA, scalp acupuncture.

3.3. Risk of Bias in Studies

For RCTs, a total of four studies [36–39] with proper randomization methods, such as using a random number table, were evaluated as low risk in the random sequence generation domain. Only one study [37] used a special envelope to perform allocation concealment, which was assessed to have low risk in the domain of allocation concealment. None of the included studies used sham acupuncture as a control, suggesting that double blinding was impossible. Therefore, all studies were evaluated as having high risk in the domain of performance bias. Only one study [37] described the blinding of the outcome assessor, and the domain of detection bias was evaluated as having a low risk of bias. All studies were evaluated as low risk in the domain of incomplete outcome data, because there were no dropouts [35,36,38,39] or the number of dropouts was not expected to have a significant effect on the results because it was small [37]. Most studies [36–39] were evaluated as having a low risk of reporting bias in the domain of selective reporting using an objective and validated evaluation tool related to BPSD. However, one study [35] did not present the results of some outcomes as numerical values, so the domain was evaluated as high risk. As all studies reported baseline statistical homogeneity of participants' mean age, sex, disease period, or disease severity, the domains of other sources of bias were evaluated as low risk (Figure 2). In two before-after studies [40,41], both clearly stated the study questions, eligibility criteria for the study population, and outcome measures. In addition, these studies [40,41] were lost to follow-up after a baseline of 20% or less, and a statistical test using *p*-value was performed, and two or more results of assessment after baseline were reported. However, both studies [40,41] were small with a sample size of less than 60 [42], there was no previously published protocol, no assessor blinding was reported, and individual-level data were not considered. In addition, one study [40] lacked detailed descriptions related to the acupuncture method, such as stimulation method and needle retention time (Supplement 4).

3.4. Effectiveness and Safety of Acupuncture in Included RCTs

3.4.1. Acupuncture as a Monotherapy

Jia [37], comparing manual acupuncture and donepezil (first 4 weeks: 5 mg/day; thereafter: 10 mg/day) in 87 AD patients for 12 weeks, reported that there was no statistically significant difference using the AD Cooperative Study—ADL, 23-item scale (after 12 weeks: 47.85 (mean) ± 11.22 (standard deviation) vs. 48.20 ± 13.16, $p > 0.05$; 12-week follow-up: 48.18 ± 11.32 vs. 49.43 ± 13.45, $p > 0.05$) and NPI total score (after 12 weeks: 7.25 ± 2.69 vs. 7.61 ± 2.30, $p > 0.05$; 12-week follow-up: 8.13 ± 2.78 vs. 9.31 ± 2.42, $p > 0.05$). There were five cases of AE in the acupuncture group, including four cases of punctate hemorrhage and one case of bruising. In the donepezil group, there were seven cases of AE, including dizziness, nausea, loss of appetite, diarrhea, constipation, fatigue, and agitation. Interestingly, the authors reported that the acupuncture group unexpectedly improved the following symptoms: insomnia (five cases), constipation (four cases), elderly male patients with benign prostatic hyperplasia (six cases), and knee arthritis (two cases).

3.4.2. Acupuncture as an Adjunctive Therapy

Meta-analysis was possible only for TER for BPSD symptoms. As a result, TER in the acupuncture combined with psychotropic drugs group was significantly higher than that in the psychotropic drugs group (three studies [35,36,38]; RR, 1.27; 95% CI, 1.11 to 1.45; $I^2 = 51\%$) (Figure 3).

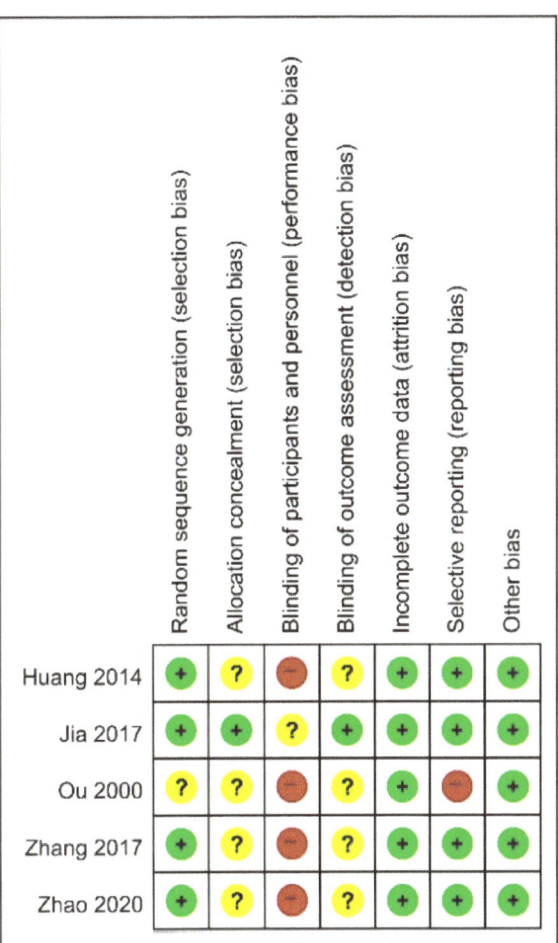

Figure 2. Risk of bias for all included studies. Low, unclear, and high risk, respectively, are represented with the following symbols: "+," "?", and "−".

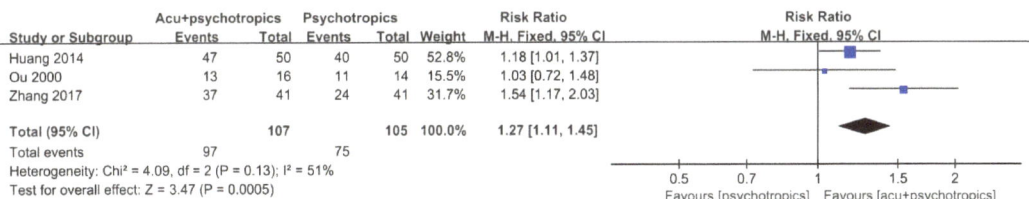

Figure 3. Forest plot of total effective rate comparing acupuncture plus psychotropic drugs and psychotropic drugs alone.

Ou [35], comparing electroacupuncture combined with perphenazine (4-30 mg/day) and perphenazine (8–40 mg/day) in 30 AD patients with BPSD for 8 weeks, reported no statistically significant difference on BPRS between the groups (27.14 ± 7.91 vs. 28.23 ± 8.42, $p > 0.05$). There was no statistically significant difference in the Rating Scale for Extrapyramidal Side Effects score after 1 week of treatment (1.3 ± 1.0, 2.1 ± 0.4, $p > 0.05$). Huang (2014) [36], comparing scalp acupuncture combined with fluoxetine (20 mg/day) and fluoxetine (20 mg/day) alone in 100 AD patients with depression for 8 weeks, reported that compared to the control group, the treatment group showed a statistically significantly lower Hamilton depression rating scale (HAMD) score (9.32 ± 4.93 vs. 11.89 ± 5.97, $p < 0.05$) and higher ADL score (36.76 ± 3.29 vs. 34.92 ± 4.33, $p < 0.05$). Zhang [38] compared electroacupuncture combined with midazolam (7.5 mg/day) and midazolam (7.5 mg/day) alone in 82 AD patients with sleep disorder for 30 days and reported that compared to the control group, the treatment group showed a statistically significantly lower global score of the Pittsburgh sleep quality index (PSQI) (1.59 ± 2.15 vs. 4.15 ± 1.77, $p < 0.05$).

Zhao [39], comparing electroacupuncture combined with passive music therapy and routine care (i.e., routine nursing, psychological comfort, daily cognitive training, diet modification) and routine care in 120 AD patients for 4 weeks, reported that compared to the control group, the treatment group showed a statistically significantly higher ADL score (64.92 ± 8.29 vs. 47.07 ± 10.18, $p < 0.05$) and BEHAVE-AD total score (37.45 ± 4.40 vs. 27.21 ± 4.20, $p < 0.05$). Moreover, they found that all subscales of SF-36 for the treatment group were statistically significantly higher than that of control group, including physical functioning (71.39 ± 6.58 vs. 55.13 ± 7.14, $p < 0.05$), body pain (73.22 ± 7.82 vs. 59.61 ± 7.31, $p < 0.05$), general health perception (68.77 ± 6.16 vs. 50.33 ± 5.24, $p < 0.05$), vitality (71.82 ± 6.64 vs. 55.64 ± 5.67, $p < 0.05$), social functioning (80.27 ± 7.89 vs. 69.55 ± 8.10, $p < 0.05$), emotional role functioning (71.46 ± 6.21 vs. 60.24 ± 6.59, $p < 0.05$), and mental health (73.62 ± 7.46 vs. 62.31 ± 5.88, $p < 0.05$).

3.5. Results in Included Before-After Studies

Lombardo [40], performing manual acupuncture in 11 patients with AD or VD for 9-12 weeks, reported that the anxiety subscale of the Profile of Mood States (POMS) (8.8 ± 6.3 to 4.6 ± 3.4, $p = 0.05$), state anxiety of State-Trait Anxiety Inventory (STAI) (49.5 ± 8.4 to 40.1 ± 8.0, $p = 0.005$), and Cornell Scale for Depression in Dementia (CSDD) (6.4 ± 5.0 to 3.1 ± 3.0, $p = 0.011$) were significantly improved. In addition, some subscales of SF-36 in caregivers were significantly improved, including vitality (4.1 ± 1.2 to 3.4 ± 0.9, $p = 0.003$) and anxiety (3.2 ± 0.7 to 2.5 ± 0.8, $p = 0.006$), but not depression (2.8 ± 0.7 to 2.7 ± 1.0, $p = 0.394$). There was no statistically significant difference in the Geriatric Depression Scale (GDS) (7.4 ± 3.9 to 6.7 ± 7.0, $p = 0.358$) and subscales of SF-36 in participants, including vitality (2.7 ± 0.8, 2.6 ± 0.9, $p = 0.416$), anxiety (2.5 ± 0.7 to 2.1 ± 0.6, $p = 0.441$), and depression (2.6 ± 1.0 ± 2.2 ± 0.7, $p = 0.350$).

Ying [41], performing manual acupuncture in 33 AD patients with BPSD for 8 weeks, reported that the BEHAVE-AD total score (18.90 ± 6.67 to 15.37 ± 7.42, $p < 0.001$), and some subscales including paranoid and delusional ideation (5.22 ± 2.60 to 4.51 ± 2.50, $p < 0.01$), activity disturbances (3.80 ± 2.11 to 3.38 ± 2.28, $p = 0.002$), affective disturbances (2.17 ± 1.34 to 1.27 ± 0.98, $p < 0.01$), and anxieties and phobias (3.00 ± 1.88 to 1.50 ± 1.43, $p < 0.01$) were statistically significantly improved. However, other subscales of BEHAVE-AD including hallucinations (1.40 ± 1.43 to 1.43 ± 1.30, $p = 0.12$), aggressiveness (1.43 ± 1.83 to 1.50 ± 1.85, $p = 0.53$), and diurnal rhythm disturbances (1.90 ± 0.93 to 2.00 ± 0.98, $p = 0.58$) as well as ADL (47.67 ± 8.50 to 47.03 ± 9.91, $p = 0.141$) showed no statistically significant difference.

4. Discussion

4.1. Summary of Evidence

This systematic review is the most comprehensive review and meta-analysis to date conducted to analyze the effectiveness, safety, and research status of acupuncture for BPSD. A total of seven clinical studies, including five RCTs [35–39] and two before-after studies [40,41], mainly on patients with AD, were included in this review. In these studies, RCTs were analyzed to evaluate the effectiveness and safety of BPSD. On the other hand, the before-after studies were used as the basis for understanding the current status of research in this field, considering the low level of evidence. Meta-analysis was only possible for

TER based on BPSD symptoms from three RCTs [35,36,38]. According to the meta-analysis results, acupuncture combined with psychotropic drugs showed statistically significant superiority in terms of TER compared to the psychotropic drugs alone group. For the other outcomes, only qualitative synthesis was conducted. First, in terms of outcomes related to BPSD, acupuncture as an adjunctive therapy, but not as monotherapy, was associated with significant benefits in most included studies. One study [35] compared electroacupuncture combined with perphenazine and perphenazine and reported that there was no significant difference in the effect of the two interventions on the BPRS score. However, considering that the dose of perphenazine was used less in the combined therapy group (4–30 mg/day) than in the control group (8–40 mg/day), the results of this study suggest that EA may be helpful in BPSD management. Similarly, the other two RCTs, comparing acupuncture combined with psychotropic drugs and psychotropic drugs, found the significant benefits of acupuncture as an adjunctive therapy for HAMD [36] and PSQI [38]. One RCT [39], which investigated the additional benefits of acupuncture and music therapy based on routine care, reported the BEHAVE-AD score as a BPSD-related outcome, but the value was suspicious. The BEHAVE-AD score increased significantly after treatment in both groups, but the authors explained that BPSD symptoms were reduced in this study. Given that higher BEHAVE-AD scores reflect more severe symptoms of BPSD [23], these explanations seem unusual; therefore, we contacted the corresponding author of the paper via e-mail, but did not receive a reply. Second, in terms of ADL, two RCTs reported additional benefits of acupuncture as an adjunctive therapy to midazolam [36] or routine care [39]. However, acupuncture as a monotherapy did not show statistically significant superiority in ADL compared to donepezil [38]. Third, in one RCT [39], the patient's QOL was evaluated using the SF-36. The results showed that acupuncture and music therapy added to routine care significantly improved participants' QOL in terms of physical functioning, body pain, general health perception, vitality, social functioning, emotional functioning, and mental health. Fourth, only two RCTs [35,37] reported the safety data of the interventions. Acupuncture was mainly associated with mild local AEs such as punctate hemorrhage and bruising and did not have a significant effect on safety concerns of drug treatment such as extrapyramidal side effects. On the other hand, there were two before-after studies [40,41] included in this review, both of which used manual acupuncture, and significant improvements were reported in BPSD-related outcomes such as POMS, STAI, CSDD, and BEHAVE-AD. However, no significant improvement was observed in the GDS, the anxiety and depression subscales of SF-36, and hallucinations, aggressiveness, and diurnal rhythm disturbance subscales of BEHAVE-AD. In addition, one study [41] that reported ADL found no statistically significant change. In summary, in the included studies, improvements in individual BPSD after acupuncture were reported, in particular, for depression, anxiety, sleep quality, paranoid and delusional ideation, and activity disturbances. Among them, the improved individual symptoms of BPSD after acupuncture in the included RCTs were depression and sleep quality.

Overall, the included studies did not have optimal methodological quality. In particular, most studies were small-scale, and few studies reported blinding of outcome assessors. Considering that blinding of participants and personnel in the perfect sense is almost impossible due to the nature of acupuncture, the lack of blinding in outcome assessors could potentially affect the reliability of each study result. These blinding issues and small-scale limitations also apply to the two before-after studies.

4.2. Implications of the Results

This review presents the most comprehensive literature review conducted to evaluate the effectiveness and safety of acupuncture for BPSD. Although studies have shown that acupuncture, primarily as a form of adjuvant therapy in patients with AD, has the potential to improve overall BPSD as well as individual BPSD symptoms such as depression and sleep quality, these results were not supported by a sufficient number of studies or evidence of sufficient quality. However, given that the establishment of a non-pharmacological approach to the management of BPSD is important [6,7] and that effective and safe non-pharmacological strategies should be implemented in a viable manner [8–10], acupuncture may still be an attractive intervention. This is because the potential of acupuncture has been continuously reported for conditions, especially in the elderly, regarding the limitations of conventional pharmacological treatment, such as poly-pharmacy [43,44].

Although the underlying therapeutic mechanism of acupuncture for BPSD in patients with AD has not been fully elucidated, the results of pre-clinical and clinical experiments can be referred to. Lu that manual acupuncture on ST36 for 30 days in a rat AD model activated brain areas including the orbital cortex, medulla oblongata, and pontine tegmentum [45]. Moreover, Shan found that manual acupuncture on LI4 and LR3 in patients with AD was related to enhanced activations in cognitive-related areas, including the inferior frontal gyrus, as well as sensorimotor-related areas, the basal ganglia, and the cerebellum, by using functional magnetic resonance imaging (fMRI) [46]. A review investigating changes in acupuncture-related brain activity in fMRI concluded that acupuncture stimuli could promote activity changes in a wide range of brain regions, including the somatosensory cortices, limbic system, basal ganglia, brain stem, and cerebellum [47]. Acupuncture-induced changes in local brain activity in AD patients may be related to the therapeutic effect of acupuncture on BPSD. Among them, the possible impact of acupuncture on the orbitofrontal cortex seems to be promising. A previous systematic review suggested that volume reductions or decreased metabolism in the orbital cortex, especially the orbitofrontal cortex, are related to BPSD symptoms, particularly apathy and psychosis [48]. Furthermore, gray matter volume loss in the medial orbital frontal cortex was seen in patients with frontotemporal lobar degeneration, with symptoms of disinhibition [49]. As part of the temporo-amygdala-orbitofrontal network, the orbitofrontal cortex may be associated with semantic deficits, language difficulties, personality changes, aggression, and disinhibition in patients with advanced AD [50]. Effects on other brain regions are also likely to be related to the potential effects of acupuncture on BPSD. The pontine tegmentum contains numerous serotonergic neurons, and abnormalities in this region could potentially be related to low mood and low self-esteem in patients with AD [51]. White matter changes in the frontal or parieto-occipital region and basal ganglia may be associated with psychotic symptoms, particularly delusional misidentification, in AD patients [52]. Modulation of some neurotransmitters may also explain the potential therapeutic effect of acupuncture on BPSD, and a recent review summarized the effect of acupuncture on glutamatergic neurotransmission in depression, anxiety, schizophrenia, and AD [53]. According to the results of the review [53], glutamatergic neurotransmission may be a common therapeutic pathway of acupuncture for BPSD symptoms (i.e., depression, anxiety, and psychotic symptoms) as well as the pathology (i.e., glutamate excitotoxicity) of AD. However, further research in this field is still needed, and the therapeutic mechanism of acupuncture for BPSD in AD patients has not been fully elucidated.

Although this systematic review allowed all of the original clinical studies that reported the effect of acupuncture on BPSD regardless of the study type, the fact that only seven studies were included suggests that research in this field is lacking. Therefore, in terms of EBM, to formally recommend that acupuncture be used as a supplement to BPSD management, more high-quality research in this field is needed in the future. In particular, dementia is currently becoming a social, national, and global problem beyond the individual or family level, so research support for non-pharmacological treatments including acupuncture for BPSD management of dementia patients is needed at the national level.

4.3. Limitations

This review presents some promising results of acupuncture as an adjuvant therapy for BPSD, but the following limitations should be considered:

(1) Because the number of studies included in this review was small, quantitative synthesis was limited, and the results for each outcome were dependent on either one or two RCTs. In this situation, each RCT was implemented on a small scale, which

may cause small-study effects, and its methodological quality is poor. Therefore, the reliability of the results obtained in this review was limited, and the level of evidence could be evaluated as weak.

(2) The subgroup analysis planned in this review protocol [21] was not performed because of the lack of included studies. However, the characteristics of the participants and interventions in the included studies were not sufficiently homogeneous, so differences in effect estimates according to the severity of dementia, the severity of BPSD, and the duration of treatment should be further investigated in future studies.

(3) The included studies also lacked the homogeneity of the evaluation tools used for BPSD evaluation. In particular, some studies used evaluation tools for individual BPSD symptoms such as HAMD, STAI, and PSQI and did not use an evaluation tool specific to BPSD such as BEHAVE-AD or NPI. Therefore, future studies require the uniformity of these evaluation tools, and the use of evaluation tools specific to BPSD is recommended.

(4) Most of the included studies were conducted in China. In particular, all the included RCTs were implemented in China. Although publication bias using funnel plots was not evaluated in this review, studies implemented only in certain countries could potentially contribute to publication bias. In addition, as China has been using acupuncture for a long time, participants of acupuncture studies usually exhibit a favorable attitude toward this treatment method. These factors can act as obstacles to generalizing the results of this review to other countries.

5. Conclusions

Our review highlights the limited evidence supporting the effectiveness and safety of acupuncture for BPSD in patients with AD. Although some clinical studies have reported the potential benefits of acupuncture as an adjuvant therapy in managing BPSD or improving ADL, the evidence is weak and based on small studies. Although the development of effective non-pharmaceutical therapies for the management of BPSD is important, high-quality research on acupuncture seems to be lacking, and research in this field is needed.

Supplementary Materials: The following are available online at https://www.mdpi.com/article/10.3390/jcm10143087/s1, Supplement 1: PRISMA 2020 Checklist, Supplement 2: Search terms used in each database, Supplement 3: Excluded studies after full-text review, Supplement 4: Methodological quality of the included before-after studies.

Author Contributions: Conceptualization: C.-Y.K. Methodology: C.-Y.K. and B.L. Formal analysis: C.-Y.K. and B.L. Writing—Original Draft: C.-Y.K. and B.L. Writing—Review & Editing: C.-Y.K. and B.L. Supervision: C.-Y.K. Funding acquisition: C.-Y.K. All authors have read and agreed to the published version of the manuscript.

Funding: This research was supported by a grant from the Korea Health Technology R&D Project through the Korea Health Industry Development Institute (KHIDI), funded by the Ministry of Health & Welfare, Republic of Korea (grant number: HF20C0207).

Institutional Review Board Statement: This study is a systematic review targeting previously published studies, and does not require institutional review board approval.

Informed Consent Statement: This study is a systematic review targeting previously published studies, and does not require patient consent.

Data Availability Statement: The data extracted from included studies and data used for all analyses were all included in this manuscript.

Acknowledgments: In this section, you can acknowledge any support given which is not covered by the author contribution or funding sections. This may include administrative and technical support, or donations in kind (e.g., materials used for experiments).

Conflicts of Interest: The authors declare no conflict of interest.

References

1. Livingston, G.; Huntley, J.; Sommerlad, A.; Ames, D.; Ballard, C.; Banerjee, S.; Brayne, C.; Burns, A.; Cohen-Mansfield, J.; Cooper, C.; et al. Dementia prevention, intervention, and care: 2020 report of the Lancet Commission. *Lancet* **2020**, *396*, 413–446. [CrossRef]
2. Hebert, L.E.; Weuve, J.; Scherr, P.A.; Evans, D.A. Alzheimer disease in the United States (2010–2050) estimated using the 2010 census. *Neurology* **2013**, *80*, 1778–1783. [CrossRef] [PubMed]
3. Prince, M.; Bryce, R.; Albanese, E.; Wimo, A.; Ribeiro, W.; Ferri, C. The global prevalence of dementia: A systematic review and metaanalysis. *Alzheimers Dement.* **2013**, *9*, 63–75. [CrossRef] [PubMed]
4. Arthur, P.B.; Gitlin, L.N.; Kairalla, J.A.; Mann, W.C. Relationship between the number of behavioral symptoms in dementia and caregiver distress: What is the tipping point? *Int. Psychogeriatr.* **2018**, *30*, 1099–1107. [CrossRef]
5. Beeri, M.S.; Werner, P.; Davidson, M.; Noy, S. The cost of behavioral and psychological symptoms of dementia (BPSD) in community dwelling Alzheimer's disease patients. *Int. J. Geriatr. Psychiatry* **2002**, *17*, 403–408. [CrossRef]
6. Tible, O.P.; Riese, F.; Savaskan, E.; von Gunten, A. Best practice in the management of behavioural and psychological symptoms of dementia. *Ther. Adv. Neurol. Disord.* **2017**, *10*, 297–309. [CrossRef]
7. Kales, H.C.; Lyketsos, C.G.; Miller, E.M.; Ballard, C. Management of behavioral and psychological symptoms in people with Alzheimer's disease: An international Delphi consensus. *Int. Psychogeriatr.* **2019**, *31*, 83–90. [CrossRef]
8. Masopust, J.; Protopopová, D.; Vališ, M.; Pavelek, Z.; Klímová, B. Treatment of behavioral and psychological symptoms of dementias with psychopharmaceuticals: A review. *Neuropsychiatr. Dis. Treat.* **2018**, *14*, 1211–1220. [CrossRef]
9. White, N.; Leurent, B.; Lord, K.; Scott, S.; Jones, L.; Sampson, E.L. The management of behavioural and psychological symptoms of dementia in the acute general medical hospital: A longitudinal cohort study. *Int. J. Geriatr. Psychiatry* **2016**, *32*, 297–305. [CrossRef]
10. Lee, K.S.; Kim, S.-H.; Hwang, H.-J. Behavioral and Psychological Symptoms of Dementia and Antipsychotic Drug Use in the Elderly with Dementia in Korean Long-Term Care Facilities. *Drugs-Real World Outcomes* **2015**, *2*, 363–368. [CrossRef]
11. Cohen-Mansfield, J.; Thein, K.; Marx, M.S.; Dakheel-Ali, M. What Are the Barriers to Performing Nonpharmacological Interventions for Behavioral Symptoms in the Nursing Home? *J. Am. Med Dir. Assoc.* **2012**, *13*, 400–405. [CrossRef]
12. Rubin, R. Medicare Proposes Coverage of Acupuncture for Lower Back Pain. *JAMA* **2019**, *322*, 716. [CrossRef]
13. Harris, M.L.; Titler, M.G.; Struble, L.M. Acupuncture and Acupressure for Dementia Behavioral and Psychological Symptoms: A Scoping Review. *West. J. Nurs. Res.* **2019**, *42*, 867–880. [CrossRef]
14. Ma, Y.; Dong, M.; Zhou, K.; Mita, C.; Liu, J.; Wayne, P.M. Publication Trends in Acupuncture Research: A 20-Year Bibliometric Analysis Based on PubMed. *PLoS ONE* **2016**, *11*, e0168123. [CrossRef]
15. Birch, S. Treating the patient not the symptoms: Acupuncture to improve overall health–Evidence, acceptance and strategies. *Integr. Med. Res.* **2019**, *8*, 33–41. [CrossRef]
16. Chan, M.W.C.; Wu, X.Y.; Wu, J.C.Y.; Wong, S.Y.-S.; Chung, V.C.H. Safety of Acupuncture: Overview of Systematic Reviews. *Sci. Rep.* **2017**, *7*, 1–11. [CrossRef]
17. Casanova, M.F.; Starkstein, S.E.; Jellinger, K.A. Clinicopathological correlates of behavioral and psychological symptoms of dementia. *Acta Neuropathol.* **2011**, *122*, 117–135. [CrossRef]
18. Guo, X.; Ma, T. Effects of Acupuncture on Neurological Disease in Clinical- and Animal-Based Research. *Front. Integr. Neurosci.* **2019**, *13*, 47. [CrossRef]
19. Bensamoun, D.; Guignard, R.; Furst, A.J.; Derreumaux, A.; Manera, V.; Darcourt, J.; Benoit, M.; Robert, P.H.; David, R.; Initiative, F.T.A.D.N. Associations between Neuropsychiatric Symptoms and Cerebral Amyloid Deposition in Cognitively Impaired Elderly People. *J. Alzheimers Dis.* **2015**, *49*, 387–398. [CrossRef]
20. Chen, Y.; Dang, M.; Zhang, Z. Brain mechanisms underlying neuropsychiatric symptoms in Alzheimer's disease: A systematic review of symptom-general and –specific lesion patterns. *Mol. Neurodegen.* **2021**, *16*, 1–22. [CrossRef]
21. Kwon, C.-Y.; Lee, B. Acupuncture for behavioral and psychological symptoms of dementia. *Medicine* **2021**, *100*, e24341. [CrossRef] [PubMed]
22. Page, M.J.; McKenzie, J.E.; Bossuyt, P.M.; Boutron, I.; Hoffmann, T.C.; Mulrow, C.D.; Shamseer, L.; Tetzlaff, J.M.; Akl, E.A.; Brennan, S.E.; et al. The PRISMA 2020 statement: An updated guideline for reporting systematic reviews. *BMJ* **2021**, *372*, n71. [CrossRef] [PubMed]
23. Sclan, S.G.; Saillon, A.; Franssen, E.; Hugonot-Diener, L.; Saillon, A.; Reisberg, B. The behavior pathology in Alzheimer's disease rating scale (Behave-AD): Reliability and analysis of symptom category scores. *Int. J. Geriatr. Psychiatry* **1996**, *11*, 819–830. [CrossRef]
24. Cummings, J.L.; Mega, M.; Gray, K.; Rosenberg-Thompson, S.; Carusi, D.A.; Gornbein, J. The Neuropsychiatric Inventory: Comprehensive assessment of psychopathology in dementia. *Neurology* **1994**, *44*, 2308. [CrossRef]
25. Overall, J.E.; Gorham, D.R. The brief psychiatric rating scale. *Psychol. Rep.* **1962**, *10*, 799–812. [CrossRef]
26. Mahoney, F.I.; Barthel, D.W. Functional evaluation: The Barthel Index: A simple index of independence useful in scoring improvement in the rehabilitation of the chronically ill. *Md. State Med. J.* **1965**, *14*, 61–65.
27. Galasko, D.; Bennett, D.A.; Sano, M.; Marson, D.; Kaye, J.; Edland, S.D. ADCS Prevention Instrument Project: Assessment of Instrumental Activities of Daily Living for Community-dwelling Elderly Individuals in Dementia Prevention Clinical Trials. *Alzheimer Dis. Assoc. Disord.* **2006**, *20*, S152–S169. [CrossRef]

28. Kasper, J.D.; Black, B.S.; Shore, A.D.; Rabins, P.V. Evaluation of the validity and reliability of the Alzheimer's Disease-Related Quality of Life (ADRQL) assessment instrument. *Alzheimer Dis. Assoc. Disord.* **2009**, *23*, 275. [CrossRef]
29. Novak, M.; Guest, C. Application of a multidimensional caregiver burden inventory. *Gerontologist* **1989**, *29*, 798–803. [CrossRef]
30. Ware, J.E., Jr.; Sherbourne, C.D. The MOS 36-item short-form health survey (SF-36). I. Conceptual framework and item selection. *Med. Care* **1992**, *30*, 473–483. [CrossRef]
31. Higgins, J.; Altman, D. Assessing Risk of Bias in Included Studies. In *Cochrane Handbook for Systematic Reviews of Interventions*; John Wiley & Sons, Ltd.: Hoboken, NJ, USA, 2008.
32. National Heart, Lung, and Blood Institute (NHLBI). Study Quality Assessment Tools. Available online: https://www.nhlbi.nih.gov/health-topics/study-quality-assessment-tools (accessed on 25 February 2021).
33. Guyatt, G.; Rennie, D.; Meade, M.; Cook, D. *Users' Guides to the Medical Literature: A Manual for Evidence-Based Clinical Practice*; AMA Press: Chicago, IL, USA, 2002; Volume 706.
34. Balshem, H.; Helfand, M.; Schünemann, H.J.; Oxman, A.D.; Kunz, R.; Brozek, J.; Vist, G.E.; Falck-Ytter, Y.; Meerpohl, J.; Norris, S.L. GRADE guidelines: 3. Rating the quality of evidence. *J. Clin. Epidemiol.* **2011**, *64*, 401–406. [CrossRef]
35. Ou, Y.-Q. Clinical observation of electric acupuncture combined with fentazin in treating mental symptom of alzheimer's disease. *Shanghai J. Acupunct. Moxibustion* **2000**, *19*, 16.
36. Huang, D.; Pang, S.; Lu, Y.; Liao, L.; Jiang, R.; Jiang, W. Study on the effect of scalp-point cluster needling method on depression caused by Alzheimer's disease and its rehabilitation. *Guangxi Med. J.* **2014**, *36*, 1279–1280. [CrossRef]
37. Jia, Y.; Zhang, X.; Yu, J.; Han, J.; Yu, T.; Shi, J.; Zhao, L.; Nie, K. Acupuncture for patients with mild to moderate Alzheimer's disease: A randomized controlled trial. *BMC Complement. Altern. Med.* **2017**, *17*, 1–8. [CrossRef]
38. Zhang, L.; Li, F.; Ma, L.; Cao, M. Clinical Observation of Electroacupuncture Combined with Midazolam Maleate in Improving Alzheimer's Disease Sleep Disorder. *Shaanxi J. Tradit. Chin. Med.* **2017**, *38*, 1471–1472. [CrossRef]
39. Zhao, Y.; Ge, L.; Zhao, L.; Zhang, J.; Yang, T.; Li, G. Effects of Acusector Combined with Music Therapy on Cognitive Function and Activities of Daily Living in Patients with Mild and Moderate Alzheimer's Disease. *World Chin. Med.* **2020**, *15*, 1998–2001. [CrossRef]
40. Lombardo, N.B.E.; Dresser, M.V.B.; Malivert, M.; McManus, C.A.; Vehvilainen, L.; Ooi, W.L.; Xu, G.; Rosowsky, E.; Drebing, C.; Sheridan, P.L.; et al. Acupuncture as treatment for anxiety and depression in persons with dementia: Results of a feasibility and effectiveness study. *Alzheimers Care Q.* **2001**, *2*, 28–41.
41. Ying, J. Clinical Study on the Effect of Acupuncture on Mental and Behavioral Symptoms of Alzheimer's Disease. Master's Thesis, Chengdu University of Traditional Chinese Medicine, Chengdu, China, 2006.
42. Teare, M.D.; Dimairo, M.; Shephard, N.; Hayman, A.; Whitehead, A.; Walters, S.J. Sample size requirements to estimate key design parameters from external pilot randomised controlled trials: A simulation study. *Trials* **2014**, *15*, 264. [CrossRef]
43. Pagones, R.; Lee, J.L.; Hurst, S. Long-Term Acupuncture Therapy for Low-Income Older Adults with Multimorbidity: A Qualitative Study of Patient Perceptions. *J. Altern. Complement. Med.* **2018**, *24*, 161–167. [CrossRef]
44. Çevik, C.; Anıl, A.; İşeri, S. Özlem Effective chronic low back pain and knee pain treatment with acupuncture in geriatric patients. *J. Back Musculoskelet. Rehabil.* **2015**, *28*, 517–520. [CrossRef]
45. Huang, Y.; Tang, C.-Z.; Lu, Y.-J.; Cai, X.-W.; Zhang, G.-F.; Shan, B.-C.; Cui, S.-Y.; Chen, J.-Q.; Qu, S.-S.; Zhong, Z.; et al. Long-term acupuncture treatment has a multi-targeting regulation on multiple brain regions in rats with Alzheimer's disease: A positron emission tomography study. *Neural Regen. Res.* **2017**, *12*, 1159–1165. [CrossRef]
46. Shan, Y.; Wang, J.; Wang, Z.-Q.; Zhao, Z.-L.; Zhang, M.; Xu, J.-Y.; Han, Y.; Li, K.-C.; Lu, J. Neuronal Specificity of Acupuncture in Alzheimer's Disease and Mild Cognitive Impairment Patients: A Functional MRI Study. *Evid. Based Complement. Altern. Med.* **2018**, *2018*, 1–10. [CrossRef]
47. Huang, W.; Pach, D.; Napadow, V.; Park, K.; Long, X.; Neumann, J.; Maeda, Y.; Nierhaus, T.; Liang, F.; Witt, C.M. Characterizing Acupuncture Stimuli Using Brain Imaging with fMRI-A Systematic Review and Meta-Analysis of the Literature. *PLoS ONE* **2012**, *7*, e32960. [CrossRef]
48. Alves, G.; Carvalho, A.; Carvalho, L.; Sudo, F.; Siqueira-Neto, J.; Oertel-Knöchel, V.; Jurcoane, A.; Knöchel, C.; Boecker, H.; Laks, J.; et al. Neuroimaging Findings Related to Behavioral Disturbances in Alzheimer's Disease: A Systematic Review. *Curr. Alzheimer Res.* **2016**, *14*, 61–75. [CrossRef]
49. Massimo, L.; Powers, C.; Moore, P.; Vesely, L.; Avants, B.; Gee, J.; Libon, D.J.; Grossman, M. Neuroanatomy of Apathy and Disinhibition in Frontotemporal Lobar Degeneration. *Dement. Geriatr. Cogn. Disord.* **2009**, *27*, 96–104. [CrossRef]
50. Van Dam, D.; Vermeiren, Y.; Dekker, A.; Naudé, P.J.; De Deyn, P.P. Neuropsychiatric Disturbances in Alzheimer's Disease: What Have We Learned from Neuropathological Studies? *Curr. Alzheimer Res.* **2016**, *13*, 1145–1164. [CrossRef]
51. Šimić, G.; Babić Leko, M.; Wray, S.; Harrington, C.R.; Delalle, I.; Jovanov-Milošević, N.; Bažadona, D.; Buée, L.; De Silva, R.; Di Giovanni, G.; et al. Monoaminergic neuropathology in Alzheimer's disease. *Prog. Neurobiol.* **2017**, *151*, 101–138. [CrossRef]
52. Lee, N.Y.; Choo, I.H.; Kim, K.W.; Jhoo, J.H.; Youn, J.C.; Lee, U.Y.; Woo, J.I. White Matter Changes Associated With Psychotic Symptoms in Alzheimer's Disease Patients. *J. Neuropsychiatry Clin. Neurosci.* **2006**, *18*, 191–198. [CrossRef]
53. Tu, C.-H.; Macdonald, I.; Chen, Y.-H. The Effects of Acupuncture on Glutamatergic Neurotransmission in Depression, Anxiety, Schizophrenia, and Alzheimer's Disease: A Review of the Literature. *Front. Psychiatry* **2019**, *10*, 14. [CrossRef]

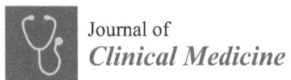

Article

Multidimensional Prognostic Index and Outcomes in Older Patients Undergoing Transcatheter Aortic Valve Implantation: Survival of the Fittest

Jeannette A. Goudzwaard [1,*], Sadhna Chotkan [1], Marjo J. A. G. De Ronde-Tillmans [2], Mattie J. Lenzen [2], Maarten P. H. van Wiechen [2], Joris F. W. Ooms [2], Harmke A. Polinder-Bos [1], Madelon de Beer-Leentfaar [1], Nicolas M. Van Mieghem [2], Joost Daemen [2], Alberto Pilotto [3,4], Peter P. T. de Jaegere [2] and Francesco U. S. Mattace-Raso [1]

[1] Section of Geriatrics, Department of Internal Medicine, Erasmus MC University Medical Center, 3015 GD Rotterdam, The Netherlands; chotkan.sa@gmail.com (S.C.); h.polinder-bos@erasmusmc.nl (H.A.P.-B.); m.debeer-leentfaar@erasmusmc.nl (M.d.B.-L.); f.mattaceraso@erasmusmc.nl (F.U.S.M.-R.)

[2] Department of Cardiology, Thoraxcenter, Erasmus MC University Medical Center, 3015 GD Rotterdam, The Netherlands; m.j.a.g.deronde@erasmusmc.nl (M.J.A.G.D.R.-T.); m.lenzen@erasmusmc.nl (M.J.L.); m.vanwiechen@erasmusmc.nl (M.P.H.v.W.); j.f.w.ooms@erasmusmc.nl (J.F.W.O.); n.vanmieghem@erasmusmc.nl (N.M.V.M.); j.daemen@erasmusmc.nl (J.D.); p.dejaegere@erasmusmc.nl (P.P.T.d.J.)

[3] Department of Geriatric Care, Orthogeriatrics and Rehabilitation, E.O. Galliera Hospital, 16128 Genoa, Italy; alberto.pilotto@galliera.it

[4] Department of Interdisciplinary Medicine, University of Bari, 70121 Bari, Italy

* Correspondence: j.goudzwaard@erasmusmc.nl; Tel.: +31-64-576-8716

Abstract: Selecting patients with a high chance of endured benefit from transcatheter aortic valve implantation (TAVI) is becoming relevant with changing indications and increasing number of TAVI being performed. The aim of our study was to investigate the association of the multidimensional prognostic index (MPI) based on a comprehensive geriatric assessment (CGA) on survival. The TAVI Care & Cure program is a prospective, observational registry of patients referred for TAVI at the Erasmus MC University Medical Center. Consecutive patients who underwent a complete CGA and TAVI were included. CGA components were used to calculate the MPI score. The impact of the MPI score on survival was evaluated using Cox regression. Furthermore, 376 patients were included, 143 (38.0%) patients belonged to the MPI-1 group and 233 (61.9%) patients to the MPI-2–3 group. After 3 years, 14.9% of the patients in the MPI-1 group and 30.5% of the patients in the MPI-2–3 group died ($p = 0.001$). Patients in MPI-1 had increased chances of overall survival in comparison with patients in MPI group 2–3 Hazard Ratio (HR) 0.57, (95% Confidence Interval (CI) 0.33–0.98)). In this study we found that the MPI tool could be useful to assess frailty and to predict which patient will have a higher chance of enduring benefit from a TAVI procedure.

Keywords: aortic stenosis (AS); transcatheter aortic valve implantation (TAVI); multidimensional prognostic index; outcome; mortality; frailty

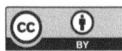

1. Introduction

The indications for transcatheter aortic valve implantation (TAVI) for treating symptomatic aortic stenosis are expanding from older patients who are frail and have high surgical risk to patients with low surgical risk [1–4]. With the rapid uptake of TAVIs being performed [5], selection of patients who can benefit from TAVI is becoming more relevant. Performing a comprehensive geriatric assessment (CGA) is a growing routine practice and the impact of frailty status of patients on outcomes after TAVI is increasingly described [6–9]. The multidimensional prognostic index (MPI) is based on a CGA and has been shown to predict mortality in older patients with acute and chronic conditions [10], including cardiovascular diseases, i.e., heart failure [11] and acute myocardial infarction [12]. In a large, multicenter, longitudinal study, the MPI has shown to be predictive of mortality and negative health outcomes in older, hospitalized patients [13]. Recent studies in relatively small groups of patients, have suggested that the MPI can predict death and stroke for up to three months after TAVI, and mortality for up to one year after TAVI [14–16]. Since the population of patients qualifying for a TAVI is changing and growing, late outcomes are also becoming important. There has been limited research on the effect of frailty and long-term survival after TAVI [17,18]. The aim of this study was therefore to investigate the association between the MPI and survival at 1 and 3 years in older patients undergoing TAVI.

2. Materials and Methods

2.1. Study Population

The study population consists of patients who underwent TAVI (November 2013–July 2018) within the framework of the TAVI Care & Cure program [19]. The TAVI Care & Cure program is a collaboration between the departments of geriatrics and interventional cardiology to optimize care for older patients. Patients referred for severe aortic valve stenosis are seen by the interventional cardiologist for a cardiac assessment, followed by a consultation by the geriatrician to complete a comprehensive geriatric assessment (CGA). Predefined cardiovascular and non-cardiovascular characteristics, procedural and postoperative data of all patients referred for and treated with TAVI were collected [19]. There were no specific exclusion criteria. Treatment decision and strategy were decided during the multidisciplinary heart team meeting (interventional cardiologists, cardiac surgeons, anesthesiologists, geriatricians and a TAVI-nurse coordinator) [19–21]. The study was approved by the Medical Ethics Committee of the Erasmus MC University Medical Center and was conducted according to the Helsinki Declaration. All participants provided written informed consent.

2.2. Cardiology Assessment

Cardiology assessment included determining symptoms using the New York Heart Association (NYHA) classification and the Canadian Cardiovascular Society (CCS) grading of angina pectoris, medical history, physical examination, laboratory assessment and electrocardiogram [19]. Echocardiography, coronary angiography and multislice computed tomography (MSCT) were examined to evaluate the condition of the aortic valve and to determine access site [22].

2.3. Comprehensive Geriatric Assessment

The MPI is based on a standardized CGA and includes eight domains [10]. We calculated the MPI as described in previous studies [11,14,23], with some modifications based on availability of data. We used five of the eight original MPI domains: Activities of Daily Living (ADL) [24], instrumental activities of daily living (IADL) [25], cumulative illness rating scale and comorbidity index (CIRS-CI) [26], the number of medications and social support network. For the cognition, malnutrition and pressure risk domain scores we used different, validated instruments, which have been used previously in calculating the MPI [23]. For the cognition domain we used the mini mental state examination (MMSE) [27], for the domain malnutrition we used the malnutrition screening tool (MUST) [28] and for the pressure risk domain score we used the Waterlow score [29]. The cumulative illness rating scale for geriatrics (CIRS-G) measures chronic medical illness burden while taking into account the severity of the chronic disease across 14 items representing individual body systems. The cumulative final score can vary theoretically from 0 to 56. The severity index is calculated by dividing the total score through the total number of categories endorsed [26].

For each of the eight domains, a three-level score was assigned with score 0 indicating no problem, score 0.5 indicating a minor problem and score 1 indicating a severe problem, as established in previous studies [10,14,23]. The categorization of each domain can be found in Table 1. The sum of all domain values is then divided by 8 to obtain the final MPI score ranging between 0 and 1. Since our aim was to verify the effectiveness of the previously established index in this specific cohort, we used the previously defined cut-off points for the risk of mortality: MPI-1 score 0–0.33, indicating low risk, MPI-2 score 0.34–0.66, indicating medium risk and MPI-3 score 0.67–1.0, indicating high risk [10].

Table 1. Multidimensional prognostic index score assigned to each domain based on severity of the problem.

Assessment	No Problem (Value = 0)	Minor Problem (Value = 0.5)	Severe Problem (Value = 1)
ADL	0	1–6	7–12
IADL	0–1	2–7	8–14
MMSE	28–30	25–27	0–24
CIRS-CI	0	1–2	≥ 3
MUST	0	1	≥ 2
Waterlow score	3–9	10–14	15–45
Number of medications	0–3	4–6	≥ 7
Social support network	Living with family	Institutionalized	Living alone

Abbreviations used: ADL, activities of daily living; IADL, instrumental activities of daily living; MMSE, mini mental state examination; CIRS-CI, cumulative illness rating scale and comorbidity index; MUST, malnutrition screening tool.

As complementary functional tests we used two validated tests for mobility: the 5 meter gait speed test and the timed up and go test. A gait speed of ≤ 1 m/s is suspect of moderate or severe limitation of mobility [30]. Slowness was evaluated with the timed up and go test. A timed up and go test of ≥ 20 s confirms moderate or severe limitation of mobility [31].

2.4. Outcome Measures

Primary outcomes were survival at 1 year and 3 years after TAVI. Secondary outcomes included vascular complications (in-hospital life-threatening or major bleeding or other vascular complications), in-hospital stroke, infection, delirium and 30-day mortality. Delirium was defined according to the Diagnostic and Statistical Manual of Mental Disorders, Fourth Edition (DSM-IV). Life-threatening or major bleeding, vascular complications and stroke were assessed according to the guidelines of the Valve Academic Research Consortium [32]. Procedural outcomes and mortality were assessed prospectively by consulting medical files and the Dutch Civil Registry.

2.5. Statistical Analysis

Categorical variables are presented as numbers and corresponding percentages and differences between MPI groups with the chi-square or Fisher's exact tests as appropriate. Continuous variables are expressed as means $\pm$ SD or median values with corresponding interquartile ranges (IQR) and differences between MPI groups were compared using the independent t-test or its non-parametric equivalents, respectively. A Cox regression analysis was performed for the primary outcome survival. Hazard ratios (HR) and corresponding 95% confidence intervals (CI) were computed. Univariate analyses were performed, every variable with a p value < 0.10 was entered in the multivariate regression model. Variables in the multivariate regression analysis included: age, sex, MPI score, diabetes mellitus, limitation of mobility (5MGST), limitation of mobility (TUGT), reduced grip strength, logistic Euroscore, STS score and post procedural stroke. A logistic univariate regression analysis was performed for secondary outcome measures. p value of 0.05 was considered statistically significant. Data was analyzed with statistic program IBM Statistical Package for Social Science for Windows version 25, Rotterdam, The Netherlands (SPSS).

3. Results

3.1. Patient Characteristics

In total 895 patients underwent TAVI. Within this group, 376 patients completed baseline CGA and were included in this study. According to the MPI score, 143 (38.0%) patients belonged to the MPI-1 group, 221 (58.8%) patients to the MPI-2 group and 12 (3.2%) to the MPI-3 group (Table 2). As only 12 patients belonged to the MPI-3 group we combined this group with the MPI-2 group for further analyses. The baseline characteristics of the MPI group 1 and MPI group 2–3 are shown in Table 2. Patients in the MPI-2-3 group were older (82.0 ± 6.4 vs. 80.7 ± 5.7, p = 0.04) than patients in the MPI-1 group and less men belonged to MPI-2-3 group (38.2% vs. 68.1%, p < 0.001). Hypertension (82.8% vs. 71.6%, p = 0.013), diabetes mellitus (40.9% vs. 19.9%, p < 0.001), previous stroke (21.1% vs. 14.9%, p = 0.028) and renal dysfunction (49.4% vs. 33.3%, p = 0.002) were more prevalent in the MPI-2-3 group compared to the MPI-1 group. The mean logistic Euroscore was 16.8 (±11.0)%, with 111 (29.7%) patients considered to have a high surgical risk according to a logistic Euroscore ≥ 20%. Mean MPI score was 0.39 (±0.14) points.

Table 2. Baseline patient characteristics (n = 376).

Characteristic	Total (377)	MPI-1 N = 141	MPI-2–3 N = 233	p Value
Age (y)	81.54 (±6.1)	80.68 (±5.7)	82.03 (±6.4)	0.040
Men (%)	189 (49.7%)	96 (68.1%)	89 (38.2%)	<0.001
BMI (kg/m^2)	27.2 (±4.8)	27.35 (±4.25)	27.14 (±5.20)	0.697
Cardiovascular risk factors				
Hypertension (%)	294 (78.2%)	101 (71.6%)	192 (82.8%)	0.013
Hypercholesterolemia (%)	231 (61.4%)	83 (58.9%)	147 (63.9%)	0.378
Diabetes mellitus (%)	124 (33.1%)	28 (19.9%)	95 (40.9%)	<0.001
Current smoker (%)	30 (8.0%)	13 (9.2%)	17 (7.3%)	0.558
Comorbidities				
Previous myocardial infarction (%)	73 (19.4%)	27 (19.1%)	46 (19.7%)	1.00
Previous stroke (%)	82 (21.8%)	21 (14.9%)	49 (21.1%)	0.028
COPD (%)	82 (21.8%)	35 (24.8%)	47 (20.4%)	0.367
Renal dysfunction (%)	162 (43.5%)	47 (33.3%)	115 (49.4%)	0.002
CIRS index	1.91 (±0.27)	1.84 (±0.26)	1.96 (±0.26)	<0.001
Symptoms				
NYHA Class 3 or 4 (%)	244 (64.9%)	73 (51.8%)	171 (73.4%)	<0.001
Angina CCS classification 3 or 4 (%)	43 (11.4%)	13 (9.4%)	30 (13.2%)	0.318
Vertigo (%)	143 (41.4%)	53 (40.5%)	90 (42.5%)	0.736
Echocardiography				
AV area (cm^2)	0.76 (±0.24)	0.8 (±0.23)	0.74 (±0.25)	0.052
Peak AoV, (m/s)	4.0 (±0.70)	4.0 (±0.69)	4.0 (±0.71)	0.923
Cardiovascular risk scores				
Logistic Euroscore	16.82 (±11.03)	14.80 (±9.55)	18.02 (±11.70)	0.006
STS score	5.47 (±3.03)	4.29 (±2.19)	6.17 (±3.25)	0.228
CGA domains				
Cognitive impairment probable (%)	111 (29.5%)	20 (14.2%)	91 (39.1%)	<0.001
Malnutrition probable (%)	41 (10.9%)	5 (3.5%)	36 (15.5%)	<0.001
Limitation of mobility, TUGT (%)	48 (12.8%)	5 (3.9%)	43 (21.6%)	<0.001
Limitation of mobility, 5MGS (%)	219 (58.2%)	61 (48.8%)	158 (77.5%)	<0.001
Reduced muscle strength, male (%)	65 (17.3%)	24 (17%)	39 (16.7%)	0.004
Reduces muscle strength, female (%)	100 (26.6%)	17 (12.1%)	83 (35.6%)	0.016
Limitation in ADL activity (%)	111 (29.5%)	9 (6.4%)	102 (43.8%)	<0.001
Limitation in IADL activity (%)	200 (53.2%)	35 (24.8%)	165 (70.8%)	<0.001

Abbreviations used: BMI, body mass index; COPD, chronic obstructive pulmonary disease; CIRS, cumulative illness rating scale; NYHA, New York Heart Association; CCS, Canadian Cardiovascular Society; AoV, aortic valve; STS, Society for Thoracic Surgeons; TUGT, timed up and go test; 5MGS, 5 meter gait speed; ADL, activities of daily living; IADL, instrumental activities of daily living.

3.2. Primary Outcomes

One year after TAVI, 87% of the total study population survived. The one-year survival rate in the MPI-1 group was 92% compared to 84% in the MPI-2–3 group ($p = 0.018$). In multivariate Cox regression analysis, the presence of renal dysfunction ($p = 0.004$) and limitation of mobility (5MGST) ($p = 0.01$) were associated with mortality one year after TAVI.

Three years after TAVI, 85.1% of patients belonging to MPI-1 group compared to 69.5% in the MPI-2–3 group were still alive ($p = 0.001$). In multivariate logistic regression analysis, belonging to the MPI group 2–3 was associated with mortality at 3 years after TAVI (HR 1.99 95% CI 1.13–3.50) (Figure 1).

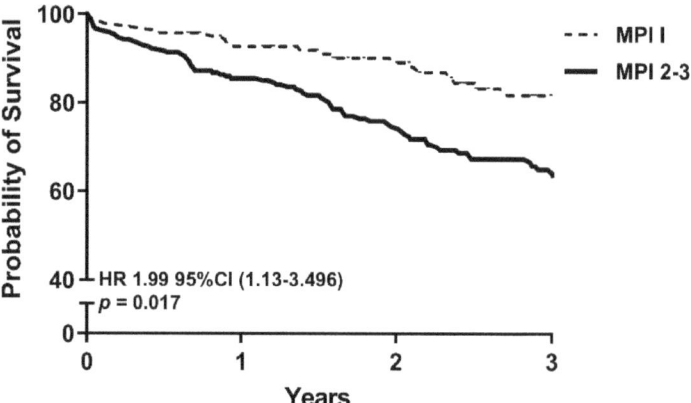

Figure 1. Cox regression survival curve stratified by MPI groups. Model adjusted for age, sex, diabetes mellitus, hypercholesterolemia, peripheral artery disease, renal dysfunction, limitation of mobility, logistic Euroscore, post-procedural stroke and delirium. Abbreviations used: MPI, Multiple Prognostic Index; HR, Hazard Ratio; CI, Confidence Interval.

Other factors associated with 3-year mortality were the presence of renal dysfunction (HR 1.85, 95% CI 1.19–2.87), reduced gait speed (HR 2.05, 95% CI 1.49–3.65) and the occurrence of post-procedural stroke (HR 2.96, 95% CI 1.26–6.99). The presence of hypercholesterolemia (HR 0.52, 95% CI 0.33–0.81) was associated with reduced overall mortality (Table 3).

Table 3. Multivariable Cox analysis for primary outcome 3-year mortality.

Variable	HR	95% CI	*p*-Value
Age	0.99	0.95–1.03	0.51
Sex (men)	0.63	0.84–1.03	0.07
MPI-1 vs. MPI-2–3	1.99	1.13–3.50	0.02
Diabetes mellitus	1.16	0.71–1.90	0.56
Hypercholesterolemia	0.80	0.50–0.32	0.003
Peripheral artery disease	1.34	0.84–2.12	0.23
Renal dysfunction	1.85	1.19–2.87	0.006
Limitation of mobility (5MGST)	2.09	1.15–3.65	0.02
Logistic Euroscore	1.01	0.99–1.03	0.43
Post procedural stroke	2.96	1.26–6.99	0.01
Delirium	1.22	0.71–2.10	0.48

Abbreviations used: MPI, multidimensional prognostic index; 5MGS, 5 meter gait speed.

Within the MPI-2–3 group women (HR 2.09 95% CI 1.230–3.562), patients with renal dysfunction before TAVI (HR 2.03 95% CI 1.21–3.40) and limitation of mobility (5MGST) (HR 2.00 95% CI 1.02–3.93) had the highest risk of 3-year mortality (Table 4).

Table 4. Multivariable Cox analysis for 3-year mortality in the MPI-2–3 group.

Variable	HR	95% CI	p-Value
Age	0.99	0.95–1.04	0.66
Sex (women)	2.09	1.23–3.56	0.006
Diabetes mellitus	0.88	0.51–1.50	0.63
Hypercholesterolemia	0.47	0.28–0.80	0.005
Peripheral artery disease	1.42	0.82–2.46	0.21
Renal dysfunction	1.98	1.18–3.33	0.01
Limitation of mobility (5MGST)	1.19	0.97–3.79	0.06
Logistic Euroscore	1.01	0.98–1.03	0.66
Post procedural stroke	3.98	1.59–10.05	0.003
Delirium	0.97	0.52–1.81	0.93

Abbreviations used: MPI, multidimensional prognostic index; 5MGS, 5 meter gait speed.

3.3. Secondary Outcomes

There were 56 (14.9%) vascular complications in the 30 days after the procedure. Patients with a high risk MPI score (MPI score 2 or 3) had a higher risk of vascular complications in comparison to those in the MPI-1 group (OR 2.00, 95% CI 1.05–3.80, $p = 0.04$) in univariate regression analysis. When adjusted for age and sex, estimates were no longer statistically significant (OR 1.81, 95% CI 0.92–3.53). There were no differences found between the MPI groups for the other procedural outcomes (Table A1). Thirteen (3.5%) patients died within 30 days after the procedure; 2 (0.5%) within MPI-1 group and 11 (3.0%) patients within MPI-2–3 group ($p = 0.26$).

4. Discussion

In this study we found that the MPI tool is useful to assess frailty and could be able to predict survival after TAVI. One- and three-year survival rates were 92% and 85% in patients belonging to MPI-1, corresponding survival rates were 85% and 69.5% in patients belonging to MPI-2–3, respectively. Patients in MPI-1 had a 50% higher chance of long-term survival in comparison with patients in MPI-2–3.

The selection of older patients who will benefit the most from TAVI still remains a challenge. This study shows that the MPI tool could be helpful in the decision-making process. The traditional risk scores commonly used to predict surgical mortality (e.g., logistic Euroscore or the Society of Thoracic Surgeons (STS)) are not sufficient to predict mortality for TAVI procedure in high-risk patients of 80 years and older with substantial comorbidity [33,34]. The incorporation of frailty can have an additional prognostic role as a geriatric biomarker, as studies have shown that frailty is a predictive factor for negative health outcomes after TAVI [6,7,9]. Frailty is defined as a state of reduced physical, cognitive and social functioning, resulting in a reduction of reserve capacity for dealing with stressors [35]. Several conceptual models of frailty have been described; a general agreement exists, however, on the concept that frailty is a multidimensional condition, with physical and psychosocial factors playing a part in its development [35]. Accordingly, the use of the CGA, i.e., a multidimensional diagnostic process for evaluating clinical, functional, cognitive, nutritional and social characteristics of individuals, has been suggested as a clinically useful tool to guarantee a multidimensional approach to frailty [36], even in older patients with aortic stenosis [37]. The incorporation of CGA measures into clinical assessment of patients opting for TAVI procedure is becoming more routine in a growing number of centers [15,19]. The MPI is derived from a standard CGA [10] and has shown to predict mortality in older hospitalized patients, including patients with heart failure, acute myocardial infarction and transient ischemic attack [11,13,23,38]. The value of the MPI in predicting outcomes in TAVI patients has previously been investigated. In a study performed on behalf of the MPI_AGE Project, investigators found that CGA based on the MPI tool predicted prognosis in older patients undergoing TAVI procedure where mortality rate was significantly different between MPI groups at six and twelve months [14]. The MPI tool was also used in a multi-center TAVI registry and found that the MPI showed value for predicting the likelihood of death and a combination of either death, fatal stroke, or both, by one year after TAVI [16]. However, the number of patients included in previous studies was relatively small (116 patients and 71 patients, respectively). To the best of our knowledge this is the first study that investigated the role of the MPI tool for predicting long-term outcomes in a large population of older patients undergoing TAVI.

The incorporation of information derived from a CGA can predict frailty in patients. The assessment of frailty in older patients with comorbidities can give a clear vision of the individual reserve capacity defining the somatic, cognitive and functional situation secondary to the damage due to chronic and intercurrent diseases and the individual capacity to react to external stressors. With growing numbers of TAVI being performed and the growing amount of evidence that being frail is not only predictive of reduced survival, but also on other relevant outcomes such as periprocedural outcomes [39] and health-related quality of life [40], the incorporation of a CGA-based tool can help assess frailty and therefore aid in selecting patients who are less frail with a higher chance of endured benefit from TAVI. When decisions are made concerning therapeutic interventions, the estimation of patient survival is crucial to assess the balance of benefits and risks of performing TAVI.

This study has several limitations. First, results should be interpreted within the framework of a single center and therefore cannot be extrapolated to other groups of patients. Second, the MPI tool investigated in the present study is a somewhat modified version of the original. However, the same modifications have been used in other studies [23], with the same range of predictive value as the original MPI. Third, although the sample size of the complete population was relatively large, there was a low sample size in the MPI-3 group (3.2%), therefore we could not draw any conclusions about the prognosis after TAVI in this specific group.

Further research should focus on the use of the MPI and other geriatric outcomes such as functionality and post-operative HRQoL, since for this specific population survival may be of less importance than improving functional status and quality of life.

In conclusion, in this study we found that the MPI tool is useful to assess frailty and predicts survival after TAVI. We found that in patients eligible for TAVI, 92% of patients belonging to the more vital group (MPI-1) are still alive one year after TAVI and 85% three years after the procedure in comparison to 84% and 69%, respectively, in the frailer MPI-2–3 group. The MPI tool could be useful to assess frailty and to predict which patients will have a higher change of enduring benefit from a TAVI procedure.

Author Contributions: Conceptualization, J.A.G., A.P., F.U.S.M.-R. and S.C.; methodology, J.A.G., S.C., A.P., N.M.V.M., P.P.T.d.J. and F.U.S.M.-R.; software, M.J.L., M.P.H.v.W., J.F.W.O., N.M.V.M. and P.P.T.d.J.; validation, J.A.G., A.P. and F.U.S.M.-R.; formal analysis, J.A.G., S.C., F.U.S.M.-R. and M.J.L.; investigation, J.A.G., S.C., M.J.A.G.D.R.-T., M.J.L., N.M.V.M., P.P.T.d.J., A.P. and F.U.S.M.-R.; resources, M.J.L., N.M.V.M., M.P.H.v.W., J.F.W.O., J.D., H.A.P.-B., M.d.B.-L., M.J.A.G.D.R.-T. P.P.T.d.J. and F.U.S.M.-R.; data curation, J.A.G., S.C., M.J.L., M.J.A.G.D.R.-T., M.P.H.v.W., J.F.W.O., H.A.P.-B., M.d.B.-L., N.M.V.M., J.D, P.P.T.d.J. and F.U.S.M.-R.; writing—original draft preparation, J.A.G. and S.C.; writing—review and editing, J.A.G., S.C., M.J.A.G.D.R.-T., M.J.L., M.P.H.v.W., J.F.W.O., H.A.P.-B., M.d.B.-L., N.M.V.M., J.D, A.P., P.P.T.d.J. and F.U.S.M.-R.; visualization, J.A.G. and S.C.; supervision, N.M.V.M., P.P.T.d.J. and F.U.S.M.-R.; project administration, J.A.G. All authors have read and agreed to the published version of the manuscript.

Funding: This research received no external funding.

Institutional Review Board Statement: The study was conducted according to the guidelines of the Declaration of Helsinki, and approved by the Institutional Review Board (or Ethics Committee) of Erasmus Medical Center (MEC-2014-277).

Informed Consent Statement: Informed consent was obtained from all subjects involved in the study.

Conflicts of Interest: The authors declare no conflict of interest.

Appendix A

Table A1. Univariate logistic regression analysis for secondary outcomes.

Complication	Total	MPI-1	MPI-2–3	Univariable OR (95% CI)	p Value
Post procedural stroke	12/374 (3.2%)	3/141 (2.1%)	9/233 (3.9%)	1.85 (0.49–6.95)	0.36
New pacemaker	63/376 (16.8%)	25/141 (17.7%)	38/233 (16.3%)	0.90 (0.52–1.57)	0.72
Vascular complication	56/376 (14.9%)	14/141 (9.9%)	42/233 (18.0%)	2.00 (1.05–3.80)	0.04
Infection	32/376 (8.5%)	8/141 (5.7%)	24/233 (10.3%)	1.91 (0.83–4.37)	0.13
MI postprocedural	1/323 (85.9%)	1/119 (0.7%)	0/233	-	-
Delirium	55/375 (14.6%)	15/141 (10.6%)	40/233 (17.2%)	1.75 (0.93–3.30)	0.08
Any Complication	145/322 (45.0%)	47/119 (39.4%)	98/201 (48.7%)	1.15 (0.92–2.31)	0.11

MPI: Multiple Prognostic Index; CI: confidence intervals; MI postprocedural: Myocardial Infarction postprocedural; Univariable OR: Univariable Odds Ratio.

References

1. Grimard, B.H.; Larson, J.M. Aortic stenosis: Diagnosis and treatment. *Am. Fam. Physician* **2008**, *78*, 717–724. [PubMed]
2. Popma, J.J.; Adams, D.H.; Reardon, M.J.; Yakubov, S.J.; Kleiman, N.S.; Heimansohn, D.; Hermiller, J.; Hughes, G.C.; Harrison, J.K.; Coselli, J.; et al. Transcatheter aortic valve replacement using a self-expanding bioprosthesis in patients with severe aortic stenosis at extreme risk for surgery. *J. Am. Coll. Cardiol.* **2014**, *63*, 1972–1981. [CrossRef]
3. Mack, M.J.; Leon, M.B.; Thourani, V.H.; Makkar, R.; Kodali, S.K.; Russo, M.; Kapadia, S.R.; Malaisrie, S.C.; Cohen, D.J.; Pibarot, P.; et al. Transcatheter aortic-valve replacement with a balloon-expandable valve in low-risk patients. *N. Engl. J. Med.* **2019**, *380*, 1695–1705. [CrossRef] [PubMed]
4. Voigtländer, L.; Seiffert, M. Expanding TAVI to low and intermediate risk patients. *Front. Cardiovasc. Med.* **2018**, *5*. [CrossRef] [PubMed]
5. Barbanti, M.; Webb, J.; Gilard, M.; Capodanno, D.; Tamburino, C. Transcatheter aortic valve implantation in 2017: State of the art. *EuroIntervention* **2017**, *13*, AA11–AA21. [CrossRef]
6. Schoenenberger, A.W.; Stortecky, S.; Neumann, S.; Moser, A.; Jüni, P.; Carrel, T.; Huber, C.; Gandon, M.; Bischoff, S.; Schoenenberger, C.-M.; et al. Predictors of functional decline in elderly patients undergoing transcatheter aortic valve implantation (TAVI). *Eur. Heart J.* **2013**, *34*, 684–692. [CrossRef]
7. Stortecky, S.; Schoenenberger, A.W.; Moser, A.; Kalesan, B.; Jüni, P.; Carrel, T.; Bischoff, S.; Schoenenberger, C.-M.; Stuck, A.E.; Windecker, S.; et al. Evaluation of multidimensional geriatric assessment as a predictor of mortality and cardiovascular events after transcatheter aortic valve implantation. *JACC Cardiovasc. Interv.* **2012**, *5*, 489–496. [CrossRef]
8. Green, P.; Woglom, A.E.; Genereux, P.; Daneault, B.; Paradis, J.-M.; Schnell, S.; Hawkey, M.; Maurer, M.S.; Kirtane, A.J.; Kodali, S. The impact of frailty status on survival after transcatheter aortic valve replacement in older adults with severe aortic stenosis: A single-center experience. *JACC Cardiovasc. Interv.* **2012**, *5*, 974–981. [CrossRef]
9. Goudzwaard, J.A.; de Ronde-Tillmans, M.J.; El Faquir, N.; Acar, F.; Van Mieghem, N.M.; Lenzen, M.J.; de Jaegere, P.P.; Mattace-Raso, F.U. The Erasmus Frailty Score is associated with delirium and 1-year mortality after Transcatheter Aortic Valve Implantation in older patients. The TAVI Care & Cure program. *Int. J. Cardiol.* **2019**, *276*, 48–52. [CrossRef]
10. Pilotto, A.; Ferrucci, L.; Franceschi, M.; D'Ambrosio, L.P.; Scarcelli, C.; Cascavilla, L.; Paris, F.; Placentino, G.; Seripa, D.; Dallapiccola, B.; et al. Development and validation of a multidimensional prognostic index for one-year mortality from comprehensive geriatric assessment in hospitalized older patients. *Rejuvenation Res.* **2008**, *11*, 151–161. [CrossRef]
11. Pilotto, A.; Addante, F.; Franceschi, M.; Leandro, G.; Rengo, G.; D'Ambrosio, P.; Longo, M.G.; Rengo, F.; Pellegrini, F.; Dallapiccola, B.; et al. Multidimensional prognostic index based on a comprehensive geriatric assessment predicts short-term mortality in older patients with heart failure. *Circ. Heart Fail.* **2010**, *3*, 14–20. [CrossRef]
12. Cammalleri, V.; Bonanni, M.; Bueti, F.M.; Matteucci, A.; Cammalleri, L.; Stifano, G.; Muscoli, S.; Romeo, F. Multidimensional Prognostic Index (MPI) in elderly patients with acute myocardial infarction. *Aging Clin. Exp. Res.* **2021**, *33*, 1875–1883. [CrossRef]
13. Pilotto, A.; Veronese, N.; Daragjati, J.; Cruz-Jentoft, A.J.; Polidori, M.C.; Mattace-Raso, F.; Paccalin, M.; Topinkova, E.; Siri, G.; Greco, A.; et al. Using the multidimensional prognostic index to predict clinical outcomes of hospitalized older persons: A prospective, multicenter, international study. *J. Gerontol. Ser. A Biol. Sci. Med. Sci.* **2018**, *74*, 1643–1649. [CrossRef]
14. Bureau, M.-L.; Liuu, E.; Christiaens, L.; Pilotto, A.; Mergy, J.; Bellarbre, F.; Ingrand, P.; Paccalin, M.; Cruz-Jentoft, A.J.; Maggi, S.; et al. Using a multidimensional prognostic index (MPI) based on comprehensive geriatric assessment (CGA) to predict mortality in elderly undergoing transcatheter aortic valve implantation. *Int. J. Cardiol.* **2017**, *236*, 381–386. [CrossRef]
15. Ungar, A.; Mannarino, G.; Van Der Velde, N.; Baan, J.; Thibodeau, M.-P.; Masson, J.-B.; Santoro, G.; Van Mourik, M.; Jansen, S.; Deutsch, C.; et al. Comprehensive geriatric assessment in patients undergoing transcatheter aortic valve implantation—results from the CGA-TAVI multicentre registry. *BMC Cardiovasc. Disord.* **2018**, *18*, 1. [CrossRef] [PubMed]

16. Van Mourik, M.S.; van der Velde, N.; Mannarinom, G.; Thibodeau, M.-P.; Masson, J.-B.; Santoro, G.; Baan, J.; Jansen, S.; Kurucova, J.; Thoenes, M. Value of a comprehensive geriatric assessment for predicting one-year outcomes in patients undergoing transcatheter aortic valve implantation: Results from the CGA-TAVI multicentre registry. *J. Geriatr. Cardiol. JGC* **2019**, *16*, 468. [PubMed]
17. Skaar, E.; Eide, L.S.P.; Norekvål, T.M.; Ranhoff, A.H.; Nordrehaug, J.E.; Forman, D.E.; Schoenenberger, A.W.; Hufthammer, K.O.; Kuiper, K.K.-J.; Bleie, Ø. A novel geriatric assessment frailty score predicts 2-year mortality after transcatheter aortic valve implantation. *Eur. Heart J. Qual. Care Clin. Outcomes* **2018**, *5*, 153–160. [CrossRef]
18. Martin, G.P.; Sperrin, M.; Ludman, P.F.; Mark, A.; Gunning, M.; Townend, J.; Redwood, S.R.; Kadam, U.T.; Buchan, I.; Mamas, M.A. Do frailty measures improve prediction of mortality and morbidity following transcatheter aortic valve implantation? An analysis of the UK TAVI registry. *BMJ Open* **2018**, *8*, e022543. [PubMed]
19. De Ronde-Tillmans, M.; Goudzwaard, J.A.; El Faquir, N.; van Mieghem, N.M.; Mattace-Raso, F.U.S.; Cummins, P.A.; Lenzen, M.J.; de Jaegere, P.P.T. TAVI Care and Cure, the Rotterdam multidisciplinary program for patients undergoing transcatheter aortic valve implantation: Design and rationale. *Int. J. Cardiol.* **2020**, *302*, 36–41. [CrossRef]
20. De Ronde-Tillmans, M.J.; Lenzen, M.J.; Abawi, M.; Van Mieghem, N.M.; Zijlstra, F.; De Jaegere, P.P. 10 years of transcatheter aortic valve implantation: An overview of the clinical applicability and findings. *Ned. Tijdschr. Voor Geneeskd.* **2013**, *158*, A7768–A7768.
21. Baumgartner, H.; Falk, V.; Bax, J.J.; De Bonis, M.; Hamm, C.; Holm, P.J.; Iung, B.; Lancellotti, P.; Lansac, E.; Muñoz, D.R.; et al. 2017 ESC/EACTS Guidelines for the management of valvular heart disease. *Eur. J. Cardiothorac. Surg.* **2017**, *52*, 616–664. [CrossRef]
22. Schultz, C.J.; Moelker, A.D.; Tzikas, A.; Rossi, A.; Van Geuns, R.-J.; De Feyter, P.J.; Serruys, P.W. Cardiac CT: Necessary for precise sizing for transcatheter aortic implantation. *EuroIntervention* **2010**, *6*, G6–G13.
23. Angleman, S.B.; Santoni, G.; Pilotto, A.; Fratiglioni, L.; Welmer, A.-K. Investigators MAP: Multidimensional prognostic index in association with future mortality and number of hospital days in a population-based sample of older adults: Results of the EU funded MPI_AGE project. *PLoS ONE* **2015**, *10*, e0133789. [CrossRef]
24. Katz, S. Studies of illness in the aged. The index of ADL: A standardized measure of biologic and psychologic function. *JaMa* **1963**, *185*, 94–99. [CrossRef] [PubMed]
25. Lawton, M.P.; Brody, E.M. Assessment of Older People: Self-Maintaining and Instrumental Activities of Daily Living. *Gerontologist* **1969**, *9*, 179–186. [CrossRef] [PubMed]
26. Parmelee, P.A.; Thuras, P.D.; Katz, I.R.; Lawton, M.P. Validation of the Cumulative Illness Rating Scale in a Geriatric Residential Population. *J. Am. Geriatr. Soc.* **1995**, *43*, 130–137. [CrossRef] [PubMed]
27. Folstein, M.F.; Folstein, S.E.; McHugh, P.R. "Mini-mental state". A practical method for grading the cognitive state of patients for the clinician. *J. Psychiatr. Res.* **1975**, *12*, 189–198. [CrossRef]
28. Elia, M. *Nutritional Screening of Adults: A Multidisciplinary Responsibility*; Malnutrition Advisory Group (MAG): Redditch, UK; BAPEN: Reditch, UK, 2003.
29. Balzer, K.; Pohl, C.; Dassen, T.; Halfens, R. The norton, waterlow, braden, and care dependency scalesl comparing their validity when identifying patients' pressure sore risk. *J. Wound Ostomy Cont. Nurs.* **2007**, *34*, 389–398. [CrossRef]
30. Steffen, T.M.; Hacker, T.A.; Mollinger, L. Age and gender-related test performance in community-dwelling elderly people: Six-minute walk test, berg balance scale, timed up & go test, and gait speeds. *Phys. Ther.* **2002**, *82*, 128–137. [CrossRef]
31. Podsiadlo, D.; Richardson, S. The timed "Up & Go": A test of basic functional mobility for frail elderly persons. *J. Am. Geriatr. Soc.* **1991**, *39*, 142–148.
32. Kappetein, A.P.; Head, S.J.; Généreux, P.; Piazza, N.; Van Mieghem, N.M.; Blackstone, E.H.; Brott, T.G.; Cohen, D.J.; Cutlip, D.E.; van Es, G.-A. Updated standardized endpoint definitions for transcatheter aortic valve implantation: The valve academic research consortium-2 consensus document. *J. Am. Coll. Cardiol.* **2012**, *60*, 1438–1454. [CrossRef]
33. Smith, C.R.; Leon, M.B.; Mack, M.J.; Miller, D.C.; Moses, J.W.; Svensson, L.G.; Tuzcu, E.M.; Webb, J.G.; Fontana, G.P.; Makkar, R.R.; et al. Transcatheter versus surgical aortic-valve replacement in high-risk patients. *N. Engl. J. Med.* **2011**, *364*, 2187–2198. [CrossRef] [PubMed]
34. Roques, F.; Nashef, S.A.M.; Michel, P.; Gauducheau, E.; De Vincentiis, C.; Baudet, E.; Cortina, J.; David, M.; Faichney, A.; Gavrielle, F.; et al. Risk factors and outcome in European cardiac surgery: Analysis of the EuroSCORE multinational database of 19030 patients. *Eur. J. Cardio-Thorac. Surg.* **1999**, *15*, 816–823. [CrossRef]
35. Hoogendijk, E.O.; Afilalo, J.; Ensrud, K.E.; Kowal, P.; Onder, G.; Fried, L.P. Frailty: Implications for clinical practice and public health. *Lancet* **2019**, *394*, 1365–1375. [CrossRef]
36. Pilotto, A.; Custodero, C.; Maggi, S.; Polidori, M.C.; Veronese, N.; Ferrucci, L. A multidimensional approach to frailty in older people. *Ageing Res. Rev.* **2020**, *60*, 101047. [CrossRef]
37. Lilamand, M.; Dumonteil, N.; Nourhashémi, F.; Hanon, O.; Marcheix, B.; Toulza, O.; Elmalem, S.; van Kan, G.A.; Raynaud-Simon, A.; Vellas, B.; et al. Gait speed and comprehensive geriatric assessment: Two keys to improve the management of older persons with aortic stenosis. *Int. J. Cardiol.* **2014**, *173*, 580–582. [CrossRef]
38. Sancarlo, D.; Pilotto, A.; Panza, F.; Copetti, M.; Longo, M.G.; D'Ambrosio, P.; D'Onofrio, G.; Ferrucci, L.; Pilotto, A. A Multidimensional Prognostic Index (MPI) based on a comprehensive geriatric assessment predicts short and long-term all-cause mortality in older hospitalized patients with transient ischemic attack. *J. Neurol.* **2011**, *259*, 670–678. [CrossRef]

39. Goudzwaard, J.A.; Ronde-Tillmans, M.J.A.G.D.; Jager, T.A.J.D.; Lenzen, M.J.; Nuis, R.-J.; van Mieghem, N.M.; Daemen, J.; de Jaegere, P.P.T.; Mattace-Raso, F.U.S. Incidence, determinants and consequences of delirium in older patients after transcatheter aortic valve implantation. *Age Ageing* **2020**, *49*, 389–394. [CrossRef]
40. Goudzwaard, J.A.; Ronde-Tillmans, M.J.A.G.D.; Hoorn, F.E.D.V.; Kwekkeboom, E.H.C.; Lenzen, M.J.; van Wiechen, M.P.H.; Ooms, J.F.W.; Nuis, R.-J.; Van Mieghem, N.M.; Daemen, J.; et al. Impact of frailty on health-related quality of life 1 year after transcatheter aortic valve implantation. *Age Ageing* **2020**, *49*, 989–994. [CrossRef] [PubMed]

outpatient setting (not institutionalised). All participants provided informed consent to take part in the study. The study population was composed of 89,615 persons living in the community in Malaga, Spain. Patients were recruited at twelve primary healthcare centres by using stratified random sampling designed to obtain a representative sample. The study population was allocated in proportion to the size of each centre. Based on a published prevalence of frailty in primary care of 30% [23–25] and assuming a 4% margin of error and a 95% confidence interval, we calculated that the minimum sample size required for this study would be 502 persons, a figure that was increased by 15% to offset possible losses.

2.2. Data Collection and Global Assessment

In order to obtain the study data for analysis, patients were interviewed using a structured questionnaire. Further data were obtained from medication packaging and digital medical records. The questionnaire was used to obtain detailed information on the patients' regular drug use, together with clinical, functional and sociodemographic data. Clinical diagnoses were examined, and the Charlson Comorbidity Index (CCI) [26] was calculated. The Spanish version (Nestlé Nutrition Institute) of the Mini Nutritional Assessment Short Form (MNA) was used for nutritional screening [27]. The patients' independence in performing instrumental activities of daily living (IADL) was assessed using the Lawton scale [28]. Cognitive function was evaluated by using the short portable mental state questionnaire by Pfeiffer (SPMSQ) [29], and mood status was determined by using the Geriatric Depression Scale (GDS-15) by Yesavage [30].

2.3. Measuring Medication Appropriateness

Data were obtained for the medication prescribed (indication, dosage and duration of treatment during the last three months or more). The presence of polymedication, defined as the regular use of five or more medications, was noted, as was that of potentially inappropriate medication (PIM) according to the STOPP v2 criteria (Screening Tool of Older Person's Potentially Inappropriate Prescriptions, version 2) [31]. The latter variable was operationalised as the percentage of patients receiving at least one PIM.

2.4. Frailty Assessment

The main study outcome was frailty, assessed by the phenotype proposed by Fried et al. [5] which consists of the following criteria: (a) unintentional weight loss of 4.5 kg or more in the previous year; (b) self-reported exhaustion, identified by two questions in the Center for Epidemiological Studies Depression (CES-D) scale; (c) weakness, defined by low handgrip strength and measured in Kg in the dominant hand by using a dynamometer (Jamar hydraulic grip hand dynamometer SP-5030J1) (highest of three consecutive measurements), adjusted for gender and body mass index (grip strength was classified as low when the force exerted was below the first quintile of the distribution) (d) slow walking speed (lowest quintile of gait speed), assessed by the walking time (in seconds) over a distance of 4.57 m, adjusted for gender and height; (e) low physical activity, measured by the weighted score of kilocalories expended per week, obtained from the Minnesota Leisure Time Activity Questionnaire and adjusted for gender. Participants were classified as non-frail (robust) if they met none of the criteria, pre-frail if they met one or two criteria, and frail if three or more criteria were met.

2.5. Statistical Analysis

Exploratory data analysis and frequency tables were used to describe the study variables. Taking into account the three possible states of frailty (frail, pre-frail and robust), a multinomial logistic regression model was used to study the relationship between the independent variables and the outcome variable, frailty [32]. All independent variables were included in the regression model. The influence of various factors on the states of frailty and pre-frailty was examined, taking robust patients as a benchmark. Odds ratios (OR) and 95% confidence intervals (CI) were calculated for each covariate included in

39. Goudzwaard, J.A.; Ronde-Tillmans, M.J.A.G.D.; Jager, T.A.J.D.; Lenzen, M.J.; Nuis, R.-J.; van Mieghem, N.M.; Daemen, J.; de Jaegere, P.P.T.; Mattace-Raso, F.U.S. Incidence, determinants and consequences of delirium in older patients after transcatheter aortic valve implantation. *Age Ageing* **2020**, *49*, 389–394. [CrossRef]
40. Goudzwaard, J.A.; Ronde-Tillmans, M.J.A.G.D.; Hoorn, F.E.D.V.; Kwekkeboom, E.H.C.; Lenzen, M.J.; van Wiechen, M.P.H.; Ooms, J.F.W.; Nuis, R.-J.; Van Mieghem, N.M.; Daemen, J.; et al. Impact of frailty on health-related quality of life 1 year after transcatheter aortic valve implantation. *Age Ageing* **2020**, *49*, 989–994. [CrossRef] [PubMed]

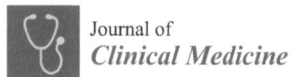

Article

Assessing Prevalence and Factors Related to Frailty in Community-Dwelling Older Adults: A Multinomial Logistic Analysis

Encarnación Blanco-Reina [1,*], Lorena Aguilar-Cano [2], María Rosa García-Merino [3], Ricardo Ocaña-Riola [4,5], Jenifer Valdellós [3], Inmaculada Bellido-Estévez [1] and Gabriel Ariza-Zafra [6]

1. Pharmacology and Therapeutics Department, Instituto de Investigación Biomédica de Málaga-IBIMA, School of Medicine, University of Málaga, 29016 Málaga, Spain; ibellido@uma.es
2. Physical Medicine and Rehabilitation Department, Hospital Regional Universitario, 29010 Málaga, Spain; loagca2011@hotmail.com
3. Health District of Málaga-Guadalhorce, 29009 Málaga, Spain; rosaballet@yahoo.es (M.R.G.-M.); jenny_dok7@hotmail.com (J.V.)
4. Escuela Andaluza de Salud Pública, 18011 Granada, Spain; ricardo.ocana.easp@juntadeandalucia.es
5. Instituto de Investigación Biosanitaria ibs.GRANADA, 18011 Granada, Spain
6. Geriatrics Department, Complejo Hospitalario Universitario, 02006 Albacete, Spain; gariza@sescam.jccm.es
* Correspondence: eblanco@uma.es; Tel.: +34-952136648

Citation: Blanco-Reina, E.; Aguilar-Cano, L.; García-Merino, M.R.; Ocaña-Riola, R.; Valdellós, J.; Bellido-Estévez, I.; Ariza-Zafra, G. Assessing Prevalence and Factors Related to Frailty in Community-Dwelling Older Adults: A Multinomial Logistic Analysis. *J. Clin. Med.* **2021**, *10*, 3576. https://doi.org/10.3390/jcm10163576

Academic Editors: Francesco Mattace Raso and Ersilia Lucenteforte

Received: 26 June 2021
Accepted: 11 August 2021
Published: 14 August 2021

Publisher's Note: MDPI stays neutral with regard to jurisdictional claims in published maps and institutional affiliations.

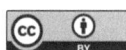

Copyright: © 2021 by the authors. Licensee MDPI, Basel, Switzerland. This article is an open access article distributed under the terms and conditions of the Creative Commons Attribution (CC BY) license (https://creativecommons.org/licenses/by/4.0/).

Abstract: Frailty is an age-related clinical condition that typically involves a deterioration in the physiological capacity of various organ systems and heightens the patient's susceptibility to stressors. For this reason, one of the main research goals currently being addressed is that of characterising the impact of frailty in different settings. The main aim of this study is to determine the prevalence of Fried's frailty phenotype among community-dwelling older people and to analyse the factors associated with frailty. In this research study, 582 persons aged 65 years or more participated in this cross-sectional study that was conducted at primary healthcare centres in Málaga, Spain. Sociodemographic, clinical, functional and comprehensive drug therapy data were compiled. The relationship between the independent variables and the different states of frailty was analysed by using a multinomial logistic regression model. Frailty was present in 24.1% of the study sample (95% CI = 20.7–27.6) of whom 54.3% were found to be pre-frail and 21.6% were non-frail. The study variable most strongly associated with frailty was the female gender (OR = 20.54, 95% CI = 9.10–46.3). Other factors found to be associated with the state of frailty included age, dependence for the instrumental activities of daily living (IADL), polymedication, osteoarticular pathology and psychopathology. This study confirms the high prevalence of frailty among community-dwelling older people. Frailty may be associated with many factors. Some of these associated factors may be preventable or modifiable and, thus, provide clinically relevant targets for intervention. This is particularly the case for depressive symptoms, the clinical control of osteoarthritis and the use of polypharmacy.

Keywords: frailty; older adults; polymedication; osteoarticular pathology; psychopathology; primary care

1. Introduction

Population ageing is a global phenomenon that is producing significant sociodemographic transformations. According to the 2015 EU Ageing Report, the age demographic of the European population will change dramatically over the coming decades, with older people accounting for an increasing proportion out of the total. By 2060, persons aged over 65 years are expected to account for 28% of the total population in Europe (currently 18%), while the proportion of individuals over 80s will increase from 5% to 12% during the same period [1]. However, there is little evidence that increased longevity is accompanied by an extended period of good health [2]. In this respect, the WHO has published a *World*

Report on Ageing and Health, reviewing current knowledge, identifying gaps and providing a public health framework for action. This report redefines healthy ageing, focusing on the notion of functional ability. In this respect, the authors remark that comprehensive assessments of functioning in older age are much better predictors of survival and other outcomes than the presence/absence of disease or even the extent of comorbidities. According to this report, the foremost condition among geriatric syndromes producing a negative impact on survival is the condition of frailty [3].

Without question, frailty will be one of the most serious public health challenges facing the world during this century [4]. Frailty is an age-related clinical condition that typically involves a deterioration in the physiological capacity of various organ systems [5–7] and heightens the patient's susceptibility to stressors [5–10]. When stressor events (such as acute illness) occur, the functional capacity of a person with frailty deteriorates rapidly. Frailty often precedes disability [5,8], although the two conditions may coexist [11]. Quite evidently, older persons with frailty are more likely to present unmet care needs, to suffer falls and/or fractures, to require hospitalisation, to have a reduced quality of life and to be subject to iatrogenic complications and early mortality [5,6,8,12,13]. Studies have shown that frailty is a dynamic entity that may be encountered on a continuum ranging from fit to frail. Moreover, an individual's level of frailty is liable to change in either direction (i.e., worsening or improving) over time [4]. In fact, a substantial proportion of the population experience at least one such transition [14–16], and thus the process is potentially reversible. Frailty is not an inevitable consequence of ageing, and therefore a strong focus on early screening and diagnosis is needed to enable optimal prevention.

Increasing numbers of persons with frailty are attending their general practitioners. Primary care is the first point of contact for most such persons. Attention is usually comprehensive and personalised, and thus this healthcare environment is very suitable for the identification, management and study of frailty [17,18]. However, the absence of a consensus on how to define and measure frailty presents challenges for research and clinical practice. Among the many operational definitions of frailty that have been proposed, the best known are Fried's Frailty Phenotype [5] and Rockwood's Frailty Index [9]. The heterogeneity of assessment instruments is one of the factors underlying the wide range of prevalence estimates that have been reported for frailty (4–59%) [19].

Frailty is an important public health issue for several reasons: Firstly, it is highly prevalent and is the condition that most commonly results in death; secondly, the process is potentially preventable and treatable, particularly with early intervention; finally, despite its prevalence, frailty is either not recognised as a clinical or diagnostic syndrome, or (on many occasions) it is not recorded in clinical charts. Accordingly, one of the main research goals currently being addressed is that of characterising the impact of frailty on the population [20]. In this respect, the ADVANTAGE initiative "Joint Action on the Prevention of Frailty", which is co-funded by the Third European Health Programme (2014–2020), has highlighted the need for studies to be undertaken in order to determine the current prevalence of frailty in different settings [21]. Moreover, due to the multidimensional nature of frailty, diverse factors may be involved in its progression. Given the real possibility that frailty may transition and/or be reversed, we consider it of interest to investigate the question of frailty among older adults living in Spain, where life expectancy is among the highest in the world [22]. In this study, we assess clinical, functional and pharmacological aspects of risk factors for frailty. We consider many variables, some of which are potentially modifiable by targeted interventions and preventive actions. Specifically, our study aim is to determine the prevalence of Fried's frailty phenotype among community-dwelling older people and to analyse the factors associated with frailty.

2. Materials and Methods

2.1. Study Design, Setting and Participants

In this cross-sectional study, all participants met the following inclusion criteria: aged 65 years or more, registered in the database of the Spanish NHS and belonging to the outpatient setting (not institutionalised). All participants provided informed consent to take part in the study. The study population was composed of 89,615 persons living in the community in Malaga, Spain. Patients were recruited at twelve primary healthcare centres by using stratified random sampling designed to obtain a representative sample. The study population was allocated in proportion to the size of each centre. Based on a published prevalence of frailty in primary care of 30% [23–25] and assuming a 4% margin of error and a 95% confidence interval, we calculated that the minimum sample size required for this study would be 502 persons, a figure that was increased by 15% to offset possible losses.

2.2. Data Collection and Global Assessment

In order to obtain the study data for analysis, patients were interviewed using a structured questionnaire. Further data were obtained from medication packaging and digital medical records. The questionnaire was used to obtain detailed information on the patients' regular drug use, together with clinical, functional and sociodemographic data. Clinical diagnoses were examined, and the Charlson Comorbidity Index (CCI) [26] was calculated. The Spanish version (Nestlé Nutrition Institute) of the Mini Nutritional Assessment Short Form (MNA) was used for nutritional screening [27]. The patients' independence in performing instrumental activities of daily living (IADL) was assessed using the Lawton scale [28]. Cognitive function was evaluated by using the short portable mental state questionnaire by Pfeiffer (SPMSQ) [29], and mood status was determined by using the Geriatric Depression Scale (GDS-15) by Yesavage [30].

2.3. Measuring Medication Appropriateness

Data were obtained for the medication prescribed (indication, dosage and duration of treatment during the last three months or more). The presence of polymedication, defined as the regular use of five or more medications, was noted, as was that of potentially inappropriate medication (PIM) according to the STOPP v2 criteria (Screening Tool of Older Person's Potentially Inappropriate Prescriptions, version 2) [31]. The latter variable was operationalised as the percentage of patients receiving at least one PIM.

2.4. Frailty Assessment

The main study outcome was frailty, assessed by the phenotype proposed by Fried et al. [5] which consists of the following criteria: (a) unintentional weight loss of 4.5 kg or more in the previous year; (b) self-reported exhaustion, identified by two questions in the Center for Epidemiological Studies Depression (CES-D) scale; (c) weakness, defined by low handgrip strength and measured in Kg in the dominant hand by using a dynamometer (Jamar hydraulic grip hand dynamometer SP-5030J1) (highest of three consecutive measurements), adjusted for gender and body mass index (grip strength was classified as low when the force exerted was below the first quintile of the distribution) (d) slow walking speed (lowest quintile of gait speed), assessed by the walking time (in seconds) over a distance of 4.57 m, adjusted for gender and height; (e) low physical activity, measured by the weighted score of kilocalories expended per week, obtained from the Minnesota Leisure Time Activity Questionnaire and adjusted for gender. Participants were classified as non-frail (robust) if they met none of the criteria, pre-frail if they met one or two criteria, and frail if three or more criteria were met.

2.5. Statistical Analysis

Exploratory data analysis and frequency tables were used to describe the study variables. Taking into account the three possible states of frailty (frail, pre-frail and robust), a multinomial logistic regression model was used to study the relationship between the independent variables and the outcome variable, frailty [32]. All independent variables were included in the regression model. The influence of various factors on the states of frailty and pre-frailty was examined, taking robust patients as a benchmark. Odds ratios (OR) and 95% confidence intervals (CI) were calculated for each covariate included in the model. A 5% significance level was assumed to indicate statistical significance. All statistical data analyses were performed using SPSS version 24.0 (IBM SPSS Statistics, Armonk, NY, USA).

2.6. Ethical Considerations

This study was conducted in accordance with the Declaration of Helsinki. The Málaga Clinical Research Ethics Committee approved the study (PI-0234-14), and informed consent was obtained from all patients prior to their inclusion.

3. Results

3.1. Characteristics of the Study Population

We included a total of 582 patients, with a mean age of 73.1 years (standard deviation 5.5, range 65–104) and slightly more than half of the sample being female. There were only eleven patients who declined to participate, which is a negligible proportion. Furthermore, as our study is based on a personal face-to-face interview in the primary care outpatient facility, there were no patients without data of our interest primary variable (frailty), and missing data were exceptional. Only 21.1% lived alone, whereas 62.4% lived with their partner (62.4%) or family (16.5%). The average CCI score was 1.48 (standard deviation 1.6, range 0–8), and 38.8% of the patients had scores greater than 2. Each patient presented 7.8 diagnoses on average (standard deviation 3.3, range 0–20). The most prevalent chronic conditions were bone and joint disorders (mainly osteoarthritis of the knee, hip, hand and shoulder) (75.3%), hypertension (70.9%) and dyslipidaemia (51.7%). Some form of psychopathology (mainly anxiety and/or depression) was present in 36% of the patients. Only 13.3% of the patients had a normal weight, while a large proportion presented overweight (40.9%) or obesity (45.7%). The mean body mass index was 30.2 (standard deviation 5.1, range 17–54.5). The mean score on the Lawton scale was 6.6 (standard deviation 1.8, range 0–8) with half of the sample being independently capable of performing IADL. Table 1 details the main characteristics of the study population. Each patient consumed on average 6.8 drugs (standard deviation 4.0; range 0–23) resulting in a polymedication prevalence pf 68.6%. Omeprazole and acetaminophen were the most prescribed drugs, followed by aspirin, simvastatin, metformin, metamizole, enalapril and bromazepam. A large proportion of patients (66.8%) presented at least one potentially inappropriate medication, according to the STOPP v2 criteria. The mean number of PIMs per patient was 2.1 (standard deviation 2.2, range 0–10). Benzodiazepines were the most frequently detected PIMs (61% of all PIMs).

Table 1. Characteristics of the study population (n = 582).

Quantitative Variables	Mean	Standard Deviation
Age (years)	73.1	5.5
Lawton (IADL)	6.6	1.8
BMI (kg/m^2)	30.2	5.1
Number of comorbidities	7.8	3.3
Number of drugs per patient	6.8	4.0
Number of PIMs per patient	2.1	2.2
Qualitative Variables	**Subjects (n)**	**Percentage (%)**
Gender		
Male	248	42.6
Female	334	57.4
Lawton (IADL)		
0–1	12	2.1
2–3	37	6.4
4–5	72	12.4
6–7	165	28.4
8	295	50.8

Table 1. Cont.

Quantitative Variables	Mean	Standard Deviation
SPMSQ (Pfeiffer)		
0–2 errors	533	91.9
3–4 errors	36	6.2
5 errors and over	11	1.9
GDS-15		
0–5	440	75.9
6–9	107	18.4
10 and over	33	5.7
BMI categories		
Underweight	1	0.2
Normal	77	13.3
Overweight	237	40.8
Obese	265	45.7
Nutritional status		
Normal	552	95.3
Malnutrition risk	20	3.5
Malnourished	7	1.2
Charlson Comorbidity Index		
0–1	356	61.2
2	106	18.2
3 and over	120	20.6
Most frequent comorbidities		
Bone and joint disorders	438	75.3
Hypertension	412	70.9
Dyslipidaemia	301	51.7
Insomnia	258	44.3
Gastrointestinal disease	249	42.4
Psychopathology	210	36.1
Diabetes mellitus	176	30.3
Heart disease	169	29.1
Respiratory disease	125	21.5
Polymedication	399	68.6
PIM prevalence	389	66.8

IADL: Instrumental activities of daily living; BMI: Body mass index; PIM: Potentially inappropriate medication (according to STOPP v2 criteria); SPMSQ: Short Portable Mental Status Questionnaire (0–2 errors: normal mental functioning; 3–4 errors: mild cognitive impairment; 5 errors and over: moderate-severe cognitive impairment); GDS-15: Geriatric Depression Scale (0–5: no depression; 6–9 suggestive of depression; 10 and over: almost always depression).

3.2. Assessment of Frailty and Analysis of Related Factors

Among the study population of older adults, frailty was present in 24.1% (95% CI = 20.7–27.6), while 54.3% were pre-frail and 21.6% were non-frail. The most prevalent Fried phenotype criterion observed in the sample was weakness (63.9%), followed by low physical activity (48%) and exhaustion (21.3%), while unintentional weight loss (7.2%) was infrequent. These results are detailed in Table 2.

In order to further examine the impact of the independent variables on the frailty states considered, a multinomial logistic regression analysis was performed (Table 3). The main factor related to being frail was the female gender. Thus, in the sample, the female frailty odds were 20-fold the male frailty odds, all other covariates being equal. Age was also related to frailty; for each additional year of life, the odds of being frail increased by 19% (OR = 1.19, 95% CI = 1.11–1.27). The presence of frailty was also associated with the level of dependence in the IADL, with polypharmacy, with osteoarticular pathology and with the presence of mental disorder. Among the sample, the odds of frailty decreased by 47% for each additional point of independence on the Lawton scale (OR = 0.53, 95% CI = 0.42–0.67). However, the odds doubled for persons receiving polymedication (OR = 2.67, 95% CI = 1.08–6.61). The OR of people with vs. without osteoarticular pathology was 3.5 (95% CI = 1.51–8.13), and the OR of patients with vs. without psychopathology was 2.23 (95% CI = 1.12–4.44). No association was found between frailty and the other prevalent pathologies considered or with the use of at least one PIM.

Table 2. Frailty states and criteria according to Fried's phenotype (n = 582).

	Subjects (n)	Percentage (%)
Frailty states		
Robust (non-frail)	126	21.6
Pre-frail	316	54.3
Frail	140	24.1
Fried criterion		
Unintentional weight loss	42	7.2
Exhaustion	124	21.3
Weakness	372	63.9
Slow walking speed	113	19.4
Low physical ctivity	279	48.0

Robust: 0 criteria present; Pre-frail: 1–2 criteria present; Frail: 3 or more criteria present.

Table 3. Factors related to frailty. Multinomial logistic regression for frail and pre-frail states (with respect to non-frail).

Independent Variable	Frail OR (95% CI)	Pre-Frail OR (95% CI)
Age	1.19 (1.11–1.27) ***	1.09 (1.04–1.16) **
Charlson comorbidity index	1.27 (0.99–1.62)	1.08 (0.85–1.31)
Lawton-Brody (IADL)	0.53 (0.42–0.67) ***	0.97 (0.81–1.17)
Gender		
Female	20.54 (9.10–46.3) ***	2.53 (1.52–4.23) ***
Male	1	1
Diabetes mellitus		
Yes	1.82 (0.83–3.96)	1.09 (0.61–1.98)
No	1	1
Heart disease		
Yes	1.74 (0.82–3.69)	1.15 (0.64–2.08)
No	1	1
Respiratory disease		
Yes	1.47 (0.50–2.85)	2.17 (1.14–4.10) *
No	1	1
Bone and joint disorder		
Yes	3.51 (1.51–8.13) **	1.36 (0.83–2.21)
No	1	1
Psychopathology		
Yes	2.23 (1.12–4.44) *	2.01 (1.17–3.46) *
No	1	1
Polypharmacy		
Yes	2.67 (1.08–6.61) *	0.94 (0.55–1.61)
No	1	1
PIM		
At least one	2.95 (0.66–3.13)	0.77 (0.46–1.26)
None	1	1

OR: odds ratio; 95% CI: 95% Confidence Interval; IADL: Instrumental activities of daily living (numerical value of the Lawton Index); PIM: Potentially inappropriate medications (according to STOPP v2 criteria). * $p < 0.05$; ** $p < 0.01$; *** $p < 0.001$.

The odds of an older person being pre-frail vs. robust remained unchanged concerning the association with the female gender (OR = 2.53, 95% CI = 1.52–4.23) and with age (OR = 1.09, 95% CI = 1.04–1.16).

4. Discussion

Overall, our results for frailty among community-dwelling older patients in Málaga (southern Spain) are consistent with those reported in similar studies conducted in other regions of Spain [33] and elsewhere in Europe [23]. The prevalence of frailty in our study population is slightly higher than the mean values reported by other studies in similar outpatient settings [34,35], and it is also higher than the mean values for Europe as a whole [21]. However, the prevalence of frailty is known to be fairly heterogeneous [19,21,25], possibly due to methodological differences that preclude direct comparison of the results obtained. The most important of these differences is the use of diverse operational definitions of frailty. Other factors that may also be relevant include the age of the persons analysed and the general characteristics of the sample (for example, the inclusion or otherwise of those who are institutionalised). In our study, the Fried frailty phenotype assessment components were used for classification because this is the most commonly used and most widely reported instrument in community settings [21]. However, the heterogeneity observed in the prevalence of frailty may also be due (at least in part) to economic and social factors or even to phenotypic diversity, i.e., expressed predominantly in the criteria associated with physical function (weakness, slowness and physical activity). In this respect, variations in the reported prevalence of frailty in Europe suggest there is a north-south gradient, producing a higher proportion of frailty and pre-frailty in Southern Europe than in northern countries [25].

Among the frailty-related criteria considered, a striking feature was the high proportion of patients who presented physical weakness, a finding consistent with the European multicentre study SHARE which reported that the prevalence of low grip strength contributed to that of frailty in Spain and Italy [25]. An earlier study of older ambulatory adults in Spain obtained results comparable to our own, namely that the most prevalent components of frailty were weakness and low physical activity [24]. According to these authors, poor muscle strength was closely associated with a lack of physical activity. In another analysis of this question, frailty has been associated with objectively-assessed sedentary behaviour patterns in older adults [36]. On the other hand, some researchers have found other criteria, such as exhaustion, to be of greater relevance [37,38]. This variability may be because the frailty syndrome does not present a single clinical course but differs according to the causes that trigger it. Differences may also arise from variations in how the dimensions of the frailty phenotype are operationalised. In our study, the original frailty phenotype criteria were applied, with the corresponding reference values, although according to some authors this approach may overestimate the prevalence of frailty [33].

In our study findings, the factor most strongly associated with frailty was the female gender, which corroborates prior longitudinal studies on ageing according to which frailty is more common among women than men, and with greater age [25]. The level of dependency for IADL was also found to be associated with frailty. According to the multinomial logistic regression model, a higher score on the Lawton scale (i.e., greater independence) significantly reduced the odds of frailty (by 47% for each additional point of independence). These data are consistent with the known relationship between frailty and disability [35,39].

With respect to comorbidities, the main variable related to frailty in our study was the presence of bone and joint disorders (especially osteoarthritis). We believe that frailty is closely linked to musculoskeletal health; indeed, musculoskeletal functioning is a key component in quantifying frailty, which is known to be associated with common age-related musculoskeletal conditions [40]. In particular, osteoarthritis, similarly to frailty, is commonly observed with increasing age. Although relatively little research has been undertaken to elucidate the mechanisms underlying the relation between osteoarthritis and frailty, potential links include elevated levels of pro-inflammatory markers in the circulatory system, age-related muscle atrophy and decreased physical activity [41]. Another factor that may provoke the development of frailty is that of chronic pain related to osteoarthritis, which could heighten the risk of physical inactivity, disability and falls [42]. The considerable prevalence of osteoarticular pathology in this sample has potentially contributed to the high frequency of the muscle weakness criterion. This criterion may therefore be overestimated with respect to populations with lower rates of said pathology, which could reduce external validity. Psychopathologies such as anxiety and/or depression may also aggravate the presence and impact of frailty among older persons. For example, a person with depressive symptoms may have a less active social life, be less physically active, consume a less healthy diet and, at the same time, be consuming psychotropic drugs. All of these consequences tend to promote or heighten frailty. In line with the above information, there are certain studies that conclude that the lack of joy and the presence of a negative attitude towards ageing can function as risk factors for frailty [43,44]. Our findings show that the presence of a psychopathology doubles the odds of an older person presenting pre-frailty. Therefore, we believe more extensive screening for depression and anxiety should be performed among older populations because these conditions tend to be under-diagnosed and because a more active approach to this question would promote healthy ageing.

Regarding medication, we observed a significant relationship between polypharmacy and frailty. This finding is consistent with previous research in which polymedication has been identified as a determinant factor of frailty [38,39,45–49]. The association between the two situations may be complex and bidirectional, but it seems evident that the chance of frailty developing is greater among patients who are receiving polymedication [45,47] and that the risk of a worsening transition in frail states is heightened by a greater consumption of medication [16]. Accordingly, it would seem reasonable to recommend that clinicians should seek to reduce polypharmacy in their older patients. However, although polypharmacy was associated with an increased risk of adverse events in pre-frail and frail older adults, this was not the case for non-frail individuals. Therefore, polypharmacy could be appropriate to treat multiple chronic diseases, and for robust older persons it should be managed as in younger populations [46]. Although further research is needed to confirm the possible benefits of reducing polymedication in the development, reversion or delay of frailty, it seems apparent that any treatment regimen should be evaluated with special care for frail older adults, since these patients have susceptibilities that can decrease medication benefit, as well as increase adverse secondary effects. Such an evaluation may not be straightforwardly achieved, and the identification of appropriate polypharmacy for these patients requires the development of more robust criteria for evaluating the net effects of complex medication regimens [50]. On the other hand, we found no evidence of any association between the use of one or more PIMs and the presence of frailty or pre-frailty. We speculate that such a relationship might not have been evident because the STOPP v2 criteria contain a large number of items of varying clinical significance (in terms of risk), and therefore the impact produced on frailty states by a single PIM might be slight impact. In other words, this means of measuring the risk might be insufficiently sensitive. At present, no conclusive results in this respect have been provided, except for specific medications such as anticholinergics [16,38,51] and the potentially inappropriate use of nonsteroidal anti-inflammatory drugs [52]. What does seem clear to us and to other authors [17,18] is that medication and treatment should be carefully personalised and that the regimen should be subject to periodic structured review.

The strengths of our study lie in the analysis conducted on a representative sample of healthcare centres, the global approach taken and the great variety of clinical, functional and treatment data compiled. Among its limitations is the cross-sectional design employed, which does not allow causal relationships to be established, although it can detect factors related to frailty. In addition, selecting a sample population from a single region or country may have resulted in a certain lack of external validity, even more so when taking into account the heterogeneous nature of the profile of older people living in the community. Nevertheless, the sample examined in this study is believed to be representative of the population of older adults in the ambulatory setting as long as they have a clinical and functional profiles similar to that of this sample. Furthermore, in our opinion it is preferable to assess frailty in the community as we have performed here rather than to focus more narrowly on an acute situation. A longer-term goal should be to establish frailty assessment as an integral part of routine primary care practice, as early identification and optimal management of this condition facilitates the patient's transition towards improvement whether from a pre-frail state or when frailty is already present. This will require new prospective studies that support the evidence and possible recommendations.

5. Conclusions

According to the Fried phenotype, frailty may be associated with many factors, including age, female gender, dependence for IADL, polymedication, the presence of osteoarticular pathology and/or mental disorder. Some of these variables may be preventable or modifiable and, thus, provide clinically relevant targets for intervention. This is particularly the case for depressive symptoms, the clinical control of osteoarthritis and the use of polypharmacy. In this respect, many of the interventions currently being proposed are based on an effective multicomponent approach, which may include physical activity, dietary intervention, structured medication reviews and strengthened social networks.

Author Contributions: Conceptualization, E.B.-R. and G.A.-Z.; R.O.-R., methodology, E.B.-R. and R.O.-R.; formal analysis, E.B.-R. and R.O.-R.; investigation, E.B.-R., R.O.-R., G.A.-Z., L.A.-C., M.R.G.-M., J.V. and I.B.-E.; resources, E.B.-R. and I.B.-E.; data curation: L.A.-C., M.R.G.-M. and J.V.; writing-original draft preparation, E.B.-R., R.O.-R. and L.A.-C.; writing—review and editing, E.B.-R., R.O.-R., L.A.-C. and I.B.-E.; visualization, E.B.-R., R.O.-R. and I.B.-E.; supervision, E.B.-R. and I.B.-E.; project administration, E.B.-R.; funding acquisition: E.B.-R. All authors have read and agreed to the published version of the manuscript.

Funding: This research was funded by the Fundación Pública Andaluza Progreso y Salud, Consejería de Salud, Junta de Andalucía, through the Programme Proyectos de Investigación Biomédica (Grant number PI 0234/14). The APC was funded by the University of Málaga. The funders had no role in the design of the study; in the collection, analyses or interpretation of data; in the writing of the manuscript or in the decision to publish the results.

Institutional Review Board Statement: The study was conducted according to the guidelines of the Declaration of Helsinki and approved by the Málaga Clinical Research Ethics Committee (protocol EBR-MED-2013-01, PI-0234-14; approval date, 25 July 2013).

Informed Consent Statement: Informed consent was obtained from all subjects involved in the study.

Data Availability Statement: The data that support the findings of this study are not publicly available due to being used for further investigational objectives and because the data contain information that could compromise the privacy of research participants. However, specific information can be obtained from the corresponding author upon reasonable request (E.B.-R.).

Acknowledgments: The authors wish to thank the Primary Care Management Team (Health District of Málaga-Guadalhorce) for providing access to the health centres and patient lists.

Conflicts of Interest: The authors declare no conflict of interest.

References

1. The 2015 Ageing Report, Economic and Budgetary Projections for the 28 EU Member States (2013–2060). 2015. Available online: https://ec.europa.eu/economy_finance/publications/european_economy/2015/ee3_en.htm (accessed on 14 June 2021).
2. Crimmins, E.M.; Beltrán-Sánchez, H. Mortality and morbidity trends: Is there compression of morbidity? *J. Gerontol. B Psychol. Sci. Soc. Sci.* **2011**, *66*, 75–86. [CrossRef]
3. Beard, J.R.; Officer, A.; de Carvalho, I.A.; Sadana, R.; Pot, A.M.; Michel, J.P. The World report on ageing and health: A policy framework for healthy ageing. *Lancet* **2016**, *387*, 2145–2154. [CrossRef]
4. Dent, E.; Martin, F.C.; Bergman, H.; Woo, J.; Romero-Ortuno, R.; Walston, J.D. Management of frailty: Opportunities, challenges, and future directions. *Lancet* **2019**, *394*, 1376–1386. [CrossRef]
5. Gottdiener, J.; Seeman, T.; Tracy, R.; Kop, W.J.; Burke, G.; McBurnie, M.A. Frailty in older adults: Evidence for a phenotype. *J. Gerontol. A Biol. Sci. Med. Sci.* **2001**, *56*, M146–M156.
6. Clegg-Young, J.A.; Iliffe, S.; Rikkert, M.O.; Rockwood, K. Frailty in elderly people. *Lancet* **2013**, *381*, 752–762. [CrossRef]
7. Xue, Q.L. The frailty syndrome: Definition and natural history. *Clin. Geriatr. Med.* **2011**, *27*, 1–15. [CrossRef]
8. Junius-Walker, U.; Onder, G.; Soleymani, D.; Wiese, B.; Albaina, O.; Bernabei, R.; Marzetti, E.; ADVANTAGE JA WP4 group. The essence of frailty: A systematic review and qualitative synthesis on frailty concepts and definitions. *Eur. J. Intern. Med.* **2018**, *56*, 3–10. [CrossRef]
9. Rockwood, K.; Mitnitski, A. Frailty defined by deficit accumulation and geriatric medicine defined by frailty. *Clin. Geriatr. Med.* **2011**, *27*, 17–26. [CrossRef] [PubMed]

10. Morley, J.E.; Vellas, B.; van Kan, G.A.; Anker, S.D.; Bauer, J.M.; Bernabei, R. Frailty consensus: A call to action. *J. Am. Med. Dir. Assoc.* **2013**, *14*, 92–97. [CrossRef] [PubMed]
11. Cheung, J.T.K.; Yu, R.; Wu, Z.; Wong, S.Y.S.; Woo, J. Geriatric syndromes, multimorbidity, and disability overlap and increase healthcare use among older Chinese. *BMC Geriatr.* **2018**, *18*, 147. [CrossRef] [PubMed]
12. Hoogendijk, E.O.; Muntinga, M.E.; van Leeuwen, K.M.; van der Horst, H.E.; Deeg, D.J.; Frijters, D.H.; Hermsen, L.A.H.; Jansen, A.P.D.; Nijpels, G.; van Hout, H.P.; et al. Self-perceived met and unmet care needs of frail older adults in primary care. *Arch Gerontol Geriatr* **2014**, *58*, 37–42. [CrossRef] [PubMed]
13. Vermeiren, S.; Vella-Azzopardi, R.; Beckwée, D.; Habbig, A.K.; Scafoglieri, A.; Jansen, B.; Bautmans, I. Gerontopole Brussels Study group. Frailty and the Prediction of Negative Health Outcomes: A Meta-Analysis. *J. Am. Med. Dir. Assoc.* **2016**, *17*, 1163.e1–1163.e17. [CrossRef]
14. Pollack, L.R.; Litwack-Harrison, S.; Cawthon, P.M.; Ensrud, K.; Lane, N.E.; Barrett-Connor, E.; Dam, T.T. Patterns and Predictors of Frailty Transitions in Older Men: The Osteoporotic Fractures in Men Study. *J. Am. Geriatr. Soc.* **2017**, *65*, 2473–2479. [CrossRef]
15. Trevisan, C.; Veronese, N.; Maggi, S.; Baggio, G.; Toffanello, E.D.; Zambon, S.; Sergi, G. Factors Influencing Transitions Between Frailty States in Elderly Adults: The Progetto Veneto Anziani Longitudinal Study. *J. Am. Geriatr. Soc.* **2017**, *65*, 179–184. [CrossRef] [PubMed]
16. Lorenzo-López, L.; López-López, R.; Maseda, A.; Buján, A.; Rodríguez-Villamil, J.L.; Millán-Calenti, J.C. Changes in frailty status in a community-dwelling cohort of older adults: The VERISAÚDE study. *Maturitas* **2019**, *119*, 54–60. [CrossRef]
17. Reeves, D.; Pye, S.; Ashcroft, D.; Clegg, A.; Kontopantelis, E.; Blakeman, T.; van Marwijk, H. The challenge of ageing populations and patient frailty: Can primary care adapt? *BMJ* **2018**, *362*, k3349. [CrossRef] [PubMed]
18. Abbasi, M.; Rolfson, D.; Khera, A.S.; Dabravolskaj, J.; Dent, E.; Xia, L. Identification and management of frailty in the primary care setting. *Can. Med Assoc. J.* **2018**, *190*, E1134–E1140. [CrossRef] [PubMed]
19. Collard, R.M.; Boter, H.; Schoevers, R.A.; Oude Voshaar, R.C. Prevalence of frailty in community-dwelling older persons: A systematic review. *J. Am. Geriatr. Soc.* **2012**, *60*, 1487–1492. [CrossRef]
20. Hendry, A.; Vanhecke, E.; Carriazo, A.M.; López-Samaniego, L.; Espinosa, J.M.; Sezgin, D.; O'Caoimh, R. Key Messages for a Frailty Prevention and Management Policy in Europe from the ADVANTAGE JOINT ACTION Consortium. *J. Nutr. Health Aging* **2018**, *22*, 892–897.
21. O'Caoimh, R.; Galluzzo, L.; Rodríguez-Laso, Á.; Van der Heyden, J.; Ranhoff, A.H.; Lamprini-Koula, M.; Liew, A. Work Package 5 of the Joint Action ADVANTAGE. Prevalence of frailty at population level in European ADVANTAGE Joint Action Member States: A systematic review and meta-analysis. *Ann. Ist. Super Sanita* **2018**, *54*, 226–238. [PubMed]
22. Foreman, K.J.; Marquez, N.; Dolgert, A.; Fukutaki, K.; Fullman, N.; McGaughey, M. Forecasting life expectancy, years of life lost, and all-cause and cause-specific mortality for 250 causes of death: Reference and alternative scenarios for 2016-40 for 195 countries and territories. *Lancet* **2018**, *392*, 2052–2090. [CrossRef]
23. Van Kempen, J.A.L.; Schers, H.J.; Jacobs, A.; Zuidema, S.U.; Ruikes, F.; Robben, S.H.M.; Melis, R.J.F.; Rikkert, M.G.M.O. Development of an instrument for the identification of frail older people as a target population for integrated care. *Br. J. Gen. Pr.* **2013**, *63*, e225–e231. [CrossRef] [PubMed]
24. Papiol, M.; Serra-Prat, M.; Vico, J.; Jerez, N.; Salvador, N.; Garcia, M.; López, J. Poor Muscle Strength and Low Physical Activity Are the Most Prevalent Frailty Components in Community-Dwelling Older Adults. *J. Aging Phys. Act.* **2016**, *24*, 363–368. [CrossRef] [PubMed]
25. Santos-Eggimann, B.; Cuénoud, P.; Spagnoli, J.; Junod, J. Prevalence of frailty in middle-aged and older community-dwelling Europeans living in 10 countries. *J. Gerontol. A Biol. Sci. Med. Sci.* **2009**, *64*, 675–681. [CrossRef]
26. Charlson, M.E.; Pompei, P.; Ales, K.L.; MacKenzie, C.R. A new method of classifying prognostic comorbidity in longitudinal studies: Development and validation. *J. Chronic. Dis.* **1987**, *40*, 373–383. [CrossRef]
27. Kaiser, M.J.; Bauer, J.M.; Ramsch, C.; Uter, W.; Guigoz, Y.; Cederholm, T.; Sieber, C.C. MNA-International Group. Validation of the Mini Nutritional Assessment short-form (MNA-SF): A practical tool for identification of nutritional status. *J. Nutr. Health Aging* **2009**, *13*, 782–788. [CrossRef]
28. Lawton, M.P.; Brody, E.M. Assessment of older people: Self-maintaining and instrumental activities of daily living. *Gerontologist* **1969**, *9*, 179–186. [CrossRef]
29. Pfeiffer, E. A short portable mental status questionnaire for the assessment of organic brain deficit in elderly patients. *J. Am. Geriatr. Soc.* **1975**, *23*, 433–441. [CrossRef]
30. Sheikh, J.I.; Yesavage, J.A. Geriatric Depression Scale (GDS): Recent evidence and development of a shorter version. *Clin. Geront.* **1986**, *5*, 165–173.
31. O'Mahony, D.; O'Sullivan, D.; Byrne, S.; O'Connor, M.N.; Ryan, C.; Gallagher, P. STOPP/START criteria for potentially inappropriate prescribing in older people: Version 2. *Age Ageing* **2015**, *44*, 213–218. [CrossRef]
32. Hosmer, D.W.; Lemeshow, S.; Sturdivant, R.X. *Applied Logistic Regression*, 3rd ed.; John Wiley & Sons: Hoboken, NJ, USA, 2013.
33. Alonso-Bouzón, C.; Carnicero, J.A.; Turín, J.G.; García-García, F.J.; Esteban, A.; Rodríguez-Mañas, L. The Standarization of Frailty Phenotype Criteria Improves Its Predictive Ability: The Toledo Study for Healthy Aging. *J. Am. Med. Dir. Assoc.* **2017**, *18*, 402–408. [CrossRef] [PubMed]
34. Abizanda, P.; Romero, L.; Sánchez-Jurado, P.M.; Martínez-Reig, M.; Gómez-Arnedo, L.; Alfonso, S.A. Frailty and mortality, disability and mobility loss in a Spanish cohort of older adults: The FRADEA study. *Maturitas* **2013**, *74*, 54–60. [CrossRef]

35. Ferrer, A.; Badia, T.; Formiga, F.; Sanz, H.; Megido, M.J.; Pujol, R.; Octabaiz Study Group. Frailty in the oldest old: Prevalence and associated factors. *J. Am. Geriatr. Soc.* **2013**, *61*, 294–296. [CrossRef] [PubMed]
36. Del Pozo-Cruz, B.; Mañas, A.; Martín-García, M.; Marín-Puyalto, J.; García-García, F.J.; Rodriguez-Mañas, L.; Guadalupe-Grau, A.; Ara, I. Frailty is associated with objectively assessed sedentary behaviour patterns in older adults: Evidence from the Toledo Study for Healthy Aging (TSHA). *PLoS ONE* **2017**, *12*, e0183911. [CrossRef]
37. Jürschik, P.; Botigué, T.; Nuin, C.; Lavedán, A. Association between Mini Nutritional Assessment and the Fried frailty index in older people living in the community. *Med. Clin.* **2014**, *143*, 191–195. [CrossRef]
38. Herr, M.; Sirven, N.; Grondin, H.; Pichetti, S.; Sermet, C. Frailty, polypharmacy, and potentially inappropriate medications in old people: Findings in a representative sample of the French population. *Eur. J. Clin. Pharmacol.* **2017**, *73*, 1165–1172. [CrossRef] [PubMed]
39. Herr, M.; Robine, J.M.; Pinot, J.; Arvieu, J.J.; Ankri, J. Polypharmacy and frailty: Prevalence, relationship, and impact on mortality in a French sample of 2350 old people. *Pharmacoepidemiol. Drug Saf.* **2015**, *24*, 637–646. [CrossRef] [PubMed]
40. McGuigan, F.E.; Bartosch, P.; Åkesson, K.E. Musculoskeletal health and frailty. *Best Pr. Res. Clin. Rheumatol.* **2017**, *31*, 145–159. [CrossRef]
41. O'Brien, M.S.; McDougall, J.J. Age and frailty as risk factors for the development of osteoarthritis. *Mech. Ageing Dev.* **2019**, *180*, 21–28. [CrossRef] [PubMed]
42. Veronese, N.; Maggi, S.; Trevisan, C.; Noale, M.; De Rui, M.; Bolzetta, F.; Sergi, G. Pain Increases the Risk of Developing Frailty in Older Adults with Osteoarthritis. *Pain Med.* **2017**, *18*, 414–427. [CrossRef]
43. Kume, Y.; Takahashi, T.; Itakura, Y.; Lee, S.; Makizako, H.; Ono, T. Polypharmacy and Lack of Joy Are Related to Physical Frailty among Northern Japanese Community-Dwellers from the ORANGE Cohort Study. *Gerontology* **2021**, *67*, 184–193. [CrossRef]
44. Gale, C.R.; Cooper, C. Attitudes to Ageing and Change in Frailty Status: The English Longitudinal Study of Ageing. *Gerontology* **2018**, *64*, 58–66. [CrossRef] [PubMed]
45. Saum, K.; Schöttker, B.; Meid, A.D.; Holleczek, B.; Haefeli, W.E.; Hauer, K.; Brenner, H. Is Polypharmacy Associated with Frailty in Older People? Results from the ESTHER Cohort Study. *J. Am. Geriatr. Soc.* **2016**, *65*, e27–e32. [CrossRef] [PubMed]
46. Bonaga, B.; Sánchez-Jurado, P.M.; Martínez-Reig, M.; Ariza, G.; Rodríguez-Mañas, L.; Gnjidic, D. Frailty, Polypharmacy, and Health Outcomes in Older Adults: The Frailty and Dependence in Albacete Study. *J. Am. Med. Dir. Assoc.* **2018**, *19*, 46–52. [CrossRef]
47. Veronese, N.; Stubbs, B.; Noale, M.; Solmi, M.; Pilotto, A.; Vaona, A.; Maggi, S. Polypharmacy Is Associated With Higher Frailty Risk in Older People: An 8-Year Longitudinal Cohort Study. *J. Am. Med. Dir. Assoc.* **2017**, *18*, 624–628. [CrossRef] [PubMed]
48. Gutiérrez-Valencia, M.; Izquierdo, M.; Cesari, M.; Casas-Herrero, Á.; Inzitari, M.; Martínez-Velilla, N. The relationship between frailty and polypharmacy in older people: A systematic review. *Br. J. Clin. Pharmacol.* **2018**, *84*, 1432–1444. [CrossRef]
49. de Breij, S.; van Hout, H.P.J.; de Bruin, S.R.; Schuster, N.A.; Deeg, D.J.H.; Huisman, M. Predictors of Frailty and Vitality in Older Adults Aged 75 years and Over: Results from the Longitudinal Aging Study Amsterdam. *Gerontology* **2021**, *67*, 69–77. [CrossRef]
50. Fried, T.R.; Mecca, M.C. Medication Appropriateness in Vulnerable Older Adults: Healthy Skepticism of Appropriate Polypharmacy. *J. Am. Geriatr. Soc.* **2019**, *67*, 1123–1127. [CrossRef]
51. Muhlack, D.C.; Hoppe, L.K.; Saum, K.U.; Haefeli, W.E.; Brenner, H.; Schöttker, B. Investigation of a possible association of potentially inappropriate medication for older adults and frailty in a prospective cohort study from Germany. *Age Ageing* **2019**, *49*, 20–25. [CrossRef]
52. Martinot, P.; Landré, B.; Zins, M.; Goldberg, M.; Ankri, J.; Herr, M. Association between Potentially Inappropriate Medications and Frailty in the Early Old Age: A Longitudinal Study in the GAZEL Cohort. *J. Am. Med. Dir. Assoc.* **2018**, *19*, 967–973. [CrossRef]

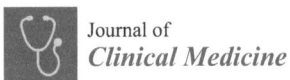

Article

Association of Acute Kidney Injury with the Risk of Dementia: A Meta-Analysis

Salman Hussain [1,*], Ambrish Singh [2], Benny Antony [2], Rolando Claure-Del Granado [3,4], Jitka Klugarová [1], Radim Líčeník [1] and Miloslav Klugar [1]

[1] Czech National Centre for Evidence-Based Healthcare and Knowledge Translation (Czech EBHC: JBI Centre of Excellence, Masaryk University GRADE Centre Cochrane, Czech Republic), Institute of Biostatistics and Analyses, Faculty of Medicine, Masaryk University, Kamenice 5, 625 00 Brno, Czech Republic; klugarova@med.muni.cz (J.K.); radim.licenik@gmail.com (R.L.); klugar@med.muni.cz (M.K.)
[2] Menzies Institute for Medical Research, University of Tasmania, 17 Liverpool Street, Hobart, TAS 7000, Australia; ambrish.singh@utas.edu.au (A.S.); benny.eathakkattuantony@utas.edu.au (B.A.)
[3] Division of Nephrology, Hospital Obrero No 2–CNS, Cochabamba, Bolivia; rclaure@yahoo.com
[4] Universidad Mayor de San Simon School of Medicine, Cochabamba, Bolivia
* Correspondence: mohammad.hussain@med.muni.cz or salmanpharma@gmail.com

Abstract: Acute kidney injury (AKI) is associated with several adverse outcomes, including new or progressive chronic kidney disease, end-stage kidney disease, and mortality. Epidemiological studies have reported an association between AKI and dementia as a long-term adverse outcome. This meta-analysis was aimed to understand the association between AKI and dementia risk. A literature search was performed in MEDLINE and Embase databases, from inception to July 2021, to identify epidemiological studies reporting the association between AKI and dementia risk. Title and abstract followed by the full-text of retrieved articles were screened, data were extracted, and quality was assessed, using the Newcastle–Ottawa scale by two investigators independently. The primary outcome was to compute the pooled risk of dementia in AKI patients. Subgroup analysis was also performed based on age and co-morbidities. Certainty of evidence was assessed using the GRADE approach. Statistical analysis was performed using Review Manager 5.4 software. Four studies (cohort ($n = 3$) and case–control ($n = 1$)) with a total of 429,211 patients, of which 211,749 had AKI, were identified. The mean age of the patients and the follow-up period were 64.15 ± 16.09 years and 8.9 years, respectively. Included studies were of moderate to high quality. The pooled estimate revealed a significantly higher risk of dementia in AKI patients with an overall relative risk/risk ratio (RR) of 1.92 (95% CI: 1.52–2.43), $p \leq 0.00001$. Dementia risk increases by 10% with one year increase in age with an RR of 1.10 (95% CI: 1.09–1.11), $p < 0.00001$. Subgroup analysis based on stroke as a co-morbid condition also revealed significantly higher dementia risk in AKI patients (RR 2.30 (95% CI: 1.62–3.28), $p = 0.009$). All-cause mortality risk was also significantly higher in AKI patients with dementia with a pooled RR of 2.11 (95% CI: 1.20–3.70), $p = 0.009$. The strength of the evidence was of very low certainty as per the GRADE assessment. Patients with AKI have a higher risk of dementia. Further large epidemiological studies are needed to confirm the mechanistic association.

Keywords: acute kidney injury; dementia; dialysis; epidemiology; systematic review; meta-analysis

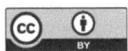

1. Introduction

Acute kidney injury (AKI) is a complex disorder characterized by an abrupt decline in kidney function over a short period of time [1]. AKI is associated with poor quality of life, decreased productivity, and adverse health economic impact [2,3]. The reported prevalence of AKI ranged from 1 to 66%, with a varied incidence between high-income and low-to-middle-income countries [3,4]. Many recent epidemiologic studies have shown that patients with AKI are at a higher risk of developing chronic kidney disease (CKD), end-stage kidney disease (ESKD), cardiovascular diseases, and acute neurological complications such as attention deficits, decreased mental status, seizures, and hyperreflexia [5–9]. Dementia is a neurodegenerative disorder characterized by progressive deterioration of intellectual function, and it is one of the leading causes of limiting the capacity for independent living for the elderly population [10,11]. Over the last few decades, the global prevalence of dementia has increased considerably [12]. It is important to identify the determinants of dementia, particularly in the absence of effective treatments [13]. Numerous studies have provided evidence on the associations between various modifiable risk factors and cognitive decline or dementia later in life [14,15]. Both AKI and dementia are significant public health concerns and are associated with poor health outcomes and rising health care costs for society [3]. The occurrence of dementia in patients with AKI is of clinical importance as dementia is associated with an increased humanistic and economic burden [12].

Studies have reported that chronic kidney conditions such as CKD and ESKD are associated with accelerated cardiovascular events and share common risk factors with dementia [16–19]. These common vascular co-morbidities such as hypertension, diabetes mellitus, or hyperlipidemia, may also have a role in the development of dementia in this population [20]. Few previous meta-analyses found the increased odds for cognitive impairment in patients with CKD and renal dysfunction [18,21]. In addition, an animal study has found that AKI-induced inflammation adversely impacts the brain, among other organs [5]. The brain and kidneys share similar hemodynamic and anatomic pathways. Vascular damage due to alteration in the blood–brain barrier, high vascular permeabilities, and inflammatory cascades could be the potential mechanism for the occurrence of dementia in AKI patients [22,23].

Although the long-term neurological effects of AKI are unclear, these factors may predispose patients with AKI to an increased risk of developing dementia, as observed in a few recent studies [24,25]. Although primary epidemiological studies exploring this association are limited, the risk of dementia in the AKI population can be assessed using meta-analytical techniques to pool the evidence from real-world data studies.

The preliminary search of existing systematic reviews or meta-analysis was performed on July 2021 in Epistemonikos, PROSPERO, Open Science Framework, Cochrane Library, and JBI Evidence Synthesis, and no reviews evaluating the association of acute kidney injury with the risk of dementia were identified. Hence, we conducted a meta-analysis of existing evidence from primary epidemiological studies that compared the risk of dementia in patients with AKI versus individuals without AKI.

2. Materials and Methods

2.1. Protocol

The present meta-analysis followed the preferred reporting items for systematic review and meta-analysis (PRISMA) and Meta-analysis of Observational Studies in Epidemiology (MOOSE) reporting guidelines [26,27]. Refer to Table S1 and S2 for the checklists. The protocol of the current study was prospectively published as a preprint at medRxiv [28].

2.2. Search Strategy

A three-step search strategy was utilized to locate both published and unpublished studies. An initial, limited search was undertaken in MEDLINE (Ovid) using keywords and index terms related to AKI and dementia. An analysis of the text words in the title and abstract as well as the index terms used to describe the articles were followed. A second search using all identified keywords and index terms was conducted in MEDLINE (Ovid) and Embase (Ovid) databases (the search period was from inception to 14 July 2021). Thirdly, the reference lists of all studies that met the inclusion criteria were checked manually for additional records. Lastly, abstract booklets of major international nephrology and neurology congress—World Congress of Nephrology, American Society of Nephrology, European Renal Association–European Dialysis and Transplant Association (ERA-EDTA), Asian Pacific Congress of Nephrology, Neuroscience, Alzheimer's Association International Conference (AAIC), and American Academy of Neurology—from the last two years were also searched. Citation tracking was also performed for all the articles qualified for inclusion. The search strategy used in this study is available in Table S3. The literature search was not restricted to any date or language; however, only the studies published in English were included.

2.3. Study Selection/Inclusion Criteria

Studies that are eligible for inclusion into the meta-analysis must be observational analytical studies (prospective, retrospective, cohort, or case–control) that assessed the risk of dementia in the AKI population compared to the risk of dementia in the population without AKI. Primary studies including individuals with AKI with dementia at the entry of the cohort were excluded from the analysis. Eligible studies must report relative risk/risk ratio (RR), hazard ratio (HR), or odds ratio (OR) with 95% confidence intervals (CI) or must provide enough raw data to calculate those ratios. In the case of insufficient information, primary study authors were contacted.

The studies retrieved from the database search were evaluated against eligibility for inclusion using the Covidence software (Covidence systematic review software, Veritas Health Innovation, Melbourne, Australia. Available at www.covidence.org, accessed on 20 September 2021) by two investigators (S.H. and A.S.) independently, firstly by title/abstract screening and secondly by full-text screening. Studies excluded from full-text screening are available in Table S4 with reasons for exclusion. In the case of discrepancies in the inclusion of a study, the agreement was reached by consensus and/or by consulting the third investigator (M.K.).

2.4. Data Extraction

An excel-based, standardized data collection form was used to extract the information: study title, first author, year of publication, country/countries where the study was conducted, study population, methods used to identify control/cohort, methods used to confirm the diagnosis of AKI and dementia, number of cases and control/cohort size, demographics of the cases and control/cohort, the average duration of follow-up, confounders that were adjusted for, and the adjusted effect estimates with 95% CI.

The data extraction was independently performed, in duplicate, by two investigators (S.H. and A.S.), ensuring the accuracy of the data extracted. The extracted data for all studies were then cross-checked by the third investigator (M.K.) for any data discrepancies which were resolved by referring to the primary source.

2.5. Quality Assessment and Certainty of the Evidence

We used Newcastle–Ottawa (NOS) quality assessment scale to evaluate the quality of the included studies. Two reviewers assessed the quality of eligible studies independently. The NOS is a standard quality assessment tool used to evaluate the quality of the observational study on the basis of three domains: (1) the recruitment of the cases and controls, (2) the comparability between cases and controls, and (3) the ascertainment of the key outcomes of interest [29]. Based on the score achieved by the individual study, a high, medium, or low quality of the study was determined. Studies were not excluded from meta-analyses based on the quality assessment; however, the influence of the quality on the results of meta-analyses was explored by the sensitivity analyses.

The Grading of Recommendations Assessment, Development and Evaluation (GRADE) tool was used to assess the certainty or quality of the evidence [30]. The GRADE working group rated the certainty of evidence as high, moderate, low, or very low certainty of evidence based on the study design, risk of bias, inconsistency, indirectness, imprecision, and other considerations.

2.6. Statistical Analysis

We used Cochrane's (London, UK) Review Manager 5.4 data analysis software to perform the meta-analysis. The dementia events in AKI patients are considered as rare;

therefore, odds ratio, RR, and hazard ratio were used interchangeably. For simplicity, RR was used for all these measures [31]. We used the generic inverse-variance method (GIVM) to combine the point estimates from each study to calculate pooled effect estimates. The GIVM of the DerSimonian and Laird assigns the weight for each study in the pooled analysis in reverse to its variance.

Considering the high probability of between-study variance due to distinction in populations and techniques used to diagnose AKI and dementia, the random-effect model was picked over the fixed-effect model. We used the Cochran's Q test, complemented with the I2 statistic, to evaluate the between-study statistical heterogeneity [32]. The I2 statistic quantifies the proportion of total variation across studies resulting from heterogeneity rather than chance. The value of I2 = 0–25% represents insignificant heterogeneity, 25–50% low heterogeneity, 50–75% moderate heterogeneity, and more than 75% high heterogeneity [33,34]. Subgroup analysis based on age, co-morbidities, and the all-cause mortality rate was performed. Sensitivity analysis was performed using the leave-one-out method to assess if pooled effect estimates were influenced by any single study alone or by the risk of bias in the included studies. Summary of findings tables were created using the GRADEpro GDT tool [35].

3. Results

3.1. Studies Characteristics

Of 976 citations retrieved, four articles [24,25,36,37], including one abstract [37], qualified for inclusion in this meta-analysis with a total of 429,211 patients, of which 211,749 had AKI. PRISMA diagram showed the detailed study inclusion process (Figure 1).

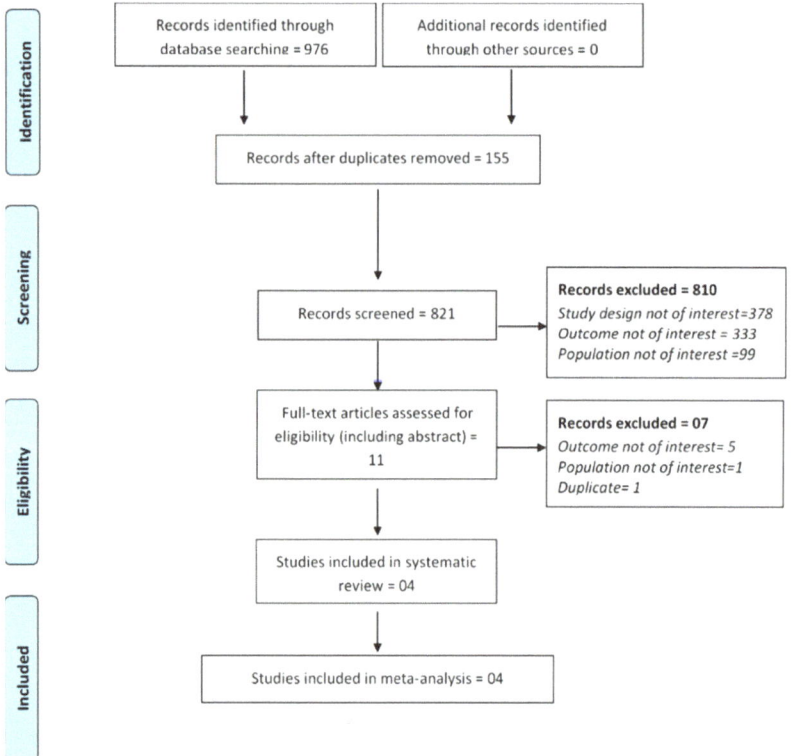

Figure 1. PRISMA flowchart showing study inclusion process.

The mean age of the patients and the follow-up period were 64.15 ± 16.09 years and 8.9 years, respectively. All the included studies were retrospective cohort in nature, except the study by Wu et al. [37], which was a case–control study. Studies were conducted in Taiwan ($n = 2$), China ($n = 1$), and the USA ($n = 1$) and published between 2017 and 2020. There were two studies from Taiwan [25,36]; Tsai et al., used the national health insurance research database (NHIRD), and Kao et al. used the longitudinal health insurance database (LHID). The study from the US [24] used clinical and administrative data from intermountain healthcare—an organization that covers patients from the Utah and Idaho region. AKI was ascertained based on the International Classification of Diseases (ICD) 9th edition codes, procedure codes, and definitions outlined in KDIGO guidelines, while dementia was confirmed using ICD-9 codes and clinical modification codes in all the included studies (Table 1).

3.2. Quality Assessment and Certainty of the Evidence

Based on NOS for non-randomized studies, the methodological quality of included studies was moderate to high quality with a mean score of 8 (range: 6–9). However, the inherent bias of observational studies design should be considered while interpreting the result. Refer to Table 2 for a detailed quality assessment.

The evidence on the association between AKI and risk of dementia was of very low certainty as per the GRADE rating system. Certainty assessment ratings and the summary of findings are presented in Table 3.

3.3. Meta-Analysis

The pooled estimate revealed a significantly higher risk of dementia in AKI patients compared to patients without AKI with an overall RR of 1.92 (95% CI: 1.52–2.43), $p \leq 0.00001$ (Figure 2).

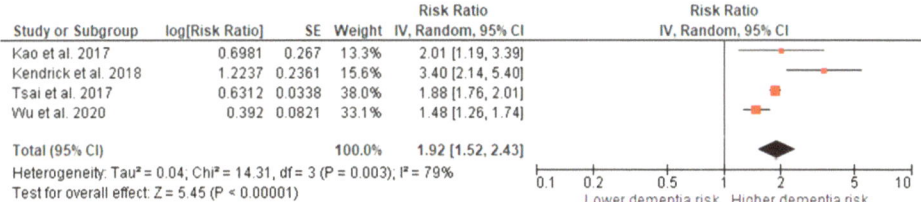

Figure 2. Meta-analysis showing the pooled risk of dementia in AKI patients compared to patients without AKI.

This pooled estimate was based on adjusted RR (adjusted for all possible confounding factors such as age, sex, previous cognitive dysfunction, and several co-morbidities including diabetes, hypertension, hyperlipidemia, head injury, depression, stroke, chronic obstructive pulmonary disease, estimated glomerular filtration rate, coronary artery disease, congestive heart failure, atrial fibrillation, cancer, liver disease, and chronic infection/inflammation). Dementia risk increases 10% with one year increase in age with an RR of 1.10 (95% CI: 1.09–1.11), $p < 0.00001$ (Figure 3).

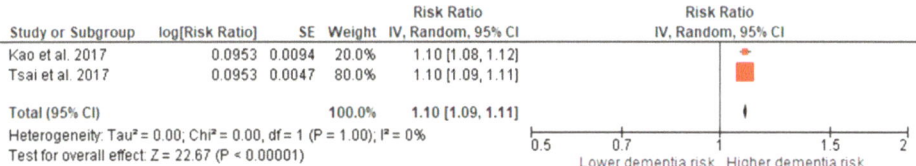

Figure 3. Risk of dementia in AKI patients with one year increase in age.

Table 1. Characteristics of included studies.

Author, Year, and Country	Study Design	Database Used	Study Duration	Follow-Up Period	Cohort Size	AKI Patients	Non-AKI Patients	Mean Age (Years)	Female (%)	Assessment of AKI	Assessment of Outcomes (Dementia)	Number of Dementia Cases in AKI/Non-AKI Group	Unadjusted Hazard Ratio/Risk Ratio	Adjusted Hazard/Risk Ratio/Odds Ratio	Study Adjusted for
Kao et al. 2017; Taiwan [36]	Cohort	Longitudinal Health Insurance Database	1999–2008	NR	3445	689	2756	63.33 ± 16.19	41.90%	Procedure code	ICD-9-CM codes (290.X, 290.XX, 294.X, 294.XX, 331.X)	44/67	NR	2.01 (95% CI: 1.19–3.39)	Adjusted for baseline co-morbidities, acute organ dysfunction, and the propensity score
Kendrick et al. 2019, USA [24]	Cohort	Intermountain Healthcare	1999–2009	5.8 years	2082	1041	1041	61 ± 16	NR	ICD-9 codes and KDIGO guidelines	ICD-9 codes (290 to 290.4 and 331)	73/24	NR	3.4 (95% CI: 2.14–5.40); composite outcome of dementia or death: 1.60 (1.40, 1.84)	Propensity matched
Tsai et al. 2017; Taiwan [25]	Cohort	Taiwan's National Health Insurance Research Database	2000–2011	12 years	415576	207788	207788	68.13 ± 16.08	39.20%	ICD-9-CM Code 584	ICD9-CM Codes 290, 294.1, 331.0	3265/4806	NR	1.88 (95% CI: 1.76–2.01)	Study adjusted for age, sex, and several co-morbidities (diabetes, hypertension, hyperlipidemia, head injury, depression, chronic obstructive pulmonary disease, coronary artery disease, congestive heart failure, atrial fibrillation, cancer, liver disease, chronic infection/inflammation, autoimmune disease, malnutrition
Wu et al. 2020 * [37]	Case–control	NR	NR	NA	8108	2231	5877	NR	NR	KDIGO guidelines	NR	NR	NR	1.48 (95% CI: 1.26–1.74)	Adjusted for estimated glomerular filtration rate, age, albumin level, hypertension, myocardial infarction, congestive heart failure, peripheral vascular disease, cerebrovascular disease, chronic lung disease, connective tissue disease, moderate/severe renal disease, tumor, and anemia

AKI: Acute Kidney Injury; ICD-9: International Classification of Disease, 9th Edition; KDIGO: Kidney Disease Improving Global Outcomes; NA: Not Applicable; NR: Not Reported; U.S: United States of America. * Represents conference abstract.

Table 2. Quality assessment of included studies.

Cohort Studies	Selection				Comparability	Outcome			
Study Author	Representation of the Exposed Cohort	Selection of the Non-Exposed Cohort	Ascertainment of Exposure	Demonstration that Outcome of Interest Was Not Present at the Start of the Study	Comparability of Cohorts on the Basis of Design or Analysis	Assessment of Outcome	Was Follow-Up Long Enough for Outcomes to Occur	Accuracy of Follow-Up of Cohorts	Overall Score
Kao, 2017, Taiwan [36]	✓	✓	✓	✓	✓✓	✓	✗	✓	High (8)
Kendrick, 2019, USA [24]	✓	✓	✓	✓	✓✓	✓	✓	✓	High (9)
Tsai, 2017, Taiwan [25]	✓	✓	✓	✓	✓✓	✓	✓	✓	High (9)
Case-Control Study	**Selection**				**Comparability**	**Outcome**			
Study author	Is the case definition adequate	Representativeness of the Cases	Selection of Controls	Definition of Controls	Comparability of Cases and Controls on the Basis of the Design or Analysis	Ascertainment of Exposure	Same method of ascertainment for cases and controls	Non-Response Rate	Overall Score
Wu, 2020, China [37]	✓	✗	✓	✓	✓✓	✗	✗	✓	Medium (6)

✓: Yes; ✗: No.

Table 3. Summary of findings table showing certainty of evidence for dementia risk in AKI compared to non-AKI patients. **Patients:** Dementia risk in AKI patients compared to non-AKI patients. **Risk factor:** Dementia incidence. **Comparisons:** Non-AKI patients.

№ of Studies	Certainty Assessment						№ of Patients		Effect		Certainty	Importance
	Study Design	Risk of Bias	Inconsistency	Indirectness	Imprecision	Other Considerations	AKI and Dementia Risk	Placebo	Relative (95% CI)	Absolute (95% CI)		
Dementia Risk												
4	observational studies	not serious	serious [a]	not serious	not serious	none	3382/211749 (1.6%)	4897/217462 (2.3%)	RR 1.92 (1.52 to 2.43)	21 more per 1000 (from 12 more to 32 more)	⊕◯◯◯ VERY LOW	High importance

CI: Confidence interval; **RR:** Risk ratio. Explanations: a. Presence of significantly high heterogeneity ($I^2 = 79\%$). **GRADE Working Group grades of evidence:** Very low certainty: The true effect is probably markedly different from the estimated effect.

Subgroup analysis based on stroke as a co-morbidity revealed significantly higher dementia risk (Figure 4) in AKI patients (RR 2.30 (95% CI: 1.62 to 3.28), $p \leq 0.00001$).

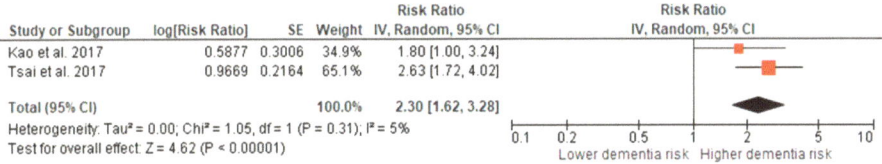

Figure 4. Risk of dementia in AKI patients with stroke.

All-cause mortality risk was also significantly higher (Figure 5) in AKI patients with dementia than patients without AKI with a pooled RR of 2.11 (95% CI: 1.20–3.70), $p = 0.009$. Only one study analyzed and reported a higher dementia risk with a hazard ratio of 2.01 (95% CI: 1.19–3.39), $p = 0.01$ in AKI patients who survived at least 90 days after recovery from acute dialysis.

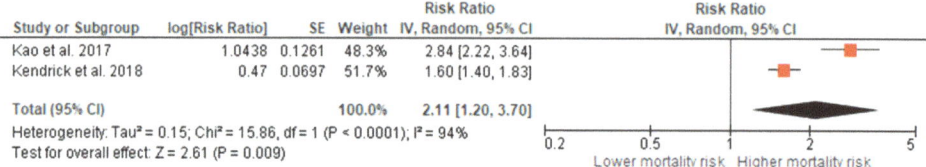

Figure 5. All-cause mortality risk in AKI patients with dementia.

3.4. Sensitivity Analysis

There was no evidence of change in significance level of effect size as confirmed through sensitivity analysis by omitting each study one by one (leave-one-out) from the pooled analysis. Refer to Table S5 for the sensitivity plot.

4. Discussion

This is the first meta-analysis to investigate the association of AKI with dementia risk. A significantly higher dementia risk was observed in patients with AKI as compared to patients without AKI in an adjusted analysis (adjusted for several possible confounding factors). Sensitivity analysis also revealed a consistently higher risk of dementia in AKI patients. All-cause mortality risk was higher in AKI patients who developed dementia.

CKD is a common risk factor for the development of dementia, and CKD following AKI might be responsible for the development of dementia. AKI increases the risk of developing new or progressive CKD (HR: 2.67) and ESKD (HR: 4.67) [38]. The studies by Tsai et al. [25] and Kao et al. [36] suggest that there may be other pathways also to develop dementia in AKI patients apart from CKD only. Furthermore, there is considerable overlap in the pathophysiology, risk factors, and outcomes between AKI and CKD [39,40]. A plethora of evidence found a higher risk of developing dementia in patients with co-morbidities [41–43]. AKI patients with co-morbidities (diabetes, hypertension, depression, chronic obstructive pulmonary disease, coronary artery disease, congestive heart failure, atrial fibrillation, malnutrition, and inflammation) were also found to have significantly higher dementia risk [42,43]. Due to the reversible nature of AKI, long-term outcomes remain ambiguous and debatable.

Cognitive impairment is a well-recognized complication of CKD [18]. Evidence from the literature found a worsening of cognitive function as the kidney function declines [44–46]. A recent cohort study using clinical practice research datalink found a co-occurrence of CKD and dementia in the real-world setting [47]. There is inconclusive research on the mechanistic association of AKI with the development of dementia. Evidence from preclinical studies suggested that AKI influences the blood–brain barrier permeability and may be responsible for various brain and hippocampal complications [48,49]. Hippocampal involvement in AKI patients could be due to the upregulation of macrophage scavenger receptor 1, serum amyloid A3, Ras homolog gene family member J, downregulation of G protein-coupled receptor 34 and 124, and others [50]. Due to dysregulation of transporters across the blood–brain barrier, AKI causes an imbalance of excitatory and inhibitory neurotransmitters [51]. According to the evidence from the clinical study, it could be assumed that AKI is an independent risk factor for CKD development and is associated with multiple organ dysfunction [52]. The kidneys and the brain share similar vascoregulatory and anatomic pathways [53]. The kidneys and the brain are more susceptible to vascular damage due to a high amount of blood flow. This damage can alter endothelial dysfunction, which leads to loss of vascoregulatory abilities [54]. This can affect the brain through inflammatory cascades generated via oxidative stress, proapoptotic pathways activation, and may lead to dementia [22,23].

Age is also a potential risk factor for the development of dementia, as we have observed in our meta-analysis that the risk of dementia increases 10% with one year increase in age. Kao et al. [36], in the extended analysis (adjusted for age and potential confounders), found an increased risk of dementia in AKI patients after the age of 58 years compared to non-AKI patients. Higher dementia risk was observed in AKI patients with stroke as a co-morbidity. Evidence from a recent meta-analysis confirms stroke as an independent and potentially modifiable risk factor based on the analysis of 1,885,536 participants [55]. In our meta-analysis, the all-cause mortality rate was higher in AKI patients with dementia. High mortality in AKI patients is not only attributable to renal failure but also to extra renal complications and its impact on other distant organs [56]. A Danish national registry-based cohort study concluded dementia as an independent risk factor for all-cause mortality, and the mortality rate further exceeds with co-morbidities [57]. In addition to that, another study from the same registry found a higher annual mortality rate ratio in patients with dementia aged ≥65 years in the last 20 years (1996–2015) [58].

The strength of the current study includes a literature search in major databases, an extensive search of major nephrology and neurology conference proceedings, and citation tracking of all the included articles. The majority of the included studies were of high-quality with a large sample size and use of the GRADE approach to rate the certainty of evidence. Pooled analysis was based on data adjusted for several possible confounding factors, which strengthen the conclusion. Furthermore, subgroup and sensitivity analysis also confirm the higher dementia risk.

This meta-analysis has few limitations, such as a diagnosis of AKI based on ICD-9 codes in the majority of the included studies, and dementia was also identified based on ICD-9 codes. Classification of disease based on ICD-9 codes may lead to misdiagnosis as the included studies collected data retrospectively. Preexisting cognitive impairment was not ruled out at the baseline of the study in two of the included studies and might have imparted influence on the overall results; however, a higher risk of developing dementia risk was consistent in the sensitivity analysis. We noticed significantly high heterogeneity among the included studies. In order to explore the heterogeneity, a random effect model was chosen, and findings from subgroup analysis were reported separately. Lastly, retrospective studies are typically a source of inherent bias, which decreased the certainty of the evidence.

Overall, this meta-analysis showed a higher dementia risk in AKI patients. Future studies should look to establish the mechanistic association of AKI with dementia and stratification of dementia risk as per AKI stages. Furthermore, future, large prospective studies should adjust the findings for potential clinical (patients with non-recovery/partial recovery vs. complete recovery) and other associated covariates.

5. Conclusions

In conclusion, this meta-analysis demonstrated a significantly higher risk of dementia among patients with AKI compared with individuals without AKI. The strength of evidence was of very low certainty as per the GRADE assessment. Further large epidemiological studies are needed to confirm the mechanistic association. We recommend close monitoring of patients for dementia after AKI to curtail morbidity.

Supplementary Materials: The following are available online at https://www.mdpi.com/article/10.3390/jcm10194390/s1, Table S1: PRISMA checklist; Table S2: MOOSE checklist; Table S3: Complete search strategy; Table S4: List of articles excluded with reasons during full-text screening; Table S5: Sensitivity plot.

Author Contributions: Conceptualization, S.H.; methodology, S.H. and A.S.; software, S.H.; validation, S.H.; formal analysis, S.H.; resources, M.K. and J.K.; data curation, S.H. and A.S.; writing—original draft preparation, S.H. and A.S.; writing—review and editing, B.A., R.C.-D.G., J.K., R.L. and M.K.; visualization, S.H.; supervision, S.H. and M.K.; project administration, S.H.; funding acquisition, M.K. All authors have read and agreed to the published version of the manuscript.

Funding: S.H. was supported by Operational Programme Research, Development and Education –Project, Postdoc2MUNI "(No. CZ.02.2.69/0.0/0.0/18_053/0016952)". J.K., R.L., and M.K. were supported by the INTER-EXCELLENCE grant number LTC20031—"Towards an International Network for Evidence-based Research in Clinical Health Research in the Czech Republic".

Institutional Review Board Statement: Ethical review and approval were waived for this study due to its observational nature and its use of publicly accessible data.

Conference Presentation: Abstract from this work was presented by the first author (Salman Hussain) in the form of an oral presentation at the 3rd AKI CRRT Congress 2019 held at Kuala Lumpur, Malaysia. The presenter received a meritorious award for this oral presentation.

Informed Consent Statement: Not applicable.

Data Availability Statement: The data that support the findings of this study are available from the corresponding author upon reasonable request.

Conflicts of Interest: The authors declare no conflict of interest.

References

1. Levey, A.S.; Levin, A.; Kellum, J.A. Definition and classification of kidney diseases. *Am. J. Kidney Dis.* **2013**, *61*, 686–688. [CrossRef] [PubMed]
2. Lameire, N.H.; Bagga, A.; Cruz, D.; De Maeseneer, J.; Endre, Z.; Kellum, J.A.; Liu, K.D.; Mehta, R.L.; Pannu, N.; Biesen, W.V. Acute kidney injury: An increasing global concern. *Lancet* **2013**, *382*, 170–179. [CrossRef]
3. Luyckx, V.A.; Tonelli, M.; Stanifer, J.W. The global burden of kidney disease and the sustainable development goals. *Bull. World Health Organ.* **2018**, *96*, 414. [CrossRef]
4. Hoste, E.A.J.; Kellum, J.A.; Selby, N.M.; Zarbock, A.; Palevsky, P.M.; Bagshaw, S.M.; Goldstein, S.L.; Cerdá, J.; Chawla, L.S. Global epidemiology and outcomes of acute kidney injury. *Nat. Rev. Nephrol.* **2018**, *14*, 607–625. [CrossRef] [PubMed]
5. Grams, M.E.; Rabb, H. The distant organ effects of acute kidney injury. *Kidney Int.* **2012**, *81*, 942–948. [CrossRef] [PubMed]
6. Fortrie, G.; de Geus, H.R.; Betjes, M.G. The aftermath of acute kidney injury: A narrative review of long-term mortality and renal function. *Crit. Care* **2019**, *23*, 1–11. [CrossRef] [PubMed]
7. Crowson, C.S.; Liao, K.P.; Davis, J.M., III; Solomon, D.H.; Matteson, E.L.; Knutson, K.L.; Hlatky, M.A.; Gabriel, S.E. Rheumatoid arthritis and cardiovascular disease. *Am. Heart J.* **2013**, *166*, 622–628.e1. [CrossRef]
8. Cioffi, G.; Ognibeni, F.; Dalbeni, A.; Giollo, A.; Orsolini, G.; Gatti, D.; Rossini, M.; Viapiana, O. High prevalence of occult heart disease in normotensive patients with rheumatoid arthritis. *Clin. Cardiol.* **2018**, *41*, 736–743. [CrossRef] [PubMed]
9. Ungprasert, P.; Srivali, N.; Kittanamongkolchai, W. Risk of incident atrial fibrillation in patients with rheumatoid arthritis: A systematic review and meta-analysis. *Int. J. Rheum. Dis.* **2017**, *20*, 434–441. [CrossRef] [PubMed]
10. Uzun, S.; Kozumplik, O.; Folnegović-Šmalc, V. Alzheimer's dementia: Current data review. *Coll. Antropol.* **2011**, *35*, 1333–1337. [PubMed]
11. WHO. Dementia. Available online: https://www.who.int/news-room/fact-sheets/detail/dementia (accessed on 25 August 2021).
12. Nichols, E.; Szoeke, C.E.I.; Vollset, S.E.; Abbasi, N.; Abd-Allah, F.; Abdela, J.; Aichour, M.T.E.; Akinyemi, R.O.; Alahdab, F.; Asgedom, S.W. Global, regional, and national burden of Alzheimer's disease and other dementias, 1990–2016: A systematic analysis for the Global Burden of Disease Study 2016. *Lancet Neurol.* **2019**, *18*, 88–106. [CrossRef]
13. Duggan, S.; Blackman, T.; Martyr, A.; Van Schaik, P. The impact of early dementia on outdoor life: Ashrinking world'? *Dementia* **2008**, *7*, 191–204. [CrossRef]
14. Norton, S.; Matthews, F.E.; Barnes, D.E.; Yaffe, K.; Brayne, C. Potential for primary prevention of Alzheimer's disease: An analysis of population-based data. *Lancet Neurol.* **2014**, *13*, 788–794. [CrossRef]
15. Plassman, B.L.; Williams, J.W., Jr.; Burke, J.R.; Holsinger, T.; Benjamin, S. Systematic review: Factors associated with risk for and possible prevention of cognitive decline in later life. *Ann. Intern. Med.* **2010**, *153*, 182–193. [CrossRef]
16. Schiffrin, E.L.; Lipman, M.L.; Mann, J.F. Chronic kidney disease: Effects on the cardiovascular system. *Circulation* **2007**, *116*, 85–97. [CrossRef]
17. Tamura, M.K.; Yaffe, K. Dementia and cognitive impairment in ESRD: Diagnostic and therapeutic strategies. *Kidney Int.* **2011**, *79*, 14–22. [CrossRef] [PubMed]
18. Etgen, T.; Chonchol, M.; Förstl, H.; Sander, D. Chronic kidney disease and cognitive impairment: A systematic review and meta-analysis. *Am. J. Nephrol.* **2012**, *35*, 474–482. [CrossRef] [PubMed]
19. Bugnicourt, J.-M.; Godefroy, O.; Chillon, J.-M.; Choukroun, G.; Massy, Z.A. Cognitive disorders and dementia in CKD: The neglected kidney-brain axis. *J. Am. Soc. Nephrol.* **2013**, *24*, 353–363. [CrossRef] [PubMed]
20. Kalaria, R.N.; Maestre, G.E.; Arizaga, R.; Friedland, R.P.; Galasko, D.; Hall, K.; Luchsinger, J.A.; Ogunniyi, A.; Perry, E.K.; Potocnik, F. Alzheimer's disease and vascular dementia in developing countries: Prevalence, management, and risk factors. *Lancet Neurol.* **2008**, *7*, 812–826. [CrossRef]
21. Deckers, K.; Camerino, I.; van Boxtel, M.P.; Verhey, F.R.; Irving, K.; Brayne, C.; Kivipelto, M.; Starr, J.M.; Yaffe, K.; de Leeuw, P.W. Dementia risk in renal dysfunction: A systematic review and meta-analysis of prospective studies. *Neurology* **2017**, *88*, 198–208. [CrossRef] [PubMed]
22. Liu, M.; Liang, Y.; Chigurupati, S.; Lathia, J.D.; Pletnikov, M.; Sun, Z.; Crow, M.; Ross, C.A.; Mattson, M.P.; Rabb, H. Acute kidney injury leads to inflammation and functional changes in the brain. *J. Am. Soc. Nephrol.* **2008**, *19*, 1360–1370. [CrossRef] [PubMed]

23. Verma, S.K.; Molitoris, B.A. Renal endothelial injury and microvascular dysfunction in acute kidney injury. *Semin. Nephrol.* **2015**, *35*, 96–107. [CrossRef] [PubMed]
24. Kendrick, J.; Holmen, J.; Srinivas, T.; You, Z.; Chonchol, M.; Jovanovich, A. Acute kidney injury is associated with an increased risk of dementia. *Kidney Int. Rep.* **2019**, *4*, 1491. [CrossRef] [PubMed]
25. Tsai, H.-H.; Yen, R.-F.; Lin, C.-L.; Kao, C.-H. Increased risk of dementia in patients hospitalized with acute kidney injury: A nationwide population-based cohort study. *PLoS ONE* **2017**, *12*, e0171671.
26. Page, M.J.; McKenzie, J.E.; Bossuyt, P.M.; Boutron, I.; Hoffmann, T.C.; Mulrow, C.D.; Shamseer, L.; Tetzlaff, J.M.; Moher, D. The PRISMA 2020 statement: An updated guideline for reporting systematic reviews. *BMJ* **2021**, *372*, n71. [CrossRef] [PubMed]
27. Stroup, D.F.; Berlin, J.A.; Morton, S.C.; Olkin, I.; Williamson, G.D.; Rennie, D.; Moher, D.; Becker, B.J.; Sipe, T.A.; Thacker, S.B. Meta-analysis of observational studies in epidemiology: A proposal for reporting. Meta-analysis Of Observational Studies in Epidemiology (MOOSE) group. *JAMA* **2000**, *283*, 2008–2012. [CrossRef] [PubMed]
28. Hussain, S.; Singh, A.; Antony, B.S.E.; Kulgarova, J.; Licenik, R.; Klugar, M. Association of acute kidney injury with the risk of dementia: A meta-analysis protocol. *medRxiv* **2021**. [CrossRef]
29. Hussain, S.; Singh, A.; Zameer, S.; Jamali, M.C.; Baxi, H.; Rahman, S.O.; Alam, M.; Altamish, M.; Singh, A.K.; Anil, D.; et al. No association between proton pump inhibitor use and risk of dementia: Evidence from a meta-analysis. *J. Gastroenterol. Hepatol.* **2020**, *35*, 19–28. [CrossRef] [PubMed]
30. GRADE Working Group. Grading quality of evidence and strength of recommendations. *BMJ* **2004**, *328*, 1490. [CrossRef] [PubMed]
31. Shi, F.; Sun, L.; Kaptoge, S. Association of beta-2-microglobulin and cardiovascular events and mortality: A systematic review and meta-analysis. *Atherosclerosis* **2021**, *320*, 70–78. [CrossRef]
32. Higgins, J.P.; Thomas, J.; Chandler, J.; Cumpston, M.; Li, T.; Page, M.J.; Welch, V.A. *Cochrane Handbook for Systematic Reviews of Interventions*; John Wiley & Sons: Hoboken, NJ, USA, 2019.
33. Higgins, J.P.; Thompson, S.G.; Deeks, J.J.; Altman, D.G. Measuring inconsistency in meta-analyses. *BMJ* **2003**, *327*, 557–560. [CrossRef] [PubMed]
34. Singh, A.; Hussain, S.; Najmi, A.K. Number of studies, heterogeneity, generalisability, and the choice of method for meta-analysis. *J. Neurol. Sci.* **2017**, *381*, 347. [CrossRef] [PubMed]
35. *GRADEpro GDT: GRADEpro Guideline Development Tool [Software]*. McMaster University; Evidence Prime, Inc.: Hamilton, ON, Canada, 2020; Available online: https://gradepro.org (accessed on 25 August 2021).
36. Kao, C.-C.; Wu, C.-H.; Lai, C.-F.; Huang, T.-M.; Chen, H.-H.; Wu, V.-C.; Chen, L.; Wu, M.-S.; Wu, K.-D.; The NSARF Group. Long-term risk of dementia following acute kidney injury: A population-based study. *Tzu-Chi Med. J.* **2017**, *29*, 201.
37. Wu, Y. Dementia as an independent risk factor for acute kidney injury in elderly patients: A propensity-score matching study. *Nephrology* **2020**, *25*, 24.
38. See, E.J.; Jayasinghe, K.; Glassford, N.; Bailey, M.; Johnson, D.W.; Polkinghorne, K.R.; Toussaint, N.D.; Bellomo, R. Long-term risk of adverse outcomes after acute kidney injury: A systematic review and meta-analysis of cohort studies using consensus definitions of exposure. *Kidney Int.* **2019**, *95*, 160–172. [CrossRef]
39. Bedford, M.; Farmer, C.; Levin, A.; Ali, T.; Stevens, P. Acute kidney injury and CKD: Chicken or egg? *Am. J. Kidney Dis.* **2012**, *59*, 485–491. [CrossRef]
40. CKD increases risk of acute kidney injury during hospitalization. *Nat. Clin. Pract. Nephrol.* **2008**, *4*, 408. Available online: https://www.nature.com/articles/ncpneph0850#citeas (accessed on 25 August 2021). [CrossRef]
41. Chen, T.-B.; Yiao, S.-Y.; Sun, Y.; Lee, H.-J.; Yang, S.-C.; Chiu, M.-J.; Chen, T.-F.; Lin, K.-N.; Tang, L.-Y.; Lin, C.-C. Comorbidity and dementia: A nationwide survey in Taiwan. *PLoS ONE* **2017**, *12*, e0175475. [CrossRef] [PubMed]
42. Peters, R.; Booth, A.; Rockwood, K.; Peters, J.; D'Este, C.; Anstey, K.J. Combining modifiable risk factors and risk of dementia: A systematic review and meta-analysis. *BMJ Open* **2019**, *9*, e022846. [CrossRef]
43. Bunn, F.; Burn, A.-M.; Goodman, C.; Rait, G.; Norton, S.; Robinson, L.; Schoeman, J.; Brayne, C. Comorbidity and dementia: A scoping review of the literature. *BMC Med.* **2014**, *12*, 1–15. [CrossRef]
44. Zijlstra, L.E.; Trompet, S.; Mooijaart, S.P.; van Buren, M.; Sattar, N.; Stott, D.J.; Jukema, J.W. The association of kidney function and cognitive decline in older patients at risk of cardiovascular disease: A longitudinal data analysis. *BMC Nephrol.* **2020**, *21*, 1–10. [CrossRef]
45. Yaffe, K.; Ackerson, L.; Tamura, M.K.; Le Blanc, P.; Kusek, J.W.; Sehgal, A.R.; Cohen, D.; Anderson, C.; Appel, L.; DeSalvo, K. Chronic kidney disease and cognitive function in older adults: Findings from the chronic renal insufficiency cohort cognitive study. *J. Am. Geriatr. Soc.* **2010**, *58*, 338–345. [CrossRef]
46. Hailpern, S.M.; Melamed, M.L.; Cohen, H.W.; Hostetter, T.H. Moderate chronic kidney disease and cognitive function in adults 20 to 59 years of age: Third National Health and Nutrition Examination Survey (NHANES III). *J. Am. Soc. Nephrol.* **2007**, *18*, 2205–2213. [CrossRef]
47. Hiramatsu, R.; Iwagami, M.; Nitsch, D. Association between chronic kidney disease and incident diagnosis of dementia in England: A cohort study in Clinical Practice Research Datalink. *BMJ Open* **2020**, *10*, e033811. [CrossRef]
48. Fleegal-DeMotta, M.A.; Doghu, S.; Banks, W.A. Angiotensin II modulates BBB permeability via activation of the AT(1) receptor in brain endothelial cells. *J. Cereb. Blood Flow Metab.* **2009**, *29*, 640–647. [CrossRef]

49. Bernardo-Castro, S.; Sousa, J.A.; Brás, A.; Cecília, C.; Rodrigues, B.; Almendra, L.; Machado, C.; Santo, G.; Silva, F.; Ferreira, L. Pathophysiology of Blood–Brain Barrier Permeability Throughout the Different Stages of Ischemic Stroke and Its Implication on Hemorrhagic Transformation and Recovery. *Front. Neurol.* **2020**, *11*, 1605. [CrossRef] [PubMed]
50. Malek, M. Brain consequences of acute kidney injury: Focusing on the hippocampus. *Kidney Res. Clin. Pract.* **2018**, *37*, 315. [CrossRef]
51. Nongnuch, A.; Panorchan, K.; Davenport, A. Brain–kidney crosstalk. *Crit. Care* **2014**, *18*, 1–11. [CrossRef] [PubMed]
52. Nie, S.; Feng, Z.; Tang, L.; Wang, X.; He, Y.; Fang, J.; Li, S.; Yang, Y.; Mao, H.; Jiao, J. Risk factor analysis for AKI including laboratory indicators: A Nationwide multicenter study of hospitalized patients. *Kidney Blood Press. Res.* **2017**, *42*, 761–773. [CrossRef] [PubMed]
53. Mogi, M.; Horiuchi, M. Clinical interaction between brain and kidney in small vessel disease. *Cardiol. Res. Pract.* **2011**, *2011*. [CrossRef] [PubMed]
54. Sutton, T.A.; Fisher, C.J.; Molitoris, B.A. Microvascular endothelial injury and dysfunction during ischemic acute renal failure. *Kidney Int.* **2002**, *62*, 1539–1549. [CrossRef]
55. Kuźma, E.; Lourida, I.; Moore, S.F.; Levine, D.A.; Ukoumunne, O.C.; Llewellyn, D.J. Stroke and dementia risk: A systematic review and meta-analysis. *Alzheimer's Dement. J. Alzheimer's Assoc.* **2018**, *14*, 1416–1426. [CrossRef] [PubMed]
56. Chertow, G.M.; Lazarus, J.M.; Paganini, E.P.; Allgren, R.L.; Lafayette, R.A.; Sayegh, M.H. Predictors of mortality and the provision of dialysis in patients with acute tubular necrosis. The Auriculin Anaritide Acute Renal Failure Study Group. *J. Am. Soc. Nephrol.* **1998**, *9*, 692–698. [CrossRef] [PubMed]
57. Taudorf, L.; Nørgaard, A.; Brodaty, H.; Laursen, T.M.; Waldemar, G. Dementia increases mortality beyond effects of comorbid conditions: A national registry-based cohort study. *Eur. J. Neurol.* **2021**, *28*, 2174–2184. [CrossRef] [PubMed]
58. Taudorf, L.; Nørgaard, A.; Waldemar, G.; Laursen, T.M. Mortality in Dementia from 1996 to 2015: A National Registry-Based Cohort Study. *J. Alzheimer's Dis.* **2021**, *79*, 289–300. [CrossRef]

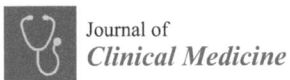

Article

Polypharmacy Is Significantly and Positively Associated with the Frailty Status Assessed Using the 5-Item FRAIL Scale, Cardiovascular Health Phenotypic Classification of Frailty Index, and Study of Osteoporotic Fractures Scale

Chi-Di Hung [1,2,3,4], Chen-Cheng Yang [1,2,3,4,*], Chun-Ying Lee [4], Stephen Chu-Sung Hu [5], Szu-Chia Chen [6], Chih-Hsing Hung [7], Hung-Yi Chuang [2], Ching-Yu Chen [8] and Chao-Hung Kuo [6]

1. Department of Occupational and Environmental Medicine, Kaohsiung Municipal Siaogang Hospital, Kaohsiung Medical University, Kaohsiung City 812, Taiwan; ciem273555@gmail.com
2. Department of Occupational and Environmental Medicine, Kaohsiung Medical University Hospital, Kaohsiung Medical University, Kaohsiung City 807, Taiwan; ericch@kmu.edu.tw
3. Department of Family Medicine, Kaohsiung Municipal Siaogang Hospital, Kaohsiung Medical University, Kaohsiung City 812, Taiwan
4. Department of Family Medicine, Kaohsiung Medical University Hospital, Kaohsiung Medical University, Kaohsiung City 807, Taiwan; june.lee@gap.kmu.edu.tw
5. Department of Dermatology, Kaohsiung Municipal Siaogang Hospital, Kaohsiung Medical University, Kaohsiung City 812, Taiwan; stephenhu30@hotmail.com
6. Department of Internal Medicine, Kaohsiung Municipal Siaogang Hospital, Kaohsiung Medical University, Kaohsiung City 812, Taiwan; scarchenone@yahoo.com.tw (S.-C.C.); kjh88kmu@gmail.com (C.-H.K.)
7. Environmental and Occupational Medicine Center, Kaohsiung Municipal Siaogang Hospital, Kaohsiung Medical University, Kaohsiung City 812, Taiwan; pedhung@gmail.com
8. Department of Family Medicine, National Taiwan University Hospital, Taipei City 100, Taiwan; cycchen@ntu.edu.tw
* Correspondence: u106800001@kmu.edu.tw or abcmacoto@gmail.com.tw; Tel.: +886-7-8036783 (ext. 3460)

Abstract: The aim of this study was to investigate the association between frailty and polypharmacy using three different frailty screening tools. This was a cross-sectional study of people aged ≥65 years. Participants were included and interviewed using questionnaires. Polypharmacy was defined as the daily use of eight or more pills. Frailty was assessed using a screening tool, including (1) the Fatigue, Resistance, Ambulation, Illness and Loss of Weight Index (5-item FRAIL scale), (2) the Cardiovascular Health Phenotypic Classification of Frailty (CHS_PCF) index (Fried's Frailty Phenotype), and (3) the Study of Osteoporotic Fracture (SOF) scale. A total of 205 participants (mean age: 71.1 years; 53.7% female) fulfilled our inclusion criteria. The proportion of patients with polypharmacy was 14.1%. After adjustments were made for comorbidity or potential confounders, polypharmacy was associated with frailty on the 5-item FRAIL scale (adjusted odds ratio [aOR]: 9.12; 95% confidence interval [CI]: 3.6–23.16), CHS_PCF index (aOR: 8.98; 95% CI: 2.51–32.11), and SOF scale (aOR: 6.10; 95% CI: 1.47–25.3). Polypharmacy was associated with frailty using three frailty screening tools. Future research is required to further enhance our understanding of the risk of frailty among older adults.

Keywords: polypharmacy; frailty; Cardiovascular Health Study; Study of Osteoporotic Fracture

Citation: Hung, C.-D.; Yang, C.-C.; Lee, C.-Y.; Hu, S.C.-S.; Chen, S.-C.; Hung, C.-H.; Chuang, H.-Y.; Chen, C.-Y.; Kuo, C.-H. Polypharmacy Is Significantly and Positively Associated with the Frailty Status Assessed Using the 5-Item FRAIL Scale, Cardiovascular Health Phenotypic Classification of Frailty Index, and Study of Osteoporotic Fractures Scale. *J. Clin. Med.* 2021, 10, 4413. https://doi.org/10.3390/jcm10194413

Academic Editor: Francesco Mattace-Raso

Received: 5 August 2021
Accepted: 23 September 2021
Published: 26 September 2021

Publisher's Note: MDPI stays neutral with regard to jurisdictional claims in published maps and institutional affiliations.

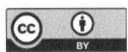

Copyright: © 2021 by the authors. Licensee MDPI, Basel, Switzerland. This article is an open access article distributed under the terms and conditions of the Creative Commons Attribution (CC BY) license (https://creativecommons.org/licenses/by/4.0/).

1. Introduction

Frailty is a clinical syndrome characterized by physical activities, cognition and emotional impairment [1]. It is a state of increased vulnerability to stressors, especially in older adults [1], that leads to adverse health outcomes such as falls, disability, hospitalization, institutionalization and mortality [2–4]. As people of advanced age are gradually increasing in many countries, frailty is considered of growing importance in geriatric population.

Previous studies estimated that the prevalence of frailty varied from 3.9% to 51.4% [5–7]. This variance is influenced by the differences in countries and socioeconomic status and, more importantly, screening tools. Because there is no gold standard for assessing frailty, multiple assessment methods have been developed, such as Fried's phenotype model [8], and the frailty index of Rockwood's cumulated deficit model [9]. These screening tools help to identify frail patients at high risk for negative health outcomes and provide an opportunity to prevent the progression of comorbidity [10].

Polypharmacy refers to multiple use of medications and/or unnecessary drug use, commonly defined by five or more medications daily [11,12]. A systematic review [11] reported that even if the most common definition of polypharmacy was the numerical definition of five or more medications daily ($n = 51$, 46.4% of articles), some articles [13,14] use definitions with ten or more medicines. Polypharmacy is common in older adults especially with multimorbidity, as one or more medications may be used in each condition. The patient may suffer from increased risk of various adverse effects and harm. A retrospective study demonstrated that larger numbers of medications used among 259 patients attending a cardiovascular outpatient department were associated with faster declines in renal function and may have worsened the prognosis [15]. Additionally, potential adverse outcomes included declines in cognition and mobility as well as drug-drug interactions and drug-disease interactions [16,17].

Since both frailty and polypharmacy have been considered as common geriatric syndromes, they have gained increasing interest and attention. However, the association between frailty evaluation and polypharmacy is still scarce. Therefore, we aim to investigate the association between frailty and polypharmacy.

2. Materials and Methods

2.1. Subjects

The study was a cross-sectional study. Participants were included, after informed consent, from the outpatient clinic and the health examination department in a single center located in the urban area of Kaohsiung City. The inclusive criterion was adults aged 65 years old or more. The exclusive criteria were (1) less than 65 years old, (2) mental disability or psychological disease, and (3) who were unwilling to agree to the informed consent form or were unable to cooperate with the study. During October 2020 to April 2021, 205 participants were included. The IRB number was KMUHIRB-F(I)-20200052.

2.2. Measurement and Questionnaire

Participants were interviewed by questionnaire. One-on-one interviews were conducted by well-trained interviewers. Participants could complete the questionnaire with the assistance of interviewers or their family. The demographic characteristics included gender, age, living environment, education level, and smoking and alcohol habits. Low education was defined as elementary school or no education. Daily use of more than eight pills was consider as polypharmacy. Evaluation tools for frailty included (1) Fatigue, Resistance, Ambulation, Illness and Loss of Weight Index (FRAIL model) [18]; (2) Cardiovascular Health Phenotypic Classification of Frailty index (CHS-PCF, Fried's Frailty Phenotype) [19]; and (3) Study of Osteoporotic Fracture Index (SOF) [20]. All questionnaires were input into the computer twice by two independent personnel and the input correction was checked.

2.3. Frailty Evaluation

The 5-item FRAIL scale represented the abbreviation of Fatigue, Resistance, Ambulation, Illness, and Loss of weight, which was established at the International Nutrition, Health and Ageing Group. The scale consists of five items: (1) exhaustion, (2) weakness, (3) slowness while walking, (4) low activity, and (5) weight loss. These factors represent biological factors (fatigue and weight loss), functional factors (resistance and ambulation), and deficit accumulation by illness. The 5-item FRAIL scale classification was defined as frail (3–5), pre-frail (1–2), and robust health status (0) [18].

Fried's phenotype model of frailty is also known as the Cardiovascular Health Phenotypic Classification of Frailty (CHS_PCF) index, a biological model of frailty comprising five components: unintentional weight loss, feelings of exhaustion, decreased physical activity, slow walking speed, and weakness. CHS_PCF scores were categorized as frail (3–5), pre-frail (1–2), and robust health status (0) [8,19].

The Study of Osteoporotic Fractures (SOF) scale comprised two factors with three components, including biological factors (inability to complete five chair rises, weight loss) and functional factors (reduced energy level). SOF scale scores were categorized as frail (2–3), pre-frail (1), and robust health status (0) [20].

2.4. Statistics

Descriptive statistics were used to analyze the means and dispersion of the continuous variables, including the age and the scores of the three frailty assessment tools. For the categorical variables, such as gender and smoking and alcohol consumption, numbers and proportions were used for this evaluation. Furthermore, we divided the participants into different groups according to different frail conditions. The 5-item FRAIL scale was divided into robust health, pre-frail and frail groups. CHS_PCF was classified into robust health, prefrail, and frail groups. SOF was divided into robust health, pre-frail and frail groups. Analysis of variance was performed to analyze the differences in polypharmacy among the frail groups. The non-frail groups (robust health and pre-frail participants) were selected as a reference. The crude logistic regression model of frail condition and polypharmacy, or frail condition and other variables including age, body mass index (BMI), gender, education level, living situation, and smoking and alcohol habits were performed. Finally, two adjusted logistic regression models (one by the Hosmer–Lemeshow goodness-of-fit test and the other by the exact logistic regression model) were conducted. IBM-SPSS version 20 statistical software (IBM Corp. Released 2011. IBM SPSS Statistics for Windows, Version 20.0. Armonk, NY, USA: IBM Corp.) was used, with a significant p value of 0.05, two-tailed tests.

3. Results

During the period of October 2020 to April 2021 we had registered 400 participants, of whom 205 fulfilled our inclusion criteria. Table 1 shows key descriptive analysis of the study baseline. We classified these participants into robust health, pre-frail, and frail groups by the 5-item FRAIL scale, CHS_PCF, and SOF scale according to these scale definitions, respectively. In FRAIL model, 105 (51.22%) were robust health, 54 (26.34%) were pre-frail, and 46 (22.43%) were frail; in CHS_PCF, 38 (18.53%) were robust health, 73 (35.61%) were pre-frail, and 94 (45.85%) were frail; in SOF model, 138 (67.31%) were robust health, 54 (26.34%) were pre-frail, and 13 (6.34%) were frail. Detailed demographic data on the different scales is shown in Table 1. Of these 205 participants, their average age was 71.1 years and average BMI was 26.06 kg/m^2. The participants included 95 males (46.3%) and 110 females (53.7%). Moreover, 42.9% (88 participants) of all participants were of low education (elementary school only or no education), 18% (37 participants) lived alone, 4.4% (nine participants) were smokers, 8.8% (18 participants) consumed alcohol and 14.1% (29 participants) were polypharmaceutical.

Table 1. Demographics of the participants according to their frail status (n = 205).

	Robust Health	Pre-Frail	Frail
	n (%)/Mean ± SD	n (%)/Mean ± SD	n (%)/Mean ± SD
5-item FRAIL			
n (%)	105 (51.22)	54 (26.34)	46 (22.43)
Age, mean (SD), years	70.8 ± 5.6	71.0 ± 5.1	71.9 ± 5.3
BMI, mean (SD), kg/m^2	26.0 ± 4.1	25.7 ± 3.4	26.6 ± 4.4
Gender, Male, n (%)	56 (53.3)	21 (38.9)	18 (39.1)
Education (low), n (%)	33 (31.4)	32 (59.3)	23 (50)

Table 1. Cont.

	Robust Health	Pre-Frail	Frail
	n (%)/Mean ± SD	n (%)/Mean ± SD	n (%)/Mean ± SD
5-item FRAIL			
Living alone, n (%)	19 (18.1)	9 (16.7)	9 (19.6)
Smoking, n (%)	6 (5.7)	2 (3.7)	1 (2.2)
Consuming alcohol, n (%)	13 (12.4)	3 (5.6)	2 (4.3)
Polypharmacy, n (%)	1 (1.0)	9 (16.7)	19 (41.3)
Comorbidity			
0	14 (13.3)	4 (7.4)	3 (6.5)
1	66 (62.9)	27 (50.0)	19 (41.3)
2	25 (23.8)	23 (42.6)	24 (52.2)
CHS_PCF			
n (%)	38 (18.53)	73 (35.61)	94 (45.85)
Age, mean (SD), years	69.7 ± 3.6	70.4 ± 5.3	72.1 ± 5.8
BMI, mean (SD), kg/m²	25.6 ± 3.9	25.9 ± 3.9	26.4 ± 4.1
Gender, Male, n (%)	19 (50.0)	30 (41.1)	46 (48.9)
Education (low), n (%)	8 (21.1)	30 (41.1)	50 (53.2)
Living alone, n (%)	7 (18.4)	17 (23.3)	13 (13.8)
Smoking, n (%)	1 (2.6)	4 (5.5)	4 (4.3)
Consuming alcohol, n (%)	4 (10.5)	7 (9.6)	7 (7.4)
Polypharmacy, n (%)	1 (2.6)	2 (2.7)	26 (27.7)
Comorbidity			
0	4 (10.5)	11 (15.1)	6 (6.4)
1	24 (63.2)	47 (64.4)	41 (43.6)
2	10 (26.3)	15 (20.5)	47 (50.0)
SOF			
n (%)	138 (67.31)	54 (26.34)	13 (6.341)
Age, mean (SD), years	70.8 ± 5.2	71.4 ± 5.9	72.3 ± 5.5
BMI, mean (SD), kg/m²	26.0 ± 4.2	26.1 ± 3.2	26.2 ± 4.1
Gender, Male, n (%)	67 (48.6)	23 (42.6)	5 (38.5)
Education (low), n (%)	52 (37.7)	29 (53.7)	7 (53.8)
Living alone, n (%)	25 (18.1)	10 (18.5)	2 (15.4)
Smoking, n (%)	6 (4.3)	3 (5.6)	0 (0.0)
Consuming alcohol, n (%)	15 (10.9)	3 (5.6)	0 (0.0)
Polypharmacy, n (%)	15 (10.9)	9 (16.7)	5 (38.5)
Comorbidity			
0	16 (11.6)	3 (5.6)	2 (15.4)
1	79 (57.2)	27 (50.0)	6 (46.2)
2	43 (31.2)	24 (44.4)	5 (38.5)

FRAIL, Fatigue, Resistance, Ambulation, Illness, and Loss of Weight. CHS_PCF, Cardiovascular Health Phenotypic Classification of Frailty. SOF, Study of Osteoporotic Fracture. SD, standard deviation. BMI, body mass index. Comorbidity: 0, no disease; 1, one to two diseases; 2, three or more diseases. Disease category: hypertension, diabetes mellitus, hyperlipidemia, cerebral vascular disease, cardiovascular disease, pulmonary disease, liver disease, urologic disease, neurology disease, and malignant cancer.

We defined these non-frail participants as the reference group and a logistic regression model was created to analyze the variance of differences and odd ratio in polypharmacy as well as other potential confounders between the frail group and the reference groups. Moreover, the regression model was adjusted by potential confounders, including age, BMI, gender, education level, whether or not patients lived alone, and smoking and alcohol habits, in case these potential confounders and frailty revealed a significant association in the crude regression model. Comorbidity was considered as an important risk factor of frailty, so we adjusted it in the adjusted regression model. Table 2 shows that in the crude regression model of the FRAIL scale, the factor most strongly associated with 5-item FRAIL scale frail status was polypharmacy (odd ratio [OR] 10.49, 95% confidence interval [CI]

4.40–24.99, p-value < 0.001). Otherwise, parameters such as age, BMI, gender, education level, living environment, and smoking and alcohol habits were not associated with frailty in 5-item FRAIL scale. Furthermore, the adjusted model and the exact logistic regression shown a consistent trend; frailty was significantly and positively associated with polypharmacy after adjusting comorbidity (aOR * 9.12, 95% CI 3.6–23.16, p-value < 0.001; the exact logistic regression model aOR † 9.02, 95% CI 3.32–26.16, p-value < 0.001, respectively).

Table 2. Regression model of the 5-item Fatigue, Resistance, Ambulation, Illness, and Loss of Weight scale.

	Crude (95% CI)	p-Value	Adjusted (95% CI) *	p-Value	Adjusted (95% CI) †	p-Value
Age	1.04 (0.98–1.10)	0.220				
BMI	1.05 (0.96–1.13)	0.275				
Gender (male)	0.68 (0.35–1.34)	0.267				
Education (high)	0.69 (0.36–1.34)	0.272				
Live alone	1.14 (0.49–2.62)	0.762				
Smoke	0.42 (0.05–3.44)	0.419				
Alcohol	0.41 (0.09–1.84)	0.242				
Polypharmacy	10.49 (4.40–24.99)	<0.001	9.12 (3.6–23.16)	<0.001	9.02 (3.32–26.16)	<0.001
Comorbidity						
0	1.00		1.00			
1–2	1.23 (0.33–4.58)	0.762	0.98 (0.26–3.73)	0.9819		
>2	3.00 (0.80–11.19)	0.102	1.35 (0.34–5.44)	0.6708		
Per category	2.07 (1.18–3.64)	0.012			1.24 (0.63–2.46)	0.603
Goodness-of-fit statistic *			$\chi^2 = 0.30, p = 0.859$			

Crude odds ratio (OR) was calculated using the logistic regression model. * Adjusted polypharmacy and comorbidity; the Hosmer–Lemeshow goodness-of-fit test was used. † Adjusted OR was calculated using the exact logistic regression model. Comorbidity: 0, no disease; 1, one to two diseases; 2, three or more diseases.

In Table 3, the crude regression model of CHS_PCF identified the factors, including polypharmacy (OR 13.76, 95% CI 4.01–47.23, p-value < 0.001), age (OR 1.07, 95% CI 1.02–1.13, p-value 0.010) and low education level (high education versus low education OR 0.46, 95% CI 0.26–0.80, p-value 0.007) which were associated with frail status in CHS_PCF model. Compared with participants with non-comorbidity, participants with three or more comorbidities were significantly and positively associated with frailty (OR 4.70, 95% CI 1.62–13.62, p-value 0.004). However, after adjusting for comorbidity, polypharmacy revealed consistent significantly positive association with CHS PCF frailty (aOR * 8.98, 95% CI 2.51–32.11, p-value < 0.001; aOR † 8.81, 95% CI 2.42–48.81, p-value < 0.001, respectively). Finally, the regression model of SOF in Table 4 determined that the factor associated with frailty was polypharmacy (crude OR 4.38, 95% CI 1.32–14.47, p-value 0.016; aOR * 6.10, 95% CI 1.47–25.3, p-value 0.013; and aOR † 6.31, 95% CI 1.21–33.29, p-value 0.027). Age, BMI, gender, education level, and living environment were not associated with frail status in the SOF model.

Table 3. Regression model of Cardiovascular Health Phenotypic Classification of Frailty (CHS_PCF) index.

	Crude (95% CI)	p-Value	Adjusted (95% CI) *	p-Value	Adjusted (95% CI) †	p-Value
Age	1.07 (1.02–1.13)	0.010	1.06 (0.99–1.12)	0.058	1.06 (0.99–1.12)	0.054
BMI	1.04 (0.97–1.11)	0.330				
Gender (male)	1.21 (0.70–2.10)	0.493				
Education (high)	0.46 (0.26–0.80)	0.007	0.50 (0.26–0.96)	0.036	0.45 (0.23–0.87)	0.015
Live alone	0.58 (0.28–1.22)	0.151				
Smoke	0.94 (0.25–3.61)	0.931				
Alcohol	0.73 (0.27–1.97)	0.536				
Polypharmacy	13.76 (4.01–47.23)	<0.001	8.98 (2.51–32.11)	<0.001	8.81 (2.42–48.81)	<0.001

Table 3. Cont.

	Crude (95% CI)	p-Value	Adjusted (95% CI) *	p-Value	Adjusted (95% CI) †	p-Value
Comorbidity						
0	1.00		1.00			
1	1.44 (0.52–4.01)	0.481	1.32 (0.46–3.83)	0.605		
2	4.70 (1.62–13.62)	0.004	3.28 (1.06–10.15)	0.034		
Per category	2.57 (1.59–4.18)	<0.001			2.02 (1.17–3.56)	0.001
Goodness-of-fit statistic *			$\chi^2 = 3.03, p = 0.882$			

Crude odds ratio (OR) was calculated using the logistic regression model. * Adjusted age, education, polypharmacy, and comorbidity; the Hosmer–Lemeshow goodness-of-fit test was used. † Adjusted OR was calculated using the exact logistic regression model. Comorbidity: 0, no disease; 1, one to two diseases; 2, three or more diseases.

Table 4. Regression model of Study of Osteoporotic Fracture (SOF) scale.

	Crude (95% CI)	p-Value	Adjusted (95% CI) *	p-Value	Adjusted (95% CI) †	p-Value
Age	1.04 (0.95–1.15)	0.395				
BMI	1.01 (0.87–1.16)	0.929				
Gender (male)	0.71 (0.22–2.24)	0.558				
Education (high)	0.63 (0.2–1.93)	0.415				
Live alone	0.82 (0.17–3.84)	0.797				
Polypharmacy	4.38 (1.32–14.47)	0.016	6.10 (1.47–25.3)	0.013	6.31 (1.21–33.29)	0.027
Comorbidity						
0	1.00		1.00			
1	0.54 (0.1–2.87)	0.467	0.43 (0.08–2.35)	0.326		
2	0.71 (0.13–3.95)	0.695	0.29 (0.04–2.12)	0.225		
Per category	0.95 (0.39–2.33)	0.915			0.57 (0.18–1.78)	0.396
Goodness-of-fit statistic *			$\chi^2 = 0.23, p = 0.892$			

Crude odds ratio (OR) was calculated using the logistic regression model. * Adjusted polypharmacy and comorbidity; the Hosmer–Lemeshow goodness-of-fit test was used. † Adjusted OR was calculated using the exact logistic regression model. Comorbidity: 0, no disease; 1, one to two diseases; 2, three or more diseases.

4. Discussion

To our knowledge, this is the first study comparing three different frailty models to examine the association between frailty and polypharmacy. This cross-sectional study explored the association of polypharmacy and frailty using the 5-item FRAIL scale, CHS_PCF index, and the SOF scale. The results showed that polypharmacy was strongly associated with frailty in each tool. Previous studies demonstrated similar results [21–24]. In Korea, Jung et al. [21] reported that frailty using the 5-item FRAIL scale was associated with the use of an increased number of medications. Furthermore, Jung et al. [22] reported that polypharmacy with five drugs or more was associated with physical frailty (OR 1.61, 95% CI 1.13–2.30) among 2907 adults aged 70–84 years in Korea, using the CHS_PCF index. In France, Herr et al. [23] reported that polypharmacy with five to nine drugs (OR 1.77, 95% CI 1.20–2.61) and excessive polypharmacy with ten drugs or more (OR 4.47, 95% CI 2.37–8.42) were associated with physical frailty among 2350 adults aged 70 years and over in France, also using the CHS_PCF index. Another cross-sectional study in France reported that polypharmacy with five drugs or more and inappropriateness of medications were both associated with the CHS_PCF index score in people aged 65 and over [24]. Additionally, an eight-year longitudinal cohort study which involved 4402 participants in North America using the SOF scale also demonstrated that using four to six medications had a higher risk of frailty of 55% (hazard ratio [HR] 1.55; 95%CI 1.22–1.96), and using more than seven drugs increased this to approximately 147% (HR 2.47; 95% CI 1.78–3.43) [25]. A systematic review evaluated the correlation between frailty and polypharmacy and demonstrated that frailty was associated with polypharmacy, especially with an increasing number of medications used; however, the definitions of frailty and polypharmacy varied between each article [26]. We used three tools for the frailty evaluation and found a consistent trend in our study which matched these previous publications.

Polypharmacy is strongly associated with multi-morbidity, since one or more medications may be used for each illness [27]. However, polypharmacy has potential adverse effects including falls, cognitive impairment, adverse drug events, increased health care utilization, hospitalization, and mortality [28,29]. The potential mechanisms of these adverse outcomes were multidimensional. As age increases, changes in metabolism may result in drug toxicity and drug-drug interaction [30]. Decreased body weight, decreased blood pressure and dehydration are common in older people [31–33]. Overtreatment by antihypertensive medicines and diuretics may cause hypotension or dehydration, which are associated with frailty, falls, syncope, poor cognition, disability and mortality [30].

Frailty results from an accumulation of multiple age-related health issues, and not surprisingly is associated with increased pharmaceutical intervention [34]. Since more and more importance is attached to inappropriate polypharmacy, determining interventions to improve appropriate polypharmacy is essential. Davies [29] reported that polypharmacy was significantly associated with both prefrailty (pooled OR 1.52; 95% CI 1.32–1.79) and frailty (pooled OR 2.62, 95% CI 1.81–3.79). However, it was also found that almost all reviews identified polypharmacy by medication count; few examined the relationship between disease states and drug groups. Another systematic review found that there were no studies examining the negative effects of single drugs on frailty, and some specific medications had benefits and improvements with respect to physical performance, muscle strength or body composition [35]. Nwadiugwu [34] stated that person-centered care for frail people may provide better engagement with individuals to reduce the occurrence of polypharmacy. Providing the frail patients with a comprehensive geriatric assessment and using medication prescription aid with Beers criteria and the STOPP/START criteria may decrease unnecessary medication usage and reduce the extent of frailty and polypharmacy [36,37]. Furthermore, alternative prescriptive interventions such as regular exercise and social participation could reduce medication use as well as treat frailty [38].

This study found that low education level was associated with frailty status in the CHS_PCF model. Previous studies have examined the impact of educational level on frailty [39,40]. In a Dutch 13-year longitudinal study, Hoogendijk et al. demonstrated that low education levels in older adults had a higher OR of being frail compared with those with a high educational level (relative index of inequality OR 2.94; 95% CI 1.84–4.71) [39]. Another study in Brazil investigated patients with limited formal education (defined by 0–4 years of formal schooling) and found that having no formal education increased the odds ratio of being categorized as frail (OR 2.0; 95% CI 1.0–3.9) [40]. Furthermore, limited education was also associated with cognitive performance and functional disability [40]. Similar results have been reported by several studies [41,42]. Explanations for educational effects on frailty may be based on shared associated factors such as socioeconomic differences and low income which can result in lack of access to healthy food, obesity and living in deprived neighborhoods [43,44].

Living alone was not associated with frailty in our study in any of the three models. Multiple previous studies have reported that living alone had adverse health effects, such as social isolation, loneliness, as well as depression [45,46]. However, living alone was barely considered a risk factor for frailty. A systematic review found that living alone is associated with physical frailty in cross-sectional studies but not significant in longitudinal studies; furthermore, men living alone are more likely to be frail than women [47]. In a cross-sectional study that investigated 1602 Japanese men and women living on isolated islands reported that living alone was associated with frailty in men (OR 3.85; 95% CI 1.94–7.65), but not in women (OR 1.08; 95% CI 0.72–1.63) [48]. Another cross-sectional study also demonstrated that living alone is associated with frailty in Hong Kong men, but not in Hong Kong women or Taiwanese people [49]. A potential explanation is that women are thought to have larger or more diverse social networks than men [50]. Social networks may be an important confounding factor that influences the effect of living alone and multiple adverse effects [51]. Our study was conducted in a Taiwanese urban area, and the relationship between living alone and frailty may be affected by social networks which depend on differences in local policy and culture.

There are several limitations in this study. First, this is a cross-sectional study that could only demonstrate associations and could not infer causality. Further longitudinal study is required for the demonstration of causality between polypharmacy and frailty. Second, we used self-reported questionnaires, and the results may be influenced by recall biases involving memory, mood or cognition. Finally, we specially investigated a single area in an urban locale, which might not present the whole picture of Taiwan.

5. Conclusions

This study demonstrated that polypharmacy is associated with frailty under the 5-item FRAIL scale, CHS_PCF index, and SOF scale. Low educational level was associated with frailty using the Fried's phenotype model. More studies investigating the risk factors of frailty using different screening tools are needed, in order to further enhance our understanding of the risk of frailty among older adults and to design appropriate interventions.

Author Contributions: Conceptualization, C.-C.Y., C.-Y.L. and C.-Y.C.; Methodology, C.-C.Y. and C.-H.H.; Software, C.-C.Y. and H.-Y.C.; Formal analysis, C.-D.H., C.-C.Y. and H.-Y.C.; Investigation, C.-C.Y., S.C.-S.H. and S.-C.C.; Writing–original draft preparation, C.-D.H. and C.-C.Y.; Writing–review & editing, C.-C.Y., C.-H.H. and C.-H.K.; Supervision, C.-H.K. All authors have read and agreed to the published version of the manuscript.

Funding: This study was supported by grant from the Kaohsiung Municipal Siaogang Hospital (grant number: S-110-03).

Institutional Review Board Statement: The study was conducted according to the guidelines of the Declaration of Helsinki and approved by the Kaohsiung Medical University Hospital Institutional Review Board. The IRB number is KMUHIRB-F(I)-20200052.

Informed Consent Statement: Informed consent was obtained from all subjects involved in the study.

Data Availability Statement: The data presented in this study are available on request from the corresponding author. The data are not publicly available due to privacy issues.

Acknowledgments: We would like to thank all the participants, Hung-Pin Tu (Kaohsiung Medical University), and Yuh-Jyh Jong (Kaohsiung Medical University) for their cooperation.

Conflicts of Interest: The authors declare no conflict of interest.

References

1. Xue, Q.L. The frailty syndrome: Definition and natural history. *Clin. Geriatr. Med.* **2011**, *27*, 1–15. [CrossRef]
2. Makizako, H.; Shimada, H.; Doi, T.; Tsutsumimoto, K.; Suzuki, T. Impact of physical frailty on disability in community-dwelling older adults: A prospective cohort study. *BMJ Open* **2015**, *5*, e008462. [CrossRef] [PubMed]
3. Boyd, C.M.; Xue, Q.L.; Simpson, C.F.; Guralnik, J.M.; Fried, L.P. Frailty, hospitalization, and progression of disability in a cohort of disabled older women. *Am. J. Med.* **2005**, *118*, 1225–1231. [CrossRef] [PubMed]
4. McKenzie, K.; Ouellette-Kuntz, H.; Martin, L. Frailty as a Predictor of Institutionalization Among Adults With Intellectual and Developmental Disabilities. *Intellect. Dev. Disabil.* **2016**, *54*, 123–135. [CrossRef] [PubMed]
5. Siriwardhana, D.D.; Hardoon, S.; Rait, G.; Weerasinghe, M.C.; Walters, K.R. Prevalence of frailty and prefrailty among community-dwelling older adults in low-income and middle-income countries: A systematic review and meta-analysis. *BMJ Open* **2018**, *8*, e018195. [CrossRef] [PubMed]
6. O'Caoimh, R.; Galluzzo, L.; Rodríguez-Laso, Á.; Van der Heyden, J.; Ranhoff, A.H.; Lamprini-Koula, M.; Ciutan, M.; López-Samaniego, L.; Carcaillon-Bentata, L.; Kennelly, S.; et al. Prevalence of frailty at population level in European ADVANTAGE Joint Action Member States: A systematic review and meta-analysis. *Ann. Ist. Super. Sanita* **2018**, *54*, 226–238. [CrossRef]
7. Coelho-Junior, H.J.; Marzetti, E.; Picca, A.; Calvani, R.; Cesari, M.; Uchida, M.C. Prevalence of Prefrailty and Frailty in South America: A Systematic Review of Observational Studies. *J. Frailty Aging* **2020**, *9*, 197–213. [CrossRef]
8. Fried, L.P.; Tangen, C.M.; Walston, J.; Newman, A.B.; Hirsch, C.; Gottdiener, J.; Seeman, T.; Tracy, R.; Kop, W.J.; Burke, G.; et al. Frailty in older adults: Evidence for a phenotype. *J. Gerontol. A Biol. Sci. Med. Sci.* **2001**, *56*, M146–M157. [CrossRef] [PubMed]

9. Mitnitski, A.B.; Mogilner, A.J.; Rockwood, K. Accumulation of deficits as a proxy measure of aging. *Sci. World J.* **2001**, *1*, 323–336. [CrossRef] [PubMed]
10. Walston, J.; Buta, B.; Xue, Q.L. Frailty Screening and Interventions: Considerations for Clinical Practice. *Clin. Geriatr. Med.* **2018**, *34*, 25–38. [CrossRef] [PubMed]
11. Masnoon, N.; Shakib, S.; Kalisch-Ellett, L.; Caughey, G.E. What is polypharmacy? A systematic review of definitions. *BMC Geriatr.* **2017**, *17*, 230. [CrossRef]
12. Kim, J.; Parish, A.L. Polypharmacy and Medication Management in Older Adults. *Nurs. Clin. N. Am.* **2017**, *52*, 457–468. [CrossRef]
13. Onder, G.; Liperoti, R.; Foebel, A.; Fialova, D.; Topinkova, E.; van der Roest, H.G.; Gindin, J.; Cruz-Jentoft, A.J.; Fini, M.; Gambassi, G.; et al. Polypharmacy and mortality among nursing home residents with advanced cognitive impairment: Results from the SHELTER study. *J. Am. Med. Dir. Assoc.* **2013**, *14*, 450.e7-2. [CrossRef]
14. Glans, M.; Kragh Ekstam, A.; Jakobsson, U.; Bondesson, Å.; Midlöv, P. Risk factors for hospital readmission in older adults within 30 days of discharge—A comparative retrospective study. *BMC Geriatr.* **2020**, *20*, 467. [CrossRef] [PubMed]
15. Sakamoto, J.I.; Shikata, T.; Ito, S.; Kimura, T.; Takamoto, K.; Manabe, E.; Asakura, M.; Ishihara, M.; Tsujino, T. Polypharmacy Is Associated with Accelerated Deterioration of Renal Function in Cardiovascular Outpatients. *Cardiol. Res.* **2020**, *11*, 15–21. [CrossRef]
16. Rodrigues, M.C.; Oliveira, C. Drug-drug interactions and adverse drug reactions in polypharmacy among older adults: An integrative review. *Rev. Lat. Am. Enfermagem.* **2016**, *24*, e2800. [CrossRef] [PubMed]
17. Nobili, A.; Garattini, S.; Mannucci, P.M. Multiple diseases and polypharmacy in the elderly: Challenges for the internist of the third millennium. *J. Comorb.* **2011**, *1*, 28–44. [CrossRef]
18. Wu, Y.H.; Lee, H.N.; Chang, Y.S.; Wu, C.H.; Wang, C.J. Depressive symptoms were a common risk factor for pre-frailty and frailty in patients with Alzheimer's disease. *Arch. Gerontol. Geriatr.* **2020**, *89*, 104067. [CrossRef] [PubMed]
19. Chan, D.C.; Tsou, H.H.; Yang, R.S.; Tsauo, J.Y.; Chen, C.Y.; Hsiung, C.A.; Kuo, K.N. A pilot randomized controlled trial to improve geriatric frailty. *BMC Geriatr.* **2012**, *12*, 58. [CrossRef] [PubMed]
20. Ensrud, K.E.; Ewing, S.K.; Taylor, B.C.; Fink, H.A.; Cawthon, P.M.; Stone, K.L.; Hillier, T.A.; Cauley, J.A.; Hochberg, M.C.; Rodondi, N.; et al. Comparison of 2 frailty indexes for prediction of falls, disability, fractures, and death in older women. *Arch. Intern. Med.* **2008**, *168*, 382–389. [CrossRef] [PubMed]
21. Jung, H.W.; Yoo, H.J.; Park, S.Y.; Kim, S.W.; Choi, J.Y.; Yoon, S.J.; Kim, C.H.; Kim, K.I. The Korean version of the FRAIL scale: Clinical feasibility and validity of assessing the frailty status of Korean elderly. *Korean J. Intern. Med.* **2016**, *31*, 594–600. [CrossRef] [PubMed]
22. Jung, H.; Kim, M.; Lee, Y.; Won, C.W. Prevalence of Physical Frailty and Its Multidimensional Risk Factors in Korean Community-Dwelling Older Adults: Findings from Korean Frailty and Aging Cohort Study. *Int. J. Environ. Res. Public Health* **2020**, *17*, 7883. [CrossRef] [PubMed]
23. Herr, M.; Robine, J.M.; Pinot, J.; Arvieu, J.J.; Ankri, J. Polypharmacy and frailty: Prevalence, relationship, and impact on mortality in a French sample of 2350 old people. *Pharmacoepidemiol. Drug Saf.* **2015**, *24*, 637–646. [CrossRef] [PubMed]
24. Herr, M.; Sirven, N.; Grondin, H.; Pichetti, S.; Sermet, C. Frailty, polypharmacy, and potentially inappropriate medications in old people: Findings in a representative sample of the French population. *Eur. J. Clin. Pharmacol.* **2017**, *73*, 1165–1172. [CrossRef] [PubMed]
25. Veronese, N.; Stubbs, B.; Noale, M.; Solmi, M.; Pilotto, A.; Vaona, A.; Demurtas, J.; Mueller, C.; Huntley, J.; Crepaldi, G.; et al. Polypharmacy Is Associated With Higher Frailty Risk in Older People: An 8-Year Longitudinal Cohort Study. *J. Am. Med. Dir. Assoc.* **2017**, *18*, 624–628. [CrossRef]
26. Gutiérrez-Valencia, M.; Izquierdo, M.; Cesari, M.; Casas-Herrero, A.; Inzitari, M.; Martínez-Velilla, N. The relationship between frailty and polypharmacy in older people: A systematic review. *Br. J. Clin. Pharmacol.* **2018**, *84*, 1432–1444. [CrossRef]
27. Mannucci, P.M.; Nobili, A. Multimorbidity and polypharmacy in the elderly: Lessons from REPOSI. *Intern. Emerg. Med.* **2014**, *9*, 723–734. [CrossRef]
28. Hilmer, S.N.; Gnjidic, D. The effects of polypharmacy in older adults. *Clin. Pharmacol. Ther.* **2009**, *85*, 86–88. [CrossRef]
29. Davies, L.E.; Spiers, G.; Kingston, A.; Todd, A.; Adamson, J.; Hanratty, B. Adverse Outcomes of Polypharmacy in Older People: Systematic Review of Reviews. *J. Am. Med. Dir. Assoc.* **2020**, *21*, 181–187. [CrossRef]
30. Rolland, Y.; Morley, J.E. Editorial: Frailty and Polypharmacy. *J. Nutr. Health Aging* **2016**, *20*, 645–646. [CrossRef]
31. Morley, J.E. Weight loss in older persons: New therapeutic approaches. *Curr. Pharm. Des.* **2007**, *13*, 3637–3647. [CrossRef]
32. Morley, J.E. Treatment of hypertension in older persons: What is the evidence? *Drugs Aging* **2014**, *31*, 331–337. [CrossRef]
33. Thomas, D.R.; Cote, T.R.; Lawhorne, L.; Levenson, S.A.; Rubenstein, L.Z.; Smith, D.A.; Stefanacci, R.G.; Tangalos, E.G.; Morley, J.E. Understanding clinical dehydration and its treatment. *J. Am. Med. Dir. Assoc.* **2008**, *9*, 292–301. [CrossRef] [PubMed]
34. Nwadiugwu, M.C. Frailty and the Risk of Polypharmacy in the Older Person: Enabling and Preventative Approaches. *J. Aging Res.* **2020**, *2020*, 6759521. [CrossRef]
35. Pazan, F.; Petrovic, M.; Cherubini, A.; Onder, G.; Cruz-Jentoft, A.J.; Denkinger, M.; van der Cammen, T.J.M.; Stevenson, J.M.; Ibrahim, K.; Rajkumar, C.; et al. Current evidence on the impact of medication optimization or pharmacological interventions on frailty or aspects of frailty: A systematic review of randomized controlled trials. *Eur. J. Clin. Pharmacol.* **2021**, *77*, 1–12. [CrossRef] [PubMed]

36. Stange, K.C. The problem of fragmentation and the need for integrative solutions. *Ann. Fam. Med.* **2009**, *7*, 100–103. [CrossRef] [PubMed]
37. Turner, G.; Clegg, A. Best practice guidelines for the management of frailty: A British Geriatrics Society, Age UK and Royal College of General Practitioners report. *Age Ageing* **2014**, *43*, 744–747. [CrossRef]
38. Morley, J.E.; Vellas, B.; van Kan, G.A.; Anker, S.D.; Bauer, J.M.; Bernabei, R.; Cesari, M.; Chumlea, W.C.; Doehner, W.; Evans, J.; et al. Frailty consensus: A call to action. *J. Am. Med. Dir. Assoc.* **2013**, *14*, 392–397. [CrossRef]
39. Hoogendijk, E.O.; van Hout, H.P.; Heymans, M.W.; van der Horst, H.E.; Frijters, D.H.; Broese van Groenou, M.I.; Deeg, D.J.; Huisman, M. Explaining the association between educational level and frailty in older adults: Results from a 13-year longitudinal study in the Netherlands. *Ann. Epidemiol.* **2014**, *24*, 538–544.e2. [CrossRef]
40. Brigola, A.G.; Alexandre, T.D.S.; Inouye, K.; Yassuda, M.S.; Pavarini, S.C.I.; Mioshi, E. Limited formal education is strongly associated with lower cognitive status, functional disability and frailty status in older adults. *Dement. Neuropsychol.* **2019**, *13*, 216–224. [CrossRef]
41. Torres, J.L.; Dias, R.C.; Ferreira, F.R.; Macinko, J.; Lima-Costa, M.F. Functional performance and social relations among the elderly in Greater Metropolitan Belo Horizonte, Minas Gerais State, Brazil: A population-based epidemiological study. *Cad. Saude Publica* **2014**, *30*, 1018–1028. [CrossRef] [PubMed]
42. Groffen, D.A.; Bosma, H.; Tan, F.E.; van den Akker, M.; Kempen, G.I.; van Eijk, J.T. Material vs. psychosocial explanations of old-age educational differences in physical and mental functioning. *Eur. J. Public Health* **2012**, *22*, 587–592. [CrossRef] [PubMed]
43. Stringhini, S.; Sabia, S.; Shipley, M.; Brunner, E.; Nabi, H.; Kivimaki, M.; Singh-Manoux, A. Association of socioeconomic position with health behaviors and mortality. *JAMA* **2010**, *303*, 1159–1166. [CrossRef] [PubMed]
44. Lang, I.A.; Hubbard, R.E.; Andrew, M.K.; Llewellyn, D.J.; Melzer, D.; Rockwood, K. Neighborhood deprivation, individual socioeconomic status, and frailty in older adults. *J. Am. Geriatr. Soc.* **2009**, *57*, 1776–1780. [CrossRef]
45. Grenade, L.; Boldy, D. Social isolation and loneliness among older people: Issues and future challenges in community and residential settings. *Aust. Health Rev.* **2008**, *32*, 468–478. [CrossRef]
46. Xiu-Ying, H.; Qian, C.; Xiao-Dong, P.; Xue-Mei, Z.; Chang-Quan, H. Living arrangements and risk for late life depression: A meta-analysis of published literature. *Int. J. Psychiatry Med.* **2012**, *43*, 19–34. [CrossRef]
47. Kojima, G.; Taniguchi, Y.; Kitamura, A.; Fujiwara, Y. Is living alone a risk factor of frailty? A systematic review and meta-analysis. *Ageing Res. Rev.* **2020**, *59*, 101048. [CrossRef]
48. Yamanashi, H.; Shimizu, Y.; Nelson, M.; Koyamatsu, J.; Nagayoshi, M.; Kadota, K.; Tamai, M.; Ariyoshi, K.; Maeda, T. The association between living alone and frailty in a rural Japanese population: The Nagasaki Islands study. *J. Prim. Health Care* **2015**, *7*, 269–273. [CrossRef]
49. Yu, R.; Wu, W.C.; Leung, J.; Hu, S.C.; Woo, J. Frailty and Its Contributory Factors in Older Adults: A Comparison of Two Asian Regions (Hong Kong and Taiwan). *Int. J. Environ. Res. Public Health* **2017**, *14*, 1096. [CrossRef]
50. Ajrouch, K.J.; Blandon, A.Y.; Antonucci, T.C. Social networks among men and women: The effects of age and socioeconomic status. *J. Gerontol. B Psychol. Sci. Soc. Sci.* **2005**, *60*, S311–S317. [CrossRef]
51. Sakurai, R.; Kawai, H.; Suzuki, H.; Kim, H.; Watanabe, Y.; Hirano, H.; Ihara, K.; Obuchi, S.; Fujiwara, Y. Poor Social Network, Not Living Alone, Is Associated With Incidence of Adverse Health Outcomes in Older Adults. *J. Am. Med. Dir. Assoc.* **2019**, *20*, 1438–1443. [CrossRef] [PubMed]

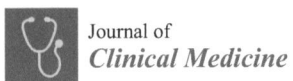

Article

Predictive Model for the Assessment of Preoperative Frailty Risk in the Elderly

Sang-Wook Lee [1], Jae-Sik Nam [1], Ye-Jee Kim [2], Min-Ju Kim [2], Jeong-Hyun Choi [3], Eun-Ho Lee [1], Kyoung-Woon Joung [1,*] and In-Cheol Choi [1]

[1] Asan Medical Center, Department of Anesthesiology and Pain Medicine, University of Ulsan College of Medicine, Seoul 05505, Korea; sangwooklee20@gmail.com (S.-W.L.); jaesik_nam@naver.com (J.-S.N.); leho@naver.com (E.-H.L.); icchoi@amc.seoul.kr (I.-C.C.)

[2] Asan Medical Center, Department of Clinical Epidemiology and Biostatistics, University of Ulsan College of Medicine, Seoul 05505, Korea; kimyejee@amc.seoul.kr (Y.-J.K.); minjukim@amc.seoul.kr (M.-J.K.)

[3] Department of Anesthesiology and Pain Medicine, College of Medicine, Kyung Hee University, Seoul 02453, Korea; choikhang@gmail.com

* Correspondence: baram0403@naver.com; Tel.: +82-2-3010-1516; Fax: +82-2-3010-6790

Abstract: Adequate preoperative evaluation of frailty can greatly assist in the efficient allocation of hospital resources and planning treatments. However, most of the previous frailty evaluation methods, which are complicated, time-consuming, and can have inter-evaluator error, are difficult to apply in urgent situations. Thus, the authors aimed to develop and validate a predictive model for pre-operative frailty risk of elderly patients by using diagnostic and operation codes, which can be obtained easily and quickly from electronic records. We extracted the development cohort of 1762 people who were hospitalized for emergency operations at a single institution between 1 January 2012 and 31 December 2016. The temporal validation cohort from 1 January 2017 to 31 December 2018 in the same center was set. External validation was conducted on 6432 patients aged 75 years or older from 2012 to 2015 who had emergency surgery in the Korean national health insurance database. We developed the Operation Frailty Risk Score (OFRS) by assessing the association of Operation Group and Hospital Frailty Risk Score with the 90-day mortality through logistic regression analysis. We validated the OFRS in both the temporal validation cohort and two external validation cohorts. In the temporal validation cohort and the external validation cohort I and II, the c-statistics for OFRS to predict 90-day mortality were 0.728, 0.626, and 0.619, respectively. OFRS from these diagnostic codes and operation codes may help evaluate the peri-operative frailty risk before emergency surgery for elderly patients where history-taking and pre-operative testing cannot be performed.

Keywords: frailty; emergency operation; elderly; hospital frailty risk score

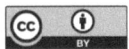

1. Introduction

Aging is an inevitable process that is measured by chronological age. There are no definite criteria for an age at which one becomes "elderly", but according to the WHO, people aged 65 or older are classified as elderly. The number of elderly patients who undergo surgery has increased rapidly, and their age is increasing dramatically as the proportion of elderly in the population increases [1,2]. Some elderly patients with more serious adverse outcomes than in the usual clinical course have come to be called frail. Frailty describes decreased physiological reserves across multiple organ systems and increased vulnerability to disability, but it happens at different rates in different people; hence, there is a high risk for poor results given an apparently innocuous stimulus in geriatric patients [3]. Surgical stress can be a clinically significant issue for the frail in geriatric medicine [4]. Frailty in elderly surgical patients increases not only postoperative mortality and morbidity, but also the likelihood of experiencing postoperative complications and the tendency to incur more hospital costs [5–7]. In particular, pre-operative frailty in the emergency setting has a greater impact on poor clinical outcomes [8–12].

Pre-operative assessment of frailty can be helpful for the efficient application of hospital resources and planning treatments [13]. However, most of the previous evaluation systems for frailty, which can be complicated, time-consuming, and subject to inter-operator error, are difficult to apply in urgent situations requiring emergency surgery [14,15]. There are currently no relevant tools to measure peri-operative frailty risk for elderly patients undergoing emergency surgery. Almost all emergency operations have been performed without proper assessment of frailty risk; there was not enough time to do so, as previous methods of frailty risk assessment required many laboratory or clinical test results. In a previous study, there was a rapid frailty-risk evaluation method called Hospital Frailty Risk Score (HFRS) that used International Statistical Classification of Diseases and Related Health Problems, Tenth Revision (ICD-10) codes, which are diagnostic codes, but it was not a model designed for surgical patients [16].

Therefore, we aimed to create a predictive model to assess the pre-operative frailty risk of elderly patients by using diagnostic codes and operation codes that can be easily and quickly obtained from the electronic medical recording system in situations where pre-operative clinical information is insufficient, such as emergency surgery.

2. Materials and Methods

This study was a nationwide cohort study using the Korean National Health Insurance Database (KNHID) and a dataset from the electronic medical records of a tertiary academic center. This study was approved by the Ethics Committee (AMC IRB 2019-1145), and written informed consent was waived for retrospective data analysis. In this study, datasets from four cohorts were needed. Figure 1 shows the flow chart of the patients in this study.

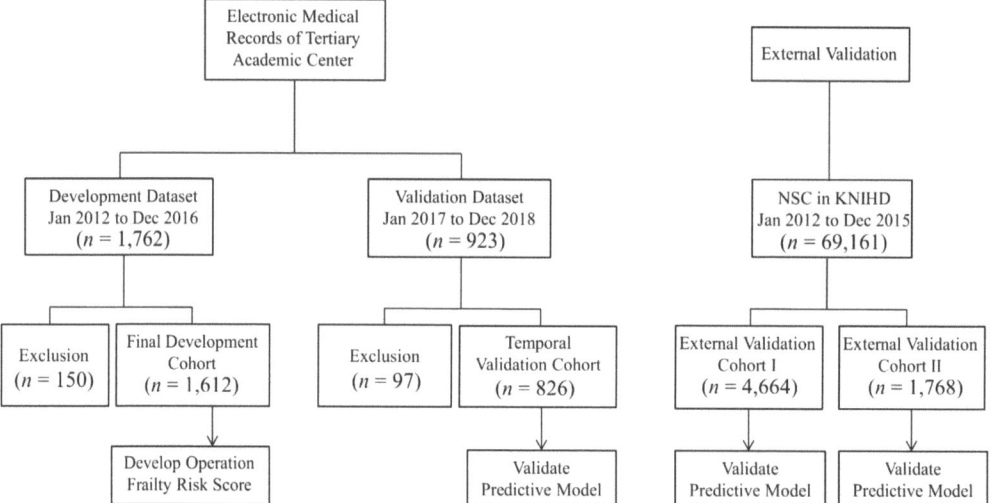

Figure 1. Diagram of the study dataset analysis. Four cohort datasets for the development and validation of predictive models. NSC, Normal Sample Cohort; KNHID, Korean National Health Insurance Database.

2.1. Development Cohort and Temporal Validation Cohort

We extracted the development cohort of people who were hospitalized for emergency operations at a single institution between 1 January 2012 and 31 December 2016. We also extracted the temporal validation cohort of people aged 75 years and older who were admitted for emergency surgeries performed from 1 January 2017 to 31 December 2018 in the same center. In this study, emergency operations were defined as an operation that can claim emergency medical management fees for patients who were admitted to the hospital through the emergency department to undergo emergency surgery or an additional charge on the night or holiday/weekend if the surgery was performed after the evening of the week or during the holiday/weekend.

We included 1612 patients aged 75 years and older from the electronic medical records of our hospital as the development cohort, excluding those whose follow-up was lost or those who lacked a pre-operative operation code. We limited elderly patients to patients 75 years and older as the HFRS presented in the previous study was created for patients 75 years of age and older [16], and it is intended to be used in our study. The operation codes were claiming codes for claiming health insurance fees from the Korean National Health Insurance Service (KNHIS).

The authors of this study classified all operation codes extracted from the development cohort into a total of 8 Operation Groups (OG) according to surgical risk. The classification of operation codes was created by two clinical experts (SWL and EHL) using their clinical experience, pre-existing studies related to surgical risk, and the American College of Surgeons National Surgical Quality Improvement Program (ACS NSQIP) surgical risk calculators [17], and another clinical expert (JSN) independently checked and verified the classification of the operation codes. In the case of different opinions among experts in the classification of operation codes, the decision was made in the direction recognized by more experts by further reflecting the verification and opinions of other experts. Operations with a higher risk were classified as an increase from OG 1 to OG 8. For example, an operation code with low risk, such as "N7133" (Mastectomy) or "P4551" (Total thyroidectomy), was classified in Group 1, while an operation code with high risk, such as "O2033" (Resection of thoracic aorta aneurysm), was classified as Group 8. Table S1 shows the operation codes classified into 8 groups. The dataset of the development cohort included information about the operation codes, diagnostic codes, and death after surgery. The primary clinical outcome of this study was 90-day all-cause mortality, which was defined as the death rate within 90 days after surgery regardless of discharge.

2.2. Operation Frailty Risk Score

In the previous study, the HFRS was developed by using cluster analysis in such a way that scores were given for ICD-10 codes that were at least twice as prevalent in the frail group as in the other groups [16]. In this study, we created an Operation Frailty Risk Score (OFRS) by performing univariate and multivariable logistic regression analysis of the mortality within 90 days after surgery according to the operation codes of the 8 groups classified as described above, the HFRS score calculated from the diagnosis codes, age, and sex. A simple scoring system was developed using the penalized maximum likelihood estimates of the covariates in models that followed the method of Sullivan et al. [18]. After selecting a reference group of each variable, we used regression coefficients as weights and the distance from the reference group to generate each point value. Score 1 was defined as the effect of a 10-year increase in age. Through this analysis, we developed a risk scoring system of the predictive model for pre-operative frailty based on the mortality within 90 days after the operation. Based on this defined score, scores were assigned to each of the eight operation risk groups, age, and HFRS by comparing and analyzing the effects of each variable on mortality within 90 days after the operation. Table 1 summarizes the OFRS points for each variable.

2.3. External Validation on the Korean National Health Insurance Database

The KNHID cohort used in this study was extracted from the National Sample Cohort provided by KNHIS version 2.0 (NHIS-NSC v2.0). The NHIS-NSC v2.0 is a population-based cohort database containing clinical data of about one million patients, 2% of the sample data, which represents all national health insurance subscribers in South Korea. For external validation, we extracted patients aged 75 years or older from 2012 to 2015 who had emergency surgery in the NHIS-NSC v2.0. For external validation dataset I, we selected data considering the type of medical institutions and excluded data from clinics, which are the primary care providers. For external validation dataset II, we applied further restrictions considering the location of the medical institution, including the capital area of Seoul and Gyeonggi-do. We extracted information about the diagnostic code based on the ICD-10 and the operation code from NHIS-NSC v2.0 and evaluated the predicted model.

Table 1. Operation frailty risk scoring system for prediction of 90-day mortality.

Variables	Categories	Point
Age	75–79	0
	80–89	1
	≥90	2
HFRS	0	0
	1–4	1
	≥5	2
Operation Group	Group 1	0
	Group 2	1
	Group 3	0
	Group 4	2
	Group 5	4
	Group 6	4
	Group 7	4
	Group 8	6

HFRS—hospital frailty risk score.

2.4. Statistical Analysis

Categorical variables are represented by numbers and percentages, while continuous variables are represented by means and standard deviations or median and interquartile range. We constructed univariate and multivariable logistic regression models to assess the association with other variables, including the HFRS and the 90-day mortality rate. Internal and external validations of the risk scoring system model were performed separately by measuring the calibration and discrimination ability. The c-statistic was used to estimate the predictive performance of the models. The calibration plot and Hosmer-Lemeshow goodness-of-fit statistic was used to evaluate the agreement between the observed and expected number of 90-days mortality across all strata, based on the probabilities of 90-day mortality estimated from the prediction model. We compared the prediction of OFRS for the pre-operative frailty risk in each dataset. For all analyses, a $p < 0.05$ was considered significant. All statistical analyses were completed using the "R" statistical language (R version 3.5.1, R Foundation for Statistical Computing, Vienna, Austria) and "SAS" Enterprise Guide ver. 7.1 (SAS Institute Inc., Cary, NC, USA).

3. Results

The data characteristics of the four cohorts are shown in Table 2. Comparing the four cohort groups reveals that the 90-day mortality rates of the four groups were different at a statistically significant level (p-value < 0.001). The 90-day mortality rate of the development cohort was 8.9%, whereas the 90-day mortality rate of the temporal validation cohort and the external validation cohort I and II was 8.4%, 13.8%, and 12.3%, respectively. In addition, the distribution of HFRS was also different in each data group. The HFRS distribution of cohort 1 and 2 showed a leftward skewed distribution pattern compared to the HFRS distribution of cohort 3 and 4.

We analyzed the distribution of emergency operations by surgical department received by the elderly patients, along with the analysis of the operation codes. According to the results for the distribution of emergency operations, an operation in the general surgery department was the most frequent in the development and temporal datasets, whereas the proportion of orthopedic surgeries was the highest in the external validation datasets. Figure S1 shows the distribution of emergency operations by surgical department in each dataset.

Table 2. Characteristics of the four cohorts.

	Cohort 1	Cohort 2	Cohort 3	Cohort 4	p Value
N	1612	826	4664	1768	
Age, years	78 (76–82)	78 (76–82)	80 (77–84)	80 (77–84)	<0.001
Male	862 (53.5)	445 (53.9)	2777 (59.5)	1047 (59.2)	<0.001
90-day death	143 (8.9)	69 (8.4)	643 (13.8)	217 (12.3)	<0.001
HFRS					<0.001
0	718 (44.5)	416 (50.4)	413 (8.9)	186 (10.5)	
1–4	683 (42.4)	335 (40.6)	2033 (43.6)	780 (44.1)	
≥5	211 (13.1)	75 (9.1)	2218 (47.6)	802 (45.4)	

Data are presented as the median (interquartile range) or number (percentage). Cohort 1, development cohort; Cohort 2, temporal validation cohort; Cohort 3, external validation cohort I; Cohort 4, external validation cohort II; HFRS—hospital frailty risk score.

In the development cohort, the distribution of HFRS scores was less than 5 points by 86.9%, and most were classified into the low-risk group. Therefore, due to this skewed distribution, risk stratification was performed by classifying the HFRS score with the new criteria instead of the risk classification suggested in the previous study. We re-categorized HFRS as low risk for 0 points, intermediate risk between 1 and 4 points, and high risk if above 5 points. The results of the logistic regression analyses of the risk scores for the 90-day mortality rate are summarized in Table S2. As a result of the multivariable regression analysis based on the 90-day mortality rate of the HFRS, group 2, with 1 to 4 points of HFRS, had an odds ratio increased to 1.55 compared to risk group 1 with 0 points of HFRS. However, in the risk group 3, with 5 points or more of HFRS, the risk of a poor outcome increased with an odds ratio of 2.06 compared to the risk group 1. Table 1 summarizes the points assigned to each variable.

The OFRS is distributed in the range of 0 to 10, and it is skewed to the left in the distribution graph for each score in four cohorts (Figure 2). Additionally, Figure S2 shows the distribution of OFRS for each surgical departments. According to the distribution of mortality rate according to OFRS, OFRS was classified as low risk if it was less than 2, high risk if it was greater than 4, and intermediate risk if it was between them (Table 3). Table 3 shows the overall predictive performance of the OFRS model proposed in this study in each cohort. In the temporal validation dataset, 237 (28.7%) were categorized as low risk, 355 (43.0%) as intermediate risk, and 234 (28.3%) as high risk. In the external validation dataset I, 644 (13.8%) were categorized as low risk, 3027 (64.9%) as intermediate risk, and 993 (21.3%) as high risk. In external validation dataset II, 251 (14.2%) were categorized as low risk, 1132 (64.0%) as intermediate risk, and 385 (21.8%) as high risk. From the results, it can be seen that the OFRS of the intermediated risk is more distributed in the external validation dataset than in the development and internal validation dataset. Different distributions of OFRS in these datasets affect predictive performance, and calibration performance declines.

Table 3. Characteristics and prediction performance of OFRS for 90-day mortality in each cohort.

		Cohort 1	Cohort 2	Cohort 3	Cohort 4
OFRS	Low risk (0–1)	458 (28.4)	237 (28.7)	644 (13.8)	251 (14.2)
	Intermediate risk (2–4)	759 (47.1)	355 (43.0)	3027 (64.9)	1132 (64.0)
	High risk (≥ 5)	395 (24.5)	234 (28.3)	993 (21.3)	385 (21.8)
Discrimination ability, c-statics (CI)		0.682 (0.635–0.728)	0.728 (0.665–0.791)	0.626 (0.602–0.649)	0.619 (0.580–0.658)
Calibration ability, Hosmer and Lemeshow Test	χ^2	3.80	4.88	102.63	20.47
	DF	5	5	5	5
	p value	0.579	0.430	<0.001	0.001

Data are presented as the number (percentage). OFRS—operation frailty risk score; Cohort 1, development cohort; Cohort 2, temporal validation cohort; Cohort 3, external validation cohort I; Cohort 4, external validation cohort II; CI—confidence interval; and DF—degrees of freedom.

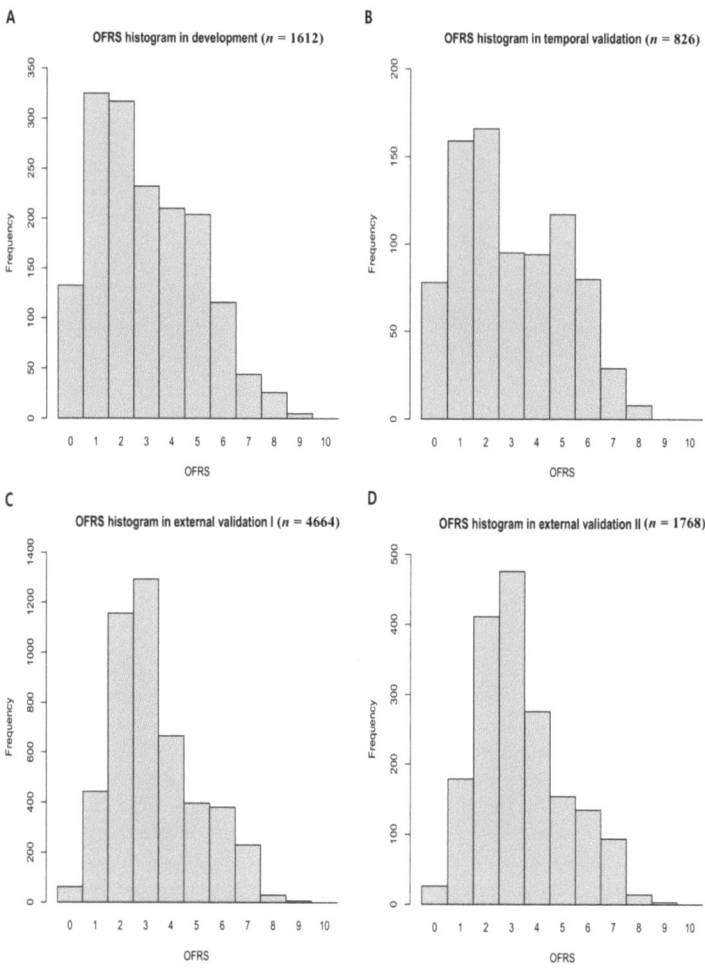

Figure 2. Distribution of the OFRS in (**A**) development cohort, (**B**) temporal validation cohort, (**C**) external validation cohort I, and (**D**) external validation cohort II. The OFRS is distributed in the range of 0 to 10. OFRS, operation frailty risk score.

Internal and External Validation

We calculated the OFRS by using the operation code and HFRS calculated from the diagnosis code in each cohort. Table 3 shows the prediction performance of OFRS in each cohort. The c-statistic for internal validation of the OFRS to predict 90-day mortality was 0.682, while the c-statistic for OFRS in the temporal validation cohort and the external validation cohort I and II was 0.728, 0.626, and 0.619, respectively. Figure 3 shows the calibration of the developed OFRS model to predict outcomes in each cohort. These graphs are calibration plots showing the relationship between the real values and the predicted values of the developed OFRS model for 90-day mortality (Figure 3). Figure 4 shows the relationship between these OFRS and the 90-day mortality rate by plotting the 90-day mortality rate according to the risk scores in each validation cohort. It can be seen that the mortality rate increases as the risk scores increase.

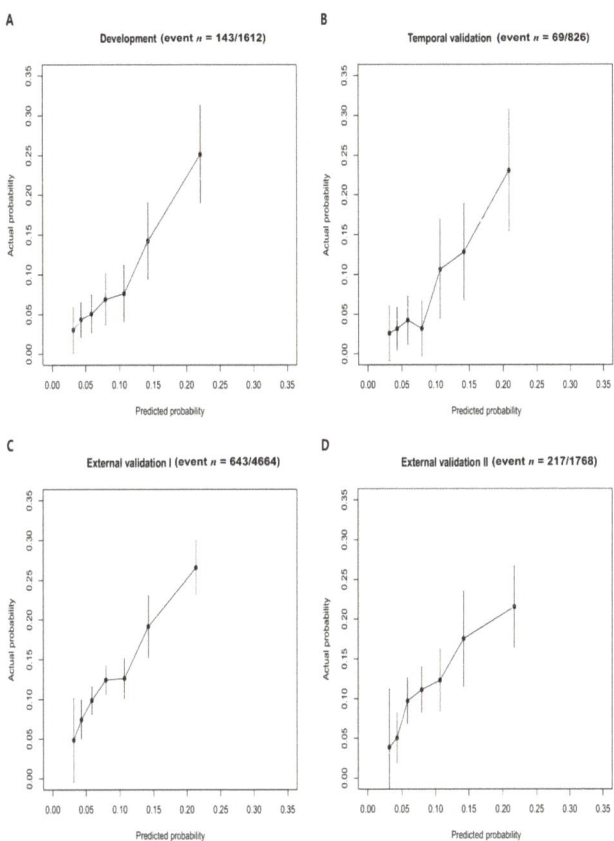

Figure 3. Calibration plot of OFRS in (**A**) development cohort, (**B**) temporal validation cohort, (**C**) external validation cohort I, and (**D**) external validation cohort II. OFRS, operation frailty risk score.

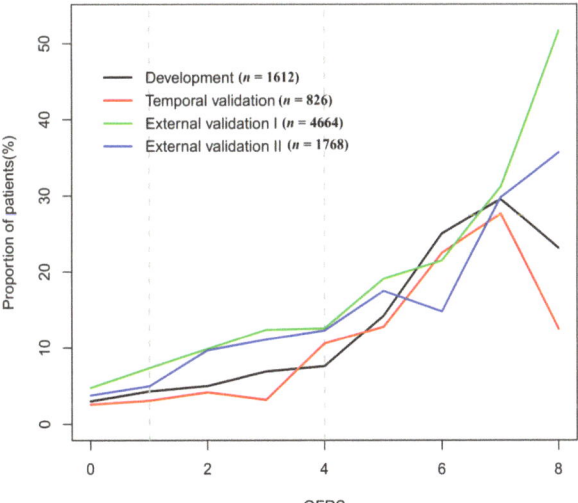

Figure 4. Association between OFRS and 90-day mortality by plotting the 90-day mortality rate according to the risk scores in each cohort. OFRS, operation frailty risk score.

4. Discussion

The main findings of this study are that OFRS, developed by using diagnostic codes and operation code information, can help predict the 90-day postoperative mortality rate, one of the indicators for pre-operative frailty when elderly patients undergo emergency surgery. Although functional improvement and decline have recently been suggested as important outcomes in elderly patients undergoing surgery, 90-day all-cause mortality rate, which has been dealt with a major postoperative clinical outcome, was set as the primary outcome in our study [19]. In the national validation cohort used for external validation, those with a higher OFRS score had higher rates of 90-day mortality, although the discriminative ability of the predictive model was low.

For elderly patients undergoing emergency surgery, pre-operative risk assessment is very important in clinical practice. In elderly patients, a high prevalence of frailty is likely to lead to postoperative adverse outcomes and vulnerability to surgical stress [4,13]. Two main models previously suggested for evaluating frailty are the phenotype model [20], and the cumulative deficit model [21]. The phenotype model proposed by Fried and colleagues was developed with five phenotypes that are largely related to frailty, and they defined "frail" as when the phenotype has more than three factors. The cumulative deficit model was defined as the proportion of each variable to the total deficits related to frailty, and they showed the correlation between the index and adverse outcomes by evaluating frailty based on this model [22]. All of these models are too complex and difficult to apply in an actual clinical setting, as it is not easy to obtain the values of each variable.

In patients undergoing emergency surgery, there have been previous studies that have tried to measure the pre-operative frailty and to determine its correlation with the postoperative outcome [8–11]. Pre-operative frailty in emergency surgical settings mostly increased the risk of postoperative mortality and longer hospital stays. Some of the previous studies on frailty in emergency surgical settings have measured frailty using the Clinical Frailty Scale [9,12,15]. It is a relatively easy and fast frailty measurement tool in the clinical setting, but it has limitations in terms of inter-operator reliability [23]. Some other studies measured pre-operative frailty in emergency surgical patients by using assessment tools such as the Modified Fried's Frailty Criteria, the Modified Frailty Index-11, the FRAIL scale, the Triage Risk Screening Tool, and the Share-Frailty Index, and tried to determine the relationship between the measured frailty and the clinical outcome [24,25]. However, all of these tools are difficult to apply when the patient is unconscious or without present caregivers, as the methods previously proposed rely on questionnaires or require direct tests such as measurement of grip strength or walking speed.

There was a previous attempt to measure the frailty risk by using hospital electronic medical records, called HFRS, and it may be useful for measuring the frailty risk for application in acute care settings [16]. However, as the HFRS is a model developed for patients hospitalized through an emergency department, there are some limitations to applying it to surgical patients. Therefore, in order to overcome these limitations, more generally applicable frailty measurement tools are required in the emergency surgical setting. A recent study showed that both pre-operative frailty and operative stress increased postoperative mortality [6,26]. Thus, the factors of operative stress must be reflected in the pre-operative frailty risk assessment of surgical patients.

Therefore, we created an integrated frailty risk assessment tool that reflects these surgical stress factors. The OFRS proposed in this study has the advantage that it can be applied easily and quickly in emergency situations as it utilizes diagnostic codes and operation code information that can be automatically extracted from the hospital database. It is an automatic risk score that can be systematically obtained by using information from both codes without relying on the subjectivity of the clinician. It is a very useful model for elderly patients that need emergency surgery as it does not require clinical information other than the diagnostic and operation codes. Additionally, we made it possible to use the risk predictive model more reliably with wide applicability by using the insurance claiming code, which is one of the criteria commonly used by all hospitals, rather than inspection items with different standards for different hospitals.

The c-statistics of the final model in the temporal validation cohort and both external validation cohorts are 0.728, 0.626, and 0.619, respectively, in predicting the clinical outcome. Thus, our model did not show a better prediction performance than the previous model for acute-care settings showing c-statistics ranging from 0.54 to 0.73 [14,27]. Similar to the previous study [16], our scores did not have strong discriminative ability as there are unpredictable factors that affect individual outcomes in emergency situations. However, it is a predictor, which is designed for risk stratification, worth considering for application in an emergency situation where it is difficult to predict a patient's clinical outcomes.

As the clinical setting changes according to the size and location of the hospital, it affects the clinical outcome [28,29]. In this study, the external validation of the OFRS was corrected according to the clinical environment change according to the size of the hospital and the location of the hospital. External validation dataset I extracted only hospital-level data, excluding data from clinics, and external validation dataset II applied further restrictions considering the location of the medical institution by extracting data from the capital area, geographically close to the hospital from which the dataset used to develop OFRS was extracted. In the two external datasets, the c-statistics of this model did not show significant gains in prediction performance, despite corrections according to hospital size and region. However, even within the same region, there is a considerable difference in the size of hospitals and the severity of patients, so it is expected that better predictive performance can be achieved if corrections are made for these areas in future studies.

The clinical significance of this study is that if the information about the patient is extremely limited in an urgent situation, such as emergency surgery, the patient's risk can be grasped in advance by using the hospital's computerized system quickly and promptly. The strength of our model is that no test results are required before surgery. There is also no need for complicated calculations to estimate the risk. As far as we know, this study is the first to predict the pre-operative risk by using only diagnostic and operation codes for surgical patients.

This study has limitations in several areas. First, it cannot safely be generalized to other clinical settings and other locations, as this model was constructed from the clinical data of a single center. As there may be differences in postoperative outcomes depending on the hospital environment, it is necessary to verify the model in various medical institutions and upgrade the model in order to have more value. In addition, developing a predictive model based on data from as many different medical institutions as possible in future studies could be a useful pre-operative risk-predictive model with broader applicability. Furthermore, it was not known whether this predictive model could be applied to other countries, especially other races, as it was developed in South Korea, which is known as an ethnically homogenous country. As the operation code in this study is the insurance claiming code commonly used in South Korea, it is difficult to apply the operation code to other countries. In order to apply this model to other countries, operation codes should be the codes that are commonly used worldwide, such as the ICD-Procedure Coding System code [30]. Therefore, future studies using this worldwide operation code for wider usability will need to verify whether the model is validated globally by using data from different races and countries. Second, another limitation of this study is that, although three clinical experts classified the OG by referring to their clinical experience, pre-existing risk prediction models, and previous studies on clinical outcomes, the subjective opinion of the clinician influenced the classification of the OG. It is expected that better results will be produced if more clinical experts participate in classifying the OG in future studies or if it is performed in a more objective fashion [31]. Additionally, in this study, the risk of all emergency surgery was classified as one criterion. However, it is difficult to classify the risk simply based on one criterion, as there may be a difference in risk according to the type of emergency operations. Therefore, in future studies, subdivision of the risk classification according to the type of emergency operation might increase predictive power. Third, another limitation of our study was that it was retrospective. Therefore, further works are needed to validate the performance and clinical usability of our predictive model in prospective multi-center studies.

5. Conclusions

In conclusion, the OFRS using ICD-10 diagnostic and operation codes may help to evaluate the peri-operative risk of elderly patients in emergency surgery where history-taking and pre-operative testing cannot be performed. It is expected that additional studies will broaden the applicability of the score, and the use of this score can help with decision making in various clinical settings.

Supplementary Materials: The following are available online at https://www.mdpi.com/article/10.3390/jcm10194612/s1, Figure S1: Distribution of emergency operations by surgical departments, Figure S2: Distribution of operation frailty risk score by surgical departments, Table S1: Operation group classified by clinical experts, Table S2: Univariate and multivariable regression analysis model for 90-day mortality in the development cohort.

Author Contributions: Conceptualization, S.-W.L., E.-H.L. and K.-W.J.; data curation, S.-W.L. and J.-S.N.; formal analysis, S.-W.L., J.-S.N., Y.-J.K. and M.-J.K.; investigation, S.-W.L.; methodology, S.-W.L., Y.-J.K. and M.-J.K.; project administration, E.-H.L. and K.-W.J.; resources, Y.-J.K. and M.-J.K.; software, Y.-J.K. and M.-J.K.; supervision, E.-H.L. and K.-W.J.; validation, Y.-J.K. and M.-J.K.; visualization, Y.-J.K. and M.-J.K.; writing—original draft preparation, S.-W.L.; and writing—review and editing, S.-W.L., J.-S.N., Y.-J.K., M.-J.K., J.-H.C., E.-H.L., K.-W.J. and I.-C.C. All authors have read and agreed to the published version of the manuscript.

Funding: There was no funding source for this study.

Institutional Review Board Statement: This study was approved by the Ethics Committee of Asan medical center, University of Ulsan College of Medicine, Republic of Korea (AMC IRB 2019-1145).

Informed Consent Statement: Written informed consent was waived for retrospective data analysis by the Ethics Committee of Asan medical center.

Data Availability Statement: The data presented in this study are available on request from the corresponding author (Kyoung-Woon Joung).

Acknowledgments: This work is attributed to, and was solely supported by, the Department of Anesthesiology and Pain Medicine, Asan Medical Center, University of Ulsan College of Medicine, Seoul, Korea. This study used data from the NHIS-NSC version 2.0 (NHIS-2020-2-058), which was released by the KNHIS. The authors alone are responsible for the content and writing of this manuscript.

Conflicts of Interest: All authors declare no competing interests.

References

1. Dall, T.M.; Gallo, P.D.; Chakrabarti, R.; West, T.; Semilla, A.P.; Storm, M.V. An aging population and growing disease burden will require a large and specialized health care workforce by 2025. *Health Aff. (Millwood)* **2013**, *32*, 2013–2020. [CrossRef]
2. Lim, B.G.; Lee, I.O. Anesthetic management of geriatric patients. *Korean J. Anesthesiol.* **2020**, *73*, 8–29. [CrossRef]
3. Clegg, A.; Young, J.; Iliffe, S.; Rikkert, M.O.; Rockwood, K. Frailty in elderly people. *Lancet* **2013**, *381*, 752–762. [CrossRef]
4. Partridge, J.S.; Harari, D.; Dhesi, J.K. Frailty in the older surgical patient: A review. *Age Ageing* **2012**, *41*, 142–147. [CrossRef] [PubMed]
5. Saxton, A.; Velanovich, V. Preoperative frailty and quality of life as predictors of postoperative complications. *Ann. Surg.* **2011**, *253*, 1223–1229. [CrossRef] [PubMed]
6. Shinall, M.C., Jr.; Arya, S.; Youk, A.; Varley, P.; Shah, R.; Massarweh, N.N.; Shireman, P.K.; Johanning, J.M.; Brown, A.J.; Christie, N.A.; et al. Association of Preoperative Patient Frailty and Operative Stress With Postoperative Mortality. *JAMA Surg.* **2019**, e194620. [CrossRef] [PubMed]
7. Wilkes, J.G.; Evans, J.L.; Prato, B.S.; Hess, S.A.; MacGillivray, D.C.; Fitzgerald, T.L. Frailty Cost: Economic Impact of Frailty in the Elective Surgical Patient. *J. Am. Coll. Surg.* **2019**, *228*, 861–870. [CrossRef] [PubMed]
8. Farhat, J.S.; Velanovich, V.; Falvo, A.J.; Horst, H.M.; Swartz, A.; Patton, J.H., Jr.; Rubinfeld, I.S. Are the frail destined to fail? Frailty index as predictor of surgical morbidity and mortality in the elderly. *J. Trauma Acute. Care Surg.* **2012**, *72*, 1526–1530. [CrossRef]

9. Hewitt, J.; Moug, S.J.; Middleton, M.; Chakrabarti, M.; Stechman, M.J.; McCarthy, K. Prevalence of frailty and its association with mortality in general surgery. *Am. J. Surg.* **2015**, *209*, 254–259. [CrossRef]
10. Joseph, B.; Zangbar, B.; Pandit, V.; Fain, M.; Mohler, M.J.; Kulvatunyou, N.; Jokar, T.O.; O'Keeffe, T.; Friese, R.S.; Rhee, P. Emergency general surgery in the elderly: Too old or too frail? *J. Am. Coll. Surg.* **2016**, *222*, 805–813. [CrossRef]
11. Orouji Jokar, T.; Ibraheem, K.; Rhee, P.; Kulvatunyou, N.; Haider, A.; Phelan, H.A.; Fain, M.; Mohler, M.J.; Joseph, B. Emergency general surgery specific frailty index: A validation study. *J. Trauma Acute Care Surg.* **2016**, *81*, 254–260. [CrossRef]
12. Hewitt, J.; Carter, B.; McCarthy, K.; Pearce, L.; Law, J.; Wilson, F.V.; Tay, H.S.; McCormack, C.; Stechman, M.J.; Moug, S.J.; et al. Frailty predicts mortality in all emergency surgical admissions regardless of age: An observational study. *Age Ageing* **2019**, *48*, 388–394. [CrossRef]
13. Chan, S.P.; Ip, K.Y.; Irwin, M.G. Peri-operative optimisation of elderly and frail patients: A narrative review. *Anaesthesia* **2019**, *74*, 80–89. [CrossRef]
14. McCusker, J.; Bellavance, F.; Cardin, S.; Trepanier, S.; Verdon, J.; Ardman, O. Detection of older people at increased risk of adverse health outcomes after an emergency visit: The ISAR screening tool. *J. Am. Geriatr. Soc.* **1999**, *47*, 1229–1237. [CrossRef] [PubMed]
15. Rockwood, K.; Song, X.; MacKnight, C.; Bergman, H.; Hogan, D.B.; McDowell, I.; Mitnitski, A. A global clinical measure of fitness and frailty in elderly people. *CMAJ* **2005**, *173*, 489–495. [CrossRef]
16. Gilbert, T.; Neuburger, J.; Kraindler, J.; Keeble, E.; Smith, P.; Ariti, C.; Arora, S.; Street, A.; Parker, S.; Roberts, H.C.; et al. Development and validation of a Hospital Frailty Risk Score focusing on older people in acute care settings using electronic hospital records: An observational study. *Lancet* **2018**, *391*, 1775–1782. [CrossRef]
17. Bilimoria, K.Y.; Liu, Y.; Paruch, J.L.; Zhou, L.; Kmiecik, T.E.; Ko, C.Y.; Cohen, M.E. Development and evaluation of the universal ACS NSQIP surgical risk calculator: A decision aid and informed consent tool for patients and surgeons. *J. Am. Coll. Surg.* **2013**, *217*, 833–842.e3. [CrossRef]
18. Sullivan, L.M.; Massaro, J.M.; D'Agostino Sr, R.B. Presentation of multivariate data for clinical use: The Framingham Study risk score functions. *Stat. Med.* **2004**, *23*, 1631–1660. [CrossRef]
19. Bertschi, D.; Moser, A.; Stortecky, S.; Zwahlen, M.; Windecker, S.; Carrel, T.; Stuck, A.E.; Schoenenberger, A.W. Evolution of Basic Activities of Daily Living Function in Older Patients One Year After Transcatheter Aortic Valve Implantation. *J. Am. Geriatr. Soc.* **2021**, *69*, 500–505. [CrossRef] [PubMed]
20. Fried, L.P.; Tangen, C.M.; Walston, J.; Newman, A.B.; Hirsch, C.; Gottdiener, J.; Seeman, T.; Tracy, R.; Kop, W.J.; Burke, G.; et al. Frailty in older adults: Evidence for a phenotype. *J. Gerontol. A Biol. Sci. Med. Sci.* **2001**, *56*, M146–M156. [CrossRef] [PubMed]
21. Mitnitski, A.B.; Mogilner, A.J.; Rockwood, K. Accumulation of deficits as a proxy measure of aging. *ScientificWorldJournal* **2001**, *1*, 323–336. [CrossRef]
22. Rockwood, K.; Mitnitski, A. Frailty defined by deficit accumulation and geriatric medicine defined by frailty. *Clin. Geriatr. Med.* **2011**, *27*, 17–26. [CrossRef]
23. Aucoin, S.D.; Hao, M.; Sohi, R.; Shaw, J.; Bentov, I.; Walker, D.; McIsaac, D.I. Accuracy and feasibility of clinically applied frailty instruments before surgery: A systematic review and meta-analysis. *Anesthesiology* **2020**, *133*, 78–95. [CrossRef] [PubMed]
24. Tan, H.L.; Chia, S.T.X.; Nadkarni, N.V.; Ang, S.Y.; Seow, D.C.C.; Wong, T.H. Frailty and functional decline after emergency abdominal surgery in the elderly: A prospective cohort study. *World J. Emerg. Surg.* **2019**, *14*, 62. [CrossRef]
25. Arteaga, A.S.; Aguilar, L.T.; Gonzalez, J.T.; Boza, A.S.; Munoz-Cruzado, V.D.; Ciuro, F.P.; Ruiz, J.P. Impact of frailty in surgical emergencies: A comparison of four frailty scales. *Eur. J. Trauma Emerg. Surg.* **2020**, *42*, 119–126. [CrossRef]
26. Shinall, M.C., Jr.; Youk, A.; Massarweh, N.N.; Shireman, P.K.; Arya, S.; George, E.L.; Hall, D.E. Association of Preoperative Frailty and Operative Stress With Mortality After Elective vs Emergency Surgery. *JAMA Netw. Open* **2020**, *3*, e2010358. [CrossRef]
27. Soong, J.; Poots, A.J.; Scott, S.; Donald, K.; Bell, D. Developing and validating a risk prediction model for acute care based on frailty syndromes. *BMJ Open* **2015**, *5*, e008457. [CrossRef] [PubMed]
28. Begg, C.B.; Cramer, L.D.; Hoskins, W.J.; Brennan, M.F. Impact of hospital volume on operative mortality for major cancer surgery. *JAMA* **1998**, *280*, 1747–1751. [CrossRef] [PubMed]
29. Chaudhary, M.A.; Shah, A.A.; Zogg, C.K.; Changoor, N.; Chao, G.; Nitzschke, S.; Havens, J.M.; Haider, A.H. Differences in rural and urban outcomes: A national inspection of emergency general surgery patients. *J. Surg. Res.* **2017**, *218*, 277–284. [CrossRef]
30. Averill, R.F.; Mullin, R.L.; Steinbeck, B.A.; Goldfield, N.I.; Grant, T.M. Development of the ICD-10 procedure coding system (ICD-10-PCS). *Top. Health Inf. Manag.* **2001**, *21*, 54–88.
31. Corey, K.M.; Kashyap, S.; Lorenzi, E.; Lagoo-Deenadayalan, S.A.; Heller, K.; Whalen, K.; Balu, S.; Heflin, M.T.; McDonald, S.R.; Swaminathan, M.; et al. Development and validation of machine learning models to identify high-risk surgical patients using automatically curated electronic health record data (Pythia): A retrospective, single-site study. *PLoS Med.* **2018**, *15*, e1002701. [CrossRef] [PubMed]

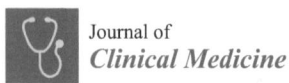

Article

The Interplay between Anticholinergic Burden and Anemia in Relation to 1-Year Mortality among Older Patients Discharged from Acute Care Hospitals

Andrea Corsonello [1,2], Luca Soraci [1,*], Francesco Corica [3], Valeria Lago [3], Clementina Misuraca [4], Graziano Onder [5], Stefano Volpato [6], Carmelinda Ruggiero [7], Antonio Cherubini [8] and Fabrizia Lattanzio [9]

1. Geriatric Medicine, IRCCS INRCA, 87100 Cosenza, Italy; a.corsonello@inrca.it
2. Unit of Geriatric Pharmacoepidemiology and Biostatistics, IRCCS INRCA, 87100 Cosenza, Italy
3. Department of Clinical and Experimental Medicine, University of Messina, 98124 Messina, Italy; coricaf@unime.it (F.C.); valeria.lago2@gmail.com (V.L.)
4. Respiratory Unit, IRCCS INRCA, 23880 Casatenovo, Italy; c.misuraca@inrca.it
5. Department of Cardiovascular, Endocrine-Metabolic Diseases and Aging, Istituto Superiore di Sanitá, 00100 Rome, Italy; graziano.onder@iss.it
6. Center for Clinical Epidemiology, Department of Medical Sciences, School of Medicine, University of Ferrara, 44122 Ferrara, Italy; stefano.volpato@unife.it
7. Geriatric and Orthogeriatric Units, Geriatric and Gerontology Section, Department of Medicine and Surgery, University of Perugia, 06156 Perugia, Italy; carmelinda.ruggiero@unipg.it
8. Geriatria, Accettazione Geriatrica e Centro di Ricerca per l'invecchiamento, IRCCS INRCA, 60124 Ancona, Italy; a.cherubini@inrca.it
9. Scientific Direction, IRCCS INRCA, 60124 Ancona, Italy; f.lattanzio@inrca.it
* Correspondence: l.soraci@inrca.it; Tel.: +39-0984-682005

Abstract: Anticholinergic burden (ACB) and anemia were found associated with an increased risk of death among older patients. Additionally, anticholinergic medications may contribute to the development of anemia. Therefore, we aimed at investigating the prognostic interplay of ACB and anemia among older patients discharged from hospital. Our series consisted of 783 patients enrolled in a multicenter observational study. The outcome of the study was 1 year mortality. ACB was assessed by an Anticholinergic Cognitive Burden score. Anemia was defined as hemoglobin < 13 g/dL in men and <12 g/dL in women. The association between study variables and mortality was investigated by Cox regression analysis. After adjusting for several potential confounders, ACB score = 2 or more was significantly associated with the outcome in anemic patients (HR = 1.93, 95%CI = 1.13–3.40), but not non anemic patients (HR = 1.51, 95%CI = 0.65–3.48). An additive prognostic interaction between ACB and anemia was observed ($p = 0.02$). Anemia may represent a relevant effect modifier in the association between ACB and mortality.

Keywords: anticholinergic burden; anemia; hospital; older patients

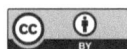

1. Introduction

Anticholinergic medications are commonly used among older patients, despite the fact they are known to cause relevant side effects, including cognitive impairment and delirium, functional decline, disability and falls [1–5]. Older patients are particularly vulnerable to adverse reactions to anticholinergic drugs due to age-related changes in pharmacokinetics and pharmacodynamics [6], deficit of cholinergic transmission [7], comorbidity, polypharmacy, use of potentially inappropriate medications, and drug interactions [8,9]. Despite these potential risks, selected medications with some degree of anticholinergic activity, such as furosemide, digoxin, laxatives, and ranitidine are frequently taken in up to 37% of older people [10]. Even if each of the above example medications have weak anticholinergic properties, their co-administration frequently results in cumulative effects that are frequently unrecognized or misattributed as geriatric syndromes, frailty or simply changes due to ageing [11].

During the last decade, anticholinergic medications were repeatedly reported to be associated with reduced survival in several different populations, including community-dwelling individuals [1], nursing home residents [12], older hospitalized patients [13], and general older population [14]. More recently, several prognostic interactions involving anticholinergic burden were observed with risk factors relevant to the older population, including dependency in basic activities of daily living (BADL) [15], depression [16], physical [17] and cognitive impairment [18]. These findings are relevant from clinical point of view because they may help to identify patients carrying high risk of mortality in relation to cumulative exposure to anticholinergic medications who are likely to benefit of anticholinergic deprescribing.

Anemia is another relevant predictor of prognosis among older patients [19,20], and especially among hospitalized ones [21,22]. Low serum hemoglobin has shown to be a risk factor for 1 year mortality and increased hospitalization rates [23,24]. Additionally, anemia was previously shown to affect both cognitive [25,26] and physical performance [27,28] over time; indeed, persistence of low serum hemoglobin concentrations may induce a state of chronic brain hypoxia and reduce aerobic capacity, which may affect cognitive reserve and increase the risk of cognitive impairment and dementia [25]; moreover, anemia was also associated with a decline in physical performance [28,29] and sarcopenia [30]. Additionally, both cognitive and functional impairment were shown to increase the risk of 1 year mortality among older hospitalized patients with high ACB [15,18]. As a consequence, anemia may potentially mediate the negative effects of anticholinergic medications on cognitive, physical performance, and survival.

On the other hand, anticholinergic medications may contribute to the development of anemia by several different mechanisms, mainly represented by inhibition of iron absorption in the stomach and disruption of transferrin signaling [31,32]. Besides their effects on iron metabolism and transport, recent evidence suggests that nonselective anticholinergic medications may exert some detrimental effects on red blood cell (RBCs) turnover mainly by nonneuronal acetylcholine (Ach)-mediated modulation of hemorheological and oxygen-carrying properties of human erythrocytes [33] through M1 muscarinic receptors on RBCs [34] and bone marrow early erythroid progenitors [35]. However, despite biological plausibility, the potential prognostic interaction between anticholinergic burden and anemia has not been studied until now.

Therefore, the aim of this study was to investigate the prognostic interplay between anticholinergic burden and anemia in relationship with 1 year mortality. This study may help discover whether anticholinergic burden acts synergically with anemia and whether levels of circulating hemoglobin modulate the effect of anticholinergic burden on survival of older patients.

2. Materials and Methods

This present study was carried out using data from the CRiteria to assess Inappropriate Medication use among Elderly complex patients (CRIME) project, a multicenter prospective observational study involving seven geriatric and internal medicine acute wards in Italy. Methodology of CRIME project was described elsewhere [36]. Given that the CRIME study aimed at enrolling a real-world population of older in-patients, all patients aged 65 or older consecutively admitted to participating wards between June 2010 and May 2011 were asked to participate. The only exclusion criteria were being aged < 65 years and unwillingness to participate in the study. All study participants were asked to sign a written informed consent and were assessed within the first 24 hours from hospital admission and followed until discharge. Collected information included demographic, socioeconomic, and clinical characteristics, as well as detailed data about drug treatment and comprehensive geriatric assessment (CGA). Medications were coded according to the Anatomical Therapeutic and Chemical (ATC) classification [37]. All the drugs taken by the patients were carefully recorded before admission, during hospital stay and at discharge. Complete data about medications were also collected at 3-month follow-up visit. After discharge, patients were reassessed at 3, 6, and 12 months. The study was conducted in accordance with the Declaration of Helsinki, and the protocol was approved by the Ethics Committee of the Catholic University of Rome (Project identification code: P/582/CE/2009).

Overall, 1123 patients were enrolled in the present study. Patients with incomplete baseline data ($n = 3$) and those who died during hospitalization ($n = 39$) were excluded from the present analysis. Patients with incomplete follow-up data ($n = 298$) were also excluded, leaving a final sample of 783 patients to be included in the analysis.

Patients excluded from the study were older (82.7 ± 7.3 vs. 80.9 ± 7.4, $p < 0.001$), more frequently females (60.8 % vs. 53.8 %, $p = 0.034$) and with lower number of medications (6.3 ± 3.5 vs. 7.5 ± 2.8, $p < 0.001$) compared to those included in the study. Additionally, they were also characterized by higher rates of cognitive impairment (68.5 % vs. 40.1%, $p < 0.001$), depression (48.1 % vs. 25.5%, $p = 0.003$), and BADL disability (51.6% vs. 32.8%, $p < 0.001$).

2.1. Outcome

The outcome of the present study was 1 year mortality. Data on living status during the follow-up were obtained by interviewing the patients and/or their formal and/or informal caregivers. For patients who died during the follow-up period, the date and place of death were retrieved by relatives or caregivers. The municipal registers were consulted when neither patients nor relatives or caregivers could be contacted.

2.2. Exposure Variables

Cumulative exposure to anticholinergic medications was assessed by the anticholinergic cognitive burden (ACB) score at discharge [38]. ACB score was chosen because of the availability of external validation and the greater accuracy in the assessment of central anticholinergic burden in comparison with other tools [39]. The main exposure variable was calculated as follows: ACB score at discharge, (1) low (ACB = 0, no ACB medications), (2) medium (ACB = 1), and (3) high burden (ACB = 2 or more). Anemia was defined by using WHO definition based on serum hemoglobin levels at discharge lower than 12 g/dL for females and 13 g/dL for males [40]. To investigate the impact of anemia on the relationship between ACB and prognosis, the ACB score at discharge was stratified by the presence or absence of anemia.

2.3. Covariates

Age, sex, number of diagnoses, history of falls, and number of medications prescribed at discharge were considered as potential confounders in the analysis. CGA data were collected at the time of discharge. Patients with age- and education-adjusted Mini-Mental State Examination score of <24 were considered as cognitively impaired [41]. Geriatric Depression Scale score > 5 was used to identify patients with depression [42]. Dependency in at least 1 BADL was also considered as a potential confounder [43]. Selected diagnoses known to affect prognosis in older populations, including hypertension, heart failure, diabetes mellitus, atrial fibrillation, coronary artery disease (CAD), stroke, peripheral arterial disease (PAD), chronic obstructive pulmonary disease (COPD), chronic kidney disease (CKD), and cancer were also included in the analysis. Given the availability of complete data about medications at 3 months, ACB score at the 3-month follow-up visit was also considered as a potential confounder in order to explore the potential impact of changes in the exposure to anticholinergic medications over time.

2.4. Analytic Approach

First, we analyzed the characteristics of patients according to ACB score at discharge among patients with or without anemia. The χ^2 test was used for categorical variables and one-way analysis of variance (ANOVA) for continuous ones. The association between exposure variables and the outcome was explored by Kaplan-Meier curves with log-rank test. Three different Cox proportional hazard model were used to estimate the HR and 95%CI for the effect of anemia and ACB score on 1 year mortality. The baseline model A was adjusted for age and sex; the multivariable model B was adjusted for all the variables associated with mortality in the preliminary analysis (age, sex, cognitive impairment, depression, history of falls, BADL disability, number of diagnoses, and number of medications); and model C including all variables from model B but specific diagnoses (hypertension, atrial fibrillation, heart failure, diabetes, CKD, PAD, CAD, COPD, cerebrovascular disease, and cancer) instead of number of comorbidities. Model C was also repeated after adjusting for ACB score at the 3-month follow-up or hemoglobin values. We used multivariable models to select predictors of mortality. To account for the impact of the severity of anemia on the observed associations, the analysis was also repeated using different cut-offs of hemoglobin [44]: mild anemia was defined as having hemoglobin of 11.0–12.9 g/dL for men or 11.0–11.9 g/dL for women; moderate-severe anemia as having hemoglobin values < 11.0 g/dL in both men and women. The interaction term ACB score at discharge*anemia was then formally investigated in Cox regression analysis; separate analyses were conducted among men and women to account for the impact of sex on the interaction term. Attrition bias was investigated by age- and sex-adjusted logistic regression analysis of ACB exposure to loss at the follow-up.

Statistical analysis was carried out using R version 4.0 (R Foundation for Statistical Computing, Vienna, Austria, https://www.r-project.org/ (accessed on 8 October 2021)).

3. Results

Overall, anemia was diagnosed in 420 out of 783 patients (53.6%). The average ACB score at discharge was similar among patients with anemia and without anemia (median (IQR): 1 (0–2) vs. 1 (0–2), $p = 0.19$). ACB score categories (0, 1, 2 or more) were observed in 118 (28.1%), 154 (36.7%), and 148 (35.2%) patients with anemia, and in 130 (35.8%), 124 (34.2%), and 109 (30.0%) patients without anemia ($p = 0.06$). Among patients without anemia, those with ACB score =2 or more at discharge were older and more frequently affected by heart failure, atrial fibrillation, CAD, PAD, COPD, and cancer compared to patients with ACB = 0. BADL dependency, overall comorbidity and number of prescribed medications were also higher among patients with ACB score = 2 or more (Table 1).

Among patients with anemia, those with ACB score = 2 or more had a greater prevalence of hypertension, heart failure, atrial fibrillation, and chronic kidney disease (CKD) and were characterized by a higher number of prescribed medications, a higher overall comorbidity, and a greater prevalence of cognitive impairment compared to those with ACB score = 0 (Table 1).

ACB medications prescribed at discharge among patients with or without anemia are reported in Table 2.

ACB score showed a clear dose-response association with mortality in the whole study population (Table 3). ACB score at the 3-month follow-up was similar to that measured at discharge (no anemia: 1 (0–2); anemia: 1 (0–2), $p = 0.25$).

The graded increase in mortality in relation to ACB score at discharge was more evident among anemic compared to non-anemic patients (Figure 1).

The association between ACB score at discharge and mortality in patients with anemia was confirmed after adjusting for potential confounders (Table 4). Furthermore, age (Hazard Ratio (HR) = 1.05, 95% Confidence Interval (CI) = 1.02–1.08), male sex (HR = 1.88, 95%CI = 1.30–2.74), and BADL dependency (HR = 3.15, 95%CI = 2.10–4.76) qualified as predictors of mortality in patients with anemia in model B; additional predictors of mortality in model C were CAD (HR = 1.74, 95%CI = 1.17–2.60), cancer (HR = 2.68, 95%CI = 1.78–4.03), and diabetes (HR = 1.52, 95%CI = 1.01–2.29).

Table 1. Demographic and clinical characteristics of patients stratified by anemia and ACB score at discharge.

| | | No Anemia (n = 363) | | | | Anemia (n = 420) | | | |
| | | ACB score at discharge | | | | ACB score at discharge | | | |
	All patients (n = 783)	0 (n = 130)	1 (n = 124)	2 or more (n = 109)	p value [a]	0 (n = 118)	1 (n = 154)	2 or more (n = 148)	p value [a]
Age, mean (± SD)	80.9 ± 7.4	76.9 ± 6.9	78.8 ± 7.3	80.7 ± 7.6	<0.001	82.5 ± 7.5	83.3 ± 6.6	82.6 ± 6.7	0.98
Male sex, n (%)	362 (46.2)	55 (42.3)	66 (53.2)	51 (46.8)	0.22	48 (40.7)	76 (49.3)	66 (44.6)	0.36
Cognitive impairment, n (%)	314 (40.1)	41 (31.5)	51 (41.1)	49 (45.0)	0.09	45 (38.1)	76 (49.3)	52 (35.1)	0.03
Depression, n (%)	200 (25.5)	31 (23.8)	29 (23.4)	31 (28.4)	0.62	24 (20.3)	43 (27.9)	42 (28.4)	0.26
History of falls, n (%)	198 (25.3)	25 (19.2)	27 (21.8)	33 (30.3)	0.12	28 (23.8)	50 (32.5)	35 (23.6)	0.15
BADL disability, n (%)	257 (32.8)	22 (16.9)	22 (17.7)	38 (34.9)	0.001	43 (36.4)	65 (42.2)	67 (45.3)	0.34
Number of diseases, mean (± SD)	5.2 ± 2.7	3.7 ± 2.0	4.7 ± 2.0	5.7 ± 2.7	<0.001	4.7 ± 2.7	5.8 ± 2.7	6.4 ± 2.8	<0.001
Hypertension, n (%)	595 (76.0)	106 (81.5)	103 (83.1)	82 (75.2)	0.29	68 (57.6)	117 (76.0)	119 (80.4)	<0.001
Heart failure, n (%)	223 (28.5)	6 (4.6)	30 (24.2)	42 (38.5)	<0.001	11 (9.3)	64 (41.6)	70 (47.3)	<0.001
Diabetes, n (%)	234 (29.9)	26 (20.0)	36 (29.0)	31 (28.4)	0.19	41 (34.7)	46 (29.9)	54 (36.5)	0.45
Atrial fibrillation, n (%)	144 (18.4)	5 (3.8)	14 (11.3)	22 (20.2)	<0.001	11 (9.3)	33 (21.4)	59 (39.9)	<0.001
CAD, n (%)	245 (31.3)	17 (13.1)	38 (30.6)	44 (40.4)	<0.001	29 (24.6)	55 (35.7)	62 (41.9)	0.01
Cerebrovascular disease, n (%)	157 (20.0)	24 (18.5)	25 (20.1)	23 (21.1)	0.87	22 (18.6)	32 (20.8)	31 (20.9)	0.88
PAD, n (%)	64 (8.2)	3 (2.3)	14 (11.3)	8 (7.3)	0.02	7 (5.9)	16 (10.4)	16 (10.8)	0.33
CKD, n (%)	409 (53.3)	42 (33.1)	56 (46.7)	52 (49.1)	0.02	56 (49.1)	101 (66.0)	102 (69.4)	0.002
COPD, n (%)	303 (38.7)	42 (32.3)	59 (47.6)	45 (41.3)	0.04	37 (31.3)	54 (35.1)	66 (44.6)	0.06
Cancer, n (%)	109 (13.9)	4 (3.1)	8 (6.4)	18 (16.5)	<0.001	25 (21.2)	28 (18.2)	26 (17.6)	0.73
Number of medications, mean (± SD)	7.5 ± 2.8	5.8 ± 2.4	8.0 ± 2.3	8.6 ± 2.7	<0.001	5.6 ± 2.6	7.7 ± 2.5	9.0 ± 2.6	<0.001

Notes: BADL = Basic Activity of Daily Living; CAD= Coronary artery disease; CKD = Chronic Kidney Disease; COPD = Chronic Obstructive Pulmonary Disease; PAD = Peripheral Arterial Disease; SD = Standard Deviation. ([a]) p values are from Chi-square or ANOVA 1-way test as appropriate.

Table 2. Anticholinergic Cognitive Burden (ACB) listed medications prescribed at discharge in the study population according to diagnosis of anemia.

	No Anemia (n = 363)	Anemia (n = 420)
ACB score 1	Furosemide 156 (43.0%) Prednisone 25 (6.9%) Metoprolol 23 (6.3%) Digoxin 14 (3.8%) Isosorbide 20 (5.5%) Codeine 17 (4.7%) Warfarin 9 (2.5%) Alprazolam 10 (2.8%) Atenolol 10 (2.7%) Trazodone 7 (1.9%) Ranitidine 6 (1.6%) Chlortalidone 2 (0.5%) Cetirizine 2 (0.5%) Haloperidol 2 (0.5%) Diazepam 3 (0.8%) Theophylline 2 (0.5%) Colchicine 1 (0.2%) Risperidone 1 (0.2%) Captopril 1 (0.2%) Aripiprazole 1 (0.2%)	Furosemide 243 (57.8%) Prednisone 41 (9.8%) Digoxin 44 (10.5%) Metoprolol 28 (6.7%) Isosorbide 20 (4.8%) Codeine 12 (2.9%) Warfarin 12 (2.9%) Trazodone 12 (2.9%) Atenolol 9 (2.1%) Alprazolam (1.9%) Ranitidine 7 (1.7%) Haloperidol 5 (1.2%) Fentanyl 4 (0.9%) Risperidone 2 (0.5%) Hydrocortisone 2 (0.5%) Chlortalidone 1 (0.2%) Cetirizine 1 (0.2%) Diazepam 1 (0.2%) Theophyilline 1 (0.2%) Aripiprazole 1 (0.2%)
ACB score 2	Carbamazepine 4 (1.1%) Oxcarbazepine 1 (0.2%)	Carbamazepine 4 (0.9%) Oxcarbazepine 1 (0.2%) Meperidine 1 (0.2%)
ACB score 3	Quetiapine 16 (9.6%) Paroxetine 6 (1.6%) Promazine 5 (1.4 %) Amitryptiline 3 (0.8%) Scopolamine 1 (0.2%) Clomipramine 1 (0.2%) Oxybutynin 1 (0.2%) Orphenadrine 1 (0.2%)	Quetiapine 16 (3.8%) Promazine 5 (1.2%) Paroxetine 3 (0.7%) Scopolamine 1 (0.2%)

Table 3. Cox regression analysis exploring dose-response relationship between ACB score and mortality in the whole study population.

ACB Score at Discharge	Mortality Rate [a]	HR (95%CI) [b]
0	36 (14.5%)	1.0
1	56 (20.1%)	1.29 (0.82–2.01)
2	38 (27.7%)	1.63 (0.98–2.71)
3	21 (31.3%)	1.96 (1.09–3.52)
4	14 (37.8%)	2.34 (1.21–4.53)
5	8 (53.3%)	5.49 (2.42–12.44)

Notes: [a]. Data are number of cases (percentages). [b]. Cox regression model was adjusted for age, sex, cognitive impairment, depression, BADL disability, history of falls, number of drugs and number of diseases.

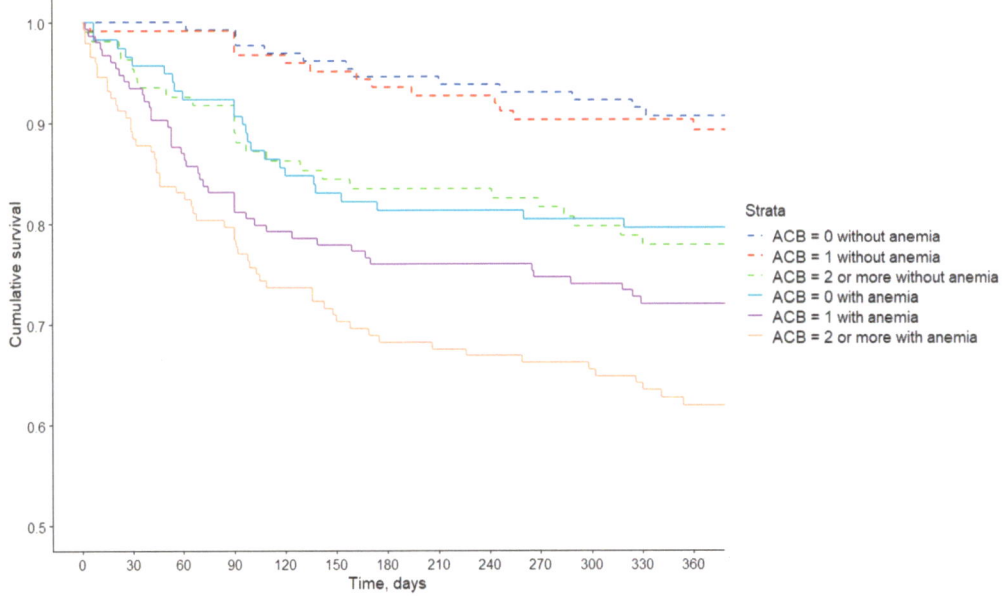

Figure 1. Kaplan Meier curves showing survival associated with ACB score and anemia.

Table 4. Cox proportional hazard models of the relationship between ACB score at discharge and 1 year mortality stratified by the presence of anemia.

	Mortality Rate (%)	Model A HR (95%CI)	Model B HR (95%CI)	Model C HR (95%CI)
ACB score at discharge				
No anemia (n = 363)				
0	12 (9.2)	1.0	1.0	1.0
1	13 (10.5)	0.96 (0.43–2.11)	0.96 (0.40.2.28)	1.02 (0.39–2.64)
2 or more	25 (22.9)	1.88 (0.93–3.81)	1.51 (0.65–3.48)	1.27 (0.49–3.25)
Anemia (n = 420)				
0	24 (20.3)	1.0	1.0	1.0
1	43 (27.9)	1.35 (0.82–2.23)	1.35 (0.79–2.29)	1.39 (0.77–2.50)
2 or more	56 (37.8)	2.20 (1.36–3.55)	1.96 (1.13–3.40)	1.97 (1.06–3.67)

Notes: ACB = Anticholinergic Cognitive Burden. CI = Confidence Interval; HR = Hazard Ratio. Model A, adjusted for age and sex; model B, adjusted for age, sex, cognitive impairment, depression, history of falls, BADL disability, number of diagnoses, and number of medications; and model C, adjusted for age, sex, cognitive impairment, depression, history of falls, BADL disability, number of medications, and specific diagnoses (hypertension, atrial fibrillation, heart failure, diabetes, CKD, PAD, CAD, COPD, cerebrovascular disease, cancer) instead of number of diagnoses.

The association between ACB score of 2 or more and mortality in patients with anemia was also confirmed after adjusting model C for hemoglobin values at discharge (HR = 2.82, 95%CI = 1.29–6.12). Finally, after adjusting for ACB score at the 3 month follow-up, the association with mortality remained unchanged in patients with anemia and ACB score of 2 or more (HR = 2.91, 95%CI:1.34–5-68). Investigation of the prognostic impact of anemia severity on the observed associations showed that risk of mortality related to ACB score = 2 or more was similar among patients with mild anemia (HR = 1.73, 95%CI = 1.11–2.70) and those with moderate-severe anemia (HR = 1.88, 95%CI = 1.15–2.81).

The ACB score was not significantly associated with survival among patients without anemia in adjusted analyses (Table 4). Predictors of mortality among patients without anemia were age (HR = 1.08, 95%CI = 1.03–1.13), and BADL dependency (HR = 4.46, 95%CI = 2.28–8.73) in model B, and age (HR = 1.07, 95%CI = 1.02–1.13), BADL dependency (HR = 5.76, 95%CI = 2.76–12.04), atrial fibrillation (HR = 2.45, 95%CI = 1.14–5.24), and cancer (HR = 4.61, 95%CI = 2.09–10.18) in model C.

When we repeated the analysis using ACB score at discharge as a continuous variable instead of categorical one in the fully adjusted model C, the association with mortality was confirmed among patients with anemia (HR = 1.32, 95%CI = 1.12–1.55) and not among patients without anemia (HR = 1.20, 95%CI = 0.92–1.57).

A mild but significant additive interaction between the ACB score at discharge and anemia was observed in the whole study population (p = 0.02). After stratifying Cox regression models by sex, the interaction between ACB score and anemia resulted to be strong and multiplicative among men (p < 0.001), and mild and additive among women (p = 0.03). The ACB score was not significantly associated with dropout rate, either in patients without anemia (ACB score = 1, odds ratio (OR) = 0.91; 95%CI = 0.83–1.00; ACB score = 2 or more, OR = 0.9; 95%CI = 0.88–1.06) or patients with anemia (ACB score = 1, OR = 0.98; 95%CI = 0.90–1.07; ACB score = 2 or more, OR = 1.05; 95%CI = 0.96–1.14).

4. Discussion

Findings from the present study show that anticholinergic burden may be associated with reduced survival among older patients with anemia discharged from acute care wards in participating hospitals. Thus, anemia may have an additive effect on mortality risk in patients with ACB score = 2 or more, with a greater impact among men compared with women. The slightly high prevalence of ACB score = 2 or more among anemic patients may have also contributed to the observed findings.

Anticholinergic medications share several central and peripheral adverse effects [45]. Mechanisms which may potentially account for ACB-associated adverse effects include cardiovascular (e.g., arrhythmias, syncope, ischemia) and neurologic (eg, hallucinations, confusion, seizure) side effects [46]. Moreover, age-related changes in pharmacokinetics and pharmacodynamics, as well as increased permeability of the blood-brain barrier and age-related acetylcholine depletion may favor the occurrence of adverse effects from anticholinergic medications among older patients [6,47]. Non-neuronal cholinergic system is disseminated on immunocompetent cells and the stimulation of nicotinic receptors may inhibit adaptive and innate immune reactions [48]. Consequently, anticholinergic drugs may harm by counteracting these immuno-modulatory actions leading to inflammation and increasing risk of death.

It is worth noting that the prevalence of anemia was 53.6% in our study, which was higher than that formerly observed in the hospital setting (about 40%) [49], but very similar to the 53.5% prevalence recently observed among hospitalized patients aged 65 or older (48.3% among patients aged 65–80 years and 59.2% among patients aged > 80 years) [21].

Anticholinergic medications may potentially favor the development of anemia through several mechanisms: in general, anticholinergic substances may inhibit the absorption of iron at the gastric level [31], thus predisposing to hypochromic sideropenic anemia; additionally, several antipsychotics with strong anticholinergic properties may favor the development of anemia [50], via both direct and immune-mediated toxic actions upon the bone marrow or RBCs, and by decreasing body iron stores. Furthermore, the commonly used antiarrhythmic digoxin has anticholinergic properties and may predispose to development of anemia mainly disturbing transferrin signaling and iron storing [32].

On the other hand, anemia itself has negative prognostic outcomes in older people [20–22]. The findings of an increased risk of mortality among patients with either ACB score = 2 or more and anemia suggests that anemia may increase vulnerability to negative prognostic effects of anticholinergic drugs and/or anemia may mediate their negative prognostic effects.

Potential reasons explaining the impact of anemia on the observed associations may be related to detrimental effects of nonselective anticholinergic medications on RBCs turnover. RBCs are in fact very effective scavengers of nonneuronal acetylcholine (ACh) escaping into the bloodstream [34]. Nonneuronal ACh is able to modulate the hemorheological and oxygen-carrying properties of human erythrocytes [33] mainly through muscarinic receptors of type M1 which have been found in high density on surface of RBCs [34] and bone marrow early erythroid progenitors [35]. Changes in the RBCs' hemorheological properties may trigger changes in blood viscosity and modulate tissue oxygenation and the distribution of blood to the peripheral tissues [33,34]. It is thought that acetylcholine down-regulates the self-renewal of RBCs and bone marrow erythroid precursors, since pharmacologic inhibition or genetic suppression of cholinergic receptors, muscarinic 4 (CHRM4) has shown to improve RBCs production in both in vitro and in vivo studies [35]. ACh action is limited to the internal environment of erythrocytes by the activity of acetylcholinesterase (AChE), an enzyme involved in its breakdown, that is highly expressed on the RBC membrane, and contribute to maintaining the size and shape of RBCs [51]. AChE seems also to mediate erythroid differentiation, working in association with erythropoietin (EPO) with a feedback-loop mechanisms: on one hand, EPO induces the transcription of AChE genes, while AChE increases the responsiveness of erythroid cells to EPO [52]; the final effect of this interaction is the increase in RBCs production. However, AChE overexpression is a reliable marker of aging, inflammatory states, and several diseases, such as hypertension, glaucoma, dementia, and anemia [51,53]. Additionally, scopolamine (i.e., a nonselective anticholinergic medication) was found to increase AChE activity in several different experimental models [54,55], though the role of anticholinergic-induced AChE overexpression in the pathophysiology of anemia is still to be elucidated.

Patients with anemia may have also high susceptibility to negative iatrogenic events. In fact, anemia is often associated with sarcopenia [56], which may in turn change the volume of distribution of several drugs, thus affecting pharmacokinetics and pharmacodynamics response to selected drugs and increasing the risk of iatrogenic adverse reactions. Moreover, both anemia and high anticholinergic burden are risk factors for cognitive impairment [57,58], which may in turn increase patient's vulnerability to iatrogenic side effects of anticholinergic drugs mainly by decreasing individual autonomy and adherence to drug regimens [59]. Additionally, ACB score was found associated with BADL dependency [15] and depression [16], that may both increase mortality of older patients and were proved to be associated with anemia [60].

Awareness of the excessive mortality risk associated with the use of anticholinergic medications should lead physicians to limit their prescription, especially among older patients with anemia. The association between ACB score = 2 or more and mortality among anemic patients was mainly driven by cumulative use of drugs with low anticholinergic effect in our study. However, it is worth noting that a not negligible proportion of patients (39 out of 363 in non-anemic group and 30 out of 420 in anemic group) were prescribed medications with moderate-high anticholinergic activity.

Thus, deprescribing of anticholinergic medications warrants further investigations. Meanwhile, hospitalization should always be considered a clue to identify anemia and to select drugs with no or less anticholinergic burden whenever possible (e.g., avoiding tricyclics, trazodone, or paroxetine). A slow and gradual withdrawal of anticholinergic medications should always be started when indications to their use are no longer present, especially among anemic patients.

Limitations of our study deserve to be mentioned. Given the observational design, confounding by indication cannot be ruled out. Patients excluded from the analysis because of incomplete follow-up had greater overall comorbidity and number of medications, as well as higher prevalence of selected diagnoses, cognitive and functional impairment. However, attrition bias analysis showed that ACB score was not associated with drop-out rate. Additionally, our results identify variables that by themselves may influence the outcome, and we could not account for illness severity, duration and management of individual diagnoses, and life expectancy. Furthermore, we cannot rule out that measures of cumulative anticholinergic burden other than ACB may yield different findings. Similarly, anemia was defined on the basis of circulating hemoglobin, and lack of data on RBCs quantity and morphology, other laboratory parameters, as well as duration of anemia, did not allow us to explore the impact of different forms of anemia on study outcomes. The short duration of the follow-up, up to 12 months, limited the study of the association between ACB and prognosis. Our dataset did not allow to investigate competing risk related to readmissions and/or emergency department visits during follow-up. Similarly, our dataset did not allow us to investigate the prognostic weight of frailty or IADL, as BADL scale was the only available measure to investigate physical dependency. Additionally, ACB data during follow-up were only available at 3 months, which limits the exploration of longer exposure to anticholinergics. Furthermore, the small sample size may reduce the precision of estimates and does not allow to preform dose-response analysis after stratification by anemia. Thus, the finding of a not significant trends for association between ACB score and mortality among patients without anemia does not mean that ACB drugs can be considered safe in these patients. Finally, our results apply to a population of older patients discharged from acute care hospitals with a diagnosis of anemia and could not be generalized or applied to other settings. Thus, further research using larger population samples with extended follow-up periods, as well as confirmatory studies with other different measures of anticholinergic burden are needed. Nevertheless, the inclusion of a real-world population of hospitalized older patients, the detailed assessment of drugs taken by each individual patients, as well as the systematic use of CGA which allowed us to adjust the analysis for a wide set of potential confounders should be considered as relevant strengths.

5. Conclusions

ACB score at discharge is a relevant predictor of 1 year mortality among older patients discharged from acute care hospitals; anemia was found to modulate the relationship between ACB score and mortality. For this reason, hospital physicians should be aware that prescribing anticholinergic medications in such a vulnerable population may have a negative prognostic impact. Thus, hospitalization should be a clue to identify patients with anemia and to revise overall drug treatment to reduce ACB at discharge whenever possible.

Author Contributions: Conceptualization, A.C. (Andrea Corsonello), L.S., F.C., V.L., F.L., C.M.; Data curation, L.S.; Formal analysis, L.S.; Funding acquisition, G.O., S.V., C.R., A.C. (Antonio Cherubini), A.C. (Andrea Corsonello), and F.L.; Investigation, G.O., S.V., C.R., A.C. (Antonio Cherubini), and A.C. (Andrea Corsonello); Methodology, G.O. and F.L.; Supervision, G.O. and F.L.; Writing–original draft, A.C. (Andrea Corsonello), L.S., V.L., F.L., C.M.; Writing–review and editing, F.C., G.O., S.V., C.R., A.C. (Antonio Cherubini), A.C. (Andrea Corsonello), and F.L. All authors have read and agreed to the published version of the manuscript.

Funding: The CRiteria to assess Inappropriate Medication use among Elderly complex patients (CRIME) project was partially supported by a grant from the Italian Ministry of Health (GR-2007 685638). The present paper was funded by Italian National Research Center on Aging (IRCCS INRCA) intramural research funds (Ricerca Corrente).

Institutional Review Board Statement: The study was conducted in accordance with the Declaration of Helsinki, and the protocol was approved by the Ethics Committee of the Catholic University of Rome (Project identification code: P/582/CE/2009).

Informed Consent Statement: Informed consent was obtained from all subjects involved in the study.

Data Availability Statement: Data are available for CRIME study researcher at IRCCS INRCA (www.inrca.it (accessed on 8 October 2021)).

Acknowledgments: The CRIME study group: Gemelli Hospital, Centro Medicina dell'Invecchiamento, Università Cattolica del Sacro Cuore, Rome, Italy; University of Perugia; University of Ferrara; Italian National Research Center on Aging (IRCCS INRCA) Ancona, Cosenza, Fermo, and Rome. The authors are grateful to Romano Firmani and Moreno Nacciariti for their skillful technical support.

Conflicts of Interest: The authors declare no conflict of interest. The funders had no role in the design of the study; in the collection, analyses, or interpretation of data; in the writing of the manuscript, or in the decision to publish the results.

References

1. Fox, C.; Richardson, K.; Maidment, I.D.; Savva, G.M.; Matthews, F.E.; Smithard, D.; Coulton, S.; Katona, C.; Boustani, M.A.; Brayne, C. Anticholinergic medication use and cognitive impairment in the older population: The medical research council cognitive function and ageing study. *J. Am. Geriatr. Soc.* **2011**, *59*, 1477–1483. [CrossRef]
2. Naja, M.; Zmudka, J.; Hannat, S.; Liabeuf, S.; Serot, J.M.; Jouanny, P. In geriatric patients, delirium symptoms are related to the anticholinergic burden. *Geriatr. Gerontol. Int.* **2016**, *16*, 424–431. [CrossRef] [PubMed]
3. Wouters, H.; Hilmer, S.N.; Gnjidic, D.; Van Campen, J.P.; Teichert, M.; Van Der Meer, H.G.; Schaap, L.A.; Huisman, M.; Comijs, H.C.; Denig, P.; et al. Long-Term Exposure to Anticholinergic and Sedative Medications and Cognitive and Physical Function in Later Life. *J. Gerontol. A Biol. Sci. Med. Sci.* **2020**, *75*, 357–365. [CrossRef] [PubMed]
4. Zia, A.; Kamaruzzaman, S.; Myint, P.K.; Tan, M.P. Anticholinergic burden is associated with recurrent and injurious falls in older individuals. *Maturitas* **2016**, *84*, 32–37. [CrossRef] [PubMed]
5. Brombo, G.; Bianchi, L.; Maietti, E.; Malacarne, F.; Corsonello, A.; Cherubini, A.; Ruggiero, C.; Onder, G.; Volpato, S. Association of Anticholinergic Drug Burden with Cognitive and Functional Decline Over Time in Older Inpatients: Results from the CRIME Project. *Drugs Aging* **2018**, *35*, 917–924. [CrossRef] [PubMed]
6. Corsonello, A.; Pedone, C.; Incalzi, R.A. Age-related pharmacokinetic and pharmacodynamic changes and related risk of adverse drug reactions. *Curr. Med. Chem.* **2010**, *17*, 571–584. [CrossRef]
7. Gibson, G.E.; Peterson, C.; Jenden, D.J. Brain acetylcholine synthesis declines with senescence. *Science* **1981**, *213*, 674–676. [CrossRef] [PubMed]
8. Onder, G.; Landi, F.; Liperoti, R.; Fialova, D.; Gambassi, G.; Bernabei, R. Impact of inappropriate drug use among hospitalized older adults. *Eur. J. Clin. Pharmacol.* **2005**, *61*, 453–459. [CrossRef]
9. Cherubini, A.; Laroche, M.L.; Petrovic, M. Mastering the complexity: Drug therapy optimization in geriatric patients. *Eur. Geriatr. Med.* **2021**, *12*, 431–434. [CrossRef]
10. Ness, J.; Hoth, A.; Barnett, M.J.; Shorr, R.I.; Kaboli, P.J. Anticholinergic medications in community-dwelling older veterans: Prevalence of anticholinergic symptoms, symptom burden, and adverse drug events. *Am. J. Geriatr. Pharmacother.* **2006**, *4*, 42–51. [CrossRef]
11. Nishtala, P.S.; Salahudeen, M.S.; Hilmer, S.N. Anticholinergics: Theoretical and clinical overview. *Expert Opin. Drug Saf.* **2016**, *15*, 753–768. [CrossRef] [PubMed]
12. Vetrano, D.L.; La Carpia, D.; Grande, G.; Casucci, P.; Bacelli, T.; Bernabei, R.; Onder, G.; Italian Group for Appropriate Drug Prescription in the Elderly. Anticholinergic Medication Burden and 5-Year Risk of Hospitalization and Death in Nursing Home Elderly Residents With Coronary Artery Disease. *J. Am. Med. Dir. Assoc.* **2016**, *17*, 1056–1059. [CrossRef] [PubMed]
13. Mangoni, A.A.; van Munster, B.C.; Woodman, R.J.; de Rooij, S.E. Measures of anticholinergic drug exposure, serum anticholinergic activity, and all-cause postdischarge mortality in older hospitalized patients with hip fractures. *Am. J. Geriatr. Psychiatry* **2013**, *21*, 785–793. [CrossRef] [PubMed]
14. Myint, P.K.; Fox, C.; Kwok, C.S.; Luben, R.N.; Wareham, N.J.; Khaw, K.T. Total anticholinergic burden and risk of mortality and cardiovascular disease over 10 years in 21,636 middle-aged and older men and women of EPIC-Norfolk prospective population study. *Age Ageing* **2015**, *44*, 219–225. [CrossRef] [PubMed]
15. Lattanzio, F.; Onder, G.; La Fauci, M.M.; Volpato, S.; Cherubini, A.; Fabbietti, P.; Ruggiero, C.; Garasto, S.; Cozza, A.; Crescibene, L.; et al. Anticholinergic Burden is Associated With Increased Mortality in Older Patients With Dependency Discharged From Hospital. *J. Am. Med Dir. Assoc.* **2018**, *19*, 942–947. [CrossRef]
16. Corsonello, A.; Cozza, A.; D'Alia, S.; Onder, G.; Volpato, S.; Ruggiero, C.; Cherubini, A.; Di Rosa, M.; Fabbietti, P.; Lattanzio, F. The excess mortality risk associated with anticholinergic burden among older patients discharged from acute care hospital with depressive symptoms. *Eur. J. Intern. Med.* **2019**, *61*, 69–74. [CrossRef]

17. D'Alia, S.; Guarasci, F.; Bartucci, L.; Caloiero, R.; Guerrieri, M.L.; Soraci, L.; Colombo, D.; Crescibene, L.; Onder, G.; Volpato, S.; et al. Hand Grip Strength May Affect the Association Between Anticholinergic Burden and Mortality Among Older Patients Discharged from Hospital. *Drugs Aging* **2020**, *37*, 447–455. [CrossRef] [PubMed]
18. Lattanzio, F.; Corica, F.; Schepisi, R.; Amantea, D.; Bruno, F.; Cozza, A.; Onder, G.; Volpato, S.; Cherubini, A.; Ruggiero, C.; et al. Anticholinergic burden and 1-year mortality among older patients discharged from acute care hospital. *Geriatr. Gerontol. Int.* **2018**, *18*, 705–713. [CrossRef]
19. Patel, K.V.; Guralnik, J.M. Prognostic implications of anemia in older adults. *Haematologica* **2009**, *94*, 1–2. [CrossRef]
20. Penninx, B.W.J.H.; Pahor, M.; Woodman, R.C.; Guralnik, J.M. Anemia in Old Age Is Associated With Increased Mortality and Hospitalization. *J. Gerontol. Ser. A* **2006**, *61*, 474–479. [CrossRef]
21. Randi, M.L.; Bertozzi, I.; Santarossa, C.; Cosi, E.; Lucente, F.; Bogoni, G.; Biagetti, G.; Fabris, F. Prevalence and Causes of Anemia in Hospitalized Patients: Impact on Diseases Outcome. *J. Clin. Med.* **2020**, *9*, 950. [CrossRef]
22. Migone De Amicis, M.; Poggiali, E.; Motta, I.; Minonzio, F.; Fabio, G.; Hu, C.; Cappellini, M.D. Anemia in elderly hospitalized patients: Prevalence and clinical impact. *Intern. Emerg. Med.* **2015**, *10*, 581–586. [CrossRef]
23. Mentz, R.J.; Greene, S.J.; Ambrosy, A.P.; Vaduganathan, M.; Subacius, H.P.; Swedberg, K.; Maggioni, A.P.; Nodari, S.; Ponikowski, P.; Anker, S.D.; et al. Clinical Profile and Prognostic Value of Anemia at the Time of Admission and Discharge Among Patients Hospitalized for Heart Failure With Reduced Ejection Fraction. *Circ. Heart Fail.* **2014**, *7*, 401–408. [CrossRef]
24. Migone de Amicis, M.; Chivite, D.; Corbella, X.; Cappellini, M.D.; Formiga, F. Anemia is a mortality prognostic factor in patients initially hospitalized for acute heart failure. *Intern. Emerg. Med.* **2017**, *12*, 749–756. [CrossRef]
25. Kung, W.-M.; Yuan, S.-P.; Lin, M.-S.; Wu, C.-C.; Islam, M.M.; Atique, S.; Touray, M.; Huang, C.-Y.; Wang, Y.-C. Anemia and the Risk of Cognitive Impairment: An Updated Systematic Review and Meta-Analysis. *Brain Sci.* **2021**, *11*, 777. [CrossRef]
26. Zamboni, V.; Cesari, M.; Zuccalà, G.; Onder, G.; Woodman, R.C.; Maraldi, C.; Ranzini, M.; Volpato, S.; Pahor, M.; Bernabei, R. Anemia and cognitive performance in hospitalized older patients: Results from the GIFA study. *Int. J. Geriatr. Psychiatry* **2006**, *21*, 529–534. [CrossRef] [PubMed]
27. Penninx, B.W.; Pahor, M.; Cesari, M.; Corsi, A.M.; Woodman, R.C.; Bandinelli, S.; Guralnik, J.M.; Ferrucci, L. Anemia is associated with disability and decreased physical performance and muscle strength in the elderly. *J. Am. Geriatr. Soc.* **2004**, *52*, 719–724. [CrossRef] [PubMed]
28. Maraldi, C.; Volpato, S.; Cesari, M.; Onder, G.; Pedone, C.; Woodman, R.C.; Fellin, R.; Pahor, M. Anemia, physical disability, and survival in older patients with heart failure. *J. Card. Fail.* **2006**, *12*, 533–539. [CrossRef] [PubMed]
29. Brombo, G.; Dianin, M.; Bianchi, L.; Corsonello, A.; Cherubini, A.; Ruggiero, C.; Onder, G.; Volpato, S.J.G.C. Prognostic value of anemia in terms of disability and mortality in hospitalized geriatric patients: Results from the CRIME study. *Geriatr. Care* **2016**, *2*. [CrossRef]
30. Tseng, S.H.; Lee, W.J.; Peng, L.N.; Lin, M.H.; Chen, L.K. Associations between hemoglobin levels and sarcopenia and its components: Results from the I-Lan longitudinal study. *Exp. Gerontol.* **2021**, *150*, 111379. [CrossRef]
31. Orrego-Matte, H.; Fernandez, O.; Mena, I. Effect of anticholinergic agents on the intestinal absorption of59Fe ferrous citrate. *Am. J. Dig. Dis.* **1971**, *16*, 789–795. [CrossRef]
32. Lin, Y.; He, S.; Feng, R.; Xu, Z.; Chen, W.; Huang, Z.; Liu, Y.; Zhang, Q.; Zhang, B.; Wang, K.; et al. Digoxin-induced anemia among patients with atrial fibrillation and heart failure: Clinical data analysis and drug-gene interaction network. *Oncotarget* **2017**, *8*, 57003–57011. [CrossRef]
33. Mesquita, R.; Pires, I.; Saldanha, C.; Martins-Silva, J. Effects of acetylcholine and spermineNONOate on erythrocyte hemorheologic and oxygen carrying properties. *Clin. Hemorheol. Microcirc.* **2001**, *25*, 153–163. [CrossRef]
34. De Almeida, J.P.; Saldanha, C. Nonneuronal cholinergic system in human erythrocytes: Biological role and clinical relevance. *J. Membr. Biol.* **2010**, *234*, 227–234. [CrossRef]
35. Trivedi, G.; Inoue, D.; Chen, C.; Bitner, L.; Chung, Y.R.; Taylor, J.; Gönen, M.; Wess, J.; Abdel-Wahab, O.; Zhang, L. Muscarinic acetylcholine receptor regulates self-renewal of early erythroid progenitors. *Sci. Transl. Med.* **2019**, *11*, eaaw3781. [CrossRef]
36. Tosato, M.; Settanni, S.; Antocicco, M.; Battaglia, M.; Corsonello, A.; Ruggiero, C.; Volpato, S.; Fabbietti, P.; Lattanzio, F.; Bernabei, R.; et al. Pattern of medication use among older inpatients in seven hospitals in Italy: Results from the CRiteria to assess Appropriate Medication use among Elderly complex patients (CRIME) project. *Curr. Drug Saf.* **2013**, *8*, 98–103. [CrossRef] [PubMed]
37. Pahor, M.; Chrischilles, E.A.; Guralnik, J.M.; Brown, S.L.; Wallace, R.B.; Carbonin, P. Drug data coding and analysis in epidemiologic studies. *Eur. J. Epidemiol.* **1994**, *10*, 405–411. [CrossRef]
38. Boustani, M.; Campbell, N.; Munger, S.; Maidment, I.; Fox, C. Impact of anticholinergics on the aging brain: A review and practical application. *Aging Health* **2008**, *4*, 311–320. [CrossRef]
39. Salahudeen, M.S.; Duffull, S.B.; Nishtala, P.S. Anticholinergic burden quantified by anticholinergic risk scales and adverse outcomes in older people: A systematic review. *BMC Geriatr.* **2015**, *15*, 31. [CrossRef] [PubMed]
40. World Health Organization. Indicators and Strategies for Iron Deficiency and Anemia Programmes. In Proceedings of the Report of the WHO/UNICEF/UNU Consultation, Geneva, Switzerland, 6–10 December 1993.
41. Folstein, M.F.; Folstein, S.E.; McHugh, P.R. "Mini-mental state". *J. Psychiatr. Res.* **1975**, *12*, 189–198. [CrossRef]
42. Lesher, E.L.; Berryhill, J.S. Validation of the Geriatric Depression Scale–Short Form among inpatients. *J. Clin. Psychol.* **1994**, *50*, 256–260. [CrossRef]

43. Katz, S.; Ford, A.B.; Moskowitz, R.W.; Jackson, B.A.; Jaffe, M.W. Studies of illness in the aged. the index of adl: A standardized measure of biological and psychosocial function. *Jama* **1963**, *185*, 914–919. [CrossRef] [PubMed]
44. World Health Organization. Haemoglobin Concentrations for the Diagnosis of Anaemia and Assessment of Severity. Available online: https://apps.who.int/iris/handle/10665/85839 (accessed on 8 October 2021).
45. Mintzer, J.; Burns, A. Anticholinergic side-effects of drugs in elderly people. *J. R. Soc. Med.* **2000**, *93*, 457–462. [CrossRef]
46. Collamati, A.; Martone, A.M.; Poscia, A.; Brandi, V.; Celi, M.; Marzetti, E.; Cherubini, A.; Landi, F. Anticholinergic drugs and negative outcomes in the older population: From biological plausibility to clinical evidence. *Aging Clin. Exp. Res.* **2016**, *28*, 25–35. [CrossRef] [PubMed]
47. Leon, C.; Gerretsen, P.; Uchida, H.; Suzuki, T.; Rajji, T.; Mamo, D.C. Sensitivity to antipsychotic drugs in older adults. *Curr. Psychiatry Rep.* **2010**, *12*, 28–33. [CrossRef] [PubMed]
48. Razani-Boroujerdi, S.; Behl, M.; Hahn, F.F.; Pena-Philippides, J.C.; Hutt, J.; Sopori, M.L. Role of muscarinic receptors in the regulation of immune and inflammatory responses. *J. Neuroimmunol.* **2008**, *194*, 83–88. [CrossRef] [PubMed]
49. Gaskell, H.; Derry, S.; Andrew Moore, R.; McQuay, H.J. Prevalence of anaemia in older persons: Systematic review. *BMC Geriatr.* **2008**, *8*, 1. [CrossRef] [PubMed]
50. Wasti, A.; Zahid, S.; Ahmed, N. Antipsychotic drugs induced iron deficiency anemia in schizophrenic patients. *Int. J. Adv. Res.* **2013**, *1*, 111–118.
51. Gupta, S.; Belle, V.S.; Kumbarakeri Rajashekhar, R.; Jogi, S.; Prabhu, R.K. Correlation of Red Blood Cell Acetylcholinesterase Enzyme Activity with Various RBC Indices. *Indian J. Clin. Biochem.* **2018**, *33*, 445–449. [CrossRef]
52. Xu, M.L.; Luk, W.K.W.; Liu, E.Y.L.; Kong, X.P.; Wu, Q.Y.; Xia, Y.J.; Dong, T.T.X.; Tsim, K.W.K. Differentiation of erythroblast requires the dimeric form of acetylcholinesterase: Interference with erythropoietin receptor. *Chem. Biol. Interact.* **2019**, *308*, 317–322. [CrossRef]
53. Saldanha, C. Human Erythrocyte Acetylcholinesterase in Health and Disease. *Molecules* **2017**, *22*, 1499. [CrossRef]
54. Wang, Y.T.; Liu, Z.M. Morphometric study of neuromuscular junction in rabbits subjected to shock by superior mesenteric artery occlusion. *Crit. Care Med.* **1990**, *18*, 213–217. [PubMed]
55. Khurana, K.; Kumar, M.; Bansal, N. Lacidipine Prevents Scopolamine-Induced Memory Impairment by Reducing Brain Oxido-nitrosative Stress in Mice. *Neurotox. Res.* **2021**. [CrossRef]
56. Bani Hassan, E.; Vogrin, S.; Hernandez Viña, I.; Boersma, D.; Suriyaarachchi, P.; Duque, G. Hemoglobin Levels are Low in Sarcopenic and Osteosarcopenic Older Persons. *Calcif. Tissue Int.* **2020**, *107*, 135–142. [CrossRef] [PubMed]
57. Trevisan, C.; Veronese, N.; Bolzetta, F.; De Rui, M.; Maggi, S.; Zambon, S.; Musacchio, E.; Sartori, L.; Perissinotto, E.; Crepaldi, G.; et al. Low Hemoglobin Levels and the Onset of Cognitive Impairment in Older People: The PRO.V.A. Study. *Rejuvenation Res.* **2016**, *19*, 447–455. [CrossRef]
58. Chatterjee, S.; Bali, V.; Carnahan, R.M.; Chen, H.; Johnson, M.L.; Aparasu, R.R. Anticholinergic burden and risk of cognitive impairment in elderly nursing home residents with depression. *Res. Soc. Adm. Pharm. RSAP* **2020**, *16*, 329–335. [CrossRef] [PubMed]
59. Cho, M.H.; Shin, D.W.; Chang, S.-A.; Lee, J.E.; Jeong, S.-M.; Kim, S.H.; Yun, J.M.; Son, K. Association between cognitive impairment and poor antihypertensive medication adherence in elderly hypertensive patients without dementia. *Sci. Rep.* **2018**, *8*, 11688. [CrossRef]
60. Lucca, U.; Tettamanti, M.; Mosconi, P.; Apolone, G.; Gandini, F.; Nobili, A.; Tallone, M.V.; Detoma, P.; Giacomin, A.; Clerico, M.; et al. Association of mild anemia with cognitive, functional, mood and quality of life outcomes in the elderly: The "Health and Anemia" study. *PLoS ONE* **2008**, *3*, e1920. [CrossRef] [PubMed]

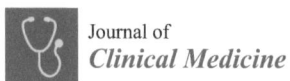

Article

Age-Related Alterations of Hyaluronan and Collagen in Extracellular Matrix of the Muscle Spindles

Chenglei Fan [1,†], Carmelo Pirri [1,*,†], Caterina Fede [1], Diego Guidolin [1], Carlo Biz [2], Lucia Petrelli [1], Andrea Porzionato [1], Veronica Macchi [1], Raffaele De Caro [1] and Carla Stecco [1,*]

[1] Department of Neurosciences, Institute of Human Anatomy, University of Padua, 35121 Padua, Italy; chenglei.fan@studenti.unipd.it (C.F.); caterina.fede@unipd.it (C.F.); diego.guidolin@unipd.it (D.G.); lucia.petrelli@unipd.it (L.P.); andrea.porzionato@unipd.it (A.P.); veronica.macchi@unipd.it (V.M.); rdecaro@unipd.it (R.D.C.)

[2] Orthopedics and Orthopedic Oncology, Department of Surgery, Oncology and Gastroenterology (DiSCOG), University of Padua, 35128 Padua, Italy; carlo.biz@unipd.it

* Correspondence: carmelop87@hotmail.it (C.P.); carla.stecco@unipd.it (C.S.); Tel.: +39-049-8272315 (C.P. & C.S.)

† These authors contributed equally to this work.

Abstract: Background: Muscle spindles (MSs) play a crucial role in proprioception and locomotor co-ordination. Although the elasticity and viscosity of the extracellular matrix (ECM) within which MSs are embedded may play a key role in MS function, the impact of aging on ECM components is unclear. The aim of the current study was to investigate the age-related physiological changes of the ECM and to verify if these could be due to alterations of the environment directly surrounding MSs. Methods: Hematoxylin Eosin and picrosirius-red staining was carried out; collagen types I (COLI) and III (COLIII) were assessed, and biotinylated hyaluronan binding protein (HABP) immunohistochemical analysis was undertaken to evaluate alterations of the ECM in the intramuscular connective tissue (IMCT) of the hindlimbs of C57BL/6J male mice. Assessments were carried out on 6-week-old (Group A), 8-month-old (Group B), and 2-year-old (Group C) laboratory mice. Results: The capsule's outer layer became progressively thicker with aging (it was 3.02 ± 0.26 μm in Group A, 3.64 ± 0.31 μm in Group B, and 5.81 ± 0.85 μm in Group C). The collagen in IMCT around and within the MSs was significantly higher in Group C, but there were no significant differences between Groups A and B. The MS capsules and continuous IMCT were primarily made up of COLI and COLIII. The average optical density (AOD) values of COLI in IMCT surrounding MS were significantly higher after aging ($p < 0.05$), but there were no significant differences in COLIII in the three groups ($p > 0.05$). HA was present in IMCT and filled the MSs capsule. The AOD of HABP of MS showed that there were lower HA levels in Group C with respect to Group A ($p = 0.022$); no significant differences were noted neither between Groups A and B nor between Groups B and C ($p > 0.05$). Conclusion: Age-related collagen accumulation and lower HA in the ECM in which the MSs were embedded may probably cause more stiffness in the ECM in vivo, which could help to partly explain the peripheral mechanisms underlying the age-related decline in functional changes related to MSs.

Keywords: aging; extracellular matrix; muscle spindle; collagen; collagen type I; collagen type III; hyaluronan; intramuscular connective tissue

Citation: Fan, C.; Pirri, C.; Fede, C.; Guidolin, D.; Biz, C.; Petrelli, L.; Porzionato, A.; Macchi, V.; De Caro, R.; Stecco, C. Age-Related Alterations of Hyaluronan and Collagen in Extracellular Matrix of the Muscle Spindles. *J. Clin. Med.* **2022**, *11*, 86. https://doi.org/10.3390/jcm11010086

Academic Editor: Francesco Mattace-Raso

Received: 10 November 2021
Accepted: 21 December 2021
Published: 24 December 2021

Publisher's Note: MDPI stays neutral with regard to jurisdictional claims in published maps and institutional affiliations.

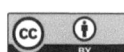

Copyright: © 2021 by the authors. Licensee MDPI, Basel, Switzerland. This article is an open access article distributed under the terms and conditions of the Creative Commons Attribution (CC BY) license (https://creativecommons.org/licenses/by/4.0/).

1. Introduction

Muscle spindles (MSs), which are detectors of muscle length and velocity, play an important role not only in proprioception but also in regulating muscle contraction [1,2]. Some time ago, a group of investigators [3] reported that the dynamic and static length sensitivities of MS primary endings in response to ramp stretch were decreased in aged rats. Age-related proprioceptive deficits have also been found to be associated with patho-physiological and morphological changes in MSs, which normally rapidly adapt to fibers in response to muscle length and speed changes. Possible morphological changes in MSs include: enlargement of the periaxial space [4], thicker spindle capsules [5–8], a lower number of intrafusal fibers [9], modifications in the myosin heavy chain content, lower sensitivity, smaller spindle diameters, changes in the shape of the MS primary endings (less helicity and vorticity), primary endings of aged MSs being less spiral or non-spiral in appearance [10], axonal swelling/expanded motor endplates due to denervation [11], and a significant increase in the number of Ia afferents with large swellings that fail to properly wrap around intrafusal muscle fibers [12]. Moreover, possible functional changes with MSs were also found. Aging is associated with alterations of MSs and their neural pathways. The muscle stiffness constant values were greater in old muscles, confirming the changes in elastic properties under passive conditions due to aging [13]. In addition, there are decreased conduction velocities and a less dynamic response of primary endings in old rats using electrophysiological experimentation [10]. Likewise, MSs containing thin muscle fibers may be intimately related to the degeneration and regeneration of extrafusal muscle fibers during aging, which may often fail to receive sensory innervation [14] and induce a decrease in the sensitivity, acuity, and integration of the proprioceptive signal [15].

New perspectives in this field recently became apparent when some investigators reported that even the intramuscular connective tissue (IMCT) of the extracellular matrix (ECM) in which MSs are embedded changes with aging [16]. The ECM refers to many proteins (collagen, elastic fibers) and ground substances (proteoglycans, multiadhesive glycoproteins, and glycosaminoglycans (GAGs)) that provide the milieu for the cells within the body [17]. Collagens are recognized as the main components of the ECM and form a family of 28 different types of collagens coded for by 44 different genes [18]. Proteoglycans can be categorized into four main families: small leucine-rich proteoglycans, hylectans, pericellular and basement membrane proteoglycans, and cell-surface proteoglycans [19]. Hyaluronan (HA) is the major extracellular GAG, which is found in many different tissues and has many roles, ranging from mechanical to chemical [19]. Cell behavior is profoundly affected by the environment in which they live, thus the aging of the ECM is central to understanding age-related changes [17]. Nowadays, ECM's role has been highlighted in different diseases and tissues [19–23].

The different ECM elements provide the mechanical properties, plasticity, and malleability of the IMCT [24]. It has been reported, for example, that immobilization results in a marked increase in the collagen fibers in the IMCT (endomysium, perimysium, epimysium) and clearly disturb the normal IMCT structure of rat skeletal muscle. The changes in the IMCT in immobilized skeletal muscle seemed to contribute to alterations in the biomechanical properties of the tissue of skeletal muscle reducing its compliance [25]. This, in turn, increased the stretch reflex of the MS as the pull is transmitted more efficiently to the MSs in a less extensible muscle [26]. The MS is covered with a strong capsule of connective tissue that is continuous with the IMCT [27,28]. A gelatinous fluid rich in GAGs probably composed of primarily hyaluronan (HA) fills the inner and outer capsule spaces [29,30]. Although the elasticity and viscosity of the ECM within which MSs are embedded may play a key role in MS function, the impact of aging on ECM components is unclear.

In light of these considerations, we hypothesized that, beyond the normal neurodegeneration and morphological alterations of the MSs, age-related physiological changes could also be explained by alterations in the environment directly surrounding them. The study set out to investigate age-related changes in MSs and the ECM that could lead to altered functional outcomes.

2. Materials and Methods

Fifteen male C57Bl/6J mice (five 6-week-old mice = Group A, five 8-month-old mice = Group B, and five 2-year-old mice = Group C) were provided by the University of Padova's Animal Center (Padova, Italy). The ages of the mice corresponded approximately to 11.5, 35, and 70 human years, respectively [31]. The mice were kept in cages in an environmentally controlled room with the temperature adjusted to 22 °C in which there were diurnal light-dark cycles and free access to water and food. The animals' accommodation and care and all experimental procedures conformed to guidelines approved by the University of Padova's Animal Care and Ethical Committee, in agreement with the guidelines of the Italian Department of Health.

Two percent isoflurane was used to anesthetize the mice. Following euthanasia, the left hindlimb (including the gastrocnemius; soleus; tibialis anterior; and posterior, fibularis longus, and brevis muscles) was collected for histological and immunohistochemistry studies. As hindlimb muscles in mice are extremely small and dissection can damage the IMCT in the skeletal muscles, the tibia and fibula bones were stored together to maintain the overall morphology and interrelationship of the hindlimb muscles and permit further specimen processing and experimental studies. The entire left hindlimb of each mouse was immediately post-fixed in 10% neutral buffered formalin (10% NBF, pH 7.4 at 4 °C for 48 h) to prepare for the decalcification procedure.

2.1. The Ethylenediaminetetraacetic Acid (EDTA) Decalcification Protocol for the Mice Hindlimbs

To preserve the antigenicity of the hindlimb sample, 10% EDTA solution at room temperature was used to decalcify the bone samples. All the samples post-fixed in 10% neutral-buffered formalin (NBF) were placed in phosphate buffered saline (PBS) (20 min × 3) and distilled water (20 min × 3). The fixed samples were then placed in 10% EDTA (at least 15 volumes), which was replaced weekly. The hindlimbs were decalcified in 10–14 days. The samples were then rinsed in distilled water (20 min × 2) for further paraffin embedding and histochemical and immunohistochemical staining.

After the samples were embedded in the paraffin wax, blocks were serially sectioned in a rostro-caudal direction and perpendicularly to the muscle fiber axis beginning under the lower edge point of the patella. Four sections at 100 μm intervals were transferred onto 2% gelatinized glass slides. A 100 μm section sampling interval was considered appropriate in light of the results of other studies [32,33], and a pilot study during which muscle tissue from two 6-week-old mice was longitudinally sectioned and the MS length was determined; it ranged between 180 and 400 μm. Sections of the muscle samples were subjected to routine histology staining (Hematoxylin Eosin, picrosirius-red) and the immunohistochemistry assessment of collagen type I (COLI), collagen type III (COLIII), and biotinylated hyaluronan binding protein (HABP) antibodies. The MS images at the equatorial region of the mice hindlimb muscle according their morphology were used to quantitatively analyze the components of the ECM in the MSs of the three mice groups.

2.2. Immunohistochemistry Staining: Analysis of Collagen Type I (COLI) and Collagen Type III (COLIII)

After formalin fixation, samples were dehydrated in graded ethanol, embedded in paraffin, and cut into 5 μm-thick sections. The sections were dewaxed in xylene 2 × 10 min and subsequently passed through 99–70–30% ethanol (10 min for each passage) and 2 × 5 min in water. Samples were treated with the blocking of endogenous peroxidases with 0.5% H_2O_2 in phosphate buffered solution (PBS; pH 7.4). The slides were then treated with 0.1% bovine serum albumin (BSA) for 1 h before being incubated with the primary antibody, the Anti-COLI, Anti-COLIII (Goat Anti-Collagen I: 1:400, SouthernBiotech, Birmingham, AL 35209, USA; Rabbit polyclonal to Collagen III: 1:400, ab7778 Sigma-Aldrich, Merk Life Science S.r.l., MI, Italy) in BSA at 4 °C overnight. After being washed three times with PBS, the sections were incubated with the secondary antibody (anti-rabbit IgG peroxidase-coniugated antibodies for COLIII and anti-Goat peroxidase-coniugated antibodies for COLI), 1:200, 1:300, respectively, for 1 h, after repeated washings; the reaction was developed with 3,3′-diaminobenzidine (Liquid DAB Substrate Chromogen System; Dako Corp, Carpinteria, CA, 93013-2921, USA). Negative controls were obtained by omitting the primary antibody. Finally, each slide was counterstained with hematoxylin, followed by dehydration in a graded ethanol series, and mounted for microscopic evaluation. The generation of the reaction product was stopped within the linear phase of the generation of the reaction product and to directly compare control (without primary antibody) with the three experimental tissues, leaving same the reaction time and solutions during the IHC [33].

2.3. Immunohistochemistry Staining: Analysis of Hyaluronic Acid Binding Protein (HABP)

Dewaxed 5 µm thick sections were treated with 0.5% H2O2 in PBS (15 min at room temperature) to block endogenous peroxidase and then washed in PBS. The specimens were incubated in 0.1% BSA solution for 1 h at room temperature, treated with biotinylated HABP (Millipore Sigma-Aldrich, Merk Life Science S.r.l., MI, Italy, 1:900 dilution), diluted in 0.1% BSA solution, and incubated overnight at 4 °C. After multiple washings with PBS, the samples were incubated with the secondary antibody, HRP-conjugated Streptavidin 1:250 for 30 min (Jackson ImmunoResearch, Cambridgeshire, UK) and washed in PBS buffer. The reaction was then developed with 3,3'-diaminobenzidine (Liquid DAB substrate Chromogen System kit Dako Corp, Carpinteria, CA, 93013-2921, USA) and it was terminated with distilled water. The nuclei were counterstained with ready-to-use hematoxylin (Dako Corp, Carpinteria, CA, 93013-2921, USA). Negative controls were checked with similarly treated sections, without the primary antibody, and the specificity of the immunostaining reaction was confirmed.

2.4. Image Analysis

The specimens were photographed using a Leica DMR microscope (Leica Microsystems, Wetzlar, Germany), and the images were analyzed with ImageJ software [34,35], which is freely available at http://rsb.info.nih.gov/ij/ (accessed on 18 August 2021).

The thickness of the outer layer of the MS capsule and the collagen were measured using a final magnification of 40×. Fields containing MSs continuous with the perimysium and endomysium stained with picrosirius red were selected (Figure 1).

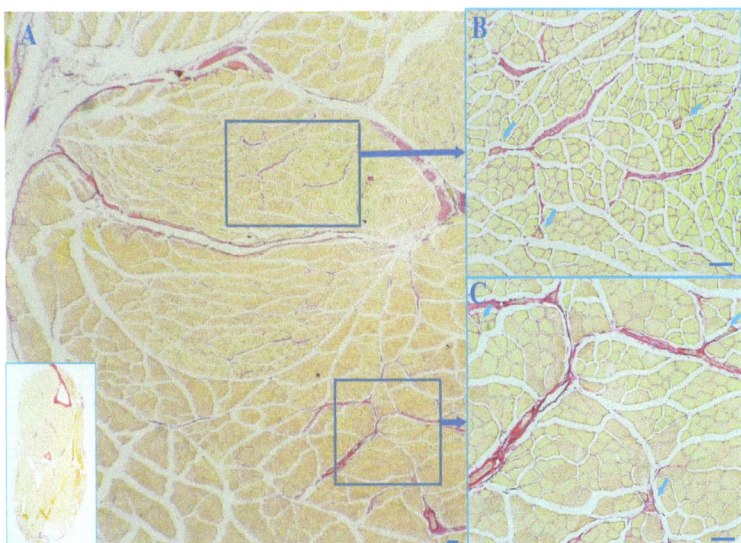

Figure 1. Picrosirius red staining of a cross section of a muscle of a mouse hindlimb. The inset in (**A**) on the bottom left corner is the whole crosse section of the mouse hindlimb. The MS capsule appears to be continuous with the perimysium, epimysium, and the endomysium. (**A**): Global view of the cross section. (**B,C**): MSs within the skeletal muscle. arrows: muscle spindles. Scale bar: 100 µm.

A minimum of 30 images, including a MS from each mouse hindlimb, were obtained, and the data were averaged to calculate representative values for the thickness of the capsule's outer layer, the area percentage of the total collagen in the cross sections of the muscle in which the MSs were embedded, and the area percentage of collagen in the MSs (Figure 2A,C,D). The results were expressed as the thickness of the outer layer of the capsule (µm) and the quantity of collagen in the MSs (%) per unit area.

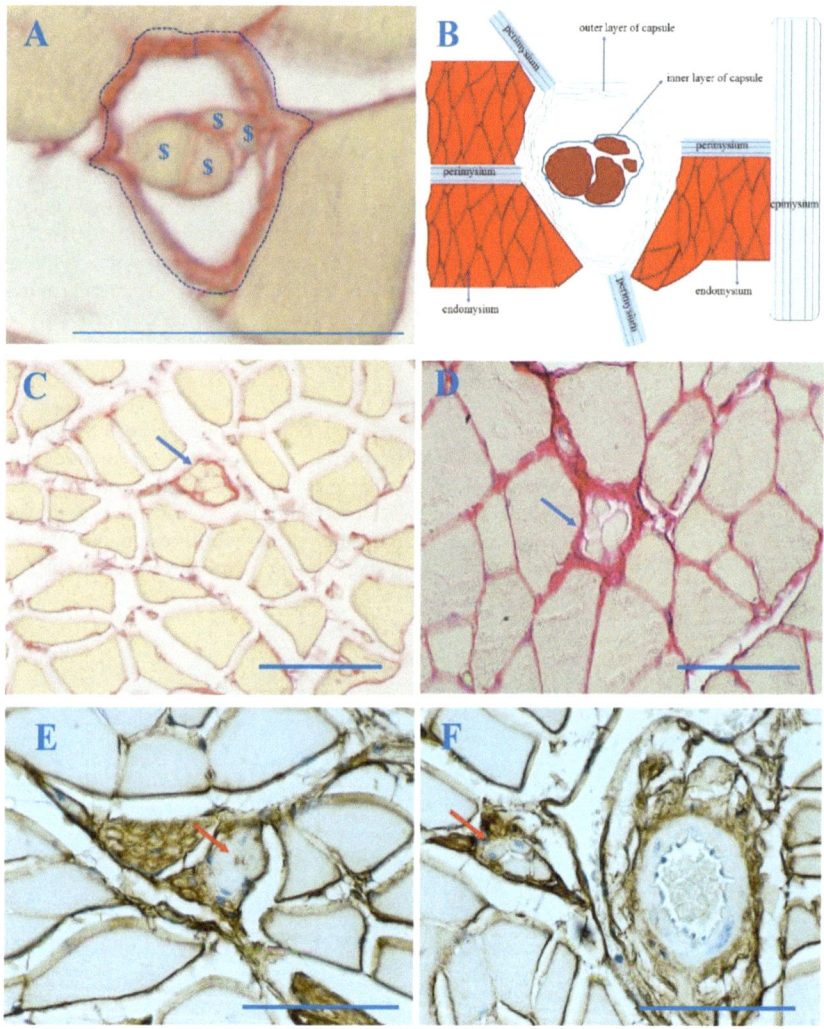

Figure 2. Picrosirius red (**A,C,D**) and biotinylated HABP immunohistochemistry staining (**E,F**) of a cross section of a muscle of a mouse hindlimb. (**A**): The MS in the skeletal muscle. $: intrafusal fiber; ↕: the thickness of the outer layer of the MS capsule; imaginary line: the area of the MS; (**B**): A drawing illustrating the MS's outer capsule's continuity with the endomysium, perimysium, and epimysium. (**C**): A MS in a muscle of the hindlimb of a 6-week-old mouse (Group A), (**D**): of a 2-year-old mouse (Group C). (**E,F**): HA is present in the MS capsule. The MS capsule was continuous with the nerve (**E**) and the blood vessel (**F**); arrows: muscle spindle; Scale bar: 50 µm.

The COLI, COLIII, and biotinylated HABP were measured using a final magnification of 40×. The average optical densities (AODs) of the COLI and COLIII of the area of the muscle cross sections in which MSs were embedded, of the area of the MS alone, and of the biotinylated HABP of the MS alone were measured. Average optical densities (AODs) = integrated optical density (IOD)/area. The semi-quantitative immunohistochemical images for analysis in the present study were taken with the same background, same exposition light for microscopy, and same background filter in Image J. In addition, the value changes with the intensity of the light source and is a part of the power ratio of the emission amplitude to the incident amplitude. In international application, the range of OD value is constant use, a scale of 0–2.71. Moreover, all the analyses are double-blinded. A minimum of 30 images was obtained, and the data regarding the AOD were averaged to calculate the representative values for the COLI, COLIII, and the biotinylated HABP. Considering that differences in any parameter need to be limited to approximately the same area of the same muscle, a minimum of 30 MS images each are from tibialis anterior, peroneus longus, peroneus brevis (10 MS images); gastrocnemius, soleus (10 MS images) and flexor digitorum longus, flexor hallucis longus, and tibialis posterior (10 MS images).

2.5. Statistical Analysis

All data management and statistical analyses were performed using IBM SPSS version 25.0 software (SPSS Inc., Chicago, IL, USA). The Shapiro–Wilks and Levene's tests were respectively performed to investigate the normality of the data distribution and the homogeneity of variance. The thickness of the capsule's outer layer, the area percentage of the total collagen in the muscle cross sections in which MSs were embedded, the area percentage of the collagen in the MS, and the AOD of the COLI and of the COLIII in the entire muscle cross sections in which MSs were embedded and in the MS alone are reported as means ± standard deviations (M ± SD) since they were found to have a normal distribution. An analysis of variance (ANOVA) with Tukey post-hoc test (normally distributed data and equal variances assumed) was carried out to compare the AOD of the COLI and the COLIII of the area of the entire muscle cross sections where the MSs were embedded and the AOD of the area of the MS alone to investigate age-related effects on collagen and subtypes (COLI, COLIII). In addition, the ANOVA with the post-hoc test of Games–Howell (normally distributed data but equality of variances not assumed) were both used to compare the thickness of the outer layer of the capsule, the area percentage of the total collagen in the entire muscle cross section in which the MSs were embedded, and the area percentage of collagen in the MS alone. The AOD of the biotinylated HABP of the MS was classified as median, minimum, and maximum, since its distribution was not normal. The Kruskal–Wallis H with Bonferroni post-hoc test was used to compare the AOD of the biotinylated HABP of the MSs of the three groups. A p-value of less than 0.05 was considered the study's limit for statistical significance.

3. Results

3.1. The Outer Capsule of MS Is Continuous with Intramuscular Connective Tissue (IMCT)

All the MSs were embedded in the IMCT, and the outer spindle capsules were found to be continuous with the endomysium, perimysium, and epimysium (Figures 1 and 2B). In addition, the outer spindle capsule was continuous with the nerve (Figure 2E) and the blood vessel (Figure 2F). The integrity of and the continuity between the different muscles and between different MSs within the same and different muscles were maintained by the IMCT.

3.2. Collagen in the MS with Aging

MSs are surrounded by a strong capsule found in the IMCT between the extrafusal fibers. The MS capsule contains outer and inner layers. The thickness of the capsule's outer layer was 3.02 ± 0.26 μm in the adolescent, 3.64 ± 0.31 μm in the middle-aged, and 5.81 ± 0.85 μm in the elderly mice. In addition, the area percentage of the total collagen in the entire cross section in which the MSs were embedded was 2.95 ± 0.46 in the adolescent, 4.42 ± 1.23 in middle-aged, and 9.29 ± 0.81 in the elderly mice. With regard to the MS alone, the area percentage of collagen was 22.97 ± 6.55 in the adolescent, 25.94 ± 2.36 in the middle-aged, and 40.80 ± 3.46 in the elderly mice. The thickness of the capsule's outer layer, the area percentage of the total collagen in the entire muscle cross sections in which the MSs were embedded, and the area percentage of collagen in the MS alone were significantly higher in Group C (the elderly group) with respect to Group A (the adolescent one) ($p < 0.01$) and Group B (the middle-aged group) ($p < 0.01$); there were no significant differences, except for the the thickness of the capsule's outer layer, in these parameters between Groups A and B ($p > 0.05$), ($p = 0.022$) (Table 1, Figures 2A,C,D and A1).

Table 1. Collagen constituting the ECM of the MSs in the mouse skeletal muscle.

Characteristic	Group A	Group B	Group C	A vs. B p-Value	A vs. C p-Value	B vs. C p-Value
$ Thickness of the outer capsule layer	3.02 ± 0.26	3.64 ± 0.31	5.81 ± 0.85	0.022 *	0.003 **	0.007 **
$ Total collagen 40× (% area)	2.95 ± 0.46	4.42 ± 1.23	9.29 ± 0.81	0.116	<0.001 ***	<0.001 ***
$ Collagen of the MS alone 40× (% area)	22.97 ± 6.55	25.94 ± 2.36	40.80 ± 3.46	0.633	0.004 **	<0.001 ***
# AOD of COLI in the whole muscle cross section	0.20 ± 0.02	0.27 ± 0.02	0.30 ± 0.01	<0.001 ***	<0.001 ***	0.032 *
# AOD of COLIII in the whole muscle cross section	0.25 ± 0.02	0.28 ± 0.01	0.26 ± 0.02	0.255	0.747	0.629
# AOD of COLI in the MS alone	0.16 ± 0.01	0.22 ± 0.01	0.28 ± 0.06	0.038 *	<0.001 ***	0.047 *
# AOD of COLIII in the MS alone	0.25 ± 0.07	0.27 ± 0.07	0.26 ± 0.05	0.849	0.968	0.950
& AOD of HABP in the MS alone	0.50 (0.45–0.67)	0.43 (0.40–0.45)	0.40 (0.33–0.47)	0.85	0.022 *	1.00

ANOVA with Tukey post-hoc test #/Games–Howell post-hoc test $; Kruskal–Wallis H with Bonferroni post-hoc test &, MS: muscle spindle, AOD: average optical density, Group A: equivalent to human adolescence (6-week-old mice), Group B: equivalent to human middle age (8-month-old mice), Group C: equivalent to old age in humans (2-year-old mice) group. The values are presented as numbers or means ± SD (normally distributed data and equal variances assumed); the values are classified as median, minimum, and maximum, since their distribution was not normal. * <0.05, ** ≤0.01, *** ≤0.001.

3.3. COLI and COLIII in MS

Collagen fibers, as fundamental components of ECM, provide a supporting framework of muscle tissues. In this study, immunohistochemistry staining uncovered that the MS capsule and the IMCT consisted of COLI and COLIII (Figure 3A–F). The AOD of COLI in the whole cross section in which MSs were embedded was 0.20 ± 0.02 in the adolescent, 0.27 ± 0.02 in the middle-aged, and 0.30 ± 0.01 in the elderly mice. The AOD of COLI in the MS alone was 0.16 ± 0.01 in the adolescent, 0.22 ± 0.01 in the middle-age, and 0.28 ± 0.06 in the elderly mice. The AOD of COLI in the whole muscle cross section in which the MSs were embedded and the AOD of COLI in the MS alone were significantly increased with aging (Group A vs. Group B: $p < 0.05$; Group A vs. Group C: $p < 0.001$; Group B vs. Group C: $p < 0.05$). The AOD of COLIII in the whole muscle cross section was 0.25 ± 0.02 in the adolescent, 0.28 ± 0.01 in the middle-aged and 0.26 ± 0.02 in the elderly mice. The AOD of COLIII in the MS alone was 0.25 ± 0.07 in the adolescent, 0.27 ± 0.07 in the middle-aged, and 0.26 ± 0.05 in the elderly mice. There were no significant differences in the COLIII neither in the whole muscle cross section in which MSs were embedded nor in the MS alone between the three groups ($p > 0.05$) (Table 1).

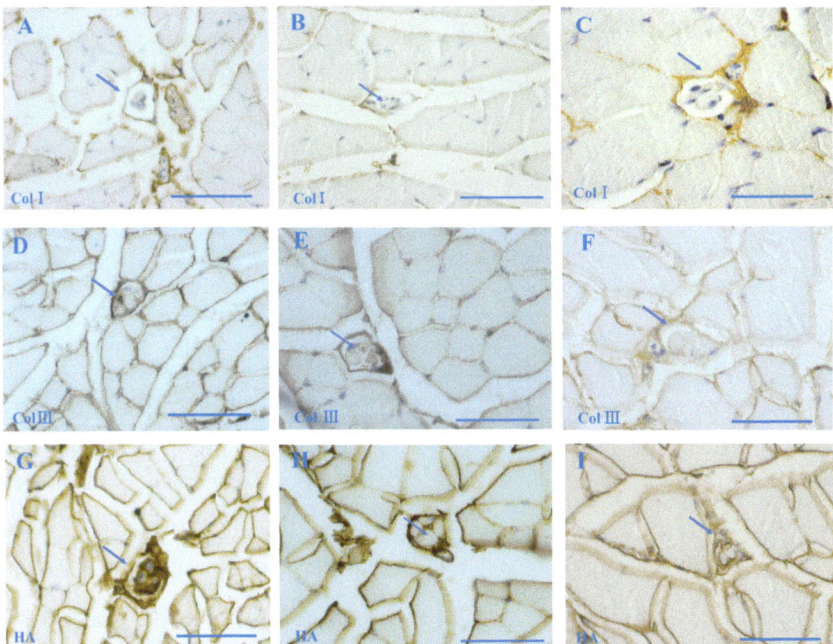

Figure 3. MS embedded in the extracellular matrix elements with immunohistochemistry staining of collagen type I (COLI) (**A–C**), collagen type III (COLIII) (**D–F**), and biotinylated HABP (**G–I**). The COLI and COLIII localized in the MS capsule. The HABP localized in the MS. (**A,D,G**): A MS in the hindlimb of a 6 week-old mouse (Group A); (**B,E,H**): a MS in the hindlimb of an 8-month-old mouse (Group B); (**C,F,I**): a MS of the hindlimb of a 2-year-old mouse (Group C). Scale bar: 50 µm.

3.4. Age-Related HA in MS According to Biotinylated HABP Immunohistochemical Staining

The ground substance of the ECM is composed of a complex mixture GAGs, most often covalently linked to proteins, forming proteoglycans and glycoproteins, in which HA appears to be the one of the most important ones. In the present study, HA was present in the IMCT (epimysium, perimysium, epimysium) and filled the MS capsule according to the biotinylated HABP immunohistochemistry staining (Figures 3E,F and A2). The AOD of the MS in the hindlimb muscle was significantly decreased in Group C (0.40, 0.33–0.47) (Figure 3I) with respect to Group A (0.50, 0.45–0.67) (Figure 3G) ($p = 0.022$); no significant differences neither between Groups A and B (0.43, 0.40–0.45) (Figure 3H) nor between Groups B and C ($p > 0.05$) were noted (Table 1).

4. Discussion

The study results outlined here have demonstrated that MSs are embedded in the IMCT and that the MS outer capsule is continuous with the perimysium, epimysium, endomysium, nerve, and blood vessel. Other studies have already demonstrated the continuity of the outer capsule with the ECM of extrafusal fibers in chicken [36] and with the perineural epithelium [37]. IMCT acts as the scaffold for muscle bundles and fiber integrity and carries the blood vessels and nerves to the muscle. IMCT continuity permits communication between different muscles, various MSs within the same muscle, and various MSs in different muscles directly and/or indirectly. This communication may play an important role in movement coordination. In addition, the intrafusal fibers of MSs possess intracapsular terminations or extend beyond the limit of the MS capsule terminating in the IMCT of adjacent extrafusal fibers [38–40]. MS distribution seems to be similar to the three-dimensional arrangement and organization of the IMCT from the fascia point of view (IMCT belongs to the fascial system). If MSs are viewed not only as isolated mechanoreceptors but also as sensory organs embedded and enclosed in the IMCT, this would explain how they can sense the tension of the IMCT as far as the fascia are concerned.

Study results also demonstrated that the capsule's outer layer, the area percentage of the total collagen in the whole cross section in which MSs were embedded and the collagen in the MSs were significantly thicker in the elderly mice and that there were no significant differences in these parameters, with the exception of the thickness of the capsule's outer layer, between the adolescent and middle-aged mice. This is in line with other studies about the thicker capsule's outer layer by Swash and Fox (1972) [9]. An analysis of our results also showed that the MS capsule and the IMCT consisted of COLI and COLIII. While the AOD of the COLI in the whole cross section where the MSs were embedded and the AOD of COLI in the MS alone were significantly increased in the aging mice, there were no significant differences in COLIII in the three groups neither in the entire cross section in which MSs were embedded nor in the MS alone. These results have confirmed the findings of another study demonstrating that older adults have thicker MS capsules [11]. Moreover, these findings are consistent with those of some studies that highlighted the role of the collagens in various diseases and tissues [21–23]. Parkes et al. [21] reported the prominent role of collagen and HA in the ECM of ovaries, suggesting their crucial activity for ovarian homeostasis, possibly through signaling events or tissue micromechanism. Numerous reports described the association between the single-nucleotide polymorphism rs12722 and rs13936 in the COL5A1 gene and injuries, such as Achilles tendon pathology, anterior cruciate ligament, and tennis elbow [41–45]. Daleswski et al. [22] studied the COL5A1 rs12722 and rs13946 polymorphisms as potential genetic factors regulating the ADDwoR-mediated soft tissue pathway in association with temporomandibular joint anterior disc displacement [22]. Pirri et al. [46] reported that:" excessive aggregation of ECM elements is present in fibrosis (e.g., in myopathies), including in fasciae, and occurs during aging [16], and diabetes, characterized by increased endomysium as well as perimysium" [47]. Diet-induced insulin resistance (IR) leads to an increase in the expression of collagens I, III, and IV [48].

However, the MS are sensitive to both the phasic and tonic stretches. When the muscle lengthens and the MS is stretched, the threshold corresponds to a tension of 3 g in humans and leads to a trigger action in the MS afferent [49]. The accumulation of collagen, especially of the COLI type, due to aging (found in elderly mice) may reduce the deformation and increase the resistance of the IMCT in the skeletal muscle, resulting in a higher threshold.

HA was found to be present in the IMCT and filled the MS capsule. Study results showed that the HA in the MS was significantly decreased in the elderly mice with respect to their adolescent counterparts. There were, however, no significant differences between the elderly and middle-aged mice nor between the middle-aged and adolescent mice. HA is not only an excellent lubricant and shock absorber [24], but also on the background discharge and the discharge in response to stretch [50]. The age-related decrease in HA could affect the mechanical properties of MSs, the background discharge, and the discharge in response to stretch, which may in turn affect age-related changes in MSs' sensitivity to the stretch and tension of skeletal muscles. As has been demonstrated by other studies, HA has many roles in the different human tissues, ranging from mechanical to chemical [19,21,48,51].

MSs also play an important role in reactive postural control, and they are also involved in producing contractile force during reflectory changes. The MSs may be unable to adapt to stretching and velocity due to the age-related alterations of the ECM in the skeletal muscle resulting in failed motor unit recruitment. Fewer motor unit activities may lead to a lower contractile strength of the muscle [52,53]. MSs also seem to participate in regulating sensitivity during the dynamic and/or static phases of stretching; this would mean that, as they become less sensitive with aging, there is a decline in postural stability and balance. During flexion of the trunk, for example, the MSs of the erector spinae muscles are lengthened. This stimulates the recruitment of motor units, resulting in the contraction of the muscles and helping the trunk return to the starting position. The same mechanism is found in the neck and other body segments [54,55]. If MSs become less sensitive to stretching due to aging, trauma, poor posture, post-surgery, or overuse, this could exacerbate changes in sensory and motor functions, leading to greater postural instability and a higher risk of falls, and the inhibition of normal MS stretching could also result in abnormal feedback to the central nervous system.

There are several limitations in this study. Firstly, aging-related changes in the musculoskeletal system included a decline not only involved in the alterations of HA and collagen in the ECM of the MSs but also a reduction in the number of MSs per muscle, a loss of intrafusal fibers, and changes in the efficacy of the fusimotor innervation. In addition, the age-related decline of the velocity of action potential propagation by sensory neurons, sarcopenia, changes in the structure of the sensory nerve terminal, and the loss of neurons in the motor cortex and cerebellum have already been demonstrated. All of these changes could potentially contribute to the decline in motor coordination, frequent falls, and unstable gait observed in elderly persons. Moreover, the inner and outer capsule contain many other ECM proteins as described in the introduction, including other proteins: laminins, nidogens, collagen type IV, fibronectin, agrin, and other proteoglycans. These molecules could also affect the biomechanical properties of the spindle capsule. Moreover, the treatment of histological sections involves tissue dehydration and thus, shrinkage. As reported by other studies [56,57], the tissue shrinkage takes place during the preparation of connective tissue specimens for histological examination. At the same time, there is likely no difference in shrinkage between young and old, as reported by Kerns et al. [58], as the decrease of shrinkage was relatively constant across age groups. Further studies are necessary to better illustrate these factors with aging, to better understand the effects of aging on locomotor ability decline.

5. Conclusions

As we found that a change in the thickness of the outer capsule, the decreased staining intensity with HA and increased staining intensity with of Col I in ECM may probably cause the MSs themselves and the surrounding microenvironment to experience more stiffness with aging in vivo. Other studies regaridng functional changes in MS have already demonstrated age-related muscle stiffness and elastic properties [13] and decreased conduction velocities and dynamic response of primary endings with aging [10]. Moreover, MSs contained thin muscle fibers that may be intimately related to the degeneration and regeneration of extrafusal muscle fibers during aging, which may often fail to receive sensory innervation [14], and that may induce a decrease in the sensitivity, acuity, and integration of the proprioceptive signal [15], which may also reduce the sensitivity of the MSs and their ability to activate motor neurons stimulating muscle contraction and to contribute to postural maintenance and positional sense, as well as to maintaining muscle tone. It has been seen, in fact, that, when the MSs cannot be activated, the regulation of muscle tone is compromised [59]. These alterations in ECM where MSs are embedded could help to explain partly the peripheral mechanisms underlying the age-related decline in functional changes related to MS.

Author Contributions: Conceptualization, C.F. (Chenglei Fan) and C.S.; methodology, C.F. (Chenglei Fan), C.P., C.B. and L.P.; software, C.F. (Chenglei Fan) and D.G.; validation, C.F. (Chenglei Fan), C.P., A.P., R.D.C. and C.S., formal analysis, C.F. (Chenglei Fan), C.P., C.F. (Caterina Fede) and D.G.; investigation, C.F. (Chenglei Fan), C.P., C.B. and V.M.; data curation, C.F. (Chenglei Fan), C.P., C.F. (Caterina Fede) and D.G.; writing—original draft preparation, C.F. (Chenglei Fan), C.P. and C.F. (Caterina Fede); writing—review and editing C.P., V.M., R.D.C. and C.S.; project administration, C.S. All authors have read and agreed to the published version of the manuscript.

Funding: The authors received no funding for the research.

Institutional Review Board Statement: The study was conducted according to the guidelines of the Declaration of Helsinki. The animals' accommodation and care and all experimental procedures conformed to guidelines approved by the University of Padova's Animal Care and Ethical Committee (Permission code: 977/2015-PR, 21 September 2015), in agreement with the guidelines of the Italian Department of Health.

Data Availability Statement: The data presented in this study are available on request from the corresponding author.

Acknowledgments: The authors thank the China Scholarship Council for Chenglei Fan (201708370097) studentship funding.

Conflicts of Interest: The authors declare no conflict of interest.

Abbreviations

Muscle spindles: MSs; extracellular matrix: ECM; collagen type I: COLI; collagen type III: COL III; hyaluronan binding protein: HABP; intramuscular connective tissue: IMCT; glycosaminoglycans: GAGs; average optical density: AOD; hyaluronan: HA.

Appendix A

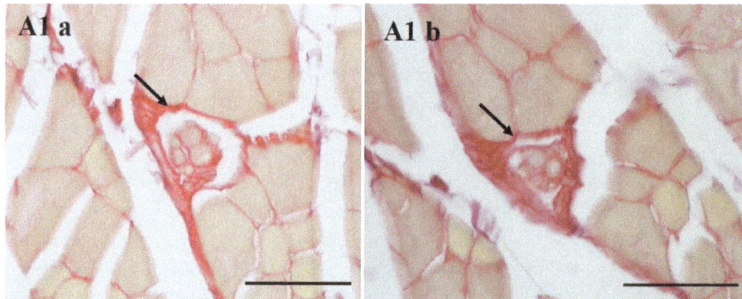

Figure A1. (a:b) MS embedded in the extracellular matrix elements with picrosirius red (**a,b**) of the hindlimb of an 8-month-old mouse (Group B). Scale bar: 50 μm.

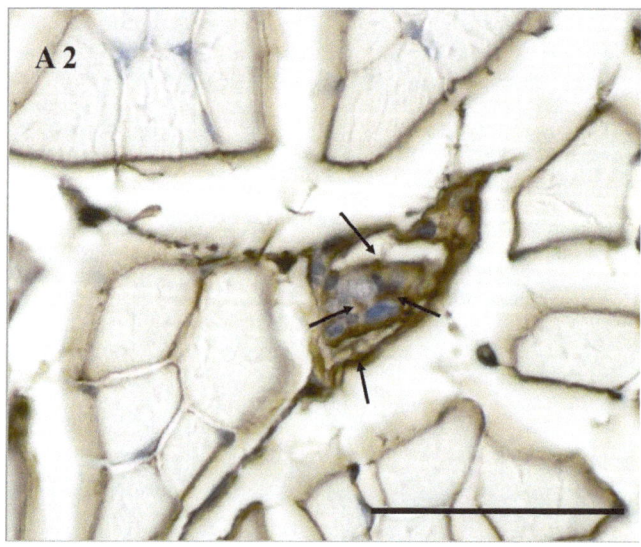

Figure A2. HA is present in the MS capsule and round intrafusal fibres. Scale bar: 50 μm.

References

1. Banks, R.W.; Ellaway, P.H.; Prochazka, A.; Proske, U. Secondary endings of muscle spindles: Structure, reflex action, role in motor control and proprioception. *Exp. Physiol.* **2021**, *106*, 2339–2366. [CrossRef]
2. Windhorst, U. Muscle proprioceptive feedback and spinal networks. *Brain Res. Bull.* **2007**, *73*, 155–202. [CrossRef] [PubMed]
3. Miwa, T.; Miwa, Y.; Kanda, K. Dynamic and static sensitivities of muscle spindle primary endings in aged rats to ramp stretch. *Neurosci. Lett.* **1995**, *201*, 179–182. [CrossRef]
4. De Reuck, J. Biometric analyses of spindles in normal human skeletal muscles. *Acta Neurol. Belg.* **1973**, *73*, 339–347. [PubMed]
5. Boyd-Clark, L.; Briggs, C.; Galea, M. Muscle spindle distribution, morphology, and density in longus colli and multifidus muscles of the cervical spine. *Spine* **2002**, *27*, 694–701. [CrossRef]
6. Boyd-Clark, L.; Galea, M.; Briggs, C.; Opeskin, K. Monitoring age-related changes of collagen content and vascularity in ganglia using unbiased stereological methods. *J. Microsc.* **2000**, *200*, 284–290. [CrossRef]
7. Roberts, N.; Cruz-Orive, L.; Reid, N.; Brodie, D.; Bourne, M.; Edwards, R. Unbiased estimation of human body composition by the Cavalieri method using magnetic resonance imaging. *J. Microsc.* **1993**, *171*, 239–253. [CrossRef] [PubMed]
8. Roberts, N.; Garden, A.; Cruz-Orive, L.; Whitehouse, G.; Edwards, R. Estimation of fetal volume by magnetic resonance imaging and stereology. *Br. J. Radiol.* **1994**, *67*, 1067–1077. [CrossRef] [PubMed]
9. Swash, M.; Fox, K.P. The effect of age on human skeletal muscle studies of the morphology and innervation of muscle spindles. *J. Neurol. Sci.* **1972**, *16*, 417–432. [CrossRef]
10. Kim, G.H.; Suzuki, S.; Kanda, K. Age-related physiological and morphological changes of muscle spindles in rats. *J. Physiol.* **2007**, *582*, 525–538. [CrossRef]
11. Goble, D.J.; Coxon, J.P.; Wenderoth, N.; Van Impe, A.; Swinnen, S.P. Proprioceptive sensibility in the elderly: Degeneration, functional consequences and plastic-adaptive processes. *Neurosci. Biobehav. Rev.* **2009**, *33*, 271–278. [CrossRef] [PubMed]
12. Vaughan, S.K.; Stanley, O.L.; Valdez, G. Impact of aging on proprioceptive sensory neurons and intrafusal muscle fibers in mice. *J. Gerontol. A Biomed. Sci. Med. Sci.* **2017**, *72*, 771–779. [CrossRef]
13. Rosant, C.; Nagel, M.-D.; Pérot, C. Aging affects passive stiffness and spindle function of the rat soleus muscle. *Exp. Gerontol.* **2007**, *42*, 301–308. [CrossRef]
14. Desaki, J.; Nishida, N. A further observation of muscle spindles in the extensor digitorum longus muscle of the aged rat. *J. Electron Microsc. (Tokyo)* **2010**, *59*, 79–86. [CrossRef] [PubMed]
15. Henry, M.; Baudry, S.J. Age-related changes in leg proprioception: Implications for postural control. *J. Neurophysiol.* **2019**, *122*, 525–538. [CrossRef] [PubMed]
16. Pavan, P.; Monti, E.; Bondí, M.; Fan, C.; Stecco, C.; Narici, M.; Reggiani, C.; Marcucci, L. Alterations of Extracellular Matrix Mechanical Properties Contribute to Age-Related Functional Impairment of Human Skeletal Muscles. *Int. J. Mol. Sci.* **2020**, *21*, 3992. [CrossRef]
17. Birch, H.L. Extracellular Matrix and Ageing. *Subcell. Biochem.* **2018**, *90*, 169–190.
18. Kadler, K.E.; Baldock, C.; Bella, J.; Boot-Handford, R.P. Collagens at a glance. *J. Cell Sci.* **2007**, *120*, 1955–1958. [CrossRef]
19. Poole, J.J.A.; Mostaço-Guidolin, L.B. Optical Microscopy and the Extracellular Matrix Structure: A Review. *Cells* **2021**, *10*, 1760. [CrossRef] [PubMed]
20. Soundararajan, A.; Ghag, S.A.; Vuda, S.S.; Wang, T.; Pattabiraman, P.P. Cathepsin K Regulates Intraocular Pressure by Modulating Extracellular Matrix Remodeling and Actin-Bundling in the Trabecular Meshwork Outflow Pathway. *Cells* **2021**, *10*, 2864. [CrossRef]
21. Parkes, W.S.; Amargant, F.; Zhou, L.T.; Villanueva, C.E.; Duncan, F.E.; Pritchard, M.T. Hyaluronan and Collagen Are Prominent Extracellular Matrix Components in Bovine and Porcine Ovaries. *Genes* **2021**, *12*, 1186. [CrossRef]
22. Burr, S.D.; Stewart, J.A., Jr. Rap1a Regulates Cardiac Fibroblast Contraction of 3D Diabetic Collagen Matrices by Increased Activation of the AGE/RAGE Cascade. *Cells* **2021**, *10*, 1286. [CrossRef]
23. Dalewski, B.; Białkowska, K.; Pałka, Ł.; Jakubowska, A.; Kiczmer, P.; Sobolewska, E. COL5A1 RS12722 Is Associated with Temporomandibular Joint Anterior Disc Displacement without Reduction in Polish Caucasians. *Cells* **2021**, *10*, 2423. [CrossRef]
24. Pawlina, W.; Ross, M.H. Connective tissue. In *Histology: A Text and Atlas: With Correlated Cell and Molecular Biology*; Lippincott Williams & Wilkins: Philadelphia, PA, USA, 2018; pp. 156–192.
25. Järvinen, T.A.; Józsa, L.; Kannus, P.; Järvinen, T.L.; Järvinen, M. Organization and distribution of intramuscular connective tissue in normal and immobilized skeletal muscles. *J. Muscle Res. Cell Motil.* **2002**, *23*, 245–254. [CrossRef]
26. Stecco, A.; Stecco, C.; Raghavan, P. Peripheral mechanisms contributing to spasticity and implications for treatment. *Curr. Phys. Med. Rehabil. Rep.* **2014**, *2*, 121–127. [CrossRef]
27. Dieler, R.; Schröder, J.M. Increase of elastic fibres in muscle spindles of rats following single or repeated denervation with or without reinnervation. *Virchows Arch. A Pathol. Anat. Histopathol.* **1990**, *417*, 213–221. [CrossRef] [PubMed]
28. Purslow, P.P. The structure and role of intramuscular connective tissue in muscle function. *Front. Physiol.* **2020**, *11*, 495. [CrossRef]
29. Koike, S.; Mukudai, Y.; Hisa, Y. Muscle Spindles and Intramuscular Ganglia. In *Neuroanatomy and Neurophysiology of the Larynx*; Springer: Berlin/Heidelberg, Germany, 2016; pp. 11–20.
30. Ovalle, W.; Dow, P. Morphological Aspects of the Muscle Spindle Capsule and Its Functional Significance. In *The Muscle Spindle*; Springer: Berlin/Heidelberg, Germany, 1985; pp. 23–28.
31. Dutta, S.; Sengupta, P. Men and mice: Relating their ages. *Life Sci.* **2016**, *152*, 244–248. [CrossRef]

32. Banks, R. The motor innervation of mammalian muscle spindles. *Prog. Neurobiol.* **1994**, *43*, 323–362. [CrossRef]
33. Bewick, G.S.; Banks, R.W. Mechanotransduction in the muscle spindle. *Pflügers Arch. Eur. J. Physiol.* **2015**, *467*, 175–190. [CrossRef]
34. Crowe, A.R.; Yue, W. Semi-quantitative determination of protein expression using immunohistochemistry staining and analysis: An integrated protocol. *Bio-Protocol* **2019**, *9*, e3465. [CrossRef] [PubMed]
35. Schneider, C.A.; Rasband, W.S.; Eliceiri, K.W. NIH Image to ImageJ: 25 years of image analysis. *Nat. Methods* **2012**, *9*, 671–675. [CrossRef] [PubMed]
36. Maier, A. Extracellular matrix and transmembrane linkages at the termination of intrafusal fibers and the outer capsule in chicken muscle spindles. *J. Morphol.* **1996**, *228*, 335–346. [CrossRef]
37. Ovalle, W.K.; Dow, P.R.; Nahirney, P.C. Structure, distribution and innervation of muscle spindles in avian fast and slow skeletal muscle. *J. Anat.* **1999**, *194*, 381–394. [CrossRef] [PubMed]
38. Eldred, E.; Maier, A.; Bridgman, C.F. Differences in intrafusal fiber content of spindles in several muscles of the cat. *Exp. Neurol.* **1974**, *45*, 8–18. [CrossRef]
39. Desaki, J.; Uehara, Y. A fine-structural study of the termination of intrafusal muscle fibres in the Chinese hamster. *Cell Tissue Res.* **1983**, *234*, 723–733. [CrossRef] [PubMed]
40. Sahgal, V.; Subramani, V.; Sahgal, S. Ultrastructure of Attachments of Human Intrafusal Fibers. In *Mechanoreceptors*; Springer: Berlin/Heidelberg, Germany, 1988; pp. 247–253.
41. Mokone, G.G.; Schwellnus, M.P.; Noakes, T.D.; Collins, M. The COL5A1 gene and Achilles tendon pathology. *Scand. J. Med. Sci. Sports* **2006**, *16*, 19–26. [CrossRef]
42. September, A.V.; Cook, J.; Handley, C.J.; Van Der Merwe, L.; Schwellnus, M.P.; Collins, M. Variants within the COL5A1 gene are associated with Achilles tendinopathy in two populations. *Br. J. Sports Med.* **2008**, *43*, 357–365. [CrossRef]
43. Posthumus, M.; September, A.V.; O'Cuinneagain, D.; Van Der Merwe, W.; Schwellnus, M.P.; Collins, M. The COL5A1 gene is associated with increased risk of anterior cruciate ligament ruptures in female participants. *Am. J. Sports Med.* **2009**, *37*, 2234–2240. [CrossRef]
44. O'Connell, K.; Knight, H.; Ficek, K.; Leonska-Duniec, A.; Maciejewska-Karlowska, A.; Sawczuk, M.; Stepien-Slodkowska, M.; O'Cuinneagain, D.; van der Merwe, W.; Posthumus, M.; et al. Interactions between collagen gene variants and risk of anterior cruciate ligament rupture. *Eur. J. Sport Sci.* **2015**, *15*, 341–350. [CrossRef]
45. Altinisik, J.; Meric, G.; Erduran, M.; Ates, O.; Ulusal, A.E.; Akseki, D. The BstUI and DpnII variants of the COL5A1 gene are associated with tennis elbow. *Am. J. Sports Med.* **2015**, *43*, 1784–1789. [CrossRef]
46. Pirri, C.; Fede, C.; Pirri, N.; Petrelli, L.; Fan, C.; De Caro, R.; Stecco, C. Diabetic Foot: The Role of Fasciae, a Narrative Review. *Biology* **2021**, *10*, 759. [CrossRef]
47. Correa-Gallegos, D.; Jiang, D.; Christ, S.; Ramesh, P.; Ye, H.; Wannemacher, J.; Gopal, S.K.; Yu, Q.; Aichler, M.; Walch, A.; et al. Patch repair of deep wounds by mobilized fascia. *Nat. Cell Biol.* **2019**, *576*, 287–292. [CrossRef]
48. Kang, L.; Ayala, J.E.; Lee-Young, R.S.; Zhang, Z.; James, F.D.; Neufer, P.D.; Pozzi, A.; Zutter, M.M.; Wasserman, D.H. Di-etinduced muscle insulin resistance is associated with extracellular matrix remodeling and interaction with integrin al-pha2beta1 in mice. *Diabetes* **2011**, *60*, 416–426. [CrossRef] [PubMed]
49. Stecco, C. *Functional Atlas of the Human Fascial System E-Book*; Elsevier Health Sciences: Amsterdam, The Netherlands, 2014.
50. Fukami, Y. Studies of capsule and capsular space of cat muscle spindles. *J. Physiol.* **1986**, *376*, 281–297. [CrossRef] [PubMed]
51. Pratt, R.L. Hyaluronan and the Fascial Frontier. *Int. J. Mol. Sci.* **2021**, *22*, 6845. [CrossRef]
52. De Luca, C.; Kline, J. Influence of proprioceptive feedback on the firing rate and recruitment of motoneurons. *J. Neural Eng.* **2012**, *9*, 016007. [CrossRef]
53. Stecco, L. *Atlas of Physiology of the Muscular Fascia*; Piccin: Padova, Italy, 2016.
54. Blecher, R.; Krief, S.; Galili, T.; Biton, I.E.; Stern, T.; Assaraf, E.; Levanon, D.; Appel, E.; Anekstein, Y.; Agar, G. The propri-oceptive system masterminds spinal alignment: Insight into the mechanism of scoliosis. *Dev. Cell* **2017**, *42*, 388–399. [CrossRef]
55. Abedi Khoozani, P.; Blohm, G. Neck muscle spindle noise biases reaches in a multisensory integration task. *J. Neurophysiol.* **2018**, *120*, 893–909. [CrossRef]
56. Langevin, H.M.; Rizzo, D.M.; Fox, J.R.; Badger, G.J.; Junru, W.; Konofagou, E.E.; Stevens-Tuttle, D.; Bouffard, N.A.; Krag, M.H. Dynamic morphometric characterization of local connective tissue network structure in humans using ultrasound. *BMC Syst. Biol.* **2007**, *5*, 25. [CrossRef] [PubMed]
57. Pirri, C.; Fede, C.; Petrelli, L.; Guidolin, D.; Fan, C.; De Caro, R.; Stecco, C. An anatomical comparison of the fasciae of the thigh: A macroscopic, microscopic and ultrasound imaging study. *J. Anat.* **2021**, *238*, 999–1009. [CrossRef] [PubMed]
58. Kerns, M.J.J.; Darst, M.A.; Olsen, T.G.; Fenster, M.; Hall, P.; Grevey, S. Shrinkage of cutaneous specimens: Formalin or other factors involved? *J. Cutan. Pathol.* **2008**, *35*, 1093–1096. [CrossRef] [PubMed]
59. Leonard, C.T. *The Neuroscience of Human Movement*; Mosby Incorporated: St. Louis, MO, USA, 1998.

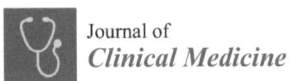

Review

Hematopoiesis, Inflammation and Aging—The Biological Background and Clinical Impact of Anemia and Increased C-Reactive Protein Levels on Elderly Individuals

Øystein Bruserud [1,2,*], Anh Khoi Vo [2] and Håkon Rekvam [1,2]

[1] Department of Clinical Science, University of Bergen, 5020 Bergen, Norway; hakon.reikvam@uib.no
[2] Department of Medicine, Haukeland University Hospital, 5021 Bergen, Norway; khoiavo93@gmail.com
* Correspondence: oystein.bruserud@helse-bergen.no

Abstract: Anemia and systemic signs of inflammation are common in elderly individuals and are associated with decreased survival. The common biological context for these two states is then the hallmarks of aging, i.e., genomic instability, telomere shortening, epigenetic alterations, loss of proteostasis, deregulated nutrient sensing, mitochondrial dysfunction, cellular senescence, stem cell exhaustion and altered intercellular communication. Such aging-associated alterations of hematopoietic stem cells are probably caused by complex mechanisms and depend on both the aging of hematopoietic (stem) cells and on the supporting stromal cells. The function of inflammatory or immunocompetent cells is also altered by aging. The intracellular signaling initiated by soluble proinflammatory mediators (e.g., IL1, IL6 and TNFα) is altered during aging and contributes to the development of both the inhibition of erythropoiesis with anemia as well as to the development of the acute-phase reaction as a systemic sign of inflammation with increased CRP levels. Both anemia and increased CRP levels are associated with decreased overall survival and increased cardiovascular mortality. The handling of elderly patients with inflammation and/or anemia should in our opinion be individualized; all of them should have a limited evaluation with regard to the cause of the abnormalities, but the extent of additional and especially invasive diagnostic evaluation should be based on an overall clinical evaluation and the possible therapeutic consequences.

Keywords: anemia; hematopoiesis; inflammation; aging; C-reactive protein; survival

Citation: Bruserud, Ø.; Vo, A.K.; Rekvam, H. Hematopoiesis, Inflammation and Aging—The Biological Background and Clinical Impact of Anemia and Increased C-Reactive Protein Levels on Elderly Individuals. *J. Clin. Med.* **2022**, *11*, 706. https://doi.org/10.3390/jcm11030706

Academic Editor: Francesco Mattace-Raso

Received: 30 December 2021
Accepted: 24 January 2022
Published: 28 January 2022

Publisher's Note: MDPI stays neutral with regard to jurisdictional claims in published maps and institutional affiliations.

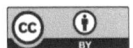

Copyright: © 2022 by the authors. Licensee MDPI, Basel, Switzerland. This article is an open access article distributed under the terms and conditions of the Creative Commons Attribution (CC BY) license (https://creativecommons.org/licenses/by/4.0/).

1. Introduction

The ageing global population is regarded as the most important present and future medical and social demographic problem worldwide by the World Health Organization [1]. Recent estimates suggest that 38% of the word population will be aged at least 65 years in 2050, and it is also estimated that in 2050 there will be a larger number of older people aged at least 60 years than adolescents aged 10–24 years (2.1 billion versus 2.0 billion). Thus, the optimal handling of medical problems in the aging population is already now a challenge and will become even more challenging during the next decades.

The complex process of aging is characterized by the modulation of fundamental cellular processes, and this is reflected in the previously described nine hallmarks of aging, which include genomic instability, telomere attrition, epigenetic alterations, loss of proteostasis, deregulated nutrient sensing, mitochondrial dysfunction, cellular senescence, stem cell exhaustion and altered intercellular communication (Figure 1) [2–11]. These cellular effects lead to aging-dependent alterations in organs and tissues, including hematopoietic cells together with their supporting stromal cells in the common bone marrow microenvironment, as well as various immunocompetent cell subsets with the modulation of their immunoregulatory interactions [2,12–16]. Aging can thus alter the regulation of both hematopoiesis and inflammation [12]. In this context we describe and discuss the effects of aging on normal hematopoiesis together with the occurrence of anemia and increased C-reactive protein

(CRP) levels in elderly individuals. We would expect the frequency and causes of anemia to differ between developed and underdeveloped countries; we therefore emphasize that the present review is mainly based on studies in developed countries.

The Cellular Hallmarks of Aging		
DNA, Transcription	**Nutrition and Metabolism**	**Cellular Proliferation and Communication**
Genomic instability. Aging is characterized by the accumulation of mutations and chromosomal aberrations within the genome [3]. *Telomere attrition.* Telomeres are the protective end complexes of human chromosomes. Telomere attrition can lead to cellular maladaptation, and greater overall telomere attrition seems to predict mortality and the risk of aging-related diseases [4]. *Epigenetic modulation.* Epigenetics can be defined as the study of the mechanisms involved in the control of gene activity without changing the DNA sequence. Epigenomic changes have important effects on several cellular functions and stress resistance in aging [5].	*Deregulated nutrient sensing.* Dietary interventions modulate aging processes; nutrient-sensing pathways represent a link between diet and aging, and several of these sensing pathways are deregulated in aging [6]. *Mitochondrial dysfunction.* Aging leads to mitochondrial dysfunction with the loss of energy homeostasis and altered cellular metabolism [7]. *Loss of proteostasis.* Proteostasis means protein homeostasis, and this requires the control of protein synthesis, conformation and degradation. The capacity of cells to maintain proteostasis declines during aging [8].	*Cellular senescence.* Cellular senescence can be defined as a stable arrest of the cell cycle coupled to defined phenotypic changes [2]. The accumulation of senescent cells during aging can reflect both increased generation and decreased removal caused by, for example, attenuated functions of immunocompetent cells [2,9]. *Stem cell exhaustion.* Stem cells are important for the optimal functions of several tissues, including bone marrow hematopoiesis as well as several other tissues (e.g., bone, muscle and gastrointestinal tract) [2,10]. *Altered intercellular communication.* Cells communicate through the release of soluble mediators and through cell–cell contact [2]. This altered communication is important for the development of inflammaging through altered communication between immunocompetent cells [11].

Figure 1. The biological hallmarks of aging: an overview and summary of biological characteristics [2–11].

2. The Biological Context of Anemia in Elderly Individuals: Hallmarks of Aging in Normal Hematopoietic Cells and Their Associations with Signs of Inflammation

The mechanisms involved in hematopoietic stem cell aging have previously been classified as stem-cell-intrinsic (i.e., alterations in the hematopoietic cells) and stem-cell-extrinsic (i.e., indirect effects mediated by aging bone marrow stromal cells) [12,14–16]. However, the various mechanisms are interconnected, and it is therefore difficult to maintain this strict classification [12]. The present article gives a relatively brief overview of the important mechanisms involved in aging hematopoiesis; for more detailed discussions and additional references we refer to several recent excellent reviews [12–17].

2.1. The Bone Marrow Microarchitecture and the Stem Cell Pool in Aging

The hematopoietic stem cell distribution in the bone marrow is altered during aging; the number of stem cell niches and hematopoietic stem cells decreases close to the bone surface (i.e., the endosteum), but they expand further away from the bone compared with younger individuals [18]. The stem cells/niches are also more distant from arterioles and megakaryocytes in aging, whereas perisinusoidal niches seem to be preserved and have a distance from sinusoids similar to younger individuals [19–21]. This altered microarchitecture is at least partly caused by decreased noradrenergic innervation in the bone marrow, where β_2-adrenergic–IL6-dependent megakaryopoiesis is important for the close localization of stem cells to megakaryocytes [19,20]. Stem cell lodging to certain non-endosteal niches thereby seems to be favored.

The number of phenotypic hematopoietic stem cells increases upon aging, but their regenerative potential decreases and they preferentially differentiate into myeloid cells and less into lymphoid cells [12,20,22–26]. The β_2/IL6 axis is also important for the regulation of the more differentiated myelopoiesis, and in experimental studies adrenergic stimulation can decrease this myeloid dominance [19,20]. Geiger and van Zand [25] suggested two decades ago that aging mainly affected hematopoietic quality rather than its quantity. Their statement was based on the observation that the hematopoietic stem cell population is increased during aging and able to maintain normal peripheral blood cell counts throughout life, but seems to lack the "functional reserve" needed during crises [25,27,28]. This may also (at least partly) explain why aging hematopoiesis with the development of anemia can be a strong comorbidity factor for several other diseases [22].

2.2. Hematopoiesis and Hematopoietic Stem Cells in Elderly Individuals: Cell-Intrinsic Mechanisms Involved in Stem Cell Aging

Several cell-intrinsic mechanisms are involved in the aging of hematopoietic cells. Table 1 presents a summarizing overview of important intrinsic mechanisms that are important in the aging of hematopoietic cells. Several of these mechanisms will also influence the regulation of inflammation and thereby contribute to the regulation of both hematopoiesis and inflammation. A more detailed discussion and additional references are included in Section 2.2.

Table 1. A summary of important cell-intrinsic mechanisms involved in aging of hematopoietic cells; for a detailed review and discussion with references we refer to Section 2.2.

Genetic: Genetic instability with accumulating DNA damage and clonal hematopoiesis; this is due to the altered function of several mechanisms involved in genomic maintenance/DNA repair.
Epigenetic: Epigenetic modulation with altered chromatin organization, posttranscriptional histone modulation and DNA methylation; transcriptional regulation is thereby altered.
Polarity: Reduced cytoplasmic and nuclear polarity, reduced ability of asymmetric cell division.
Metabolism: A shift to higher oxidative metabolism, altered proteostasis due to reduced autophagy and reduced activity of the proteasome system, reduced endoplasmic reticulum stress response with the accumulation of misfolded or damaged proteins.
Senescence, signaling and communication: Accumulation of cell-cycle-arrested senescent cells, altered intercellular communication and intracellular signaling possibly involving auto- and paracrine circuits, reduced regenerative capacity of hematopoietic stem cells.

2.2.1. Genetic Instability, Telomere Shortening, Altered Cell Communication and Inflammation

Random DNA damage accumulates in hematopoietic stem cells as a part of the aging process [3,12]; this should be regarded as a sign of genomic instability, which is one of the hallmarks of aging (Figure 1) [2,3]. Experimental studies suggest that accumulating DNA damage is an important mechanism in hematopoietic stem cell aging, and animal models suggest that altered functions of the mechanisms involved in genomic maintenance are important for this accumulation, e.g., nucleotide excision repair, telomere maintenance and non-homologous end-joining [27]. DNA damage then seems to accumulate in stem cells with age [27]. These abnormalities/deficiencies do not seem to deplete the stem cell reserve; they rather manifest as functional stem cell deficiencies under conditions of stress, e.g., wound healing, hematopoietic ablation [27,28].

DNA damage leading to telomere shortening is possibly a specific hallmark of aging that leads to stem cell aging/exhaustion/abnormalities [4], but telomere defects alone cannot explain all the signs of stem cell aging (Figure 1) [2,28]. Additional specific mutations also contribute to clonal expansion and the emergence of clonal hematopoiesis [14], an age-associated abnormality that can possibly develop later into hematological malignancies [29]. This hypothesis is supported by the observation that myelodysplastic syndromes (MDS) as well as pre-MDS stem cells show a higher degree of subclonal complexity than normal cells, including aging-associated variants [29]. However, it is controversial whether mutations associated with clonal hematopoiesis are truly oncogenic or whether they only increase self-renewal and thereby make it more likely for additional and truly oncogenic mutations to occur later in these actively self-renewing stem cells.

Patients with clonal hematopoiesis have an increased risk of atherosclerosis and cardiovascular complications [12,30,31]. This observation is consistent with the hypothesis that fully differentiated cells (especially monocytes/macrophages) in these patients have abnormal functions and thereby predispose them to inflammation with increased CRP levels and progression to atherosclerosis with clinical manifestations [32,33]. The hypothesis is supported by observations in patients with *TET2* mutations who show increased inflammasome-mediated IL1 secretion by monocytes and thereby a predisposition to inflammation and atherosclerosis [30]. Inflammation induced by clonal hematopoiesis and immune cell dysfunction thus seems to contribute to the association between CRP increase (i.e., acute-phase reaction) and cardiovascular disease [33]. However, an alternative explanation could be that mutations and clonal hematopoiesis occur more frequently in myeloid cells exposed to a chronic proinflammatory microenvironment. Whether age-dependent alterations in erythrocytes (e.g., abnormalities similar to storage lesions [34]) and/or platelets contribute to this predisposition to cardiovascular complications in patients with clonal hematopoiesis is not known. Thus, according to these observations genetic instability and altered cytokine-mediated intercellular communication (i.e., two hallmarks of aging, see Figure 1) may be involved in the association between clonal hematopoiesis and cardiovascular complications.

2.2.2. Epigenetic Abnormalities, Epigenetic Drift and Inflammation

The epigenome and the organization of chromatin differ between younger and aged hematopoietic stem cells [12,14], and mutations associated with clonal hematopoiesis are often seen in genes involved in epigenetic regulation [14]. These epigenetic changes have been discussed in detail previously [14,23,24]; they include both posttranscriptional histone modulation and chromatin organization as well as DNA methylation with site- or gene-specific modulations, e.g., the hypermethylation of genes regulated by polycomb repressive complex 2 [23,35,36]. Previous studies have described an overall increase in transcriptional activity that is at least partly caused by altered epigenetic regulation; these authors described the increased expression of genes associated with stress responses, inflammation and protein aggregation, whereas genes involved in the preservation of genomic integrity and chromatin modeling showed reduced expression [24]. Finally, age-dependent histone modifications seem to alter the expression of genes involved in the regulation of the proliferation, self-renewal, differentiation and maintenance of hematopoietic stem cells [36].

Epigenetic drift has been defined as all changes with a general effect on the epigenome and chromatin organization/architecture [37,38]; it seems to be a part of the aging process and to occur across tissues [38], and would be expected to include hematopoietic cells (Figure 1) [5,23,24,38]. Studies in animal models suggest that epigenetic drift is associated with the development of inflammation [38], and this is further supported by studies on aged human mononuclear cells [39]. Studies on aging immunocompetent cells show specific epigenetic signatures in different immunocompetent cells (T and B lymphocytes, NK cells and monocytes), and variations in signatures between individuals also seem to increase with age [39]. These histone/chromatin variations between individuals as well as cell-to-cell variations can be detected in stem, progenitor and differentiated cells, and it has been suggested that variations between mature cells arise from variations between distinct hematopoietic stem cell clones [39]. It has also been suggested that such epigenetic variations in immunocompetent cells (together with the altered balance between various lymphocyte subsets) contribute to the development of inflammaging and/or an increased risk of severe infections with increased morbidity/mortality in elderly individuals [37].

2.2.3. Cellular Polarity and Epigenetic Asymmetry in Hematopoietic Stem Cell Division

Several molecules appear to be polar in the cytoplasm and nucleus of young hematopoietic stem cells, and high levels of the two cytoplasmic molecules cell division control protein 42 (cdc42) and laminin, together with the nuclear polarity of epigenetic markers, are regarded as intrinsic markers of altered polarity and stem cell aging [18,40,41]. This polarity of the cells allows hematopoietic stem cells to undergo asymmetric cell division, i.e., one daughter cell that differentiates and another daughter cell that retains the stem cell potential [41]. This polarity seems to be reduced or lost as a part of the aging process, and this is true both for cytoskeletal and cell cycle regulatory proteins in the cytoplasm as well as epigenetic markers in the nucleus [14,18,40,41]. Hematopoietic stem cells maintain a balance between self-renewal and differentiation, and the premitotic polarity status seems to be important for this balance in addition to the outcome after hematopoietic stem cell division [41]. Aged apolar hematopoietic stem cells preferentially go through symmetric divisions, resulting in daughter cells with reduced regenerative and lymphoid potentials, whereas younger polar cells preferentially undergo asymmetric division and thereby maintain cells with stem cell potential [41].

2.2.4. Metabolic Characteristics and Regulation of Protein Homeostasis

During their development hematopoietic cells go through multiple differentiation steps and transition through several microanatomical sites that require metabolic shifts [42]. Even though quiescent and cycling hematopoietic stem cells show similar high glycolytic activities, they differ in several metabolic characteristics, e.g., quiescent cells show higher lysosomal activity and autophagy/mitophagy whereas cycling stem cells show higher protein synthesis, ATP production and intracellular levels of reactive oxygen species [42]. The metabolic balance is altered in aging hematopoietic stem cells, which show a general shift to a higher rate of oxidative metabolism [16,42]. The aged cells also show altered protein homeostasis; this process is regulated by several cellular mechanisms, including autophagy (i.e., a cellular response to stress, for example, metabolic adaptation) and the ubiquitin/proteasome system, and both these systems are reduced in aged cells (Figure 1) [7,43–45]. Aging is thereby associated with the cellular accumulation of misfolded or damaged proteins [43] because the endoplasmic reticulum stress response (also called the unfolded protein response) is reduced [44]. Finally, aging-dependent alterations in sex hormone levels seem to represent an additional systemic mechanism for the downregulation of this stress response [44].

2.2.5. Senescence and Intracellular Signaling

Cellular senescence is regarded as a stress-induced irreversible growth arrest, and it is often characterized by a distinct secretory profile, i.e., an altered communication with the neighboring cells [46]. Irreversibly cell-cycle-arrested senescent cells accumulate during normal aging, and animal models suggest that these cells actively participate in the development of aging-associated organ deterioration and may further increase the aging-dependent risk of malignant diseases (Figure 1); in these animal models the elimination of senescent cells therefore increases the life span [46]. This effect was also seen for normal hematopoietic cells, where the pharmacological elimination of senescent hematopoietic stem cells counteracted the aging-dependent reduction in the regenerative potential of hematopoietic stem cells [46,47]. Furthermore, signaling through several intracellular pathways seems to be altered during aging due to intrinsic mechanisms, e.g., TGF1β, Notch, NFκB and Wnt signaling [24,48–51]. Both the induction of senescence with an altered secretory profile and the altered intracellular signaling downstream to cell surface receptors may represent combined direct and indirect effects on hematopoiesis [12,14], including the effect of increased senescence on aging with altered mediator secretion and thereby the modulation of autocrine/paracrine circuits (Figure 1) [2,9].

2.3. Stem-Cell-Extrinsic Mechanisms Involved in Hematopoietic Aging: Stem Cell Niches, Stromal Cell Subsets and Cellular Communications

Normal hematopoietic cells have a hierarchical organization and are supported by various non-hematopoietic stromal cells that also form stem cell niches where the minor population of hematopoietic stem cells are maintained [16,17,20]. The most important stromal cells that contribute to the stem cell niches are:

- Mesenchymal stem cells (MSCs). These cells are located close to arterioles and more loosely around sinusoidal vessels [17]; they are heterogeneous, and two main populations have been identified based on their expression of platelet-derived growth factor receptor (PDGFR)α and stem cell antigen 1 [17]. The MSCs support normal hematopoiesis through several mechanisms that are modulated by MSC aging, including their supportive function in stem cell niches (Figure 2, Table 2) [16,19,52–61]. Several epigenetic mechanisms are important for MSC aging and the alterations of their hematopoiesis-supporting mechanisms, including both altered DNA methylation and histone modification (e.g., acetylation) [61]; increased senescence is also observed [19,52–61]. First, MSCs produce several soluble mediators that are important both for myelopoiesis (e.g., CXCL12) and lymphopoiesis (e.g., IL7) [52]; the release of several growth factors is thus reduced. Second, MSCs and sinusoidal endothelial cells seem to form a complex network in close contact with the extracellular matrix and pervading the marrow tissue. The structural features of stromal components are maintained during aging [53], and although central perisinusoidal MSCs are increased or maintained there is a reduction in periarteriolar MSCs [16,19,56]. Third, the MSC functions in these networks seem to be altered, especially with regard to the regulation of cell cycle progression of the stem cells, stem cell trafficking in the microenvironment and the localization of progenitors close to different MSC subsets with different perivascular localizations [57]. Finally, the adipogenic differentiation of MSCs is preferred, and another consequence of this aging effect is reduced bone formation [59].
- Osteoblasts and other osteolineage cells. Osteoblasts are the predominant bone-lining endosteal cells [54], whereas osteolineage or osteoblastic lineage cells refer to the intermediate stages of differentiation in the direction from MSCs towards osteoblasts [57]. These cells and particularly mature osteoblasts seem to be the most important for the maintenance of more committed progenitors, especially lymphoid cells [62,63]. They stimulate/regulate hematopoiesis both through cell–cell contact (e.g., expression of the Notch ligand Jagged1) and through the release of soluble mediators (e.g., the growth factors CXCL12, stem cell factor and angiopoietin 1; osteopontin) [17]. Aging causes a decrease in the number of osteoblasts and in addition decreases osteopontin release via these aging cells (Figure 2, Table 2) [19,55,62,63]. As described above, aging MSCs favor adipogenic differentiation [59], and a reduction in osteoblasts is then caused by several mechanisms, including the induction of apoptosis, the increased release of reactive oxygen species, decreased glutathione reductase activity and the increased phosphorylation of p53 and p66 [64]. Finally, animal models suggest that a reduction in/lack of osteopontin causes decreased engraftment capacity but increases long-term stem cell frequency together with loss of stem cell polarity; as would then be expected from these observations, thrombin-activated osteopontin attenuates the aging stem cell phenotype [55].
- Adipocytes. Adipocytes release factors that seem to inhibit hematopoiesis [65–67]. Aging accelerates bone marrow adipogenesis [53]. This is apparent especially in the long bones where hematopoietic marrow is gradually replaced by adipocyte-rich marrow; although adipocytes release certain supportive mediators their overall effect is a reduction in hematopoiesis (Figure 2, Table 2) [19,66,68,69]. Animal studies suggest that this aging-associated adipocyte expansion can be further increased by

dietary fat intake in aged animals [69]. The process of favored differentiation into adipocytes seems to be regulated at the transcriptional level and involves the transcriptional regulators Maf and Runx2 [58]. Furthermore, the release of adiponectin is a possible mechanism for the inhibition of hematopoiesis by adipocytes because this mediator has an antiproliferative and possibly also a proapoptotic effect, especially on myelomonocytic lineage cells [65]. The pharmacological inhibition of adipogenesis has therefore been suggested as a possible strategy to reduce the negative effects of adipogenesis on normal hematopoiesis [66,67]. However, the inhibitory effect of adipocytes may depend on the biological context, as a recent animal study has shown that adipocytes or a subset of adipocytes could release SCF and thereby promote regeneration after irradiation and myelotoxic chemotherapy [68].

- Endothelial cells. Endothelial cells and perivascular cells are intimately connected. Arteriolar and sinusoid endothelial cells seem to differ in their mechanisms with regard to supporting hematopoiesis (Figure 2) [54]; in particular, arteriolar cells release a wide range of hematopoietic growth factors [17,70,71]. The aging of endothelial cells has multiple effects on the stem cell niche and normal hematopoiesis (Table 2) [19,53–57,72,73]. First, the bone marrow endothelium shows aging-associated morphological and metabolic changes, including increased levels of reactive oxygen species that decrease their angiogenic and migratory potential, and the microvessels show a loss of integrity with augmented leakiness [70,71]. Second, the decreased release of prohematopoietic soluble mediators, including SCF and CXCL12, is one of the endothelial contributions to hematopoietic aging [70,72,74]. Third, the reduction in niche-forming vessels is likely to induce metabolic changes in the bone marrow microenvironment [70]. Finally, the niche-forming vessels in aging mice can be restored either by endothelial transplantation [72] or by the activation of endothelial Notch signaling, which seems to be altered in the aging bone marrow endothelium [56].

- Perivascular cells. This cell population is heterogeneous and includes cells expressing both pericyte and smooth muscle markers [17,70]. Aging reduces the abundance of pericytes and thereby the release of several soluble mediators that are important for the induction of quiescence of hematopoietic stem cells (e.g., SCF, bone morphogenic proteins 4 and 6) [70].

- Neural regulation. Sympathetic and sensory nerves innervate both the bone and the bone marrow [27]. Furthermore, human $CD34^+$ cells express both dopaminergic and β2 adrenergic receptors; the receptors are expressed especially by immature $CD34^+CD38^{low}$ cells and can be upregulated by G-CSF and GM-CSF [74]. Thus, adrenergic signals act directly on human hematopoietic progenitors and can increase their migration, proliferation, polarity as well as extracellular protease release, and Wnt-initiated signaling is involved in this stem cell modulation [74]. The perivascular arteriolar niche consists of specialized MSCs together with adrenergic nerves and megakaryocytes, and these cells are closely associated with quiescent stem cells [62,75–77]. Finally, nonmyelinating Schwann cells (i.e., glial fibrillary acidic protein-expressing cells) ensheath autonomic nerves, express genes that are important for the support of hematopoietic stem cells and can activate the latent form of TGFβ [76]. Thus, autonomic nerves are not only important through the direct effects of neurotransmitters on hematopoietic cells but also through their modulation of the niche cytokine network [76] and indirectly through the modulation of adrenoreceptor-expressing MSCs [77]. There is an aging-associated sympathetic denervation of the niche, and targeting this denervation with adrenoreceptor β3 agonists improves the function of aged stem cells in animal models [19,20,78]. Another effect of the denervation is the expansion of MSCs with decreased stem cell supporting capacity, a reduction in arterioles and increased stem cell numbers [16,19,54,57,74].

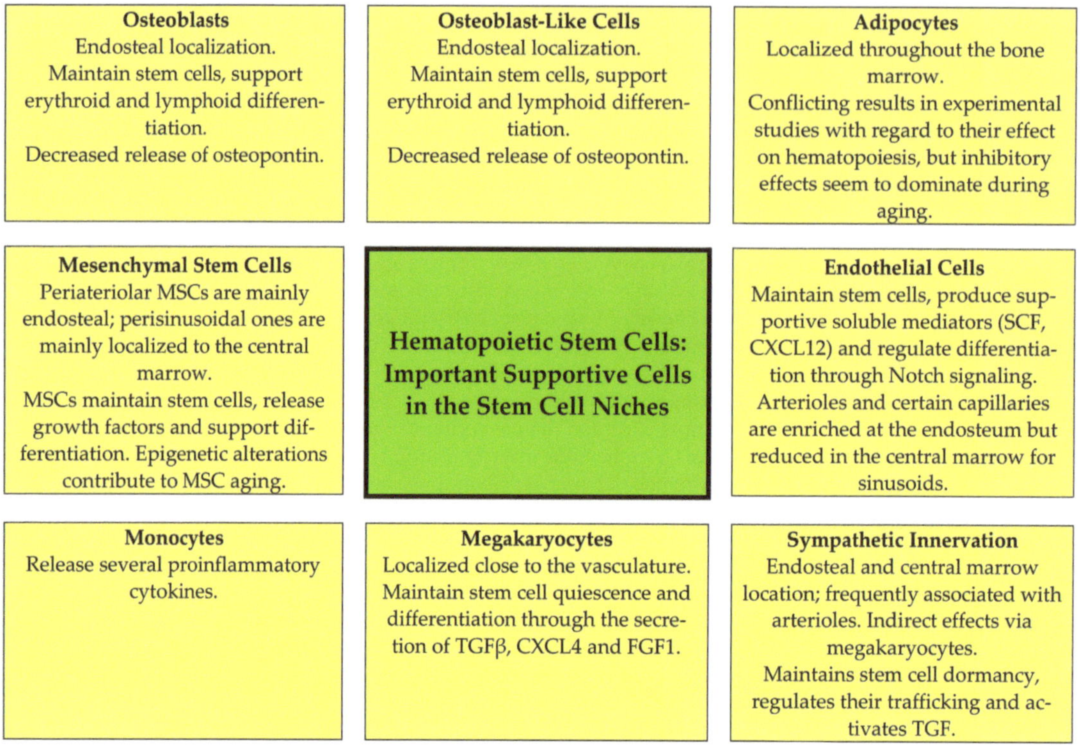

Osteoblasts Endosteal localization. Maintain stem cells, support erythroid and lymphoid differentiation. Decreased release of osteopontin.	**Osteoblast-Like Cells** Endosteal localization. Maintain stem cells, support erythroid and lymphoid differentiation. Decreased release of osteopontin.	**Adipocytes** Localized throughout the bone marrow. Conflicting results in experimental studies with regard to their effect on hematopoiesis, but inhibitory effects seem to dominate during aging.
Mesenchymal Stem Cells Periateriolar MSCs are mainly endosteal; perisinusoidal ones are mainly localized to the central marrow. MSCs maintain stem cells, release growth factors and support differentiation. Epigenetic alterations contribute to MSC aging.	**Hematopoietic Stem Cells: Important Supportive Cells in the Stem Cell Niches**	**Endothelial Cells** Maintain stem cells, produce supportive soluble mediators (SCF, CXCL12) and regulate differentiation through Notch signaling. Arterioles and certain capillaries are enriched at the endosteum but reduced in the central marrow for sinusoids.
Monocytes Release several proinflammatory cytokines.	**Megakaryocytes** Localized close to the vasculature. Maintain stem cell quiescence and differentiation through the secretion of TGFβ, CXCL4 and FGF1.	**Sympathetic Innervation** Endosteal and central marrow location; frequently associated with arterioles. Indirect effects via megakaryocytes. Maintains stem cell dormancy, regulates their trafficking and activates TGF.

Figure 2. The bone marrow stem cell niches. The figure gives an overview of important hematopoiesis-regulating members of the various stem cell niches and their main regulatory effects/mechanisms on normal hematopoiesis A detailed discussion of each cell type with corresponding references are given in Section 2.3 (abbreviations: CXCL, C-X-C motif ligand; FGF1, fibroblast growth factor; SCF, stem cell factor; and TGF, transforming growth factor).

- Megakaryocytes. The role of megakaryocytes in the regulation of normal hematopoiesis can be regarded as a feedback mechanism. Megakaryocyte precursors migrate from the endosteal microenvironment to sinusoids for maturation, and noradrenergic bone marrow innervation promotes β2-adrenergic/IL6-dependent megakaryopoiesis [20]. A subset of hematopoietic stem cells is then associated with megakaryocytes that regulate stem cell quiescence through the release of soluble mediators (especially CXCL4 and TGFβ) as well as CD41 expression (Figure 2, Table 2) [18,19,37,54,57,79–83]. Age-dependent epigenetic alterations in hematopoietic stem cells and possibly also megakaryocytes seem to modify these interactions between megakaryocytes and neighboring hematopoietic stem cells [37]. Thus, there seems to be an interaction between aging, sympathetic innervation/denervation, epigenetic modulation and megakaryopoiesis with regard to the effects of aging on hematopoiesis [37]. The effects of megakaryocyte are partly mediated through the local release of TGFβ, which is important for the regulation of quiescence and initiates SMAD signaling in stem cells [79]; additionally, megakaryocytes release thrombopoietin [80] and CXCR4 [81], which act directly on immature hematopoietic cells. The release of thrombopoietin and possibly also other mediators can be stimulated by the ligation of C-type lectin-like receptor 2 (CLEC-2), and megakaryocyte expression of this receptor thereby becomes important for the regulation of stem cell quiescence [83]. Finally, the peripheral blood platelet count will possibly modulate these megakaryocyte effects through its effects on systemic thrombopoietin levels [37].

Table 2. Extrinsic mechanisms for the aging of normal hematopoiesis: a summarizing overview of important mechanisms behind the contribution of various stromal cells to the aging of normal hematopoiesis (for additional information, see the more detailed review/discussion with corresponding references for each cell type in Section 2.3).

Stromal Component	Important Effect of Aging
MSCs [19,52–61]	Maintained or increased central MSCs with decreased hematopoietic growth factor production; loss of periarteriolar MSCs. Decreased bone formation and increased adipogenesis; MSC aging is also characterized by increased senescence (including altered mediator secretion) and epigenetic modifications.
Osteoblastic cells [19,55,62,63]	Decreased number of osteoblasts, increased differentiation in the direction of adipocytes. Decreased numbers of osteoblasts represent decreased support of lymphopoiesis. Decreased osteopontin release; this cytokine can attenuate the aging-associated phenotype of hematopoietic stem cells.
Osteoblasts [27,64]	Decreased number and release of osteopontin, decreased osteoblast number and thereby reduced support of lymphopoiesis.
Adipocytes [19,65,66,68,69]	Increased number of adipocytes during aging. The effects of adipocytes on normal hematopoiesis depend on the biological context. Hematopoiesis is often suppressive, and the release of adiponectin probably contributes to this inhibition. However, adipocytes or a subset of them also seem to facilitate regeneration after chemotherapy or irradiation through their release of SCF.
Endothelial cells [19,53–57,72,73]	Loss of certain capillaries and arterioles, decreased release of SCF and CXCL12 in addition to decreased expression of the Notch ligand Jagged1. Increased or unaltered endothelial cell pool, altered microvascular function with increased vascular leak.
Perivascular cells [17,70]	Aging of these cells is associated with reduced number of these cells and thereby reduced release of soluble stem cell-supporting mediators, e.g., SCF.
Sympathetic innervation [19,54,57,74]	Loss of sympathetic innervation in aging; this leads to expansion of medullary MSCs with decreased supportive effect, reduces the number of arterioles and increases the hematopoietic stem cell number.
Megakaryocytes [18,19,54,57,79–83]	Increased number and TGFβ release in aging.

Abbreviations: CXCL, C-X-C motif ligand; FGF1, fibroblast growth factor; HSC, hematopoietic stem cells; SCF, stem cell factor; and TGF, transforming growth factor.

- Neutrophils. Neutrophils also seem to have regulatory functions in normal hematopoiesis; the mechanisms involve the neutrophil-mediated augmentation of sympathetic nervous system effects with the release of prostaglandin E2 [63]. These observations show that neutrophils can function as a link between the sympathetic nervous system and the stem cell niches.
- Monocytes, macrophages and osteoclasts. Both monocytes and other immunocompetent cells can contribute to the aging of hematopoiesis [17], possibly through their modulation of local levels of various proinflammatory cytokines [60]. Furthermore, aging seems to be associated with a shift from the anti-inflammatory M2 phenotype to the proinflammatory M1 phenotype; this shift is associated with the increased release of proinflammatory cytokines and seems to depend on monocyte/macrophage expression of the Foxo3 transcription factor (i.e., it is probably caused by an intrinsic mechanism) [11]. This shift is associated with local inflammation in the gastrointestinal tract, and in our opinion one should further investigate whether this shift is also important for inflammaging and/or the regulation of aging normal hematopoiesis. Finally, bone-marrow-associated macrophages are also important to maintain many stem-cell-supporting characteristics of MSCs, including their release of CXCL12 and SCF [57]. Finally, osteoclasts support hematopoiesis and lymphopoiesis indirectly by increasing the osteoblast secretion of CXCL12 and IL7 [57].

- T cells. As described in a recent review, activated T cells release several cytokines involved in the regulation of normal hematopoiesis [63]. $CD4^+$ T cells thereby stimulate hematopoiesis, whereas $CD4^+CD25^+$ regulatory T cells seem to inhibit it. Furthermore, the clinical experience from allogeneic stem cell transplantation suggests that T cells facilitate engraftment, and even regulatory T cells (including $CD150^+$ Treg cells) seem to facilitate engraftment and promote stem cell quiescence [63]. Finally, animal models suggest that $CD8^+$ T cells also contribute to the regulation of hematopoiesis because IL6 and IFNγ released by $CD8^+$ T cells can trigger emergency myelopoiesis [63].

These descriptions of the various bone marrow stromal cells and their contributions to the stem cell niches are far from complete, but they clearly illustrate that many different stromal cells form an extensive and complex interacting network through the release of soluble mediators, cell–cell contact and cell–extracellular matrix contact. This hematopoiesis-supporting network is altered during aging. The age-dependent modulation of one stromal component can alter the functions of other stromal cells and will thereby have both direct and indirect effects on hematopoiesis. Furthermore, several soluble mediators released by various stromal cells are important for the aging of hematopoietic stem cells, e.g., CCL5, which shows high levels in the aging stem cell milieu and is involved in the myeloid lineage skewing [84], osteopontin that can induce a loss of cell polarity and reduced engraftment potential [55] and the T-cell- and monocyte-derived cytokines IL1α, IL1β, IL3 and IFNγ, which influence the migration and maturation of megakaryocytes (Figure 2, Table 2) [85].

2.4. Myeloid Skewing: An Intrinsic or Extrinsic Effect?

The overall effects of hematopoietic–stromal interactions in aging are illustrated by previous experimental animal studies. Transplanted young hematopoietic stem cells engraft at a lower efficiency when transplanted to aged compared with young recipients [15,84]. Furthermore, coculture experiments show that aged endothelial cells impair the function and increase the myeloid bias of younger hematopoietic stem cells, whereas endothelial cells restored the repopulating capacity of aged hematopoietic stem cells but did not alter the myeloid bias, which seems to be an intrinsic characteristic of stem cells [72]. However, other studies have shown that the IL1-mediated inflammatory (aging-associated) effects on hematopoiesis and hematopoietic stem cells are reversible [85–88]; the same is possibly true for lymphoid hematopoietic stem cells, which seem to retain their normal lymphoid potential if they are removed from the aging microenvironment that causes the myeloid skewing of hematopoiesis [89]. Thus, hematopoietic aging with myeloid skewing depends both on the aging of the hematopoietic cells themselves and on the aging of the supporting stromal cells.

2.5. Inflammation and Hematopoiesis in Aging: The Contributions of Individual Cytokines and A Focus on the Myeloid Skewing

The aging of the bone marrow microenvironment is associated with increased levels of several proinflammatory cytokines, including IL1β, IL6 and TNFα, which are also known as drivers of the acute-phase reaction together with other members of the IL6 family and various chemokines [60,86]. Experimental studies suggest that several age-associated characteristics of normal hematopoiesis are associated with increased proinflammatory cytokine activity caused by increased release by various stromal cells:

- IL1. IL1α/β exposure can induce myeloid skewing of normal hematopoietic stem cells at the expense of self-renewal [87]. Aging macrophages seem to stimulate megakaryocytic differentiation and myeloid skewing through IL1β-induced signaling [60,88]. IL1 also blocks the lymphoid differentiation of stem cells [89].
- IL6. This cytokine seems to promote thrombopoiesis (i.e., megakaryocyte modulation) [60].
- TNFα. This cytokine seems to stimulate myelopoiesis in aging [90].
- CCL5. This proinflammatory chemokine increases with age and seems to stimulate myeloid-biased differentiation [84].

- TGFβ and IFNγ. These two cytokines are also regarded as proinflammatory and contribute to megakaryocyte modulation [60,91].
- A certain subset of hematopoietic stem cells seems to respond to proinflammatory stimuli and thereby becomes particularly important for the myeloid skewing of hematopoiesis [90]. This study also suggests that young and aged long-term hematopoietic stem cells respond differently to inflammatory stress, such that the aged cells show a myeloid-biased gene expression initiated by several transcription factors, including Klf5, Ikzf1 and Stat3 [90].

These observations, together with the increased levels of proinflammatory cytokines in many elderly individuals (see Section 6), strongly suggest that there is an association between the induction of an acute-phase reaction and the development of anemia in aging.

Aging-dependent alterations in normal hematopoiesis are caused by the overall effect of a wide range of factors both in hematopoietic cells and in their supporting stromal cells. There is a complex crosstalk between hematopoietic and stromal cells as well as between various stromal cell subsets; this communication is altered in aging. Our present description of the effects of aging on hematopoiesis is definitely not complete, and for more detailed discussion and additional references we refer to recent excellent reviews [12–20,60]. However, our review shows that aging of hematopoiesis is a multifactorial process involving both immunocompetent cells and the regulation of inflammation.

2.6. Aging and Leukemic Hematopoiesis: Acute Myeloid Leukemia as an Example

Hematological malignancies are most common in elderly individuals, e.g., acute myeloid leukemia (AML) has a median age at the time of first diagnosis of 65–70 years [92,93]. As outlined above (Section 2.2), clonal hematopoiesis can be detected in elderly individuals and can be regarded as a part of the aging process. The biological characteristics of hematological malignancies seem to be determined not only by cancer-associated genetic abnormalities alone but also by the biological characteristics of the aging process that are transferred from normal to leukemic hematopoietic cells, and the experience with AML suggests that aging is associated with chemoresistance. First, favorable genetic abnormalities are less common in elderly individuals [92,93]. Second, a larger subset of elderly patients has high-risk secondary AML following previous chemotherapy or hematological disease (i.e., MDS, chronic myeloproliferative neoplasia) [92,93]. Third, the biology of AML cells from elderly individuals seems to differ from that of AML cells in younger patients even when the cells have similar AML-associated genetic abnormalities [94]. Thus, aging not only influences the risk but also the biological characteristics of AML; the same may also be true for other malignancies.

3. Anemia in Elderly Individuals

3.1. Definition of Anemi

The level of hemoglobin varies considerably between healthy individuals and depends on age as well as gender; despite these variations, the level in each individual is relatively stable [95]. The World Health Organization (WHO) definition of anemia is <13.0 g/100 mL for men and <12.0 g/100 mL for non-pregnant women (Table 3) [95]. However, whether this definition is optimal has been a topic of discussion [95,96]. Some scientists have suggested that higher levels should be used; this is supported by a Swedish epidemiological study that used different limits/definitions in analyses of the data [97]. These authors observed an association between anemia according to the WHO definition and increased mortality (hazard ratio 2.16), but excess mortality was also observed at higher hemoglobin levels. Another study described that the severity of anemia was predictive for the underlying cause [98]: mild anemia was more frequently caused by chronic disease whereas severe anemia was more common with iron deficiency. These observations illustrate that the results from scientific studies of anemia can depend on the definition of anemia [95]. Finally, it has been suggested that the same definition with a hemoglobin level <12.0 g/100 mL should be used both for men and women (Table 3) [99].

Table 3. Definition and prevalence of anemia: alternative definitions and the prevalence of anemia in subsets of elderly individuals.

Definitions of Anemia [95,96,99]		
	Definition Men	Definition Women
WHO definition of anemia (Hb)	<13 g/dL	<12 g/dL
Alternative definitions	<12 g/dL	<12 g/dL
	Decrease in Hb > 2 g/dL	Decrease in Hb > 2 g/dL
Prevalence of Hemoglobin Levels in Elderly Individuals [97]		
Percent of Individuals	Criteria Men	Criteria Women
22.0%	<14 g/dL	<13 g/dL
5.6%	<13.2 g/dL	<12.2 g/dL
3.8%	<13.0 g/dL	<12.0 g/dL
0.6%	<11.0 g/dL	<11 g/dL
Prevalence of Anemia in Various Subsets of Elderly Patients [99–101]		
Percent of Individuals	Subset of Elderly Individuals	
12%	Elderly living in private homes	
47%	Elderly living in nursery homes	
40%	Elderly admitted to hospital	

It is difficult to define an optimal hemoglobin level for elderly individuals, and by strictly using the WHO definition it is not possible to take into account individual differences in hemoglobin levels [95]. An alternative strategy is to define anemia based on a decrease from previously measured hemoglobin levels, e.g., a decrease corresponding to at least 2 g/100 mL; however, for many individuals/studies it will not be possible to compare present and previous measurements.

Taken together, the observations referred to above illustrate the importance of clearly stating the definition of anemia used in clinical studies. The use of the WHO definition is important to allow comparisons between different studies, but additional analyses using/comparing different definitions may also be useful [97,98].

3.2. Anemia Is Common but Severe Anemia Is Uncommon in Elderly Individuals

Several previous studies have shown that anemia is common among elderly individuals in developed countries. A recent Swedish population-based study included 30,447 individuals between 44 and 73 years of age [97]. This study compared the WHO definition of anemia with alternative definitions for men/women, i.e., <14.0/<13.0 g/100 mL, <13.2/<12.2 g/100 mL, <13.0/<12.0 g/100 mL (i.e., the WHO definition) and <11.0 g/100 mL. These results are summarized in Table 3, and it can be seen that even though anemia is common in elderly individuals severe anemia (i.e., Hb < 11.0 g/dL) is uncommon. However, one should emphasize that this study included many relatively young individuals that had a relatively low mortality compared with the general population. Despite this, the results illustrate how the prevalence of anemia is highly dependent on its definition; moderate anemia is quite common whereas severe anemia is uncommon.

Other studies have demonstrated that the prevalence of anemia depends on the study population. The prevalence according to the WHO definition for elderly patients above 65 years of age is 12% for individuals living in their private homes, whereas nearly half of elderly nursing home residents and elderly patients admitted to hospital are anemic (Table 3) [99–101]. Some studies also describe that anemia seems to be more common for male (52%) than for female residents (32%) [100]. Finally, the prevalence of anemia also depends on age [99,101]: a previous study described that 11.0% of men and 10.2% of women 65 years or older were anemic, but that the prevalence of anemia rose rapidly to more than 20% at 85 years of age or older [95,99].

3.3. Causes of Anemia in Elderly Individuals

The cause of anemia in elderly individuals was investigated in a prospective American study that included 190 patients above 65 years of age [102]. All the patients were referred to hematological out-patient wards and diagnosed with anemia according to the WHO criteria. They all lived at home without help, and the exclusion criteria were known hematological disease, expected survival <3 months and renal failure requiring dialysis. These individuals were compared with a matched control group without anemia. All participants were interviewed and a clinical examination was performed as was a blood sample examination, including peripheral blood cell counts, examination for iron deficiency and levels of folic acid, cobalamin, thyroid-stimulating hormone, erythropoietin and creatinine, with an estimation of the glomerular filtration rate. For most individuals protein electrophoresis (performed for 86% of the patients) and microscopy of peripheral blood smears were performed, whereas bone marrow examination was performed only for a minority. If an individual had more than one cause of anemia they were classified according to the main cause. The following observations were made:

- Six percent of the patients were diagnosed with a hematological malignancy, the most common being myelodysplastic syndrome (MDS), which was the suspected cause for 16% of the patients.
- Eleven percent had a non-hematological malignancy.
- Twelve percent had iron deficiency, but only a minority of these patients had microcytic anemia and for many patients the hemoglobin level did not normalize in response to iron supplementation. Iron deficiency was thus a possible contributing cause of anemia for many of these patients
- Renal failure was the cause of anemia for 4% of the patients.
- Long-lasting inflammation was the cause for 6% of the patients.
- Anemic patients and controls did not differ with regard to pharmacotherapy.
- For 35% of the individuals the cause of their anemia was not found. None of these individuals had hemoglobin levels below 9 g/dL (i.e., they probably did not require regular erythrocyte transfusions) and there was no association with ethnicity, age or sex. However, many of these patients had increased erythrocyte sedimentation rates and ferritin levels, i.e., they had systemic signs of an acute-phase reaction.

Many elderly individuals with anemia are probably handled by general practitioners without a diagnostic follow-up at a hematological out-patient ward, and the present patient population therefore represents a selected group compared with the general population of elderly individuals. A relatively large group of these elderly patients are characterized by an unknown cause of anemia, a moderate decrease in the hemoglobin level and systemic signs of inflammation. The cause of anemia in elderly individuals has also been investigated in other studies [99,102,103], and the overall results show that a relatively large number of elderly patients with anemia has an unknown cause after a limited evaluation based on clinical examination and blood samples (Table 4).

Table 4. Causes of anemia in elderly patients, a summary of the results from selected previous studies [98,99,102,103]. For a detailed discussion with additional references see Sections 3.5 and 3.6.

Cause of Anemia	Percent of Patients
Total fraction: malnutrition, specific deficiencies	20%
Folic acid/cobalamin deficiency	12–15%
Iron deficiency	20%
Renal failure	8–10%
Other chronic diseases, including inflammatory diseases	20%
Renal failure combined with another chronic disease	<5%
Multiple etiologies	20%
Unknown cause of anemia	30–35%

What are the possible causes of anemia for the large group of patients with anemia of an unknown cause? First, one possibility is low-risk MDS with moderate anemia as the only sign of the disease; these variants of MDS can be difficult to diagnose even after repeated examinations. Many of these patients have macrocytic anemia, and the relatively short survival of anemia patients with increased mean corpuscular volume (MCV) in a large population study is consistent with this hypothesis; in this study, macrocytic anemia was rare and associated with a higher mortality than normocytic and microcytic anemia [97]. Second, pharmacotherapy may also be a possible cause, e.g., renin–angiotensin inhibitors are commonly used in patients with cardiovascular disease and can be associated with anemia [104]. Third, inflammation/inflammaging may be the cause of anemia in these patients [102,105]. In a previous study only including individuals above 65 years of age, it was observed that (independent of age, sex and hemoglobin) the number of elevated proinflammatory markers (CRP, IL6, IL1β and TNFα) was associated with progressively higher erythropoietin levels in nonanemic individuals but with decreased erythropoietin in anemic participants [105]. These last observations were consistent across different causes of anemia, and the hemoglobin threshold at which the association between inflammation and erythropoietin reversed was approximately hemoglobin 13.0 g/100 mL. These observations suggest that inflammaging (i.e., all individuals were above 65 years of age) is associated with a pre-anemic stage of high erythropoietin followed by a decrease in erythropoietin and the development of anemia. To conclude, in our opinion the large group of elderly with anemia of an unknown cause is most likely a heterogeneous group where the anemia can be caused by preleukemic MDS, pharmacotherapy, inflammaging and probably other causes.

3.4. The Diagnostic Evaluation of Anemia in Elderly Patients

The large group of individuals with an unknown cause of anemia reflects that the diagnostic evaluation was limited in these previous epidemiological studies. A recent review has suggested that the initial laboratory evaluation of anemic elderly patients should include the samples listed in Table 5 [106]. This list is more extensive than the evaluation used in previous epidemiological/clinical studies, and one would therefore expect the group of patients with unexplained anemia to decrease if this diagnostic strategy is used. In our opinion this is a reasonable diagnostic compromise.

Table 5. Suggested initial laboratory evaluation of elderly patients with anemia [106].

Type of Marker	Recommended Single Analyses (Peripheral Blood)
Peripheral blood cells	Hemoglobin, MCV, MCH, differential blood cell count, reticulocyte count, reticulocyte hemoglobin and erythropoietin
Nutritional status	Vitamin B12, serum folate, transferrin saturation and ferritin
Hemolysis	Lactate dehydrogenase, haptoglobin and bilirubin
Organ markers	Creatinine and glomerular filtration rate Alanine aminotransferase and aspartate aminotransferase
Markers of inflammation	C-reactive protein
Others	Serum electrophoresis and thyrotropin-releasing hormone

The difficult question is how extensive the additional diagnostic evaluation should be if the cause of the anemia is still unknown after this initial examination. First, this group may include patients with androgen deficiency [107,108], vitamin D deficiency [109] or altered erythropoietin homeostasis [105,108,110]. Second, an additional evaluation may become necessary to establish the diagnosis of early vitamin B12 or folic acid deficiency. Third, the initial laboratory evaluation may suggest gastro-/colonoscopy or an ultrasound examination of the abdomen/kidneys. Finally, in our opinion the most difficult question is whether a more extensive bone marrow examination is justified, i.e., bone marrow aspiration, bone marrow biopsy, cytogenetic analysis and/or molecular genetic analyses. As will be discussed later, anemia was associated with increased mortality in the prospective NHANES III study, and 17% of the anemic patients in this study had features suggesting MDS or another myeloproliferative disease (e.g., unexplained MCV increase, additional cytopenia) [99]. An Israeli study described that 15% of cognitively impaired hospitalized patients with unexplained cytopenia had evidence of MDS [111], an American study described that mutations could be detected for 40% of patients with idiopathic cytopenia of uncertain significance when using a 22-gene mutation panel [112] and a British study described a high percentage of MDS-associated mutations in patients with nondiagnostic marrow biopsies [113]. Molecular genetic analyses are now available and in a recent review the authors concluded that clinical testing for mutations in hematopoietic cells is reasonable in cases of unexplained anemia of older patients, especially if additional cytopenias are present [114]. Other authors have suggested that bone marrow evaluation should only be considered for patients with an expected survival of at least three months [106]. In our opinion the best justified recommendation is that a bone marrow evaluation (including mutational analyses) should be considered for individual patients after a careful evaluation that includes the burden of the procedure, possible therapeutic consequences, life expectancy and the burden of the anemia.

3.5. Anemia as a Prognostic Parameter in Community-Living Elderly Individuals

As described in detail in Table 6, anemia is common for elderly individuals (approximately 10% of persons above 65 years of age) and the incidence rate increases with increasing age, but severe anemia with Hb below 11 g/100mL is seen only for 2% or less of individuals depending on the study population (Tables 2, 5 and 6) [97–99,115–127]. The incidence of anemia seems to depend on race and is higher in black Americans [99,116]. The hemoglobin level associated with increased mortality also seems to depend on race: for white non-Hispanic Americans hemoglobin levels below the WHO cut-off is associated with increased mortality, whereas the mortality is increased for black American and Mexican Americans with levels lower than 1 g/100 mL below the WHO cut-off [116]. Below these cut-off points a five-year survival of 40–45% was observed, whereas individuals without anemia had a survival exceeding 80% [116]. Finally, the association between anemia and increased mortality as well as hospitalization is also observed when only including patients without prevalent disease in the studies [117].

Several prospective studies have demonstrated significant clinical effects of anemia:
- Anemia has a negative impact on survival, but this impact seems to differ between subtypes based on the relative risk in the order nutritional > chronic kidney disease > inflammation > unknown cause [118–120].
- Mild anemia is also associated with reduced physical performance, muscle strength, cognition and quality of life [117,127].
- Anemia is associated with an increased risk of depressive symptoms [128].
- Anemia with chronic inflammation is associated with autoimmune disease but also with cancer [115].

Thus, elderly anemic patients often have complex clinical problems that have to be considered when evaluation and possible treatment of the anemia is considered.

Table 6. Anemia in elderly community-living individuals, a summary of results from representative and important population studies describing the frequency of anemia and mortality in anemic individuals [98,99,116–120].

Study	Population and Methodology	Observation
Schop et al. [98]	The study included 4152 individuals from the general population above 50 years of age (median age: 75). Newly diagnosed anemia.	After an extensive evaluation in general practice the cause was unclear for 20%, one cause was seen for 59% and multiple etiologies for 22%. The most common single etiologies were anemia of chronic disease and iron deficiency. The frequency of patients with renal anemia increased with age.
Patel et al. [116]	The study included 4089 Americans above 65 years of age.	For non-Hispanic white Americans the mortality increased with the degree of anemia, and the anemia threshold for increased mortality corresponded to 0.4 and 0.2 g/100 mL above the WHO definition of anemia (see Table 2). For black Americans the threshold for increased mortality was 0.7 g/100 mL below the WHO definition.
Guralnik et al. [99]	A population-based study including 39,695 individuals, 5252 of them being older than 65.	Anemia prevalence rates increased after 50 years of age. For individuals ≥65 years of age 11.0% of men and 10.2% of women were anemic, and 20% of individuals ≥85 years of age were anemic. Nutrient deficiency was present in one-third, one-third had renal and/or chronic inflammatory anemia and the anemia was unexplained for one-third. Hb levels <11.0 were observed for 1.6% of men and 2.8% of women. Anemia was most frequent in elderly black people (27.8%) and less frequent in Mexican Americans (10.4%) and white non-Hispanics (9.0%).
Penninx et al. [117]	The study included 3607 individuals aged 71 or older, with a mean age of 78.2.	Anemia according to the WHO criteria was observed for 12.5%. The mortality was significantly higher for anemic participants (37.0% vs. 22.1%, $p < 0.001$) and they were hospitalized more frequently and spent more days in hospital. These differences remained significant after excluding persons with prevalent disease.
Shavelle et al. [118]	The study included 7171 community-dwelling individuals (aged ≥ 50), 862 of whom were anemic according to the WHO definition.	Significant negative impact of anemia on overall survival with relative risk 1.8 ($p < 0.001$). Relative risk depended on cause: (i) nutritional (2.34, $p < 0.0001$); (ii) chronic renal disease (1.70, $p < 0.0001$); (iii) chronic inflammation (1.48, $p < 0.0001$); and (iv) unexplained (1.26, $p < 0.01$).
Zakai et al. [119]	The development of anemia was evaluated for 3758 community-dwelling individuals aged 65 or older without anemia at inclusion.	Of the individuals, 498 (8.5%) developed anemia according to the WHO criteria. Baseline increasing age, being African American and kidney disease predicted anemia development over 3 years. Both anemia development and hemoglobin decline predicted subsequent mortality in men and women.
den Enzen [120]	A population-based study of 562 individuals aged 85.	The prevalence of anemia at baseline was 26.7%, and anemic individuals had more comorbidity with more disabilities, worse cognitive function and more depressive symptoms. Both prevalent and incident anemia was significantly associated with survival in adjusted analyses, including adjustment for C-reactive protein. Mortality increased with severity of anemia.

3.6. Anemia as a Prognostic Parameter in Nursing Home Residents

Anemia is more common among elderly nursing home residents than in community-living elderly individuals; this has been demonstrated in several studies from different countries, including those representative studies summarized in Table 7 [100,121–126]. Several studies have shown that more than 50% of residents have anemia according to the WHO definition [95]. The most important causes of anemia in these patients are nutritional factors, renal failure and chronic inflammation (Table 4), and anemia becomes more frequent with increasing age [98,99,126]. This is similar to community-living elderly (see Tables 6 and 7). A large subset of the anemic patients has an unknown cause after the initial routine evaluation based on clinical examination and blood sample analyses (Table 4), and hematological malignancies were not found to be a frequent cause of anemia in elderly patients in any of the studies described in Table 7. Furthermore, it should be emphasized that anemia is frequently multifactorial [129].

Table 7. Anemia in elderly nursing home residents, a summary of results from representative and important population studies [99,121–126].

Study	Population and Methodology	Observation
Chan et al. [121]	Retrospective, cross-sectional study at nine Chinese nursing homes (812 residents, mean age of 86 years).	A total of 67% were anemic, and the anemic residents were older and had a higher incidence of renal impairment; no significant associations with other comorbidities were observed.
Resnick et al. [122]	Including 451 residents, mean age of 83.7 years.	Anemia was more common among black than white residents; physical capacity was worse in anemic patients.
Westerlind et al. [100]	Including 390 patients (mean age 85.1 years), follow-up 7 years from baseline including Hb for 220 patients.	Prevalence of anemia at baseline was 52% for men and 32% for women. Two-year mortality was 61% for men with and 29% for men without anemia ($p = 0.001$), but for women no significant difference was observed (49% vs. 43%). Increased mortality in anemic men was independent of age, BNP and eGFR. Among men, anemia correlated with BNP/eGFR/CRP; for women, anemia correlated with several inflammatory markers including CRP. Anemic men were less physically active. Reduction in Hb with more than 0.9 g/100 mL during the first 2 years of follow-up was associated with increased mortality.
Pandya et al. [124]	Including 564 residents, mean age of 81 years.	In this study, 64% of males and 53% of females were anemic. Anemia was significantly associated with being African American, low eGFR, cancer, gastrointestinal bleeding and inflammatory disease,
Landi et al. [125]	Including 372 residents admitted to nursing home, aged 65 years or older.	At enrolment 63.1% of patients were anemic according to the WHO criteria. The death rate of anemic patients (38%) was higher than for nonanemic patients (28%, $p = 0.03$). This difference was independent of frailty, cognitive impairment, eGFR, cancer, stroke, body mass index and pressure ulcer.
Robinson et al. [126]	Evaluated 6200 residents, mean age of 83.2 years.	Of the residents, 59.6% were anemic. Older age was associated with lower hemoglobin in patients without kidney disease. However, for the whole study population chronic kidney disease seemed to contribute more strongly to the development of anemia than high age.

Abbreviations: BNP, B-type natriuretic peptide; CRP, C-reactive protein; and eGFR, estimated glomerular filtration rate.

Some studies suggest that the frequency of anemia also differs between men and women for nursing home residents [100,123]. Furthermore, anemia is also dependent on race, and several studies have described higher frequencies in black residents [122,124]. Finally, several studies have described an association between anemia and survival, and the more severe the anemia the stronger the prognostic impact [100,125]. Some studies also suggest that this association is strongest for men [100].

Anemia seems to be a part of a more complex clinical situation with reduced function for these patients. First, even mild anemia and low normal levels are often associated with lower muscle strength, physical function and mobility [129]. Patients with anemia below 11 g/100 mL also have significantly decreased scores for activities of daily life and quality of life [130]. Second, even though at least one study has shown no associations between anemia and decreases for community-living elderly individuals [131], such an association has been observed for nursing home residents [132,133]. Third, frailty has been defined as a medical syndrome characterized by decreased physiological reserve and increased vulnerability, and frailty seems to be a predictor for nursing home placement of elderly community-dwelling individuals [134]. Anemia may therefore be only a part of a complex physiological reduction. Finally, being underweight is also a risk factor (in addition to anemia?) for mortality in elderly nursing home residents [135], and anemia is important for the quality of life of cancer patients [136]. Taken together, these studies show that anemia will often be a part of a complex clinical situation for elderly individuals, including other factors that are also associated with mortality.

4. Causes of Mortality in Elderly Individuals with Anemia

Anemia in the elderly is very heterogeneous with regard to its etiology, and it is therefore not surprising that different causes contribute to the increased mortality.

4.1. Increased Mortality from Stroke

The impact of anemia on the mortality of patients with stroke was addressed in a recent meta-analysis based on 13 cohort studies including 19,239 patients [137]. Anemia was associated with an increased risk of mortality in stroke. This prognostic impact of anemia is possibly seen for patients with less severe stroke in particular [138]. However, the large meta-analysis was based on studies that also included younger patients, whereas the registry study by Barlas et al. [139] included 8013 patients with a mean age of 77.8 years. In this last study anemia was present at admission in 24.5% of the patients, and increased mortality was observed both for men and women with ischemic stroke. A more recent study by Barlas et al. [140] suggested that microcytic and normocytic anemia differed with regard to mortality and disability after stroke.

4.2. Increased Mortality from Heart Disease: Studies in Patients with Chronic Heart Failure

Several studies have investigated the association between anemia and mortality in patients with chronic heart failure:

- One study included 6159 outpatients with stable chronic heart failure [141]. The prevalence of anemia was 17.2% (median age: 69 years for anemic versus 65 years for nonanemic); after six months 43% of these anemic patients at baseline had normalized Hb levels, whereas 16% of the nonanemic patients had developed anemia. After a mean follow-up of 3.9 years the mortality was higher both for patients with persistent anemia (58% vs. 31%, $p < 0.0001$) and incident anemia (45% vs. 31%, $p < 0.0001$) compared with nonanemic individuals at six months.
- A meta-analysis based on 153,180 heart failure patients included 37.2% anemic patients [142]; after a follow-up of at least six months the mortality was 46.8% for anemic and 29.5% for nonanemic patients. Lower baseline Hb was associated with higher mortality. These observations were also supported by another meta-analysis [143]: the patients in 10 of the 20 included reports had a mean age above 60 years, and an association between anemia and more severe heart failure was observed.
- The study by Kosiborod et al. [144] included 2281 patients aged 65 years or older with heart failure. This study showed that elderly patients with heart failure and anemia had higher one-year mortality.

To conclude, anemia is associated with increased mortality for patients with heart failure, including elderly patients.

4.3. Nutritional Defects and the Role of Iron Deficiency in Patients with Heart Failure

The possible role of iron deficiency alone in heart failure has been investigated in several studies [145]. By using a multivariable hazard model, iron deficiency, but not anemia, was found to be a strong and independent predictor of mortality in a study of 1506 patients with chronic heart failure [146]. These authors defined iron deficiency as ferritin <100 μg/L or ferritin 100–299 μg/L together with a transferrin saturation of <20%, and this was present for 753 patients. Thus, iron deficiency was common, was associated with the severity of heart failure and was an independent prognostic marker. The possible importance of iron deficiency is also supported by two recent clinical studies describing a reduced rehospitalization rate after iron supplementation for patients with heart failure [147,148], but none of these studies could detect any effect of iron supplementation on survival. A third study could not detect any effect of iron supplementation on physical capacity either [149]. Thus, the overall results suggest that iron supplementation has only a limited effect on patients with heart failure and iron deficiency, whereas the association between anemia and mortality has been detected in several large studies.

A previous study could not detect any association between vitamin B12 or folate deficiency and mortality for patients with chronic heart failure [150].

4.4. Anemia in Patients with Cancer

Anemia is a common symptom of cancer, and 20–60% of patients with cancer have anemia at their initial diagnosis [151]. This is often referred to as the anemia of cancer, but it should be emphasized that anemia in cancer patients can be multifactorial and that possible additional contributing factors can be nutrition, inflammation, bleeding with iron deficiency or extensive bone marrow infiltration of malignant cells [151,152]. Although very few epidemiological studies of anemia in elderly patients have investigated how undiagnosed malignant disease contributes to the increased mortality of these patients, this is suggested by several observations. First, a Korean study of 10,114 elderly and apparently healthy individuals (mean age of 64 years) described an increased risk in all-cause mortality and cancer-related mortality (especially lung cancer) in men but not in women [153]. Second, a recent population-based cohort study including 138,670 individuals aged 18–93 years investigated the impact of anemia on survival [154]. An association between anemia and survival was observed especially for elderly patients (i.e., above 80 years of age). This adverse effect on survival was associated with both anemia and signs of chronic inflammation, whereas the survival was higher for patients with nutrient deficiencies and anemia of an unknown cause. As will be discussed below, the anemia of cancer is associated with inflammation. Third, unexplained anemia can be the first sign of low-risk MDS, but small studies including relevant diagnostic procedures have concluded that MDS could be diagnosed only for a small minority (i.e., less than 15%) of patients with unexplained anemia after a limited non-invasive evaluation [155]. Finally, iron deficiency can also be associated with bleeding from an undiagnosed gastrointestinal tumor, and this is one of the reasons why upper and lower gastrointestinal endoscopy have been recommended for patients with unexplained iron deficiency anemia [156]. This clinical strategy is also supported by clinical experience showing that even elderly patients with recurrent iron deficiency anemia may have a cause of iron deficiency anemia that can be treated [157,158]. Taken together, these observations strongly suggest that undiagnosed malignancy can be a cause of anemia in elderly individuals, and that these cancer patients can hide among patients with iron deficiency, anemia with chronic inflammation and anemia with an unknown cause after a limited noninvasive diagnostic evaluation.

Anemia is a common symptom of cancer and is often referred to as the anemia of cancer [151]. The cytokine-induced inhibition of erythropoiesis is regarded as an important mechanism for the development of anemia in cancer patients, TNFα in particular but also other inflammatory regulators, including IL1β, IL6, IL10 and IFNγ, probably contribute [151,159]. As discussed in previous reviews, these mediators have direct inhibitory effects on erythroid progenitors; the mechanisms differ between the various cytokines and include the inhibition of proliferation and differentiation, the downregulation of erythropoietin receptors and the induction of apoptosis through the Fas pathway [151]. However, proinflammatory cytokines may also have indirect effects on erythropoiesis, including the inhibition of renal erythropoietin production and the production of hepcidin leading to iron retention in macrophages and decreased dietary iron absorption [151,159]. Finally, uncommon causes that contribute to anemia in cancer can be (i) immune-mediated hemolytic anemia as a paraneoplastic disease, (ii) microangiopathic anemia caused by extensive cancer metastases with pathological microvessels in the tumor, (iii) microangiopathy caused by cancer-associated thrombotic thrombocytopenic purpura, (iv) hemolytic uremic syndrome or (v) anemia as a part of cancer-associated coagulopathy with disseminated intravascular coagulation [151].

Anemia and/or blood transfusions can be adverse prognostic parameters in patients with cancer [151,160]. Preoperative anemia can be an independent risk factor associated with both survival and relapse risk in cancer patients [161,162].

The treatment of cancer-associated anemia is outside the scope of this article, but it has been addressed in several recent articles [152,163].

4.5. Increased Mortality of Anemic Patients after Surgery

A large meta-analysis investigated the association between preoperative anemia and mortality after surgery [164]. This analysis included not only studies of elderly patients: 24 eligible studies were identified and these studies included 959,445 patients, of which 371,594 patients were anemic. Anemia was then associated with increased mortality (odds ratio of 2.90/p-value < 0.001), acute kidney injury (3.75/<0.001) and infection (1.92/00.01). These findings were similar for the cardiac and non-cardiac surgery patients, but anemia was also associated with stroke for the cardiac surgery patients. Thirteen of these studies used the WHO definition of anemia, and the association between anemia and postsurgery mortality remained when the analysis was restricted to these patients. It seems justified to conclude that presurgery anemia reflects a more complex clinical situation associated with increased postsurgery mortality.

We have identified four studies investigating the postoperative mortality for elderly patients. First, one study based on a national prospective database included 31,857 elderly patients above 65 years of age undergoing an elective vascular operation [165]. Forty-seven percent of these patients had anemia, and the anemic patients had increased 30 days postoperative mortality (2.4% versus 1.2%, p < 0.0001) and cardiac event rate (2.3% versus 1.2%, p < 0.0001) compared with the nonanemic patients. The mortality was highest for the patients with severe anemia. Second, another study included 310,311 patients aged 65 years or older who underwent major noncardiac surgery [166]. This study also observed an increased mortality associated with anemia. Finally, a large study investigated the association between anemia at presentation and postoperative mortality for elderly patients with a mean age of 79.2 years [167]. At presentation, 65% of these patients were anemic, and anemia was then associated with an increased odds ratio for mortality (1.3/p = 0.004); there was no significant association between anemia and myocardial infarction or cerebrovascular events. Anemia seems to be an indicator of poor general health and thereby increased mortality after surgery for many elderly patients [168].

4.6. Summarizing Comments: Anemia, Inflammation and Mortality

Anemia is common in elderly individuals, and the increased mortality in elderly patients with anemia is multifactorial. Although anemia and inflammation are present together in many patients, several studies suggest that anemia has an effect on mortality that is independent of the concomitant inflammation. An adverse prognosis due to common disorders and comorbidities (including cardiovascular disease and cancer) seems to be most important and definitely more important than an increased frequency of uncommon diseases (e.g., hematological malignancies).

5. Inflammation in Aging

5.1. CRP as a Marker of Inflammation: Its Structure and Function

CRP is an acute-phase protein and is used as a marker of inflammation both in epidemiological studies and in routine clinical practice [169]. As described in several previous reviews, CRP exists in several isoforms [170–176]. It is synthesized as monomers; the pentamer is thereafter formed in the endoplasmic reticulum where it is also stored and from where it is released slowly during the non-inflammatory baseline situation. Thus, native CRP is a pentameric protein, but it can also be detected extracellularly as a monomer (206 amino acids and a molecular weight of 23 kDa) formed by the irreversible dissociation of the released pentameters. The pentamer is rapidly released in response to increased levels of proinflammatory cytokines. Finally, CRP can also form fibril-like structures, decamers and possibly trimers as well as tetramers; various CRP peptides can also mediate biological effects [177].

The acute-phase reaction is characterized by an acute increase in the systemic (i.e., serum/plasma) levels of several proteins in response to inflammation, infection or tissue injury [86]. However, it can also be seen in chronic diseases or be a chronic or long-lasting response [169]. The reaction is regarded as a response that is induced by cytokines produced at inflammatory sites; IL6 is then an important stimulator together with other members of the IL6 family, IL1β, TNFα, IFNγ, TGFβ and IL8/CXCL8 [86]. Several of these cytokines/chemokines are involved in the regulation of CRP gene expression, including TNFα, IL6, IL8/CXCL8 and CCL2 [169]. Thus, even though CRP is only one out of several acute-phase proteins, it should be regarded as an immunoregulator that reflects and integrates intercellular signaling mediated by several proinflammatory mediators.

The release and immunoregulatory functions of CRP have also been described in previous reviews [86,169]. Briefly, the native CRP isoform is mainly released by hepatocytes but can also be released by smooth muscle cells, macrophages, endothelial cells, lymphocytes and adipocytes. Its biological effects include [86,169,178–181]:

- Monocytes/macrophages: These cells can be polarized by CRP towards the proinflammatory M1 phenotype with increased phagocytosis and cytokine release, inhibited chemotaxis and altered metabolism with increased LDL uptake.
- Dendritic cells: CRP seems to be an important regulator of dendritic cell functions and can activate monocyte-derived dendritic cells [178–180].
- T cells: Indirect stimulation/modulation of T cell activation through the effects on dendritic cells [179,180].
- Neutrophils: The functional CRP effects depend on the biological context and can be decreased activation, inhibition of chemotaxis and/or stimulated phagocytosis [181].
- Endothelial cell activation.
- Thrombocytes: Inhibition of activation, trafficking and aggregation.
- Complement activation.

To conclude, CRP is a common target that integrates information from several upstream events/immunoregulators, but at the same time CRP itself is an important immunoregulator that influences the function of several immunocompetent cells. CRP should therefore be regarded as a key point in the network of soluble immunoregulators.

5.2. Inflammaging and Systemic CRP Levels in Elderly Patients

Aging is associated with the accumulation in many tissues of senescent cells with a secretory phenotype; these cells can release proinflammatory cytokines, chemokines and other mediators that modulate their microenvironments [46,182]. Animal models suggest that this increased release is associated with the increased activation of JAK-STAT pathways [183]. This chronic state of low-grade inflammation also seems to be reflected in the increased systemic levels of several proinflammatory cytokines/markers, including IL1β, IL1Rα, IL6, TNFα and IFNγ [184,185]. These mediators may then influence various physiological systems and contribute to the complex process of aging and the clinical situation of many elderly people, including altered hematopoiesis and neurological functions [186]. This process is often referred to as inflammaging [187]. These mediators are also initiators and drivers of the acute-phase reaction [169], and these effects may therefore at least partly explain why systemic CRP levels should be regarded to reflect the process of inflammaging. Inflammaging is probably caused by age-dependent functional alterations in various immunocompetent cell types, including both the innate and adaptive immune system [186,188].

The process of inflammaging is not necessarily associated with disease development. We recently investigated the CRP levels in a group of 85 healthy allogeneic stem cell donors [189]. After a careful evaluation none of these donors showed any signs of disease, and they were all regarded as acceptable stem cell donors. However, a subset of these stem cell donors showed increased CRP levels, and these increased levels were observed especially for elderly donors. The CRP levels of this donor subgroup were further increased by stem cell mobilization by G-CSF, and our studies suggest that IL6 and possibly other members of the IL6 family can influence this systemic low-grade inflammation associated with aging.

5.3. Inflammation-Induced Modulation of the Hematopoietic Stem Cell Niche

The various hematopoiesis-supporting stromal cells of the stem cell niches express a wide range of cytokine/chemokine receptors as well as pattern recognition receptors [190]. These receptors recognize ligands that are generated locally or systemically; their cellular functions can thereby be modulated and a new or second wave of mediators released locally in response to a systemic response/reaction. This second wave also includes prostaglandins and enzymes, e.g., prostaglandin E2 and nitric oxide synthase [191]. These locally released mediators may thereafter modulate the trafficking of hematopoietic/immunocompetent/immunomodulatory cells to the bone marrow [192,193]. Another example is the endothelial cells: these cells express multiple pattern-recognizing receptors, and the stimulation of Toll-like receptor 4 induces G-CSF release whereas proinflammatory cytokines (including IL6 released by MSCs) stimulate the release of GM-CSF by endothelial cells and modulate the endothelial cell responsiveness to proinflammatory cytokines [190,194–197]. The endothelial cells thus contribute to the translation of proinflammatory signals into the regulation of hematopoiesis. Finally, cell–cell contact through adhesion molecules or membrane-expressed ligands that induce intracellular signaling are also involved in this translation [190,196]. A complete review of the molecular mechanisms between these stromal cells as well as between stromal and hematopoietic cells is beyond the scope of this review, but our examples clearly show that inflammation affects the functional phenotype of various stromal cells in the stem cell niches and thereby indirectly modulate hematopoiesis.

5.4. Inflammation, Aging, Disease and Mortality

Several studies suggest that inflammation (i.e., increased CRP and/or cytokine levels) is associated with an increased risk of future cardiovascular events [198–203]; as discussed in detail in a previous review, this is also true for elderly patients above 65 years of age (Table 8) [204]. First, Tracy et al. [198] described an association between high CRP levels and future coronary heart disease: this association was seen especially for women with subclinical cardiovascular disease who had a cardiovascular event within one year. The association was also significant when analyzing myocardial infarction alone. Second, the two studies by Cesari et al. [199,200] also described significant associations between cardiovascular disease and CRP levels, and in addition they described associations between IL6 and TNFα levels with cardiovascular disease that seemed to be stronger than the association with CRP. However, another study concluded that CRP was less useful as a prognostic marker in elderly individuals; the associations between CRP and cardiovascular health did not reach significance after adjustment for several other cardiovascular risk factors, and there was no statistical evidence for a gender interaction either [204]. Other authors have described an association between inflammation and cardiovascular events also when using a composite indicator of inflammation [205]. Third, Makita et al. [201] detected a gender difference with a significant association between carotid plaque score and high CRP levels only for men. Finally, even though CRP may not be an independent risk factor, it seems to be a part of a clinical high-risk inflammatory phenotype with complex interactions between several risk factors in elderly individuals, including smoking, diabetes, hypertension, body mass index, lipid metabolism and inherited differences in the regulation of inflammation [202,205–210]. Gender differences with regard to the impact of CRP have been described only in some studies, but differences between men and women with regard to the associations between CRP levels and cardiovascular risk would not be unexpected because associations between CRP levels and male sex hormone levels have been described [211]. Taken together, these observations suggest that there is an association between inflammaging/CRP increase and the risk of clinical cardiovascular disease. However, as concluded by a more recent study, there may not be a causal association: increased CRP levels seem rather to reflect hidden inflammatory activity that is strongly associated with all-cause and not only cardiovascular mortality [212].

Table 8. Inflammation and cardiovascular disease. A summary of observations from important studies [198–203].

Study and Study Population	Observation
Tracy et al. [198]. Prospective, nested case–control study. There were 5201 persons in the original sample, age ≥ 65. Of these, 146 cases with incident cardiovascular events were identified and 146 control subjects were matched (mean age of 72.8 and 72.9 years, respectively).	The mean CRP level was only significantly higher for case subjects than for control subjects in women. CRP levels were generally higher in persons with subclinical disease. Among the elderly with subclinical disease, CRP was associated with myocardial infarction with an overall odds ratio (OR) of 2.67 (CI 1.04–6.81), with the association being stronger for women, with an OR of 4.50 (CI 0.97 to 20.8), than for men, with an OR of 1.75 (CI 0.51 to 5.98).
Cesari et al. [199]. Cross-sectional study including 3045 well-functioning persons with a mean age of 74.2 years (range of 70–79 years). Subclinical cardiovascular disease was defined as signs of angina or claudication according to the Rose Questionnaire, positive ankle/brachial index or electrocardiographic abnormalities.	CRP was significantly associated with congestive heart failure, with an OR of 1.64 (95% CI 1.11 to 2.41), but not with any other manifestations of cardiovascular disease. When comparing patients in the highest versus those in the lowest IL6 tertile, the OR for subclinical cardiovascular disease was 1.58 (95% CI 1.26 to 1.97) and for clinical cardiovascular disease was 2.35 (95% CI 1.79 to 3.09). This was similar for TNFα, with an OR of 1.48 (95% CI 1.16 to 1.88) and 2.05 (95% CI 1.55 to 2.72), respectively. Only soluble TNFR1 but not soluble IL6R or soluble IL2R showed a significant association with cardiovascular disease.
Cesari et al. [200]. Prospective study including 2225 persons with a mean age of 74.0 years (range of 70–79 years). Outcomes were hospitalizations for coronary heart disease (CHD), stroke or congestive heart failure (CHF).	CRP was significantly associated only with congestive heart failure. In contrast, IL6 was significantly associated with all three outcomes, and TNFα was significantly associated both with coronary heart disease and congestive heart failure. The risk of both coronary heart disease and congestive heart failure was highest for patients with levels in the highest tertile for all three markers; these patients had a two- to three-fold increase in coronary disease and heart failure compared with patients with no levels in the highest tertile. These differences also remained significant in adjusted analyses.
Makita et al. [201]. Cross-sectional study including 2056 individuals with a mean age of 58.3 years (range of 25–86 years). All examined with CRP and carotid ultrasound.	An association between plaque score and increasing CRP levels was seen only for men ($p < 0.01$); this association remained significant after being adjusted for age and other risk factors. Intima–media complex thickness and arterial dilation showed significant associations with CRP only in univariate, but not in adjusted, analyses.

Table 8. *Cont.*

Study and Study Population	Observation
Hosford-Donovan et al. [202]. Cross-sectional study of 108 elderly women with a mean age of 67.5 years (range of 65–70 years).	Body mass index (BMI), waist circumference, systolic blood pressure (SBP) and diastolic blood pressure (DBP) were significantly higher in patients with high CRP above the median level. SBP and DBP remained significantly higher in the high-CRP group after adjusting for BMI and use of antihypertensive medication. The influence of CRP on SBP was attenuated when adjusted for waist circumference ($p = 0.062$). Serum derived from high-CRP patients decreased the proliferation and the capillary tube length of in vitro cultured endothelial cells.
Labonté et al. [203]. Cross-sectional study of 801 Inuits (mean age of 36.3 years, range of 18–74 years).	Increased plasma CRP levels >2.0 mg/L were more prevalent among women. SBP was significantly and independently associated with increased CRP levels.

Abbreviations: CHD, coronary heart disease; CI, confidence interval; DBP, diastolic blood pressure; IL2R, IL2 receptor; IL6R, IL6 receptor; OR, odds ratio; RR, relative risk; SBP, systolic blood pressure; and TNFR1, TNF receptor 1.

A recent systematic review of 23 cohort studies analyzed the associations between blood biomarkers and mortality [213]. These authors included studies with a mean age between 50 and 75 years at baseline. The meta-analysis of mortality risk showed significant associations not only with cardiovascular mortality but also with all-cause mortality and cancer mortality. Twenty biomarkers showed associations with mortality risk, and among them were several markers of inflammation/acute-phase reaction, including total white blood cell count, circulating neutrophil granulocytes, erythrocyte sedimentation rate, fibrinogen and TNF receptor II.

6. Summarizing Discussion

In this review we have described the biological background and clinical aspects of anemia and inflammation in elderly individuals. Both anemia and inflammation are common in the elderly and in our opinion they should be regarded as related, although only partly overlapping processes, with regard to pathogenesis and prognostic impact.

6.1. Anemia and Aging

Aging is characterized by several cellular hallmarks, including genetic instability, telomere shortening, loss of proteostasis, deregulated nutritional sensing, mitochondrial dysfunction, cellular senescence, stem cell exhaustion and altered cellular communication [2]. These factors will also influence hematopoiesis and hematopoietic stem cells in elderly individuals. The biological context of anemia as well as inflammation will therefore be different from that of younger individuals. The ageing in hematopoiesis seems to be caused by several mechanisms and complex interactions between aging-associated alterations in hematopoietic cells (including hematopoietic stem cells) and alterations in hematopoiesis-supporting bone marrow stromal cells [14,60,78]. The inflammation itself can also be a part of the aging process, and is then referred to as inflammaging [185,187]. It should also be emphasized that inflammaging occurs in the context of complex age-associated alterations in the innate and adaptive immune systems [186]. Many of the disorders that can cause anemia and/or signs of inflammation in elderly individuals are quite common (Table 3, Section 3.3), but little is known about whether or how the treatment of such diseases should be modified in elderly individuals due to differences in the biology or pathogenesis of these disorders caused by the effects of the aging of the involved cells, e.g., aging-associated effects in immunocompetent cells for patients with autoimmune diseases.

6.2. Carcinogenesis and Cancer Treatment in Elderly Individuals

Age-associated differences also seem to be reflected in the development and biological characteristics of malignant diseases in elderly individuals, e.g., hematological malignancies [94]. This has been demonstrated by proteomic studies on favorable prognosis AML (i.e., favorable genetic abnormalities) where the proteomic profiles differ between elderly and younger patients with the same cytogenetic abnormalities [96]. In our opinion the same is probably true for other malignancies: precarcinogenic aging-associated differences probably remain after carcinogenesis in malignant cells.

Another aspect is the toxicity of anticancer therapies in the elderly. Age-dependent differences are probably the explanation as to why several forms of anticancer treatment cannot be used in elderly individuals. Toxic effects and especially hematological toxicity, often dose-limiting for anticancer treatment [214], as well as immune-related toxicity are more severe in allogeneic stem cell transplantation both when using elderly stem cell donors [215–217] and for elderly recipients [218,219]. The same may be true for radiation therapy, and in our opinion an increased mortality similar to the mortality in orthopedic surgery [164–166] would also be expected for cancer surgery.

Signs of inflammation and an acute-phase reaction is associated with an adverse prognosis and decreased survival in many cancer forms [169], but at the same time the use of various forms of immunostimulatory therapies (e.g., checkpoint inhibitors) has improved the prognosis/survival for many cancer patients [220]. The explanation for this apparent discrepancy is possibly that the acute-phase reaction can be associated with local macrophage infiltration that enhances tumor growth through the release of growth factors (e.g., the stimulation of local angiogenesis) despite the concomitant induction of a systemic acute-phase reaction [221], whereas effective anticancer immunotherapy targets and enhances anticancer T cell responses.

6.3. Inflammation and Anemia

CRP is often used as a sign of inflammation and inflammaging, and cohort studies have described associations between CRP levels and overall cardiovascular and cancer mortality. However, it should be emphasized that several mechanisms can induce the acute-phase reaction, and increased CRP levels can be associated with different soluble mediator serum/plasma profiles. This last aspect is illustrated by two recent studies on cancer patients: inflammatory markers are associated with a prognosis in both head and neck squamous cell carcinoma as well as renal cancer, but the prognostic impact of systemic levels of individual proinflammatory mediators seem to differ between the two groups [222,223]. In our opinion it will therefore be important to investigate the systemic inflammation-associated mediator profile and not only the CRP levels to further characterize individual differences as well as differences in the prognostic impact of inflammaging. The observation that systemic levels of single proinflammatory cytokines show stronger associations than CRP levels to cardiovascular health further support this hypothesis [200].

For several reasons anemia in the elderly and inflammaging should be regarded as related (i.e., events with the same upstream initiator) and/or complicating events with only overlapping but not identical molecular pathogenic mechanisms. First, patients with signs of inflammation are regarded as a specific subset of elderly anemia patients (Section 3.3). Second, proinflammatory cytokine responses involving IL1, TNFα and IL6/IL6 family members can induce the systemic acute-phase response, and the same cytokines can also contribute to the aging effect on normal hematopoiesis as well as to the development of anemia due to a specific cause, e.g., they are important in the development of cancer-associated anemia (Sections 2.4 and 6.3). Third, a subset of elderly patients with anemia is characterized by inflammation and increased CRP levels, but it should also be emphasized that anemia seems to have an impact on survival that is independent of the CRP level [120]. Finally, both anemia and inflammation are associated with the same caused of mortality, e.g., cardiovascular death and possibly cancer-related mortality (Sections 4 and 5.4).

In our opinion it seems likely that there is partly an overlap in the biology/pathogenesis and clinical impact of anemia and inflammaging. However, signs of inflammation in patients with anemia are not necessarily caused by inflammaging but can alternatively be caused by a specific disease that initiates two (partly) independent events, e.g., in malignancies or autoimmune diseases [115]. The association between anemia and inflammation seems to be relatively weak, because despite the significant correlations between CRP and hemoglobin levels in anemic patients [100] the prognostic impact of anemia seems to be significant even after correcting for CRP [120]. A better understanding of the biological/molecular mechanisms behind the prognostic impact of anemia/inflammation/inflammaging will also be a necessary scientific basis when considering possible therapeutic interventions in patients with anemia and/or inflammation.

6.4. Anemia of an Unknown Cause

Several population-based studies of elderly individuals with anemia describe a relatively large group with anemia of an unknown cause (Table 3). Some previous authors have emphasized that these patients have been inadequately investigated when taking into account the diagnostic tools that are now available (see Section 3.3). In our opinion the word inadequate is misleading: one should rather refer to these patients as having an unknown cause after a limited diagnostic evaluation. Furthermore, a recent study suggests that the cause of anemia is unknown for many patients even after a more extensive laboratory work-up [224]. The extent of the diagnostic evaluation should, in our opinion, be individualized and based on an overall clinical evaluation. For many elderly patients an extensive diagnostic evaluation will not have therapeutic or prognostic consequences, and a limited diagnostic evaluation may therefore be relevant.

7. Conclusions

Aging is associated with the intrinsic (i.e., age-associated alterations of hematopoietic cells, including the stem cells) and extrinsic modulation of hematopoiesis caused by age-associated alterations of hematopoiesis-supporting bone marrow stromal cells. Furthermore, aging-associated modulation has also been described for most subsets of immunocompetent cells. These aging-associated alterations are reflected by the frequent detection of both anemia and signs of inflammation in elderly individuals. Anemia and inflammaging should be regarded as related, as they at least partly reflect the same biological mechanisms (e.g., increased levels of several proinflammatory mediators). Both anemia and inflammation are associated with increased mortality: the background for this decreased survival is probably multifactorial but seems to include increased cardiovascular mortality. Additional biological characterization of the molecular mechanisms behind anemia and inflammation is necessary to improve the clinical handling of individual patients, and the handling of these elderly patients should, in our opinion, be individualized and based on the overall clinical situation.

Author Contributions: Conceptualization, Ø.B.; writing—original draft preparation, Ø.B. and A.K.V.; writing—review and editing, Ø.B, A.K.V. and H.R. All authors have read and agreed to the published version of the manuscript.

Funding: The authors receive funding for their research from Helse Vest (grant number 911788) and the Norwegian Cancer Society (182609, 188802, 18902 and 4449050).

Institutional Review Board Statement: Not applicable.

Informed Consent Statement: Not applicable.

Data Availability Statement: Not applicable.

Conflicts of Interest: The authors declare no conflict of interest.

References

1. Rudnicka, E.; Napierała, P.; Podfigurna, A.; Męczekalski, B.; Smolarczyk, R.; Grymowicz, M. The World Health Organization (WHO) approach to healthy ageing. *Maturitas* **2020**, *139*, 6–11. [CrossRef] [PubMed]
2. López-Otín, C.; Blasco, M.A.; Partridge, L.; Serrano, M.; Kroemer, G. The hallmarks of aging. *Cell* **2013**, *153*, 1194–1217. [CrossRef] [PubMed]
3. Vijg, J.; Dong, X.; Milholland, B.; Zhang, L. Genome instability: A conserved mechanism of ageing? *Essays Biochem.* **2017**, *61*, 305–315. [CrossRef] [PubMed]
4. Blackburn, E.H.; Epel, E.S.; Lin, J. Human telomere biology: A contributory and interactive factor in aging, disease risks, and protection. *Science* **2015**, *350*, 1193–1198. [CrossRef]
5. Morris, B.J.; Willcox, B.J.; Donlon, T.A. Genetic and epigenetic regulation of human aging and longevity. *Biochim. Biophys. Acta Mol. Basis Dis.* **2019**, *1865*, 1718–1744. [CrossRef]
6. Micó, V.; Berninches, L.; Tapia, J.; Daimiel, L. NutrimiRAging: Micromanaging Nutrient Sensing Pathways through Nutrition to Promote Healthy Aging. *Int. J. Mol. Sci.* **2017**, *18*, 915. [CrossRef]
7. Fakouri, N.B.; Hou, Y.; Demarest, T.G.; Christiansen, L.S.; Okur, M.N.; Mohanty, J.G.; Croteau, D.L.; Bohr, V.A. Toward understanding genomic instability, mitochondrial dysfunction and aging. *FEBS J.* **2019**, *286*, 1058–1073. [CrossRef]
8. Klaips, C.L.; Jayaraj, G.G.; Hartl, F.U. Pathways of cellular proteostasis in aging and disease. *J. Cell Biol.* **2018**, *217*, 51–63. [CrossRef]
9. Schmeer, C.; Kretz, A.; Wengerodt, D.; Stojiljkovic, M.; Witte, O.W. Dissecting Aging and Senescence-Current Concepts and Open Lessons. *Cells* **2019**, *8*, 1446. [CrossRef]
10. Sameri, S.; Samadi, P.; Dehghan, R.; Salem, E.; Fayazi, N.; Amini, R. Stem Cell Aging in Lifespan and Disease: A State-of-the-Art Review. *Curr. Stem Cell Res. Ther.* **2020**, *15*, 362–378. [CrossRef]
11. Becker, L.; Nguyen, L.; Gill, J.; Kulkarni, S.; Pasricha, P.J.; Habtezion, A. Age-dependent shift in macrophage polarisation causes inflammation-mediated degeneration of enteric nervous system. *Gut* **2018**, *67*, 827–836. [CrossRef]
12. de Haan, G.; Lazare, S.S. Aging of hematopoietic stem cells. *Blood* **2018**, *131*, 479–487. [CrossRef] [PubMed]
13. Akunuru, S.; Geiger, H. Aging, Clonality, and Rejuvenation of Hematopoietic Stem Cells. *Trends Mol. Med.* **2016**, *22*, 701–712. [CrossRef] [PubMed]
14. Mejia-Ramirez, E.; Florian, M.C. Understanding intrinsic hematopoietic stem cell aging. *Haematologica* **2020**, *105*, 22–37. [CrossRef] [PubMed]
15. Rossi, D.J.; Bryder, D.; Zahn, J.M.; Ahlenius, H.; Sonu, R.; Wagers, A.J.; Weissman, I.L. Cell intrinsic alterations underlie hematopoietic stem cell aging. *Proc. Natl. Acad. Sci. USA* **2005**, *102*, 9194–9199. [CrossRef] [PubMed]
16. Verovskaya, E.V.; Dellorusso, P.V.; Passegué, E. Losing Sense of Self and Surroundings: Hematopoietic Stem Cell Aging and Leukemic Transformation. *Trends Mol. Med.* **2019**, *25*, 494–515. [CrossRef]
17. Pinho, S.; Frenette, P.S. Haematopoietic stem cell activity and interactions with the niche. *Nat. Rev. Mol. Cell Biol.* **2019**, *20*, 303–320. [CrossRef]
18. Florian, M.C.; Dörr, K.; Niebel, A.; Daria, D.; Schrezenmeier, H.; Rojewski, M.; Filippi, M.D.; Hasenberg, A.; Gunzer, M.; Scharffetter-Kochanek, K.; et al. Cdc42 activity regulates hematopoietic stem cell aging and rejuvenation. *Cell Stem Cell* **2012**, *10*, 520–530. [CrossRef]
19. Maryanovich, M.; Zahalka, A.H.; Pierce, H.; Pinho, S.; Nakahara, F.; Asada, N.; Wei, Q.; Wang, X.; Ciero, P.; Xu, J.; et al. Adrenergic nerve degeneration in bone marrow drives aging of the hematopoietic stem cell niche. *Nat. Med.* **2018**, *24*, 782–791. [CrossRef]
20. Ho, Y.H.; Del Toro, R.; Rivera-Torres, J.; Rak, J.; Korn, C.; García-García, A.; Macías, D.; González-Gómez, C.; Del Monte, A.; Wittner, M.; et al. Remodeling of Bone Marrow Hematopoietic Stem Cell Niches Promotes Myeloid Cell Expansion during Premature or Physiological Aging. *Cell Stem Cell* **2019**, *25*, 407–418. [CrossRef]
21. Saçma, M.; Pospiech, J.; Bogeska, R.; de Back, W.; Mallm, J.P.; Sakk, V.; Soller, K.; Marka, G.; Vollmer, A.; Karns, R.; et al. Haematopoietic stem cells in perisinusoidal niches are protected from ageing. *Nat. Cell Biol.* **2019**, *21*, 1309–1320. [CrossRef] [PubMed]
22. Wahlestedt, M.; Bryder, D. The slippery slope of hematopoietic stem cell aging. *Exp. Hematol.* **2017**, *56*, 1–6. [CrossRef] [PubMed]
23. Beerman, I.; Bock, C.; Garrison, B.S.; Smith, Z.D.; Gu, H.; Meissner, A.; Rossi, D.J. Proliferation-dependent alterations of the DNA methylation landscape underlie hematopoietic stem cell aging. *Cell Stem Cell* **2013**, *12*, 413–425. [CrossRef] [PubMed]
24. Chambers, S.M.; Shaw, C.A.; Gatza, C.; Fisk, C.J.; Donehower, L.A.; Goodell, M.A. Aging hematopoietic stem cells decline in function and exhibit epigenetic dysregulation. *PLoS Biol.* **2007**, *5*, e201. [CrossRef]
25. Geiger, H.; Van Zant, G. The aging of lympho-hematopoietic stem cells. *Nat. Immunol.* **2002**, *3*, 329–333. [CrossRef]
26. Lazzari, E.; Butler, J.M. The Instructive Role of the Bone Marrow Niche in Aging and Leukemia. *Curr. Stem Cell Rep.* **2018**, *4*, 291–298. [CrossRef]
27. Rossi, D.J.; Bryder, D.; Seita, J.; Nussenzweig, A.; Hoeijmakers, J.; Weissman, I.L. Deficiencies in DNA damage repair limit the function of haematopoietic stem cells with age. *Nature* **2007**, *447*, 725–729. [CrossRef]
28. Rudolph, K.L.; Chang, S.; Lee, H.W.; Blasco, M.; Gottlieb, G.J.; Greider, C.; DePinho, R.A. Longevity, stress response, and cancer in aging telomerase-deficient mice. *Cell* **1999**, *96*, 701–712. [CrossRef]
29. Chen, J.; Kao, Y.R.; Sun, D.; Todorova, T.I.; Reynolds, D.; Narayanagari, S.R.; Montagna, C.; Will, B.; Verma, A.; Steidl, U. Myelodysplastic syndrome progression to acute myeloid leukemia at the stem cell level. *Nat. Med.* **2019**, *25*, 103–110. [CrossRef]

30. Fuster, J.J.; MacLauchlan, S.; Zuriaga, M.A.; Polackal, M.N.; Ostriker, A.C.; Chakraborty, R.; Wu, C.L.; Sano, S.; Muralidharan, S.; Rius, C.; et al. Clonal hematopoiesis associated with TET2 deficiency accelerates atherosclerosis development in mice. *Science* **2017**, *355*, 842–847. [CrossRef]
31. Jaiswal, S.; Natarajan, P.; Silver, A.J.; Gibson, C.J.; Bick, A.G.; Shvartz, E.; McConkey, M.; Gupta, N.; Gabriel, S.; Ardissino, D.; et al. Clonal Hematopoiesis and Risk of Atherosclerotic Cardiovascular Disease. *N. Engl. J. Med.* **2017**, *377*, 111–121. [CrossRef] [PubMed]
32. Busque, L.; Sun, M.; Buscarlet, M.; Ayachi, S.; Feroz Zada, Y.; Provost, S.; Bourgoin, V.; Mollica, L.; Meisel, M.; Hinterleitner, R.; et al. High-sensitivity C-reactive protein is associated with clonal hematopoiesis of indeterminate potential. *Blood Adv.* **2020**, *4*, 2430–2438. [CrossRef] [PubMed]
33. Yura, Y.; Sano, S.; Walsh, K. Clonal Hematopoiesis: A New Step Linking Inflammation to Heart Failure. *JACC Basic Transl. Sci.* **2020**, *5*, 196–207. [CrossRef] [PubMed]
34. Hoehn, R.S.; Jernigan, P.L.; Chang, A.L.; Edwards, M.J.; Pritts, T.A. Molecular mechanisms of erythrocyte aging. *Biol. Chem.* **2015**, *396*, 621–631. [CrossRef] [PubMed]
35. Beerman, I.; Rossi, D.J. Epigenetic regulation of hematopoietic stem cell aging. *Exp. Cell Res.* **2014**, *329*, 192–199. [CrossRef]
36. Sun, D.; Luo, M.; Jeong, M.; Rodriguez, B.; Xia, Z.; Hannah, R.; Wang, H.; Le, T.; Faull, K.F.; Chen, R.; et al. Epigenomic profiling of young and aged HSCs reveals concerted changes during aging that reinforce self-renewal. *Cell Stem Cell* **2014**, *14*, 673–688. [CrossRef]
37. Choudry, F.A.; Frontini, M. Epigenetic Control of Haematopoietic Stem Cell Aging and Its Clinical Implications. *Stem Cells Int.* **2016**, *2016*, 5797521. [CrossRef]
38. Benayoun, B.A.; Pollina, E.A.; Singh, P.P.; Mahmoudi, S.; Harel, I.; Casey, K.M.; Dulken, B.W.; Kundaje, A.; Brunet, A. Remodeling of epigenome and transcriptome landscapes with aging in mice reveals widespread induction of inflammatory responses. *Genome Res.* **2019**, *29*, 697–709. [CrossRef]
39. Cheung, P.; Vallania, F.; Warsinske, H.C.; Donato, M.; Schaffert, S.; Chang, S.E.; Dvorak, M.; Dekker, C.L.; Davis, M.M.; Utz, P.J.; et al. Single-Cell Chromatin Modification Profiling Reveals Increased Epigenetic Variations with Aging. *Cell* **2018**, *173*, 1385–1397. [CrossRef]
40. Grigoryan, A.; Guidi, N.; Senger, K.; Liehr, T.; Soller, K.; Marka, G.; Vollmer, A.; Markaki, Y.; Leonhardt, H.; Buske, C.; et al. LaminA/C regulates epigenetic and chromatin architecture changes upon aging of hematopoietic stem cells. *Genome Biol.* **2018**, *19*, 189. [CrossRef]
41. Florian, M.C.; Klose, M.; Sacma, M.; Jablanovic, J.; Knudson, L.; Nattamai, K.J.; Marka, G.; Vollmer, A.; Soller, K.; Sakk, V.; et al. Aging alters the epigenetic asymmetry of HSC division. *PLoS Biol.* **2018**, *16*, e2003389. [CrossRef] [PubMed]
42. Nakamura-Ishizu, A.; Ito, K.; Suda, T. Hematopoietic Stem Cell Metabolism during Development and Aging. *Dev. Cell* **2020**, *54*, 239–255. [CrossRef] [PubMed]
43. Vilchez, D.; Simic, M.S.; Dillin, A. Proteostasis and aging of stem cells. *Trends. Cell Biol.* **2014**, *24*, 161–170. [CrossRef] [PubMed]
44. Chapple, R.H.; Hu, T.; Tseng, Y.J.; Liu, L.; Kitano, A.; Luu, V.; Hoegenauer, K.A.; Iwawaki, T.; Li, Q.; Nakada, D. ERα promotes murine hematopoietic regeneration through the Ire1α-mediated unfolded protein response. *Elife* **2018**, *7*, e31159. [CrossRef]
45. Moran-Crusio, K.; Reavie, L.B.; Aifantis, I. Regulation of hematopoietic stem cell fate by the ubiquitin proteasome system. *Trends Immunol.* **2012**, *33*, 357–363. [CrossRef]
46. Baker, D.J.; Childs, B.G.; Durik, M.; Wijers, M.E.; Sieben, C.J.; Zhong, J.; Saltness, R.A.; Jeganathan, K.B.; Verzosa, G.C.; Pezeshki, A.; et al. Naturally occurring p16(Ink4a)-positive cells shorten healthy lifespan. *Nature* **2016**, *530*, 184–189. [CrossRef]
47. Chang, J.; Wang, Y.; Shao, L.; Laberge, R.M.; Demaria, M.; Campisi, J.; Janakiraman, K.; Sharpless, N.E.; Ding, S.; Feng, W.; et al. Clearance of senescent cells by ABT263 rejuvenates aged hematopoietic stem cells in mice. *Nat. Med.* **2016**, *22*, 78–83. [CrossRef]
48. Quéré, R.; Saint-Paul, L.; Carmignac, V.; Martin, R.Z.; Chrétien, M.L.; Largeot, A.; Hammann, A.; Pais de Barros, J.P.; Bastie, J.N.; Delva, L. Tif1γ regulates the TGF-β1 receptor and promotes physiological aging of hematopoietic stem cells. *Proc. Natl. Acad. Sci. USA* **2014**, *111*, 10592–10597. [CrossRef]
49. Mastelaro de Rezende, M.; Zenker Justo, G.; Julian Paredes-Gamero, E.; Gosens, R. Wnt-5A/B Signaling in Hematopoiesis throughout Life. *Cells* **2020**, *9*, 1801. [CrossRef]
50. King, A.M.; Van der Put, E.; Blomberg, B.B.; Riley, R.L. Accelerated Notch-dependent degradation of E47 proteins in aged B cell precursors is associated with increased ERK MAPK activation. *J. Immunol.* **2007**, *178*, 3521–3529. [CrossRef]
51. Xiao, N.; Jani, K.; Morgan, K.; Okabe, R.; Cullen, D.E.; Jesneck, J.L.; Raffel, G.D. Hematopoietic stem cells lacking Ott1 display aspects associated with aging and are unable to maintain quiescence during proliferative stress. *Blood* **2012**, *119*, 4898–4907. [CrossRef] [PubMed]
52. Fistonich, C.; Zehentmeier, S.; Bednarski, J.J.; Miao, R.; Schjerven, H.; Sleckman, B.P.; Pereira, J.P. Cell circuits between B cell progenitors and IL-7+ mesenchymal progenitor cells control B cell development. *J. Exp. Med.* **2018**, *215*, 2586–2599. [CrossRef] [PubMed]
53. Gomariz, A.; Helbling, P.M.; Isringhausen, S.; Suessbier, U.; Becker, A.; Boss, A.; Nagasawa, T.; Paul, G.; Goksel, O.; Székely, G.; et al. Quantitative spatial analysis of haematopoiesis-regulating stromal cells in the bone marrow microenvironment by 3D microscopy. *Nat. Commun.* **2018**, *9*, 2532. [CrossRef] [PubMed]
54. Crane, G.M.; Jeffery, E.; Morrison, S.J. Adult haematopoietic stem cell niches. *Nat. Rev. Immunol.* **2017**, *17*, 573–590. [CrossRef]

55. Guidi, N.; Sacma, M.; Ständker, L.; Soller, K.; Marka, G.; Eiwen, K.; Weiss, J.M.; Kirchhoff, F.; Weil, T.; Cancelas, J.A.; et al. Osteopontin attenuates aging-associated phenotypes of hematopoietic stem cells. *EMBO J.* **2017**, *36*, 840–853. [CrossRef]
56. Kusumbe, A.P.; Ramasamy, S.K.; Itkin, T.; Mäe, M.A.; Langen, U.H.; Betsholtz, C.; Lapidot, T.; Adams, R.H. Age-dependent modulation of vascular niches for haematopoietic stem cells. *Nature* **2016**, *532*, 380–384. [CrossRef]
57. Schepers, K.; Campbell, T.B.; Passegué, E. Normal and leukemic stem cell niches: Insights and therapeutic opportunities. *Cell Stem Cell* **2015**, *16*, 254–267. [CrossRef]
58. Nishikawa, K.; Nakashima, T.; Takeda, S.; Isogai, M.; Hamada, M.; Kimura, A.; Kodama, T.; Yamaguchi, A.; Owen, M.J.; Takahashi, S.; et al. Maf promotes osteoblast differentiation in mice by mediating the age-related switch in mesenchymal cell differentiation. *J. Clin. Investig.* **2010**, *120*, 3455–3465. [CrossRef]
59. Singh, L.; Brennan, T.A.; Russell, E.; Kim, J.H.; Chen, Q.; Brad Johnson, F.; Pignolo, R.J. Aging alters bone-fat reciprocity by shifting in vivo mesenchymal precursor cell fate towards an adipogenic lineage. *Bone* **2016**, *85*, 29–36. [CrossRef]
60. Ho, Y.H.; Méndez-Ferrer, S. Microenvironmental contributions to hematopoietic stem cell aging. *Haematologica* **2020**, *105*, 38–46. [CrossRef]
61. Cakouros, D.; Gronthos, S. Epigenetic Regulation of Bone Marrow Stem Cell Aging: Revealing Epigenetic Signatures associated with Hematopoietic and Mesenchymal Stem Cell Aging. *Aging Dis.* **2019**, *10*, 174–189. [CrossRef] [PubMed]
62. Kunisaki, Y.; Bruns, I.; Scheiermann, C.; Ahmed, J.; Pinho, S.; Zhang, D.; Mizoguchi, T.; Wei, Q.; Lucas, D.; Ito, K.; et al. Arteriolar niches maintain haematopoietic stem cell quiescence. *Nature* **2013**, *502*, 637–643. [CrossRef] [PubMed]
63. Wei, Q.; Frenette, P.S. Niches for Hematopoietic Stem Cells and Their Progeny. *Immunity* **2018**, *48*, 632–648. [CrossRef] [PubMed]
64. Almeida, M.; Han, L.; Martin-Millan, M.; Plotkin, L.I.; Stewart, S.A.; Roberson, P.K.; Kousteni, S.; O'Brien, C.A.; Bellido, T.; Parfitt, A.M.; et al. Skeletal involution by age-associated oxidative stress and its acceleration by loss of sex steroids. *J. Biol. Chem.* **2007**, *282*, 27285–27297. [CrossRef]
65. Yokota, T.; Oritani, K.; Takahashi, I.; Ishikawa, J.; Matsuyama, A.; Ouchi, N.; Kihara, S.; Funahashi, T.; Tenner, A.J.; Tomiyama, Y.; et al. Adiponectin, a new member of the family of soluble defense collagens, negatively regulates the growth of myelomonocytic progenitors and the functions of macrophages. *Blood* **2000**, *96*, 1723–1732. [CrossRef]
66. Naveiras, O.; Nardi, V.; Wenzel, P.L.; Hauschka, P.V.; Fahey, F.; Daley, G.Q. Bone-marrow adipocytes as negative regulators of the haematopoietic microenvironment. *Nature* **2009**, *460*, 259–263. [CrossRef]
67. Zhu, R.J.; Wu, M.Q.; Li, Z.J.; Zhang, Y.; Liu, K.Y. Hematopoietic recovery following chemotherapy is improved by BADGE-induced inhibition of adipogenesis. *Int. J. Hematol.* **2013**, *97*, 58–72. [CrossRef]
68. Zhou, B.O.; Yu, H.; Yue, R.; Zhao, Z.; Rios, J.J.; Naveiras, O.; Morrison, S.J. Bone marrow adipocytes promote the regeneration of stem cells and haematopoiesis by secreting SCF. *Nat. Cell Biol.* **2017**, *19*, 891–903. [CrossRef]
69. Ambrosi, T.H.; Scialdone, A.; Graja, A.; Gohlke, S.; Jank, A.M.; Bocian, C.; Woelk, L.; Fan, H.; Logan, D.W.; Schürmann, A.; et al. Adipocyte Accumulation in the Bone Marrow during Obesity and Aging Impairs Stem Cell-Based Hematopoietic and Bone Regeneration. *Cell Stem Cell* **2017**, *20*, 771–784. [CrossRef]
70. Stucker, S.; Chen, J.; Watt, F.E.; Kusumbe, A.P. Bone Angiogenesis and Vascular Niche Remodeling in Stress, Aging, and Diseases. *Front. Cell Dev. Biol.* **2020**, *8*, 602269. [CrossRef]
71. Ramasamy, S.K. Structure and Functions of Blood Vessels and Vascular Niches in Bone. *Stem Cells Int.* **2017**, *2017*, 5046953. [CrossRef]
72. Poulos, M.G.; Ramalingam, P.; Gutkin, M.C.; Llanos, P.; Gilleran, K.; Rabbany, S.Y.; Butler, J.M. Endothelial transplantation rejuvenates aged hematopoietic stem cell function. *J. Clin. Investig.* **2017**, *127*, 4163–4178. [CrossRef] [PubMed]
73. Kusumbe, A.P.; Ramasamy, S.K.; Adams, R.H. Coupling of angiogenesis and osteogenesis by a specific vessel subtype in bone. *Nature* **2014**, *507*, 323–328. [CrossRef] [PubMed]
74. Spiegel, A.; Shivtiel, S.; Kalinkovich, A.; Ludin, A.; Netzer, N.; Goichberg, P.; Azaria, Y.; Resnick, I.; Hardan, I.; Ben-Hur, H.; et al. Catecholaminergic neurotransmitters regulate migration and repopulation of immature human CD34+ cells through Wnt signaling. *Nat. Immunol.* **2007**, *8*, 1123–1131. [CrossRef] [PubMed]
75. Kunisaki, Y.; Frenette, P.S. Influences of vascular niches on hematopoietic stem cell fate. *Int. J. Hematol.* **2014**, *99*, 699–705. [CrossRef] [PubMed]
76. Yamazaki, S.; Ema, H.; Karlsson, G.; Yamaguchi, T.; Miyoshi, H.; Shioda, S.; Taketo, M.M.; Karlsson, S.; Iwama, A.; Nakauchi, H. Nonmyelinating Schwann cells maintain hematopoietic stem cell hibernation in the bone marrow niche. *Cell* **2011**, *147*, 1146–1158. [CrossRef] [PubMed]
77. Méndez-Ferrer, S.; Michurina, T.V.; Ferraro, F.; Mazloom, A.R.; Macarthur, B.D.; Lira, S.A.; Scadden, D.T.; Ma'ayan, A.; Enikolopov, G.N.; Frenette, P.S. Mesenchymal and haematopoietic stem cells form a unique bone marrow niche. *Nature* **2010**, *466*, 829–834. [CrossRef] [PubMed]
78. Forte, D.; Krause, D.S.; Andreeff, M.; Bonnet, D.; Méndez-Ferrer, S. Updates on the hematologic tumor microenvironment and its therapeutic targeting. *Haematologica* **2019**, *104*, 1928–1934. [CrossRef]
79. Jiang, L.; Han, X.; Wang, J.; Wang, C.; Sun, X.; Xie, J.; Wu, G.; Phan, H.; Liu, Z.; Yeh, E.T.H.; et al. SHP-1 regulates hematopoietic stem cell quiescence by coordinating TGF-β signaling. *J. Exp. Med.* **2018**, *215*, 1337–1347. [CrossRef]
80. Nakamura-Ishizu, A.; Takubo, K.; Fujioka, M.; Suda, T. Megakaryocytes are essential for HSC quiescence through the production of thrombopoietin. *Biochem. Biophys. Res. Commun.* **2014**, *454*, 353–357. [CrossRef]

81. Bruns, I.; Lucas, D.; Pinho, S.; Ahmed, J.; Lambert, M.P.; Kunisaki, Y.; Scheiermann, C.; Schiff, L.; Poncz, M.; Bergman, A.; et al. Megakaryocytes regulate hematopoietic stem cell quiescence through CXCL4 secretion. *Nat. Med.* **2014**, *20*, 1315–1320. [CrossRef] [PubMed]
82. Zhao, M.; Perry, J.M.; Marshall, H.; Venkatraman, A.; Qian, P.; He, X.C.; Ahamed, J.; Li, L. Megakaryocytes maintain homeostatic quiescence and promote post-injury regeneration of hematopoietic stem cells. *Nat. Med.* **2014**, *20*, 1321–1326. [CrossRef] [PubMed]
83. Nakamura-Ishizu, A.; Takubo, K.; Kobayashi, H.; Suzuki-Inoue, K.; Suda, T. CLEC-2 in megakaryocytes is critical for maintenance of hematopoietic stem cells in the bone marrow. *J. Exp. Med.* **2015**, *212*, 2133–2146. [CrossRef] [PubMed]
84. Ergen, A.V.; Boles, N.C.; Goodell, M.A. Rantes/Ccl5 influences hematopoietic stem cell subtypes and causes myeloid skewing. *Blood* **2012**, *119*, 2500–2509. [CrossRef]
85. Pietras, E.M. Inflammation: A key regulator of hematopoietic stem cell fate in health and disease. *Blood* **2017**, *130*, 1693–1698. [CrossRef]
86. Gabay, C.; Kushner, I. Acute-phase proteins and other systemic responses to inflammation. *N. Engl. J. Med.* **1999**, *340*, 448–454. [CrossRef]
87. Pietras, E.M.; Mirantes-Barbeito, C.; Fong, S.; Loeffler, D.; Kovtonyuk, L.V.; Zhang, S.; Lakshminarasimhan, R.; Chin, C.P.; Techner, J.M.; Will, B.; et al. Chronic interleukin-1 exposure drives haematopoietic stem cells towards precocious myeloid differentiation at the expense of self-renewal. *Nat. Cell Biol.* **2016**, *18*, 607–618. [CrossRef]
88. Frisch, B.J.; Hoffman, C.M.; Latchney, S.E.; LaMere, M.W.; Myers, J.; Ashton, J.; Li, A.J.; Saunders, J., 2nd; Palis, J.; Perkins, A.S.; et al. Aged marrow macrophages expand platelet-biased hematopoietic stem cells via Interleukin1B. *JCI Insight* **2019**, *5*, e124213. [CrossRef]
89. Montecino-Rodriguez, E.; Kong, Y.; Casero, D.; Rouault, A.; Dorshkind, K.; Pioli, P.D. Lymphoid-Biased Hematopoietic Stem Cells Are Maintained with Age and Efficiently Generate Lymphoid Progeny. *Stem Cell Rep.* **2019**, *12*, 584–596. [CrossRef]
90. Mann, M.; Mehta, A.; de Boer, C.G.; Kowalczyk, M.S.; Lee, K.; Haldeman, P.; Rogel, N.; Knecht, A.R.; Farouq, D.; Regev, A.; et al. Heterogeneous Responses of Hematopoietic Stem Cells to Inflammatory Stimuli Are Altered with Age. *Cell Rep.* **2018**, *25*, 2992–3005. [CrossRef]
91. Sakamaki, S.; Hirayama, Y.; Matsunaga, T.; Kuroda, H.; Kusakabe, T.; Akiyama, T.; Konuma, Y.; Sasaki, K.; Tsuji, N.; Okamoto, T.; et al. Transforming growth factor-beta1 (TGF-beta1) induces thrombopoietin from bone marrow stromal cells, which stimulates the expression of TGF-beta receptor on megakaryocytes and, in turn, renders them susceptible to suppression by TGF-beta itself with high specificity. *Blood* **1999**, *94*, 1961–1970. [CrossRef] [PubMed]
92. Nagel, G.; Weber, D.; Fromm, E.; Erhardt, S.; Lübbert, M.; Fiedler, W.; Kindler, T.; Krauter, J.; Brossart, P.; Kündgen, A.; et al. Epidemiological, genetic, and clinical characterization by age of newly diagnosed acute myeloid leukemia based on an academic population-based registry study (AMLSG BiO). *Ann. Hematol.* **2017**, *96*, 1993–2003. [CrossRef] [PubMed]
93. Döhner, H.; Estey, E.; Grimwade, D.; Amadori, S.; Appelbaum, F.R.; Büchner, T.; Dombret, H.; Ebert, B.L.; Fenaux, P.; Larson, R.A.; et al. Diagnosis and management of AML in adults: 2017 ELN recommendations from an international expert panel. *Blood* **2017**, *129*, 424–447. [CrossRef]
94. Hernandez-Valladares, M.; Aasebø, E.; Berven, F.; Selheim, F.; Bruserud, Ø. Biological characteristics of aging in human acute myeloid leukemia cells: The possible importance of aldehyde dehydrogenase, the cytoskeleton and altered transcriptional regulation. *Aging* **2020**, *12*, 24734–24777. [CrossRef] [PubMed]
95. Cappellini, M.D.; Motta, I. Anemia in Clinical Practice-Definition and Classification: Does Hemoglobin Change With Aging? *Semin. Hematol.* **2015**, *52*, 261–269. [CrossRef]
96. Cappellini, M.D.; Beris, P. Anemia in Clinical Practice: Introduction. *Semin. Hematol.* **2015**, *52*, 259–260. [CrossRef]
97. Martinsson, A.; Andersson, C.; Andell, P.; Koul, S.; Engström, G.; Smith, J.G. Anemia in the general population: Prevalence, clinical correlates and prognostic impact. *Eur. J. Epidemiol.* **2014**, *29*, 489–498. [CrossRef]
98. Schop, A.; Stouten, K.; Riedl, J.A.; van Houten, R.J.; Leening, M.J.G.; van Rosmalen, J.; Bindels, P.J.E.; Levin, M.D. A new diagnostic work-up for defining anemia etiologies: A cohort study in patients ≥ 50 years in general practices. *BMC Fam. Pract.* **2020**, *21*, 167. [CrossRef]
99. Guralnik, J.M.; Eisenstaedt, R.S.; Ferrucci, L.; Klein, H.G.; Woodman, R.C. Prevalence of anemia in persons 65 years and older in the United States: Evidence for a high rate of unexplained anemia. *Blood* **2004**, *104*, 2263–2268. [CrossRef]
100. Westerlind, B.; Östgren, C.J.; Mölstad, S.; Midlöv, P. Prevalence and predictive importance of anemia in Swedish nursing home residents—A longitudinal study. *BMC Geriatr.* **2016**, *16*, 206. [CrossRef]
101. Gaskell, H.; Derry, S.; Andrew Moore, R.; McQuay, H.J. Prevalence of anaemia in older persons: Systematic review. *BMC Geriatr.* **2008**, *8*, 1. [CrossRef] [PubMed]
102. Price, E.A.; Mehra, R.; Holmes, T.H.; Schrier, S.L. Anemia in older persons: Etiology and evaluation. *Blood Cells Mol. Dis.* **2011**, *46*, 159–165. [CrossRef] [PubMed]
103. Woodman, R.; Ferrucci, L.; Guralnik, J. Anemia in older adults. *Curr. Opin. Hematol.* **2005**, *12*, 123–128. [CrossRef] [PubMed]
104. Cheungpasitporn, W.; Thongprayoon, C.; Chiasakul, T.; Korpaisarn, S.; Erickson, S.B. Renin-angiotensin system inhibitors linked to anemia: A systematic review and meta-analysis. *QJM* **2015**, *108*, 879–884. [CrossRef] [PubMed]
105. Ferrucci, L.; Guralnik, J.M.; Woodman, R.C.; Bandinelli, S.; Lauretani, F.; Corsi, A.M.; Chaves, P.H.; Ershler, W.B.; Longo, D.L. Proinflammatory state and circulating erythropoietin in persons with and without anemia. *Am. J. Med.* **2005**, *118*, 1288. [CrossRef] [PubMed]

106. Stauder, R.; Valent, P.; Theurl, I. Anemia at older age: Etiologies, clinical implications, and management. *Blood* **2018**, *131*, 505–514. [CrossRef]
107. Ferrucci, L.; Maggio, M.; Bandinelli, S.; Basaria, S.; Lauretani, F.; Ble, A.; Valenti, G.; Ershler, W.B.; Guralnik, J.M.; Longo, D.L. Low testosterone levels and the risk of anemia in older men and women. *Arch. Intern. Med.* **2006**, *166*, 1380–1388. [CrossRef]
108. Waalen, J.; von Löhneysen, K.; Lee, P.; Xu, X.; Friedman, J.S. Erythropoietin, GDF15, IL6, hepcidin and testosterone levels in a large cohort of elderly individuals with anaemia of known and unknown cause. *Eur. J. Haematol.* **2011**, *87*, 107–116. [CrossRef]
109. Monlezun, D.J.; Camargo, C.A., Jr.; Mullen, J.T.; Quraishi, S.A. Vitamin D Status and the Risk of Anemia in Community-Dwelling Adults: Results from the National Health and Nutrition Examination Survey 2001–2006. *Medicine* **2015**, *94*, e1799. [CrossRef]
110. Ershler, W.B.; Sheng, S.; McKelvey, J.; Artz, A.S.; Denduluri, N.; Tecson, J.; Taub, D.D.; Brant, L.J.; Ferrucci, L.; Longo, D.L. Serum erythropoietin and aging: A longitudinal analysis. *J. Am. Geriatr. Soc.* **2005**, *53*, 1360–1365. [CrossRef]
111. Beloosesky, Y.; Cohen, A.M.; Grosman, B.; Grinblat, J. Prevalence and survival of myelodysplastic syndrome of the refractory anemia type in hospitalized cognitively different geriatric patients. *Gerontology* **2000**, *46*, 323–327. [CrossRef] [PubMed]
112. Kwok, B.; Hall, J.M.; Witte, J.S.; Xu, Y.; Reddy, P.; Lin, K.; Flamholz, R.; Dabbas, B.; Yung, A.; Al-Hafidh, J.; et al. MDS-associated somatic mutations and clonal hematopoiesis are common in idiopathic cytopenias of undetermined significance. *Blood* **2015**, *126*, 2355–2361. [CrossRef] [PubMed]
113. Cargo, C.A.; Rowbotham, N.; Evans, P.A.; Barrans, S.L.; Bowen, D.T.; Crouch, S.; Jack, A.S. Targeted sequencing identifies patients with preclinical MDS at high risk of disease progression. *Blood* **2015**, *126*, 2362–2365. [CrossRef] [PubMed]
114. Steensma, D.P. New challenges in evaluating anaemia in older persons in the era of molecular testing. *Hematol. Am. Soc. Hematol. Educ. Program* **2016**, *2016*, 67–73. [CrossRef]
115. Schop, A.; Stouten, K.; van Houten, R.; Riedl, J.; van Rosmalen, J.; Bindels, P.J.; Levin, M.D. Diagnostics in anaemia of chronic disease in general practice: A real-world retrospective cohort study. *BJGP Open* **2018**, *2*, bjgpopen18X101597. [CrossRef]
116. Patel, K.V.; Longo, D.L.; Ershler, W.B.; Yu, B.; Semba, R.D.; Ferrucci, L.; Guralnik, J.M. Haemoglobin concentration and the risk of death in older adults: Differences by race/ethnicity in the NHANES III follow-up. *Br. J. Haematol.* **2009**, *145*, 514–523. [CrossRef]
117. Penninx, B.W.; Pahor, M.; Woodman, R.C.; Guralnik, J.M. Anemia in old age is associated with increased mortality and hospitalization. *J. Gerontol. A Biol. Sci. Med. Sci.* **2006**, *61*, 474–479. [CrossRef]
118. Shavelle, R.M.; MacKenzie, R.; Paculdo, D.R. Anemia and mortality in older persons: Does the type of anemia affect survival? *Int. J. Hematol.* **2012**, *95*, 248–256. [CrossRef]
119. Zakai, N.A.; French, B.; Arnold, A.M.; Newman, A.B.; Fried, L.F.; Robbins, J.; Chaves, P.; Cushman, M. Hemoglobin decline, function, and mortality in the elderly: The cardiovascular health study. *Am. J. Hematol.* **2013**, *88*, 5–9. [CrossRef]
120. den Elzen, W.P.; Willems, J.M.; Westendorp, R.G.; de Craen, A.J.; Assendelft, W.J.; Gussekloo, J. Effect of anemia and comorbidity on functional status and mortality in old age: Results from the Leiden 85-plus Study. *CMAJ* **2009**, *181*, 151–157. [CrossRef] [PubMed]
121. Chan, T.C.; Yap, D.Y.; Shea, Y.F.; Luk, J.K.; Chan, F.H.; Chu, L.W. Prevalence of anemia in Chinese nursing home older adults: Implication of age and renal impairment. *Geriatr. Gerontol. Int.* **2013**, *13*, 591–596. [CrossRef] [PubMed]
122. Resnick, B.; Sabol, V.; Galik, E.; Gruber-Baldini, A.L. The impact of anemia on nursing home residents. *Clin. Nurs. Res.* **2010**, *19*, 113–130. [CrossRef] [PubMed]
123. Abid, S.A.; Gravenstein, S.; Nanda, A. Anemia in the Long-Term Care Setting. *Clin. Geriatr. Med.* **2019**, *35*, 381–389. [CrossRef] [PubMed]
124. Pandya, N.; Bookhart, B.; Mody, S.H.; Funk Orsini, P.A.; Reardon, G. Study of anemia in long-term care (SALT): Prevalence of anemia and its relationship with the risk of falls in nursing home residents. *Curr. Med. Res. Opin.* **2008**, *24*, 2139–2149. [CrossRef] [PubMed]
125. Landi, F.; Russo, A.; Danese, P.; Liperoti, R.; Barillaro, C.; Bernabei, R.; Onder, G. Anemia status, hemoglobin concentration, and mortality in nursing home older residents. *J. Am. Med. Dir. Assoc.* **2007**, *8*, 322–327. [CrossRef] [PubMed]
126. Robinson, B.; Artz, A.S.; Culleton, B.; Critchlow, C.; Sciarra, A.; Audhya, P. Prevalence of anemia in the nursing home: Contribution of chronic kidney disease. *J. Am. Geriatr. Soc.* **2007**, *55*, 1566–1570. [CrossRef]
127. Lucca, U.; Tettamanti, M.; Mosconi, P.; Apolone, G.; Gandini, F.; Nobili, A.; Tallone, M.V.; Detoma, P.; Giacomin, A.; Clerico, M.; et al. Association of mild anemia with cognitive, functional, mood and quality of life outcomes in the elderly: The "Health and Anemia" study. *PLoS ONE* **2008**, *3*, e1920. [CrossRef]
128. Onder, G.; Penninx, B.W.; Cesari, M.; Bandinelli, S.; Lauretani, F.; Bartali, B.; Gori, A.M.; Pahor, M.; Ferrucci, L. Anemia is associated with depression in older adults: Results from the InCHIANTI study. *J. Gerontol. A Biol. Sci. Med. Sci.* **2005**, *60*, 1168–1172. [CrossRef]
129. Sabol, V.K.; Resnick, B.; Galik, E.; Ruber-Baldini, A.; Morton, P.G.; Hicks, G.E. Anemia and its impact on function in nursing home residents: What do we know? *J. Am. Acad. Nurse Pract.* **2010**, *22*, 3–16. [CrossRef]
130. Bailey, R.A.; Reardon, G.; Wasserman, M.R.; McKenzie, R.S.; Hord, R.S. Association of anemia with worsened activities of daily living and health-related quality of life scores derived from the Minimum Data Set in long-term care residents. *Health Qual Life Outcomes* **2012**, *10*, 129. [CrossRef]
131. Hopstock, L.A.; Utne, E.B.; Horsch, A.; Skjelbakken, T. The association between anemia and falls in community-living women and men aged 65 years and older from the fifth Tromsø Study 2001-02: A replication study. *BMC Geriatr.* **2017**, *17*, 292. [CrossRef] [PubMed]

132. Dharmarajan, T.S.; Avula, S.; Norkus, E.P. Anemia increases risk for falls in hospitalized older adults: An evaluation of falls in 362 hospitalized, ambulatory, long-term care, and community patients. *J. Am. Med. Dir. Assoc.* **2007**, *8*, e9–e15. [CrossRef] [PubMed]
133. Reardon, G.; Pandya, N.; Bailey, R.A. Falls in nursing home residents receiving pharmacotherapy for anemia. *Clin. Interv. Aging* **2012**, *7*, 397–407. [CrossRef] [PubMed]
134. Kojima, G. Frailty as a Predictor of Nursing Home Placement Among Community-Dwelling Older Adults: A Systematic Review and Meta-analysis. *J. Geriatr. Phys. Ther.* **2018**, *41*, 42–48. [CrossRef]
135. Veronese, N.; Cereda, E.; Solmi, M.; Fowler, S.A.; Manzato, E.; Maggi, S.; Manu, P.; Abe, E.; Hayashi, K.; Allard, J.P.; et al. Inverse relationship between body mass index and mortality in older nursing home residents: A meta-analysis of 19,538 elderly subjects. *Obes. Rev.* **2015**, *16*, 1001–1015. [CrossRef]
136. Doni, L.; Perin, A.; Manzione, L.; Gebbia, V.; Mattioli, R.; Speranza, G.B.; Latini, L.; Iop, A.; Bertetto, O.; Ferraù, F.; et al. The impact of anemia on quality of life and hospitalisation in elderly cancer patients undergoing chemotherapy. *Crit. Rev. Oncol. Hematol.* **2011**, *77*, 70–77. [CrossRef]
137. Li, Z.; Zhou, T.; Li, Y.; Chen, P.; Chen, L. Anemia increases the mortality risk in patients with stroke: A meta-analysis of cohort studies. *Sci. Rep.* **2016**, *6*, 26636. [CrossRef]
138. Sico, J.J.; Concato, J.; Wells, C.K.; Lo, A.C.; Nadeau, S.E.; Williams, L.S.; Peixoto, A.J.; Gorman, M.; Boice, J.L.; Bravata, D.M. Anemia is associated with poor outcomes in patients with less severe ischemic stroke. *J. Stroke Cerebrovasc. Dis.* **2013**, *22*, 271–278. [CrossRef]
139. Barlas, R.S.; Honney, K.; Loke, Y.K.; McCall, S.J.; Bettencourt-Silva, J.H.; Clark, A.B.; Bowles, K.M.; Metcalf, A.K.; Mamas, M.A.; Potter, J.F.; et al. Impact of Hemoglobin Levels and Anemia on Mortality in Acute Stroke: Analysis of UK Regional Registry Data, Systematic Review, and Meta-Analysis. *J. Am. Heart Assoc.* **2016**, *5*, e003019. [CrossRef]
140. Barlas, R.S.; McCall, S.J.; Bettencourt-Silva, J.H.; Clark, A.B.; Bowles, K.M.; Metcalf, A.K.; Mamas, M.A.; Potter, J.F.; Myint, P.K. Impact of anaemia on acute stroke outcomes depends on the type of anaemia: Evidence from a UK stroke register. *J. Neurol. Sci.* **2017**, *383*, 26–30. [CrossRef]
141. Tang, W.H.; Tong, W.; Jain, A.; Francis, G.S.; Harris, C.M.; Young, J.B. Evaluation and long-term prognosis of new-onset, transient, and persistent anemia in ambulatory patients with chronic heart failure. *J. Am. Coll Cardiol.* **2008**, *51*, 569–576. [CrossRef] [PubMed]
142. Groenveld, H.F.; Januzzi, J.L.; Damman, K.; van Wijngaarden, J.; Hillege, H.L.; van Veldhuisen, D.J.; van der Meer, P. Anemia and mortality in heart failure patients a systematic review and meta-analysis. *J. Am. Coll Cardiol.* **2008**, *52*, 818–827. [CrossRef] [PubMed]
143. He, S.W.; Wang, L.X. The impact of anemia on the prognosis of chronic heart failure: A meta-analysis and systemic review. *Congest Heart Fail.* **2009**, *15*, 123–130. [CrossRef] [PubMed]
144. Kosiborod, M.; Smith, G.L.; Radford, M.J.; Foody, J.M.; Krumholz, H.M. The prognostic importance of anemia in patients with heart failure. *Am. J. Med.* **2003**, *114*, 112–119. [CrossRef]
145. Arora, N.P.; Ghali, J.K. Anemia and iron deficiency in heart failure. *Heart Fail. Clin.* **2014**, *10*, 281–294. [CrossRef] [PubMed]
146. Klip, I.T.; Comin-Colet, J.; Voors, A.A.; Ponikowski, P.; Enjuanes, C.; Banasiak, W.; Lok, D.J.; Rosentryt, P.; Torrens, A.; Polonski, L.; et al. Iron deficiency in chronic heart failure: An international pooled analysis. *Am. Heart J.* **2013**, *165*, 575–582.e3. [CrossRef] [PubMed]
147. Ponikowski, P.; Kirwan, B.A.; Anker, S.D.; McDonagh, T.; Dorobantu, M.; Drozdz, J.; Fabien, V.; Filippatos, G.; Göhring, U.M.; Keren, A.; et al. Ferric carboxymaltose for iron deficiency at discharge after acute heart failure: A multicentre, double-blind, randomised, controlled trial. *Lancet* **2020**, *396*, 1895–1904. [CrossRef]
148. Anker, S.D.; Kirwan, B.A.; van Veldhuisen, D.J.; Filippatos, G.; Comin-Colet, J.; Ruschitzka, F.; Luscher, T.F.; Arutyunov, G.P.; Motro, M.; Mori, C.; et al. Effects of ferric carboxymaltose on hospitalisations and mortality rates in iron-deficient heart failure patients: An individual patient data meta-analysis. *Eur. J. Heart Fail.* **2018**, *20*, 125–133. [CrossRef]
149. Lewis, G.D.; Malhotra, R.; Hernandez, A.F.; McNulty, S.E.; Smith, A.; Felker, G.M.; Tang, W.H.W.; LaRue, S.J.; Redfield, M.M.; Semigran, M.J.; et al. Effect of Oral Iron Repletion on Exercise Capacity in Patients with Heart Failure with Reduced Ejection Fraction and Iron Deficiency: The IRONOUT HF Randomized Clinical Trial. *JAMA* **2017**, *317*, 1958–1966. [CrossRef]
150. van der Wal, H.H.; Comin-Colet, J.; Klip, I.T.; Enjuanes, C.; Grote Beverborg, N.; Voors, A.A.; Banasiak, W.; van Veldhuisen, D.J.; Bruguera, J.; Ponikowski, P.; et al. Vitamin B12 and folate deficiency in chronic heart failure. *Heart* **2015**, *101*, 302–310. [CrossRef]
151. Anand, S.; Burkenroad, A.; Glaspy, J. Workup of anemia in cancer. *Clin. Adv. Hematol. Oncol.* **2020**, *18*, 640–646. [PubMed]
152. Gilreath, J.A.; Stenehjem, D.D.; Rodgers, G.M. Diagnosis and treatment of cancer-related anemia. *Am. J. Hematol.* **2014**, *89*, 203–212. [CrossRef] [PubMed]
153. Han, S.V.; Park, M.; Kwon, Y.M.; Yoon, H.J.; Chang, Y.; Kim, H.; Lim, Y.H.; Kim, S.G.; Ko, A. Mild Anemia and Risk for All-Cause, Cardiovascular and Cancer Deaths in Apparently Healthy Elderly Koreans. *Korean J. Fam. Med.* **2019**, *40*, 151–158. [CrossRef] [PubMed]
154. Wouters, H.J.C.M.; van der Klauw, M.M.; de Witte, T.; Stauder, R.; Swinkels, D.W.; Wolffenbuttel, B.H.R.; Huls, G. Association of anemia with health-related quality of life and survival: A large population-based cohort study. *Haematologica* **2019**, *104*, 468–476. [CrossRef] [PubMed]
155. Girelli, D.; Marchi, G.; Camaschella, C. Anemia in the Elderly. *Hemasphere* **2018**, *2*, e40. [CrossRef]

156. Goddard, A.F.; James, M.W.; McIntyre, A.S.; Scott, B.B.; British Society of Gastroenterology. Guidelines for the management of iron deficiency anaemia. *Gut* **2011**, *60*, 1309–1316. [CrossRef]
157. Nahon, S.; Lahmek, P.; Barclay, F.; Macaigne, G.; Poupardin, C.; Jounnaud, V.; Delas, N.; Lesgourgues, B. Long-term follow-up and predictive factors of recurrence of anemia in a cohort of 102 very elderly patients explored for iron-deficiency anemia. *J. Clin. Gastroenterol.* **2008**, *42*, 984–990. [CrossRef]
158. Nahon, S.; Lahmek, P.; Aras, N.; Poupardin, C.; Lesgourgues, B.; Macaigne, G.; Delas, N. Management and predictors of early mortality in elderly patients with iron deficiency anemia: A prospective study of 111 patients. *Gastroenterol. Clin. Biol.* **2007**, *31*, 169–174. [CrossRef]
159. Dicato, M.; Plawny, L.; Diederich, M. Anemia in cancer. *Ann. Oncol.* **2010**, *21*, vii167–vii172. [CrossRef]
160. Endres, H.G.; Wedding, U.; Pittrow, D.; Thiem, U.; Trampisch, H.J.; Diehm, C. Prevalence of anemia in elderly patients in primary care: Impact on 5-year mortality risk and differences between men and women. *Curr. Med. Res. Opin.* **2009**, *25*, 1143–1158. [CrossRef]
161. Lee, J.; Chin, J.H.; Kim, J.I.; Lee, E.H.; Choi, I.C. Association between red blood cell transfusion and long-term mortality in patients with cancer of the esophagus after esophagectomy. *Dis. Esophagus.* **2018**, *31*, 1–8. [CrossRef] [PubMed]
162. Zhang, Y.; Chen, Y.; Chen, D.; Jiang, Y.; Huang, W.; Ouyang, H.; Xing, W.; Zeng, M.; Xie, X.; Zeng, W. Impact of preoperative anemia on relapse and survival in breast cancer patients. *BMC Cancer* **2014**, *14*, 844. [CrossRef] [PubMed]
163. Gilreath, J.A.; Rodgers, G.M. How I treat cancer-associated anemia. *Blood* **2020**, *136*, 801–813. [CrossRef] [PubMed]
164. Fowler, A.J.; Ahmad, T.; Phull, M.K.; Allard, S.; Gillies, M.A.; Pearse, R.M. Meta-analysis of the association between preoperative anaemia and mortality after surgery. *Br. J. Surg.* **2015**, *102*, 1314–1324. [CrossRef] [PubMed]
165. Gupta, P.K.; Sundaram, A.; Mactaggart, J.N.; Johanning, J.M.; Gupta, H.; Fang, X.; Forse, R.A.; Balters, M.; Longo, G.M.; Sugimoto, J.T.; et al. Preoperative anemia is an independent predictor of postoperative mortality and adverse cardiac events in elderly patients undergoing elective vascular operations. *Ann. Surg.* **2013**, *258*, 1096–1102. [CrossRef] [PubMed]
166. Wu, W.C.; Schifftner, T.L.; Henderson, W.G.; Eaton, C.B.; Poses, R.M.; Uttley, G.; Sharma, S.C.; Vezeridis, M.; Khuri, S.F.; Friedmann, P.D. Preoperative hematocrit levels and postoperative outcomes in older patients undergoing noncardiac surgery. *JAMA* **2007**, *297*, 2481–2488. [CrossRef] [PubMed]
167. Ryan, G.; Nowak, L.; Melo, L.; Ward, S.; Atrey, A.; Schemitsch, E.H.; Nauth, A.; Khoshbin, A. Anemia at Presentation Predicts Acute Mortality and Need for Readmission Following Geriatric Hip Fracture. *JB JS Open Access* **2020**, *5*, e20:00048. [CrossRef]
168. Dubljanin-Raspopović, E.; Marković-Denić, L.; Nikolić, D.; Tulic, G.; Kadija, M.; Bumbasirevic, M. Is Anemia at admission related to short-term outcomes of elderly hip fracture patients? *Cent. Eur. J. Med.* **2011**, *6*, 483–489. [CrossRef]
169. Bruserud, Ø.; Aarstad, H.H.; Tvedt, T.H.A. Combined C-Reactive Protein and Novel Inflammatory Parameters as a Predictor in Cancer-What Can We Learn from the Hematological Experience? *Cancers* **2020**, *12*, 1966. [CrossRef]
170. Sproston, N.R.; Ashworth, J.J. Role of C-Reactive Protein at Sites of Inflammation and Infection. *Front. Immunol.* **2018**, *9*, 754. [CrossRef]
171. Boncler, M.; Wu, Y.; Watala, C. The multiple faces of C-Reactive Protein-Physiological and pathophysiological implications in cardiovascular disease. *Molecules* **2019**, *24*, 2062. [CrossRef] [PubMed]
172. Yao, Z.; Zhang, Y.; Wu, H. Regulation of C-reactive protein conformation in inflammation. *Inflamm. Res.* **2019**, *68*, 815–823. [CrossRef] [PubMed]
173. Wu, Y.; Potempa, L.A.; El Kebir, D.; Filep, J.G. C-reactive protein and inflammationEvenn: Conformational changes affect function. *Biol. Chem.* **2015**, *396*, 1181–1197. [CrossRef] [PubMed]
174. Wang, H.W.; Wu, Y.; Chen, Y.; Sui, S.F. Polymorphism of structural forms of C-reactive protein. *Int. J. Mol. Med.* **2002**, *9*, 665–671. [CrossRef]
175. Li, Q.; Xu, W.; Xue, X.; Wang, Q.; Han, L.; Li, W.; Lv, S.; Liu, D.; Richards, J.; Shen, Z.; et al. Presence of multimeric isoforms of human C-reactive protein in tissues and blood. *Mol. Med. Rep.* **2016**, *14*, 5461–5466. [CrossRef]
176. Okemefuna, A.I.; Stach, L.; Rana, S.; Buetas, A.J.; Gor, J.; Perkins, S.J. C-reactive protein exists in an NaCl concentration-dependent pentamer-decamer equilibrium in physiological buffer. *J. Biol. Chem.* **2010**, *285*, 1041–1052. [CrossRef]
177. El Kebir, D.; Zhang, Y.; Potempa, L.A.; Wu, Y.; Fournier, A.; Filep, J.G. C-reactive protein-derived peptide 201-206 inhibits neutrophil adhesion to endothelial cells and platelets through CD32. *J. Leukoc. Biol.* **2011**, *90*, 1167–1175. [CrossRef]
178. Van Vré, E.A.; Bult, H.; Hoymans, V.Y.; Van Tendeloo, V.F.; Vrints, C.J.; Bosmans, J.M. Human C-reactive protein activates monocyte-derived dendritic cells and induces dendritic cell-mediated T-cell activation. *Arterioscler. Thromb. Vasc. Biol.* **2008**, *28*, 511–518. [CrossRef]
179. Jimenez, R.V.; Wright, T.T.; Jones, N.R.; Wu, J.; Gibson, A.W.; Szalai, A.J. C-Reactive protein impairs dendritic cell development, maturation, and function: Implications for peripheral tolerance. *Front. Immunol.* **2018**, *9*, 372. [CrossRef]
180. He, W.; Ren, Y.; Wang, X.; Chen, Q.; Ding, S. C reactive protein and enzymatically modified LDL cooperatively promote dendritic cell-mediated T cell activation. *Cardiovasc. Pathol.* **2017**, *29*, 1–6. [CrossRef]
181. Bach, M.; Moon, J.; Moore, R.; Pan, T.; Nelson, J.L.; Lood, C. A Neutrophil Activation Biomarker Panel in Prognosis and Monitoring of Patients with Rheumatoid Arthritis. *Arthritis Rheumatol.* **2020**, *72*, 47–56. [CrossRef] [PubMed]
182. Grabowska, W.; Sikora, E.; Bielak-Zmijewska, A. Sirtuins, a promising target in slowing down the ageing process. *Biogerontology* **2017**, *18*, 447–476. [CrossRef] [PubMed]

183. Perner, F.; Perner, C.; Ernst, T.; Heidel, F.H. Roles of JAK2 in Aging, Inflammation, Hematopoiesis and Malignant Transformation. *Cells* **2019**, *8*, 854. [CrossRef] [PubMed]
184. Kovtonyuk, L.V.; Fritsch, K.; Feng, X.; Manz, M.G.; Takizawa, H. Inflamm-Aging of Hematopoiesis, Hematopoietic Stem Cells, and the Bone Marrow Microenvironment. *Front. Immunol.* **2016**, *7*, 502. [CrossRef]
185. Franceschi, C.; Garagnani, P.; Parini, P.; Giuliani, C.; Santoro, A. Inflammaging: A new immune-metabolic viewpoint for age-related diseases. *Nat. Rev. Endocrinol.* **2018**, *14*, 576–590. [CrossRef]
186. Müller, L.; Di Benedetto, S.; Pawelec, G. The Immune System and Its Dysregulation with Aging. *Subcell. Biochem.* **2019**, *91*, 21–43.
187. Fülöp, T.; Larbi, A.; Witkowski, J.M. Human Inflammaging. *Gerontology* **2019**, *65*, 495–504. [CrossRef]
188. Cook, E.K.; Luo, M.; Rauh, M.J. Clonal hematopoiesis and inflammation: Partners in leukemogenesis and comorbidity. *Exp. Hematol.* **2020**, *83*, 85–94. [CrossRef]
189. Tvedt, T.H.A.; Melve, G.K.; Tsykunova, G.; Ahmed, A.B.; Brenner, A.K.; Bruserud, Ø. Immunological Heterogeneity of Healthy Peripheral Blood Stem Cell Donors-Effects of Granulocyte Colony-Stimulating Factor on Inflammatory Responses. *Int. J. Mol. Sci.* **2018**, *19*, 2886. [CrossRef]
190. Takizawa, H.; Manz, M.G. Impact of inflammation on early hematopoiesis and the microenvironment. *Int. J. Hematol.* **2017**, *106*, 27–33. [CrossRef]
191. Ren, G.; Zhang, L.; Zhao, X.; Xu, G.; Zhang, Y.; Roberts, A.I.; Zhao, R.C.; Shi, Y. Mesenchymal stem cell-mediated immunosuppression occurs via concerted action of chemokines and nitric oxide. *Cell Stem Cell* **2008**, *2*, 141–150. [CrossRef] [PubMed]
192. Wang, J.; Sun, Q.; Morita, Y.; Jiang, H.; Gross, A.; Lechel, A.; Hildner, K.; Guachalla, L.M.; Gompf, A.; Hartmann, D.; et al. A differentiation checkpoint limits hematopoietic stem cell self-renewal in response to DNA damage. *Cell* **2012**, *148*, 1001–1014. [CrossRef] [PubMed]
193. Shi, C.; Jia, T.; Mendez-Ferrer, S.; Hohl, T.M.; Serbina, N.V.; Lipuma, L.; Leiner, I.; Li, M.O.; Frenette, P.S.; Pamer, E.G. Bone marrow mesenchymal stem and progenitor cells induce monocyte emigration in response to circulating toll-like receptor ligands. *Immunity* **2011**, *34*, 590–601. [CrossRef] [PubMed]
194. Luu, N.T.; McGettrick, H.M.; Buckley, C.D.; Newsome, P.N.; Rainger, G.E.; Frampton, J.; Nash, G.B. Crosstalk between mesenchymal stem cells and endothelial cells leads to downregulation of cytokine-induced leukocyte recruitment. *Stem Cells* **2013**, *31*, 2690–2702.
195. Fernandez, L.; Rodriguez, S.; Huang, H.; Chora, A.; Fernandes, J.; Mumaw, C.; Cruz, E.; Pollok, K.; Cristina, F.; Price, J.E.; et al. Tumor necrosis factor-alpha and endothelial cells modulate Notch signaling in the bone marrow microenvironment during inflammation. *Exp. Hematol.* **2008**, *36*, 545–558. [CrossRef]
196. Boettcher, S.; Gerosa, R.C.; Radpour, R.; Bauer, J.; Ampenberger, F.; Heikenwalder, M.; Kopf, M.; Manz, M.G. Endothelial cells translate pathogen signals into G-CSF-driven emergency granulopoiesis. *Blood* **2014**, *124*, 1393–1403. [CrossRef]
197. Lu, Z.; Li, Y.; Jin, J.; Zhang, X.; Lopes-Virella, M.F.; Huang, Y. Toll-like receptor 4 activation in microvascular endothelial cells triggers a robust inflammatory response and cross talk with mononuclear cells via interleukin-6. *Arterioscler. Thromb. Vasc. Biol.* **2012**, *32*, 1696–1706. [CrossRef]
198. Tracy, R.P.; Lemaitre, R.N.; Psaty, B.M.; Ives, D.G.; Evans, R.W.; Cushman, M.; Meilahn, E.N.; Kuller, L.H. Relationship of C-reactive protein to risk of cardiovascular disease in the elderly. Results from the Cardiovascular Health Study and the Rural Health Promotion Project. *Arterioscler. Thromb. Vasc. Biol.* **1997**, *17*, 1121–1127. [CrossRef]
199. Cesari, M.; Penninx, B.W.; Newman, A.B.; Kritchevsky, S.B.; Nicklas, B.J.; Sutton-Tyrrell, K.; Tracy, R.P.; Rubin, S.M.; Harris, T.B.; Pahor, M. Inflammatory markers and cardiovascular disease (The Health, Aging and Body Composition [Health ABC] Study). *Am. J. Cardiol.* **2003**, *92*, 522–528. [CrossRef]
200. Cesari, M.; Penninx, B.W.; Newman, A.B.; Kritchevsky, S.B.; Nicklas, B.J.; Sutton-Tyrrell, K.; Rubin, S.M.; Ding, J.; Simonsick, E.M.; Harris, T.B.; et al. Inflammatory markers and onset of cardiovascular events: Results from the Health ABC study. *Circulation* **2003**, *108*, 2317–2322. [CrossRef]
201. Makita, S.; Nakamura, M.; Hiramori, K. The association of C-reactive protein levels with carotid intima-media complex thickness and plaque formation in the general population. *Stroke* **2005**, *36*, 2138–2142. [CrossRef]
202. Hosford-Donovan, A.; Nilsson, A.; Wåhlin-Larsson, B.; Kadi, F. Observational and mechanistic links between C-reactive protein and blood pressure in elderly women. *Maturitas* **2016**, *89*, 52–57. [CrossRef] [PubMed]
203. Labonté, M.E.; Dewailly, E.; Chateau-Degat, M.L.; Couture, P.; Lamarche, B. Population-based study of high plasma C-reactive protein concentrations among the Inuit of Nunavik. *Int. J. Circumpolar. Health* **2012**, *71*, 1–9. [CrossRef] [PubMed]
204. Kritchevsky, S.B.; Cesari, M.; Pahor, M. Inflammatory markers and cardiovascular health in older adults. *Cardiovasc. Res.* **2005**, *66*, 265–275. [CrossRef]
205. Nadrowski, P.; Chudek, J.; Skrzypek, M.; Puzianowska-Kuźnicka, M.; Mossakowska, M.; Więcek, A.; Zdrojewski, T.; Grodzicki, T.; Kozakiewicz, K. Associations between cardiovascular disease risk factors and IL-6 and hsCRP levels in the elderly. *Exp. Gerontol.* **2016**, *85*, 112–117. [CrossRef] [PubMed]
206. Shivappa, N.; Wirth, M.D.; Hurley, T.G.; Hébert, J.R. Association between the dietary inflammatory index (DII) and telomere length and C-reactive protein from the National Health and Nutrition Examination Survey-1999–2002. *Mol. Nutr. Food Res.* **2017**, *61*. [CrossRef] [PubMed]

207. Varadhan, R.; Yao, W.; Matteini, A.; Beamer, B.A.; Xue, Q.L.; Yang, H.; Manwani, B.; Reiner, A.; Jenny, N.; Parekh, N.; et al. Simple biologically informed inflammatory index of two serum cytokines predicts 10 year all-cause mortality in older adults. *J. Gerontol. A Biol. Sci. Med. Sci.* **2014**, *69*, 165–173. [CrossRef]
208. McCabe, E.L.; Larson, M.G.; Lunetta, K.L.; Newman, A.B.; Cheng, S.; Murabito, J.M. Association of an Index of Healthy Aging With Incident Cardiovascular Disease and Mortality in a Community-Based Sample of Older Adults. *J. Gerontol. A Biol. Sci. Med. Sci.* **2016**, *71*, 1695–1701. [CrossRef]
209. Hamann, L.; Bustami, J.; Iakoubov, L.; Szwed, M.; Mossakowska, M.; Schumann, R.R.; Puzianowska-Kuznicka, M. TLR-6 SNP P249S is associated with healthy aging in nonsmoking Eastern European Caucasians—A cohort study. *Immun. Ageing* **2016**, *17*, 13:7. [CrossRef]
210. Tang, Y.; Fung, E.; Xu, A.; Lan, H.Y. C-reactive protein and ageing. *Clin. Exp. Pharmacol. Physiol.* **2017**, *44*, 9–14. [CrossRef]
211. Kupelian, V.; Chiu, G.R.; Araujo, A.B.; Williams, R.E.; Clark, R.V.; McKinlay, J.B. Association of sex hormones and C-reactive protein levels in men. *Clin. Endocrinol.* **2010**, *72*, 527–533. [CrossRef] [PubMed]
212. Zacho, J.; Tybjaerg-Hansen, A.; Nordestgaard, B.G. C-reactive protein and all-cause mortality—the Copenhagen City Heart Study. *Eur. Heart J.* **2010**, *31*, 1624–1632. [CrossRef] [PubMed]
213. Barron, E.; Lara, J.; White, M.; Mathers, J.C. Blood-borne biomarkers of mortality risk: Systematic review of cohort studies. *PLoS ONE* **2015**, *10*, e0127550. [CrossRef] [PubMed]
214. Abel, G.A.; Klepin, H.D. Frailty and the management of hematologic malignancies. *Blood* **2018**, *131*, 515–524. [CrossRef] [PubMed]
215. Gadalla, S.M.; Wang, T.; Dagnall, C.; Haagenson, M.; Spellman, S.R.; Hicks, B.; Jones, K.; Katki, H.A.; Lee, S.J.; Savage, S.A. Effect of Recipient Age and Stem Cell Source on the Association between Donor Telomere Length and Survival after Allogeneic Unrelated Hematopoietic Cell Transplantation for Severe Aplastic Anemia. *Biol. Blood Marrow. Transplant.* **2016**, *22*, 2276–2282. [CrossRef]
216. Spólnicka, M.; Piekarska, R.Z.; Jaskuła, E.; Basak, G.W.; Jacewicz, R.; Pięta, A.; Makowska, Ż.; Jedrzejczyk, M.; Wierzbowska, A.; Pluta, A.; et al. Donor age and C1orf132/MIR29B2C determine age-related methylation signature of blood after allogeneic hematopoietic stem cell transplantation. *Clin. Epigenetics* **2016**, *8*, 93. [CrossRef]
217. Fabre, C.; Koscielny, S.; Mohty, M.; Fegueux, N.; Blaise, D.; Maillard, N.; Tabrizi, R.; Michallet, M.; Socié, G.; Yakoub-Agha, I.; et al. Younger donor's age and upfront tandem are two independent prognostic factors for survival in multiple myeloma patients treated by tandem autologous-allogeneic stem cell transplantation: A retrospective study from the Société Française de Greffe de Moelle et de Thérapie Cellulaire (SFGM-TC). *Haematologica* **2012**, *97*, 482–490.
218. Lazarevic, V.L. Acute myeloid leukaemia in patients we judge as being older and/or unfit. *J. Intern. Med.* **2021**. Epub ahead of print. [CrossRef]
219. Magliano, G.; Bacigalupo, A. Allogeneic Hematopoietic Stem Cell Transplantation for Acute Myeloid Leukemia of the Elderly: Review of Literature and New Perspectives. *Mediterr. J. Hematol. Infect. Dis.* **2020**, *1*, e2020081. [CrossRef]
220. Leufven, E.; Bruserud, Ø. Immunosuppression and Immunotargeted Therapy in Acute Myeloid Leukemia—The Potential Use of Checkpoint Inhibitors in Combination with Other Treatments. *Curr. Med. Chem.* **2019**, *26*, 5244–5261. [CrossRef]
221. Chittezhath, M.; Dhillon, M.K.; Lim, J.Y.; Laoui, D.; Shalova, I.N.; Teo, Y.L.; Chen, J.; Kamaraj, R.; Raman, L.; Lum, J.; et al. Molecular profiling reveals a tumor-promoting phenotype of monocytes and macrophages in human cancer progression. *Immunity* **2014**, *41*, 815–829. [CrossRef] [PubMed]
222. Aarstad, H.H.; Moe, S.E.E.; Bruserud, Ø.; Lybak, S.; Aarstad, H.J.; Tvedt, T.H.A. The Acute Phase Reaction and Its Prognostic Impact in Patients with Head and Neck Squamous Cell Carcinoma: Single Biomarkers Including C-Reactive Protein Versus Biomarker Profiles. *Biomedicines* **2020**, *8*, 418. [CrossRef] [PubMed]
223. Aarstad, H.H.; Guðbrandsdottir, G.; Hjelle, K.M.; Bostad, L.; Bruserud, Ø.; Tvedt, T.H.A.; Beisland, C. The Biological Context of C-Reactive Protein as a Prognostic Marker in Renal Cell Carcinoma: Studies on the Acute Phase Cytokine Profile. *Cancers* **2020**, *12*, 1961. [CrossRef] [PubMed]
224. Kip, M.M.; Schop, A.; Stouten, K.; Dekker, S.; Dinant, G.J.; Koffijberg, H.; Bindels, P.J.; IJzerman, M.J.; Levin, M.D.; Kusters, R. Assessing the cost-effectiveness of a routine versus an extensive laboratory work-up in the diagnosis of anaemia in Dutch general practice. *Ann. Clin. Biochem.* **2018**, *55*, 630–638. [CrossRef]

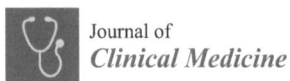

Review

Effectiveness of Interventions to Improve the Anticholinergic Prescribing Practice in Older Adults: A Systematic Review

Mohammed S. Salahudeen [1,*], Adel Alfahmi [1,2], Anam Farooq [3], Mehnaz Akhtar [4], Sana Ajaz [4], Saud Alotaibi [5], Manal Faiz [6] and Sheraz Ali [1]

1. School of Pharmacy and Pharmacology, University of Tasmania, Hobart 7001, Australia; adel.alfahmi@utas.edu.au (A.A.); sheraz.ali@utas.edu.au (S.A.)
2. Department of Pharmacy, East Jeddah General Hospital, Ministry of Health, Jeddah 22253, Saudi Arabia
3. Pharmaceutical Care Department, Dr Sulaiman Al-Habib Hospital, Riyadh 12214, Saudi Arabia; anamfarooq91@gmail.com
4. Shifa College of Pharmaceutical Sciences, Shifa Tmaeer-e-Millat University, Islamabad 44000, Pakistan; mehnaz.akhtar70@gmail.com (M.A.); sanaajaz.edu@gmail.com (S.A.)
5. Pharmaceutical Care Services, King Saud Medical City, Ministry of Health, Riyadh 12746, Saudi Arabia; saud_2007_sa@hotmail.com
6. Azra Naheed Medical College, Superior University, Lahore 55150, Pakistan; manalfaiz47@gmail.com
* Correspondence: mohammed.salahudeen@utas.edu.au

Abstract: Background: Pharmacotherapy in older adults is one of the most challenging aspects of patient care. Older people are prone to drug-related problems such as adverse effects, ineffectiveness, underdosage, overdosage, and drug interactions. Anticholinergic medications are associated with poor outcomes in older patients, and there is no specific intervention strategy for reducing drug burden from anticholinergic activity medications. Little is known about the effectiveness of current interventions that may likely improve the anticholinergic prescribing practice in older adults. Aims: This review seeks to document all types of interventions aiming to reduce anticholinergic prescribing among older adults and assess the current evidence and quality of existing single and combined interventions. Methods: We systematically searched MEDLINE, Embase, Cochrane Central Register of Controlled Trials, CINAHL, and PsycINFO from January 1990 to August 2021. Only studies that examined the effect of interventions in older people focused on improving compliance with anticholinergic prescribing guidelines with quantifiable data were included. The primary outcome of interest was to find the effectiveness of interventions that enhance the anticholinergic prescribing practice in older adults. Results: We screened 3168 records and ended up in 23 studies that met the inclusion criteria. We found only single-component interventions to reduce anticholinergic prescribing errors in older people. Pharmacists implemented interventions without collaboration in nearly half of the studies ($n = 11$). Medication review (43%) and education provision (26%) to healthcare practitioners were the most common interventions. Sixteen studies (70%) reported significant reductions in anticholinergic prescribing errors, whereas seven studies (30%) showed no significant effect. Conclusion: This systematic review suggests that healthcare practitioner-oriented interventions have the potential to reduce the occurrence of anticholinergic prescribing errors in older people. Interventions were primarily effective in reducing the burden of anticholinergic medications and assisting with deprescribing anticholinergic medications in older adults.

Keywords: anticholinergics; intervention; prescribing; older people

1. Introduction

Prescribing medications among older adults is recognised as a challenging task and an essential practice that needs to be continuously monitored, assessed, and refined accordingly. Moreover, it is based on understanding clinical pharmacology principles, knowledge about medicines, and particularly the experience and empirical knowledge of the prescribers [1,2]. Clinicians face several challenges while prescribing medications among older adults, and the prescribing of potentially inappropriate medications (PIMs) for this age group is prevalent [3]. The available epidemiological data show that up to 20% of older patients in outpatient settings and 59% of hospitalised older patients consume at least one PIM [4–8]. Adverse effects in older people due to inappropriate prescribing are prevalent, leading to increased hospital admissions and mortality [9].

Medications that possess anticholinergic activity are a class of PIMs widely prescribed for various clinical conditions in older adults [10,11]. Older people are particularly vulnerable to the adverse effects from medicines with anticholinergic-type effects [12,13]. Most medications commonly prescribed to older people are not routinely recognised as having anticholinergic activity, and empirically, clinicians prescribe these medicines based on their anticipated therapeutic benefits while overlooking the risk of cumulative anticholinergic burden [14–16]. Anticholinergic burden refers to the cumulative effect of taking multiple medications with anticholinergic activity [17,18]. There is no gold standard approach available to quantify and determine whether an acceptable range of anticholinergic drug burden exists in older adults [19,20]. The central adverse effects of anticholinergic medications are attributed to the excess blocking of cholinergic receptors within the central nervous system (CNS) [16]. The commonly reported central adverse effects are cognitive impairment, headache, reduced cognitive function, anxiety, and behavioural disturbances [16]. The common peripheral adverse effects of anticholinergic medications are hyperthermia, reduced saliva and tear production, urinary retention, constipation, and tachycardia [16].

Anticholinergic medications are associated with poor outcomes in older patients, but there is no specific intervention strategy for reducing anticholinergic drug exposure [21]. There is little evidence that medication review could be a promising strategy in reducing the drug burden in older people [22,23]. Medical practitioner-led and pharmacist-led medication reviews have earlier been reported as a standard practice for reducing anticholinergic drug exposure [24,25]. Pharmacist-led medication review has recently been found to be ineffective among older patients of the Northern Netherlands [25]. A few meta-analyses have also reported the lack of effectiveness of different types of medication reviews on mortality and hospitalisation outcomes [26–28]. Multidisciplinary strategies such as patient-centred, pharmacist–physician intervention are also recognised as promising for improving medication use in older patients at risk [29]. Another intervention strategy, i.e., the SÄKLÄK project, had some effects on the PIMs prescription and reduced potential medication-related problems [30]. The SÄKLÄK project is a multi-professional intervention model to improve medication use in older people [30], and it consists of self-assessment using a questionnaire, peer-reviewed by experienced healthcare professionals, feedback report provided by experienced healthcare professionals, and an improvement plan [30].

Interventions to improve prescribing practice more generally have been the subject of many studies and are frequently targeted according to the type of error [31,32]. It is crucial to explore which interventions have effectively changed prescribing practices and optimised patient outcomes while minimising healthcare costs. However, little is known about the effectiveness of existing interventions at improving the anticholinergic prescribing practice for older adults. Hence, this review seeks to document all types of interventions aiming to reduce anticholinergic prescribing errors among older adults and assess the evidence of existing single and combined interventions.

2. Methods

The Preferred Reporting Items for Systematic Reviews and Meta-Analyses (PRISMA) guideline was applied to report the findings of this systematic review [33].

2.1. Data Sources and Search Strategy

The following databases were examined between January 1990 and August 2021: Ovid MEDLINE, Ovid EMBASE, Ovid PsycINFO, and the Cochrane Central Register of

Controlled Trials (CENTRAL). A comprehensive electronic search was performed using appropriate keywords on anticholinergics, older people, and interventions to retrieve the relevant studies. The search was limited to the English language and humans. A detailed MEDLINE search strategy is presented in Supplementary Table S1. Citation analysis was performed in Google Scholar and Web of Science to track the prospective citing of references of the selected articles.

2.2. Study Screening and Selection

The title, abstract, and full text of each potentially relevant article were independently screened by two authors (M.S. and S.A.) for eligibility of inclusion in this review. Any discrepancies were resolved by a third author (A.A.), and decisions were made by consensus.

2.3. Inclusion Criteria

The primary outcome of interest was single and multicomponent interventions that improve anticholinergic prescribing practice or reduce adverse drug events due to the consumption of anticholinergic medications. Single-component intervention consists of only one intervention activity, such as medication review [34]. Multicomponent intervention refers to the combination of various components in a single intervention [35], such as medication review and the provision of education [34]. All interventions (e.g., medication review, educational detailing visits for physicians, nurses, and aides, pocket-sized educational cards along with clinical vignettes, educational internet site, and detailing session with physicians) performed by any healthcare professional targeting participants of either sex, mean age ≥ 65 years, and admitted to any healthcare setting were included. We included pre/post or experimental studies that employed a control group.

2.4. Exclusion Criteria

We excluded the following studies: review articles, case reports, and case series. We also excluded studies that were conducted in languages other than English.

2.5. Data Extraction and Synthesis

Two reviewers (M.S. and S.A.) independently reviewed and extracted the data from the eligible studies according to a standardised format based on variables of interest, such as the study population, study design and duration, mean age, major findings, and intervention characteristics (type of intervention and implementation). The study selection process is illustrated in Figure 1.

2.6. Quality Assessment

The quality of the included studies was critically appraised. The Cochrane Risk of Bias tool [36] was used to assess the methodological quality of the randomised controlled trials (RCTs). The Newcastle-Ottawa scale was used to assess the quality of the non-RCTs [37], which is based on three domains: the selection of study groups, comparability of cohorts and assessment of outcome (cohort studies), or comparability of case and controls and ascertainment of exposure (case-control studies). The thresholds for categorising and interpreting the Newcastle-Ottawa scale domains were described in Supplementary Table S2. The Cochrane Risk of Bias tool results for included RCTs were described in Supplementary Table S3. Studies were not excluded based on the risk of bias or quality assessment.

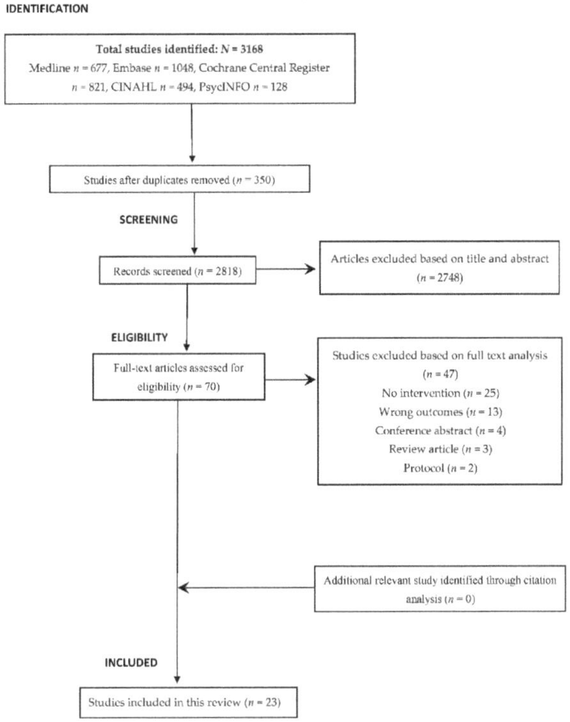

Figure 1. PRISMA flow diagram of the study selection process and citation analysis.

3. Results

The primary electronic search identified a total of 3168 studies from the five databases. Using EndNote X9 (Thomson Reuters), we eliminated 350 duplicate studies, and the remaining 2818 studies were examined to determine their relevance for inclusion. Of those, only 70 were found to be eligible for full-text analysis. Subsequently, 47 studies were excluded as they failed to meet the predefined inclusion criteria. No potential studies were identified from the citation analysis. Finally, a total of 23 studies that investigated the effectiveness of anticholinergic prescribing practice in older adults were included in this review (Figure 1).

3.1. Overview of the Included Studies

Table 1 provides the qualitative summary of the included studies, mainly showcasing the type of interventions, and Table 2 illustrates an overview of the quantitative summary of the studies based on study design, setting, sample size, study duration and follow-up, outcome measure (control/pre and intervention/post), significant association (+ or −), and statistical tests.

The countries of origin were USA ($n = 5$) [29,38–41], Australia ($n = 4$) [22,23,42,43], Finland ($n = 2$) [44,45], Norway ($n = 2$) [21,46], Ireland [47], New Zealand [48], Belgium [49], Spain [50], Sweden [51], Sweden [30], France [52], Italy [53], Taiwan [54], and The Netherlands [55].

The study settings included hospitals ($n = 7$) [40,41,44,46,50,52,53] community/primary care ($n = 7$) [22,30,38,47,49,51,55] and nursing homes/aged care facilities ($n = 9$) [21,23,29,39,42,43,45,48,54]. There were ten cross-sectional studies [22,38,40,42–44,46,51,52,54], six nonrandomised or pre/post studies [30,39,47,48,50,53], and seven RCTs [21,23,29,41,45,49,55]. The studies included in this study had sample sizes ranging from 46 to 46,078 study subjects. The average age of the participants varied between 65 and 87.5 years, and the proportion of the female subjects was 39.0–77%.

Table 1. The qualitative summary of included studies.

Author, Year, Country	Study Design	Intervention	Description of Intervention(s)	Effect on Outcome/Key Findings
Riordan et al., 2019, Ireland [47]	Convergent parallel mixed-methods design (before and after)	Academic Detailing (pharmacist-led)	Pharmacist conducted face-to-face education sessions and small focus group academic detailing sessions of 19–48 min with physicians.	Pharmacist-led academic detailing intervention was acceptable to GPs. Behavioural Change: awareness of non-pharmacological methods in treating urinary incontinence. Knowledge Gain: intervention served to refresh their knowledge
Ailabouni et al., 2019, New Zealand [48]	A single group (pre-and post-comparison) feasibility study	Medication review (de-prescribing)	A collaborative pharmacist-led medication review with GPs was employed. New Zealand registered pharmacists used peer-reviewed deprescribing guidelines. The cumulative use of anticholinergic and sedative medicines for each participant was quantified using the DBI.	Deprescribing resulted in a significant reduction in falls, depression and frailty scores, and adverse drug reactions. No improvement in cognition and quality of life. Total regular medicines use reduced statistically, by a mean difference of 2.13 medicines per patient, among patients where deprescribing was initiated.
Toivo et al., 2019, Belgium [49]	Cluster RCT	Care coordination intervention (coordinated medication risk management)	Practical nurses were trained to make the preliminary medication risk assessment during home visits and report findings to the coordinating pharmacist. The coordinating pharmacist prepared the cases for the triage meeting with the physician and home care nurse to decide further actions.	No significant impact on the medication risks between the intervention and the control group. The per-protocol analysis indicated a tendency for effectiveness, particularly in optimising central nervous system medication use.
Hernandez et al., 2020, Spain [50]	Prospective pre-and post-interventional study	Medication review	Pharmacists reviewed the medications and detected drug-related problems using the Drug Burden Index (DBI) tool. Their recommendations were communicated to the physician via telephone, weekly meetings, and email. Further review was conducted at the weekly meeting between physician and pharmacist.	Statistically significant differences were found between pre- and post-intervention in NPI at admission, drug-related problems, MAI criteria (interactions, dosage and duplication), and mean (SD) DBI score.
Lenander et al., 2018, Sweden [51]	Cross-sectional	Medication Review	Clinical Pharmacist led medication review to assess the prevalence of DRP's and recommendations to discontinue, followed by team-based discussions with general practitioners (GPs) and nurses	It shows that the medication reviews decreased the use of potentially inappropriate medication.
Weichert et al., 2018, Finland [44]	Multicentre observational study	Medication Review	Medication review was conducted for ACB in patients at the time of admission and discharge	21.1% of patients had their ACB reduced. There is considerable scope for improvement of prescribing practices in older people.

Table 1. *Cont.*

Author, Year, Country	Study Design	Intervention	Description of Intervention(s)	Effect on Outcome/Key Findings
Lenander et al., 2017, Sweden [30]	Interventional pilot study	SÅKLÅK project, a developed intervention model	Multi-professional intervention model created to improve medication safety for elderly	Significant decrease in the prescription of anticholinergic drugs indicated the SÅKLÅK intervention is effective in reducing potential DRPs
Moga et al., 2017, USA [29]	Parallel arm Randomised Interventional study	Targeted medication therapy management intervention	Targeted patient-centred pharmacist-physician team medication therapy management intervention was used to reduce the use of inappropriate anticholinergic medications in older patients.	The targeted medication therapy management intervention resulted in improvement in anticholinergic medication appropriateness and reduced the use of inappropriate anticholinergic medications in older patients.
Lagrange et al., 2017, France [52]	Retrospective study	A context-aware pharmaceutical analysis tool	A context-aware computerised decision-support system designed to automatically compare prescriptions recorded in computerised patient files against the main consensual guidelines for medical management in older adults.	Prescription of anticholinergics was significantly decreased (28%).
Carnahan et al., 2017, USA [39]	Quasi-experimental study design	Educational program on medication use	IA-ADAPT/CMS Partnership is an evidence-based training program to improve dispensing drugs for elderly	Suggests that the IA-ADAPT and the CMS Partnership improved medication use with no adverse impact on BPSD.
Hanus et al., 2016, USA [40]	Observational Pilot study	Pharmacist-led EHR-based population health initiative and ARS Service	Physicians in the primary care settings could communicate with pharmacists employing a shared EHR. As part of a quality improvement project, a pharmacist-led EHR-based medication therapy recommendation service was implemented at 2 DHS medical clinics to reduce the anticholinergic burden	High recommendation acceptance rates were achieved using objective anticholinergic risk assessment and algorithm-driven medication therapy recommendations.
McLarin et al., 2016, Australia [43]	Retrospective study	RMMR	Impact of RMMRs on anticholinergic burden quantified by sever anticholinergic risk scales	Demonstrated that RMMRs are effective in reducing ACM prescribing in elderly

Table 1. Cont.

Author, Year, Country	Study Design	Intervention	Description of Intervention(s)	Effect on Outcome/Key Findings
Kersten et al., 2015, Norway [46]	Retrospective study	Medication review	Investigated the clinical impact of PIMs in acutely hospitalised older adults.	Anticholinergic prescriptions were reduced from 39.2% to 37.9%
Juola et al., 2015, Finland [45]	Cluster RCT	Educational intervention	Nursing staff working in the intervention wards received two 4-h interactive training sessions based on constructive learning theory to recognise harmful medications and adverse drug events.	No significant differences in the change in prevalence of anticholinergic drugs.
Kersten et al., 2013, Norway [21]	RCT	Multidisciplinary drug review	Single Blind MDRD was conducted that recruited long-term nursing home residents with a total ADS score of greater than or equal to 3	After 8 weeks, the median ADS score was significantly reduced from 4 to 2 in the intervention group. The largest improvement in immediate recall after 8 weeks was observed in the five patients in the intervention group who had their ADS score reduced to 0
Ghibelli et al., 2013, Italy [53]	Pre, post-intervention study	INTERcheck CPSS	INTERcheck is a CPSS developed to optimise drug prescription for older people with multimorbidity and minimise the occurrence of adverse drug reactions.	The use of INTERCheck was associated with a significant reduction in PIMs and new-onset potentially severe DDIs.
Yeh et al., 2013, Taiwan [54]	Prospective case-control study	Educational program for primary care physicians	Educational program for primary care physicians serving in Veterans' Homes, focusing on anticholinergic adverse reactions in geriatrics and the CR-ACHS	CR-ACHS was significantly reduced in the intervention group at 12-week follow-up.
Boustani et al., 2012, USA [41]	RCT	CDSS Alert (anticholinergic discontinuation)	CDSS alert system sends an interruptive alert if any of the 18 anticholinergics were prescribed, recommending stopping the drug, suggesting an alternative, or recommending dose modification.	Physicians receiving the CDSS issued more discontinuation orders of definite anticholinergics, but the results were not statistically significant. Results suggest that human interaction may play an important role in accepting recommendations aimed at improving the care of hospitalised older adults with CI.

Table 1. Cont.

Author, Year, Country	Study Design	Intervention	Description of Intervention(s)	Effect on Outcome/Key Findings
Gnjidic et al., 2010, Australia [23]	Cluster RCT	Medication review	The study intervention included a letter and phone call to GPs, using DBI to prompt them to consider dose reduction or cessation of anticholinergic and sedative medications.	At follow-up, a DBI change was observed in 16 participants. DBI decreased in 12 participants, 6 (19%) in the control group, and 6 (32%) in the intervention group.
Castelino et al., 2010, Australia [22]	Retrospective study	Medication reviews by pharmacist	HMR by pharmacists for leads to an improvement in the use of medications	DBI and PIMs identified in 60.5% and 39.8% of the patients. Significant reduction in the cumulative DBI scores for all patients was observed following pharmacists' recommendations
Starner et al., 2009, USA [38]	Retrospective study	Educational Intervention	Intervention letters were mailed to the physicians for patients having ≥1 DAE claim	Noticeable decrease was observed after a 6-month follow-up of the intervention in the reduction of DAE claims (48.8%) specifically reduction of anticholinergics (66.7%) was highest
van Eijk et al., 2001, Netherlands [55]	RCT	Educational visits as an individual and a group for general practitioners and pharmacists	Educational visits used academic detailing to discuss prescribing of highly anticholinergic antidepressants in elderly people.	The rate of starting anticholinergic antidepressants in the elderly reduced 26% (in the individual intervention) and 45% (in the group intervention) The use of less anticholinergic antidepressants increased by 40% and 29%, respectively

MAI, medication appropriateness index; GPs, general practitioners; DBI, drug burden index; NPI, neuropsychiatry inventory; RCT, randomised controlled trial; CDSS, clinical decision support system alert; DAE, drugs to be avoided in the elderly; DRPs, drug-related problems; CI, cognitive impairment; ACB, anticholinergic burden; MDRD, modification of diet in renal disease study equation; ADS, anticholinergic drug scale; PIMs, potentially inappropriate medications; CPSS, computerised prescription support system; DDIs, drug–drug interactions; EHR, electronic health record; DHS, Department of Health Services; ARS, anticholinergic risk scale; CR-ACHS, clinician-rated anticholinergic score; HMR, home medicines review; IA-ADAPT, improving antipsychotic appropriateness in dementia patients; CMS, Centers for Medicare and Medicaid Services Partnership to Improve Dementia Care; BPSD, Behavioural and psychological symptoms of dementia; RMMRs, Residential Medication Management Reviews; ACM, anticholinergic medication.

Table 2. The quantitative summary of included studies.

Author, Year, Country	Study Design	Setting	Sample Size	Mean Age (Years)	Gender (Female %)	Study Duration	Follow-Up	Relevant Outcome(s)	Outcome Measure Control/Pre	Outcome Measure Intervention/Post	Significant Association (±)	Statistical Tests
Riordan et al., 2019, Ireland [47]	Convergent parallel mixed-methods design (before and after)	General Practice	154	75.0	72.1	5 months	6 months	Effects on DBI and ACB scores	Patients having an ACB score of 0 (34%)	Patients having an ACB score of 0 (31%) 65% of patients did not show any change in DBI over time	−	SD, Range, IQR, Frequency, Percentages
Ailabouni et al., 2020, New Zealand [48]	A single group (pre- and post-comparison) feasibility study	Residential care facilities	46	65.0	74.0	6 months	2 weeks	Reduction in DBI score	≥0.5 (median DBI)	0.34 (median DBI)	+	Wilcox-signed Rank test (WSR) t-test Fisher's exact test
Toivo et al., 2019, Belgium [49]	Cluster RCT	Primary care	129	82.8	69.8	1 year	1 year	Anticholinergic use	18.8% (Anticholinergic use at baseline) 18.8% (Anticholinergic use at 12 months)	29.6% (Anticholinergic use at baseline) 18.5% (Anticholinergic use at 12 months)	−	Binary logistic regression, two-sided statistical tests
Hernandez et al., 2020, Spain [50]	Prospective pre- and post-interventional study	Intermediate care hospital	55	84.6	60.0	12 months	NA	Anticholinergic burden per Drug Burden Index (DBI)	1.38 ± 0.7 (Mean DBI)	1.08 ± 0.7 (Mean DBI)	+	Kolmogorov–Smirnov test Student's t-test
Lenander et al., 2018, Sweden [51]	Cross-sectional	Primary care	1720	87.5	74.5	1 year	8 weeks	Discontinuation anticholinergics of DRPs	Pts with anticholinergics = 9.2%	Pts with anticholinergics = 4.2%	+	Student's t-test, Chi-square
Weichert et al., 2018, Finland [44]	Observational study	Hospital	549	79.6	58.3	1 year, 5 months	30 days	Reduction in ACB Score during the hospital stay	Patients on DAPs on admission = 60.8%	Patients on DAPs on discharge = 57.7	−	Shapiro–Wilk test, Wilcoxon signed-rank test, 2 sample t-test, Yates and Pearson's chi-square test multivariate binary logistic regression
Lenander et al., 2017, Sweden [30]	Interventional pilot study	Primary care	2400 to 13,700 patients (estimated)	65–79 (range)	63	9 months	6 months	Reduction in anticholinergic PIMs (before/after)	Anticholinergic prescriptions before intervention (4513)	Anticholinergic prescriptions after intervention (3824)	+	Chi-square test

Table 2. Cont.

Author, Year, Country	Study Design	Setting	Sample Size	Mean Age (Years)	Gender (Female %)	Study Duration	Follow-Up	Relevant Outcome(s)	Outcome Measure Control/Pre	Outcome Measure Intervention/Post	Significant Association (±)	Statistical Tests
Moga et al., 2017, USA [29]	Parallel arm Randomised Interventional study	Alzheimer's Disease Center	49	77.7 ± 6.6	70.0	1 year	8 weeks	Significant reduction in anticholinergic drug scale (ADS) Score	1.0 (0.3)	0.2 (0.3)	+	Student's t-tests (or Wilcoxon rank-sum tests for non-normally distributed variables), Chi-square or Fisher's exact tests
Lagrange et al., 2017, France [52]	Retrospective study	Hospital	187	73.9	62.1	10.5 months	33 and 37 days	Change in number of prescriptions	6538 doses (Anticholinergics)	4696 doses (Anticholinergics)	+	Descriptive statistics
Carnahan et al., 2017, USA [39]	Quasi-experimental study design	Nursing home	411	86.7	77.0	1 year 9 months	276 days	Anticholinergic use	Mean (SD) 35.9% (12.0%)	Mean (SD) 36.1% (10.9%)	−	Generalised linear mixed logistic regression
								Antipsychotic use	Mean (SD) 17.7% (10.4%)	Mean (SD) 20.7% (10.6%)	+	
Hanus et al., 2016, USA [40]	Observational Pilot study	Medical clinics	59	77 ± 9.3	51.0	2 months	2 weeks	Reduction in ACB Score, Increased medication acceptance rate	1.08 50%	0.89 95%	+	Generalised linear mixed-effects model, paired t-test
McLarin et al., 2016, Australia [43]	Retrospective study.	Aged care facilities	814	85.6	69.6	NA	NA	Reduction in anticholinergic medications after a medication review	Mean (SD) 3.73 (1.46)	Mean (SD) 3.32 (1.7)	+	Wilcoxon signed-rank test, ANOVA
Kersten et al., 2015, Norway [46]	Retrospective study	Hospital	232	86.1	59.1	8 months	1 year	Reduction in anticholinergic prescriptions	Prevalence of anticholinergic drugs was significantly reduced ($p < 0.02$)		+	Paired samples Student's t-test, McNamar's test, Mann–Whitney U tests, ANOVA, linear regression
Juola et al., 2015, Finland [45]	Cluster RCT	Assisted living facilities	227	83.0	73.9	1 year	1 year	Mean Anticholinergic drugs	1.0 (Mean Anticholinergic drugs)	1.2 (Mean Anticholinergic drugs)	−	t-tests, Mann–Whitney U tests, or Chi-square tests, GEE models, Poisson regression models
Kersten et al., 2013, Norway [21]	RCT	Nursing home	87	85.0	59.0	8 weeks	8 weeks	Marked reduction in ADS score	Median = 4	Median = 2	+	ANCOVA, Poisson regression analysis

Table 2. Cont.

Author, Year, Country	Study Design	Setting	Sample Size	Mean Age (Years)	Gender (Female %)	Study Duration	Follow-Up	Relevant Outcome(s)	Outcome Measure Control/Pre	Outcome Measure Intervention/Post	Significant Association (±)	Statistical Tests
Ghibelli et al., 2013, Italy [53]	Pre- and post-intervention study	Hospital	75 for Pre 75 for Post	81	58.3	4 months	NA	Reduction in ACB score	1.3	1.1	−	Pearson Chi-square test, Student's t-test
Yeh et al., 2013, Taiwan [54]	Prospective case-control	Veteran Home	67	83.4	NA	12 weeks	12 weeks	Anticholinergic Burden (CR-ACHS)	1.0 ± 1.1 (Mean CR-ACHS)	-0.5 ± 1.1 (Mean CR-ACHS)	+	Wilcoxon signed ranks test
Boustani et al., 2012, USA [41]	RCT	Hospital	424	74.8	68.0	21 months	At the time of discharge	Discontinuation of AC prescriptions	anticholinergic discontinued = 31.2%	anticholinergic discontinued = 48.9%	−	Fisher's exact test, t-test, logistic regression, multiple regression
Gnjidic et al., 2010, Australia [23]	Cluster RCT	Self-care retirement village	115	84.3	73.0	13 months	3 months	Drug Burden Index (DBI)	0.26 ± 0.34 (mean DBI)	0.22 ± 0.42 (mean DBI)	−	Kolmogorov–Smirnov test Mann–Whitney nonparametric test X^2 test
Castelino et al., 2010, Australia [22]	A retrospective analysis of medication reviews	Community-dwelling	372	76.1	55.0	NA	NA	Impact of pharmacist's on DBI scores	Sum of DBI scores = 206.86	Sum of DBI scores = 157.26	+	Wilcoxon signed-rank test
Starner et al., 2009, USA [38]	Retrospective study	Pharmacy claims data	10,364	65.0	NA	8 months	6 months	Rate of discontinued anticholinergics	NA	66.7%	+	NA
Nishtala et al., 2009, Australia [42]	Retrospective study	Aged care homes	500	84.0	75.0	6 months	2 months	Significant decrease in DBI score	NA	12% decrease in DBI	+	2-tailed Wilcoxon signed-rank test
van Eijk et al., 2001, Netherlands [55]	RCT	Primary care	46,078	71	58.0	1 year	NA	Reduction in the prescribing of anticholinergics	30% reduction in the rate of starting highly anticholinergic antidepressant in the individual intervention arms compared with the control arm	40% reduction in the rate of starting highly anticholinergic antidepressants in the group intervention arms compared with the control arm	+	Poisson regression model

RCT, randomised controlled trial; DBI, drug burden index; DRPs, drug-related problems; ACB, anticholinergic burden; PIM, potentially inappropriate medications; WSR, Wilcox-signed rank test; SD, standard deviation; GPs, general practitioner; CR-ACHS, clinician-rated anticholinergic score; and NA, not available.

3.2. Methodological Quality of Studies

All eligible studies were rated for their methodological quality, and many studies (*n* = 14, 61%) were identified to be of good quality based on the Newcastle-Ottawa scale [22,30,38,39,42–44,46–48,50–53] (Table S2). The quality of the RCTs was critically appraised using the Cochrane risk of bias assessment tool as shown in Supplementary Table S3. There was a general lack of adequate blinding between study subjects and healthcare practitioners, and between outcomes and assessors. Nonetheless, the follow-up duration was either not clearly specified or insufficient (less than six months) in many studies [21–23,29,40–44,48,50–55]. Altogether, the studies had a duration of follow-up ranging from 14 days [40,48] to 1 year [45,46,49] (Table 2).

3.3. Intervention Characteristics

All studies tested single-component interventions, and medication review was the most common single-component healthcare practitioner-oriented intervention [21–23,42–44,46,48,50,51,54] followed by the provision of education to the healthcare practitioners [38,39,45,47,54,55]. Healthcare practitioners conducted medication reviews using patient notes or tools such as drug burden index (DBI) and anticholinergic burden (ACB) [23,42–44,48,50]. Pharmacists implemented interventions without collaboration with other healthcare practitioners in nearly half of the studies (*n* = 11).

Healthcare practitioner-initiated education mainly consisted of professional components, such as academic detailing sessions for physicians [47,54,55], evidence-based training programs to improve dispensing [39], interactive training sessions for nurses [45], and mailing of intervention letters to the physicians [38]. In three studies [21,29,30], healthcare practitioners also performed interventions such as targeted patient-centred, pharmacist–physician team medication therapy management (MTM) intervention, SÄKLÄK project, and multidisciplinary medication review in collaborations with other healthcare practitioners. A context-aware pharmaceutical analysis tool was tested in France to automatically compare prescriptions recorded in computerised patient files against the main consensual guidelines [52]. Another study tested the clinical decision support system to discontinue orders of definite anticholinergic medications for hospitalised patients with cognitive impairment [41]. Similarly, a study tested targeted patient-centred pharmacist–physician team MTM intervention to reduce the consumption of inappropriate anticholinergic medications in older patients [29]. In Italy, researchers tested the INTERcheck computerised prescription support system to optimise drug prescriptions and minimise the occurrence of adverse drug reactions [53].

3.4. Effectiveness of Interventions at Improving Anticholinergic Prescribing Practice

Sixteen studies (70%) [21,22,29,30,38–40,42,43,46,48,50–52,54,55] investigating a healthcare practitioner-oriented intervention reported a significant reduction in anticholinergic prescribing errors, whereas seven studies (30%) [23,41,44,45,47,49,53] reported no significant effect (Table 2). Similarly, medication review (*n* = 8) and the provision of education (*n* = 4) were the most common interventions in these sixteen studies; however, these studies varied in their designs. There were 14 studies (87.5%) [22,30,38,39,42–44,46–48,50–53] that were of high quality, and of those, 11 studies [22,30,38,39,42,43,46,48,50–52] showed a significant reduction in anticholinergic prescribing errors. Seven studies had a follow-up period of $\geq$6 months, and four studies showed a significant reduction in anticholinergic prescribing errors. With a shorter follow-up period of 2 weeks to 6 months, 4 studies [42,48,51,52] out of 10 studies reported reductions in anticholinergic prescribing errors (Table 2).

Healthcare practitioner-oriented interventions that reported a significant reduction in anticholinergic prescribing errors included: medication review, education provision to healthcare practitioners, pharmacist-led electronic health record-based population health initiative and anticholinergic risk scale service, targeted patient-centred, pharmacist–physician team MTM intervention, context-aware pharmaceutical analysis tool, and SÄKLÄK project. Healthcare practitioner-oriented interventions were most effective in reducing ACB [21,29,40,54], DBI [22,42,48,50], and discontinuation or reduction of anticholinergic medications [30,38,39,43,46,51,52,55]. Hernandez et al. 2020 reported a decline in DBI from 1.38 (control group) to 1.08 (intervention group) [50]. Another study reported a reduction in ACB score from 1.08 (control group) to 0.89 (intervention group) [40]. A retrospective study by McLarin et al. [43] in Australia found a reduction in the mean scores of anticholinergic medications from 3.73 to 3.02 after implementing medication review.

4. Discussion

This is believed to be the first systematic review assessing the effectiveness of interventions to reduce anticholinergic prescribing errors in adults aged 65 and above. Previous reviews primarily evaluated the studies of pharmacist-oriented interventions on medication prescribing and the association between anticholinergic drug burden and mortality in older people [17,56,57]. We did not conduct a meta-analysis because of the methodological heterogeneity between the study designs, anticholinergic prescribing errors, types of interventions, study duration, and follow-up period. Given the high prevalence of inappropriate prescribing and polypharmacy in older people aged 65 and over, interventions to reduce anticholinergic prescribing errors in this cohort are of considerable importance. This systematic review identified 23 studies reporting interventions to reduce anticholinergic prescribing errors in older people. The interventions were mainly provided by the pharmacists using a patient-centred approach. Many studies (19 out of 23) successfully reduced the incidence of anticholinergic prescribing errors in older people. Evidence related to the pharmacist-led interventions in many studies suggests that pharmacists play a vital role in the care of older people, thus improving medication safety across the continuum of care.

In this study, medication review and education provision to the healthcare practitioners were the most common elements in many interventions. Medication review is a structured evaluation of patients' pharmacotherapy to optimise drug use and reduce the occurrence of drug-related problems [58]. Similarly, medication review is recognised as an important healthcare practitioner-oriented intervention for reducing anticholinergic prescribing errors in older people [59]. Likewise, older people benefit mostly from medication reviews as this cohort is more susceptible to adverse drug effects [60,61]. The efficacy of medication review in reducing anticholinergic prescribing errors was reported by eight studies in this review [15,21,22,43,44,46,50,62]. Previous studies inform the significant effects of structured medication review on medication prescriptions and older adults' quality of life [63–65].

Another intervention, such as the provision of education to the healthcare practitioners, was tested in eight studies, but only five studies reported the effectiveness of this intervention in reducing anticholinergic prescribing errors in older people [38,49,54,55,66]. Evidence informs that the healthcare practitioner-oriented educational intervention effectively reduces prescribing errors in older people [57,67]. The provision of education reduces the use of healthcare resources, including emergency department presentations and hospital admissions [68]. Implementing healthcare practitioner-led educational interventions encourages prescribers to change prescription practices, thus improving prescribers' clinical practice [69]. An education intervention provides precise knowledge about prescribing in older adults, medication-related errors, and prevention strategies for reducing medication-related errors [69]. This review also showed that interventions such as INTERcheck, SÄKLÄK intervention model, targeted MTM intervention, context-aware pharmaceutical analysis tool, and CDSS alert were not successful in reducing anticholinergic prescribing errors in older adults [29,41,51–53].

4.1. Implications for Clinical Practice and Future Research

Medications with anticholinergic activity are frequently prescribed in older people due to their numerous clinical benefits; however, these medications are also associated with poor clinical outcomes [70]. Implementing healthcare practitioner-oriented interventions can reduce the occurrence of anticholinergic prescribing errors in older people. This review's findings inform that healthcare practitioner-oriented interventions appear to improve medication safety in older people based on observed reductions in anticholinergic prescribing errors, particularly when the provision of care involves a medication review and an education for the physicians prescribing anticholinergic medications. The prescribing competency can be optimised through educational interventions [71], thus reducing the occurrence of anticholinergic prescribing errors. The safe and effective prescribing of medications is a challenge in older people who frequently experience multiple long-term conditions and complex polypharmacy [72]. Due to an increasing challenge to physicians when prescribing and the complexity of medication regimens taken by older people, there is a need to embed prescribing competency framework in clinical practice [72]. The prescribing competency framework engages prescribers in different stages of prescribing, such as information gathering, clinical decision making, communication, monitoring, and review [72].

The current quantification methods for anticholinergic burden tend to streamline the complexity of pharmacological mechanisms in geriatric risk assessment in older adults. However, there is no universally accepted quantification method available to estimate anticholinergic drug burden, and it is difficult to compare the study findings from distinct methods [16]. Existing tools derived from expert consensus limit the quantification of anticholinergic burden as they do not take into consideration the dose and the CNS distribution of drugs [15]. A recent review showed that the ratings of anticholinergic activity in the expert opinion scales were inconsistent [73]. Moreover, the estimation of central cognitive effects by measuring in vitro serum assay of medications with known anticholinergic activity as a composite peripheral measure still remains unclear [16]. The lack of a gold standard method for anticholinergic quantification might have a direct or indirect impact on the interpretation of the effect size of the study interventions (e.g., reduction in anticholinergic burden). In this review, many studies (69%) were either cross-sectional or nonrandomised and included a single-component intervention. Therefore, there is a need to conduct future randomised multicomponent intervention trials for evaluating the true impact of healthcare practitioner-oriented interventions on anticholinergic prescribing errors in older people.

4.2. Strengths and Limitations

This study was comprehensive in that the electronic search, conducted in four important databases, attempted to identify the complete existing body of evidence of the effectiveness of healthcare-oriented interventions aimed at reducing anticholinergic prescribing errors in older people. This is the first review that found 17 different types of healthcare-oriented interventions, and their impact on anticholinergic prescribing errors. A limitation of this study included the absence of meta-analysis and the estimation of the effect size. It was mainly due to the heterogeneity of included studies. We also excluded studies published in languages other than English, which may have introduced a language bias. However, we performed citation tracking and hand-searching of all included studies to minimise the influence of factors (e.g., inconsistent terminology or wrong indexing) that may affect the keyword-based search.

5. Conclusions

This systematic review suggests that healthcare practitioner-oriented interventions have the potential to reduce the occurrence of anticholinergic prescribing errors in older people. Medication review and the provision of education to the prescribers were the most common approaches to reducing anticholinergic prescribing errors in older people. Healthcare practitioner-oriented interventions were mostly effective in reducing the burden of anticholinergic medications and facilitating the discontinuation of anticholinergic medications in older people. In the future, there is also the need to ascertain how often the healthcare practitioner performs interventions that may reduce anticholinergic prescribing errors in older people.

Supplementary Materials: The following supporting information can be downloaded at: https://www.mdpi.com/article/10.3390/jcm11030714/s1, Table S1: MEDLINE search strategy; Table S2: The Newcastle-Ottawa scale risk of bias assessment for included cohort studies; Table S3: The Cochrane Risk of Bias tool results for included RCTs.

Author Contributions: Conceptualisation, M.S.S. and S.A. (Sheraz Ali); methodology, M.S.S. and S.A. (Sheraz Ali); validation, M.S.S. and S.A. (Sheraz Ali); formal analysis, S.A. (Sana Ajaz), M.A., A.A., S.A. (Saud Alotaibi), M.F. and A.F.; data curation, S.A. (Sana Ajaz), M.A., A.A., S.A. (Saud Alotaibi), M.F. and A.F.; writing—original draft preparation, S.A. (Sheraz Ali); writing—review and editing, S.A. (Sheraz Ali) and M.S.S.; supervision, M.S.S.; project administration, M.S.S. and S.A. (Sheraz Ali). All authors have read and agreed to the published version of the manuscript.

Funding: This research received no specific grant from any funding agency in public, commercial, or not-for-profit sectors.

Institutional Review Board Statement: Not applicable.

Informed Consent Statement: Not applicable.

Data Availability Statement: All research data generated or analysed during this review are included in this published article.

Conflicts of Interest: The authors declare no conflict of interest.

References

1. Buxton, I.L.O. Principles of Prescription Order Writing and Patient Compliance. In *Goodman &amp, Gilman's: The Pharmacological Basis of Therapeutics*, 12th ed.; Brunton, L.L., Chabner, B.A., Knollmann, B.C., Eds.; McGraw-Hill Education: New York, NY, USA, 2015.
2. Likic, R.; Maxwell, S.R. Prevention of medication errors: Teaching and training. *Br. J. Clin. Pharmacol.* **2009**, *67*, 656–661. [CrossRef] [PubMed]
3. Drag, L.L.; Wright, S.L.; Bieliauskas, L.A. Prescribing Practices of Anticholinergic Medications and Their Association with Cognition in an Extended Care Setting. *J. Appl. Gerontol.* **2012**, *31*, 239–259. [CrossRef]
4. Barton, C.; Sklenicka, J.; Sayegh, P.; Yaffe, K. Contraindicated medication use among patients in a memory disorders clinic. *Am. J. Geriatr. Pharmacother.* **2008**, *6*, 147–152. [CrossRef] [PubMed]
5. Buck, M.D.; Atreja, A.; Brunker, C.P.; Jain, A.; Suh, T.T.; Palmer, R.M.; Dorr, D.A.; Harris, C.M.; Wilcox, A.B. Potentially inappropriate medication prescribing in outpatient practices: Prevalence and patient characteristics based on electronic health records. *Am. J. Geriatr. Pharmacother.* **2009**, *7*, 84–92. [CrossRef]
6. Corsonello, A.; Pedone, C.; Lattanzio, F.; Lucchetti, M.; Garasto, S.; Di Muzio, M.; Giunta, S.; Onder, G.; Di Iorio, A.; Volpato, S.; et al. Potentially Inappropriate Medications and Functional Decline in Elderly Hospitalized Patients. *J. Am. Geriatr. Soc.* **2009**, *57*, 1007–1014. [CrossRef] [PubMed]
7. Hale, L.; Griffin, A.; Cartwright, O.; Moulin, J.; Alford, S.; Fleming, R. Potentially inappropriate medication use in hospitalized older adults: A DUE using the full Beers criteria. *Formulary* **2008**, *43*, 326–336.
8. Rajska-Neumann, A.; Wieczorowska-Tobis, K. Polypharmacy and potential inappropriateness of pharmaco-logical treatment among community-dwelling elderly patients. *Arch. Gerontol. Geriatr.* **2007**, *44* (Suppl. S1), 303–309. [CrossRef]
9. Gallagher, P.F.; Barry, P.J.; Ryan, C.; Hartigan, I.; O'Mahony, D. Inappropriate prescribing in an acutely ill population of elderly patients as determined by Beers' Criteria. *Age Ageing* **2008**, *37*, 96–101. [CrossRef]
10. Ruxton, K.; Woodman, R.J.; Mangoni, A.A. Drugs with anticholinergic effects and cognitive impairment, falls and all-cause mortality in older adults: A systematic review and meta-analysis. *Br. J. Clin. Pharmacol.* **2015**, *80*, 209–220. [CrossRef]
11. Van Eijk, M.E.; Bahri, P.; Dekker, G.; Herings, R.M.; Porsius, A.; Avorn, J.; De Boer, A. Use of prevalence and incidence measures to describe age-related prescribing of antidepressants with and without anticholinergic effects. *J. Clin. Epidemiol.* **2000**, *53*, 645–651. [CrossRef]
12. Campbell, N.; Boustani, M.; Limbil, T.; Ott, C.; Fox, C.; Maidment, I.; Schubert, C.C.; Munger, S.; Fick, D.; Miller, D.; et al. The cognitive impact of anticholinergics: A clinical review. *Clin. Interv. Aging* **2009**, *4*, 225–233. [PubMed]
13. Rudolph, J.L.; Salow, M.J.; Angelini, M.C.; McGlinchey, R.E. The anticholinergic risk scale and anticholinergic adverse effects in older persons. *Arch. Intern. Med.* **2008**, *168*, 508–513. [CrossRef]
14. Kersten, H.; Wyller, T.B. Anticholinergic drug burden in older people's brain—How well is it measured? *Basic Clin. Pharmacol. Toxicol.* **2014**, *114*, 151–159. [CrossRef] [PubMed]
15. Nishtala, P.S.; Salahudeen, M.S.; Hilmer, S.N. Anticholinergics: Theoretical and clinical overview. *Expert Opin. Drug. Saf.* **2016**, *15*, 753–768. [CrossRef] [PubMed]
16. Salahudeen, M.S.; Nishtala, P.S. Examination and Estimation of Anticholinergic Burden: Current Trends and Implications for Future Research. *Drugs Aging* **2016**, *33*, 305–313. [CrossRef] [PubMed]

17. Ali, S.; Peterson, G.M.; Bereznicki, L.R.; Salahudeen, M.S. Association between anticholinergic drug burden and mortality in older people: A systematic review. *Eur. J. Clin. Pharmacol.* **2020**, *76*, 319–335. [CrossRef] [PubMed]
18. Tune, L.E. Anticholinergic effects of medication in elderly patients. *J. Clin. Psychiatry* **2001**, *62* (Suppl. S21), 11–14.
19. Alharafsheh, A.; Alsheikh, M.; Ali, S.; Baraiki, A.A.; Alharbi, G.; Alhabshi, T.; Aboutaleb, A. A retrospective cross-sectional study of antibiotics prescribing patterns in admitted patients at a tertiary care setting in the KSA. *Int. J. Health Sci.* **2018**, *12*, 67–71.
20. Gorup, E.; Rifel, J.; Petek Šter, M. Anticholinergic Burden and Most Common Anticholinergic-acting Medicines in Older General Practice Patients. *Zdr Varst.* **2018**, *57*, 140–147. [CrossRef]
21. Kersten, H.; Molden, E.; Tolo, I.K.; Skovlund, E.; Engedal, K.; Wyller, T.B. Cognitive effects of reducing anticholinergic drug burden in a frail elderly population: A randomized controlled trial. *J. Gerontol. A. Biol. Sci. Med. Sci.* **2013**, *68*, 271–278. [CrossRef]
22. Castelino, R.L.; Hilmer, S.N.; Bajorek, B.V.; Nishtala, P.; Chen, T.F. Drug Burden Index and potentially inappropriate medications in community-dwelling older people: The impact of Home Medicines Review. *Drugs Aging* **2010**, *27*, 135–148. [CrossRef] [PubMed]
23. Gnjidic, D.; Le Couteur, D.G.; Abernethy, D.R.; Hilmer, S.N. A pilot randomized clinical trial utilizing the drug burden index to reduce exposure to anticholinergic and sedative medications in older people. *Ann. Pharmacother.* **2010**, *44*, 1725–1732. [CrossRef] [PubMed]
24. Tay, H.S.; Soiza, R.L.; Mangoni, A.A. Minimizing anticholinergic drug prescribing in older hospitalized patients: A full audit cycle. *Ther. Adv. Drug Saf.* **2014**, *5*, 121–128. [CrossRef] [PubMed]
25. van der Meer, H.G.; Wouters, H.; Pont, L.G.; Taxis, K. Reducing the anticholinergic and sedative load in older patients on polypharmacy by pharmacist-led medication review: A randomised controlled trial. *BMJ Open* **2018**, *8*, e019042. [CrossRef]
26. Christensen, M.; Lundh, A. Medication review in hospitalised patients to reduce morbidity and mortality. *Cochrane Database Syst. Rev.* **2016**, *2*, Cd008986. [CrossRef]
27. Holland, R.; Desborough, J.; Goodyer, L.; Hall, S.; Wright, D.; Loke, Y.K. Does pharmacist-led medication review help to reduce hospital admissions and deaths in older people? A systematic review and meta-analysis. *Br. J. Clin. Pharmacol.* **2008**, *65*, 303–316. [CrossRef]
28. Wallerstedt, S.M.; Kindblom, J.M.; Nylén, K.; Samuelsson, O.; Strandell, A. Medication reviews for nursing home residents to reduce mortality and hospitalization: Systematic review and meta-analysis. *Br. J. Clin. Pharmacol.* **2014**, *78*, 488–497. [CrossRef]
29. Moga, D.C.; Abner, E.L.; Rigsby, D.N.; Eckmann, L.; Huffmyer, M.; Murphy, R.R.; Coy, B.B.; Jicha, G.A. Optimizing medication appropriateness in older adults: A randomized clinical interventional trial to decrease anticholinergic burden. *Alzheimers Res. Ther.* **2017**, *9*, 36. [CrossRef]
30. Lenander, C.; Bondesson, Å.; Viberg, N.; Jakobsson, U.; Beckman, A.; Midlöv, P. Effects of an intervention (SÄKLÄK) on prescription of potentially inappropriate medication in elderly patients. *Fam. Pract.* **2017**, *34*, 213–218. [CrossRef]
31. Aronson, J.K. Medication errors: Definitions and classification. *Br. J. Clin. Pharmacol.* **2009**, *67*, 599–604. [CrossRef]
32. Velo, G.P.; Minuz, P. Medication errors: Prescribing faults and prescription errors. *Br. J. Clin. Pharmacol.* **2009**, *67*, 624–628. [CrossRef] [PubMed]
33. Moher, D.; Liberati, A.; Tetzlaff, J.; Altman, D.G. Preferred reporting items for systematic reviews and meta-analyses: The PRISMA statement. *PLoS Med.* **2009**, *6*, e1000097. [CrossRef] [PubMed]
34. Ali, S.; Salahudeen, M.S.; Bereznicki, L.R.E.; Curtain, C.M. Pharmacist-led interventions to reduce adverse drug events in older people living in residential aged care facilities: A systematic review. *Br. J. Clin. Pharmacol.* **2021**, *87*, 3672–3689. [CrossRef] [PubMed]
35. Guise, J.M.; Chang, C.; Viswanathan, M.; Glick, S.; Treadwell, J.; Umscheid, C.A.; Whitlock, E.; Fu, R.; Berliner, E.; Paynter, R.; et al. Agency for Healthcare Research and Quality Evidence-based Practice Center methods for systematically reviewing complex multicomponent health care interventions. *J. Clin. Epidemiol.* **2014**, *67*, 1181–1191. [CrossRef]
36. Higgins, J.P.T.; Altman, D.G. Assessing risk of bias in included studies. In *Cochrane Handbook for Systematic Reviews of Interventions*; Higgins, J.P.T., Green, S., Eds.; Wiley-Blackwell: Chichester, UK, 2011; pp. 187–242.
37. Wells, G.A.; O'Connell, B.S.D.; Peterson, J.; Welch, V.; Losos, M.; Tugwell, P. The Newcastle-Ottawa Scale (NOS) for Assessing the Quality of Nonrandomized Studies in Meta-Analysis. Available online: www.ohri.ca/programs/clinical_epidemiology/oxford.asp (accessed on 25 December 2021).
38. Starner, C.I.; Norman, S.A.; Reynolds, R.G.; Gleason, P.P. Effect of a retrospective drug utilization review on potentially inappropriate prescribing in the elderly. *Am. J. Geriatr. Pharmacother.* **2009**, *7*, 11–19. [CrossRef]
39. Carnahan, R.M.; Brown, G.D.; Letuchy, E.M.; Rubenstein, L.M.; Gryzlak, B.M.; Smith, M.; Reist, J.C.; Kelly, M.W.; Schultz, S.K.; Weckmann, M.T.; et al. Impact of programs to reduce antipsychotic and anticholinergic use in nursing homes. *Alzheimers Dement.* **2017**, *3*, 553–561. [CrossRef]
40. Hanus, R.J.; Lisowe, K.S.; Eickhoff, J.C.; Kieser, M.A.; Statz-Paynter, J.L.; Zorek, J.A. Evaluation of a pharmacist-led pilot service based on the anticholinergic risk scale. *J. Am. Pharm. Assoc.* **2016**, *56*, 555–561. [CrossRef]
41. Boustani, M.A.; Campbell, N.L.; Khan, B.A.; Abernethy, G.; Zawahiri, M.; Campbell, T.; Tricker, J.; Hui, S.L.; Buckley, J.D.; Perkins, A.J.; et al. Enhancing care for hospitalized older adults with cognitive impairment: A randomized controlled trial. *J. Gen. Intern. Med.* **2012**, *27*, 561–567. [CrossRef]
42. Nishtala, P.S.; Hilmer, S.N.; McLachlan, A.J.; Hannan, P.J.; Chen, T.F. Impact of residential medication management reviews on drug burden index in aged-care homes: A retrospective analysis. *Drugs Aging* **2009**, *26*, 677–686. [CrossRef]

43. McLarin, P.E.; Peterson, G.M.; Curtain, C.M.; Nishtala, P.S.; Hannan, P.J.; Castelino, R.L. Impact of residential medication management reviews on anticholinergic burden in aged care residents. *Curr. Med. Res. Opin.* **2016**, *32*, 123–131. [CrossRef]
44. Weichert, I.; Romero-Ortuno, R.; Tolonen, J.; Soe, T.; Lebus, C.; Choudhury, S.; Nadarajah, C.V.; Nanayakkara, P.; Orrù, M.; Di Somma, S.; et al. Anticholinergic medications in patients admitted with cognitive impairment or falls (AMiCI). The impact of hospital admission on anticholinergic cognitive medication burden. Results of a multicentre observational study. *J. Clin. Pharm. Ther.* **2018**, *43*, 682–694. [CrossRef] [PubMed]
45. Juola, A.L.; Bjorkman, M.P.; Pylkkanen, S.; Finne-Soveri, H.; Soini, H.; Kautiainen, H.; Bell, J.S.; Pitkala, K.H. Nurse Education to Reduce Harmful Medication Use in Assisted Living Facilities: Effects of a Randomized Controlled Trial on Falls and Cognition. *Drugs Aging* **2015**, *32*, 947–955. [CrossRef] [PubMed]
46. Kersten, H.; Hvidsten, L.T.; Gløersen, G.; Wyller, T.B.; Wang-Hansen, M.S. Clinical impact of potentially inappropriate medications during hospitalization of acutely ill older patients with multimorbidity. *Scand. J. Prim. Health Care* **2015**, *33*, 243–251. [CrossRef] [PubMed]
47. Riordan, D.O.; Hurley, E.; Sinnott, C.; Galvin, R.; Dalton, K.; Kearney, P.M.; Halpin, J.D.; Byrne, S. Pharmacist-led academic detailing intervention in primary care: A mixed methods feasibility study. *Int. J. Clin. Pharm.* **2019**, *41*, 574–582. [CrossRef]
48. Ailabouni, N.; Mangin, D.; Nishtala, P.S. DEFEAT-polypharmacy: Deprescribing anticholinergic and sedative medicines feasibility trial in residential aged care facilities. *Int. J. Clin. Pharm.* **2019**, *41*, 167–178. [CrossRef] [PubMed]
49. Toivo, T.; Airaksinen, M.; Dimitrow, M.; Savela, E.; Pelkonen, K.; Kiuru, V.; Suominen, T.; Uunimäki, M.; Kivelä, S.L.; Leikola, S.; et al. Enhanced coordination of care to reduce medication risks in older home care clients in primary care: A randomized controlled trial. *BMC Geriatr.* **2019**, *19*, 332. [CrossRef]
50. Hernandez, M.; Mestres, C.; Junyent, J.; Costa-Tutusaus, L.; Modamio, P.; Lastra, C.F.; Mariño, E.L. Effects of a multifaceted intervention in psychogeriatric patients: One-year prospective study. *Eur. J. Hosp. Pharm.* **2020**, *27*, 226–231. [CrossRef]
51. Lenander, C.; Bondesson, Å.; Viberg, N.; Beckman, A.; Midlöv, P. Effects of medication reviews on use of potentially inappropriate medications in elderly patients, a cross-sectional study in Swedish primary care. *BMC Health Serv. Res.* **2018**, *18*, 616. [CrossRef]
52. Lagrange, F.; Lagrange, J.; Bennaga, C.; Taloub, F.; Keddi, M.; Dumoulin, B. A context-aware decision-support system in clinical pharmacy: Drug monitoring in the elderly. *Le Pharmacien Hospitalier et Clinicien* **2017**, *52*, 100–110. [CrossRef]
53. Ghibelli, S.; Marengoni, A.; Djade, C.D.; Nobili, A.; Tettamanti, M.; Franchi, C.; Caccia, S.; Giovarruscio, F.; Remuzzi, A.; Pasina, L. Prevention of inappropriate prescribing in hospitalized older patients using a computerized prescription support system (INTERcheck(®)). *Drugs Aging* **2013**, *30*, 821–828. [CrossRef]
54. Yeh, Y.C.; Liu, C.L.; Peng, L.N.; Lin, M.H.; Chen, L.K. Potential benefits of reducing medication-related anticholinergic burden for demented older adults: A prospective cohort study. *Geriatr. Gerontol. Int.* **2013**, *13*, 694–700. [CrossRef] [PubMed]
55. van Eijk, M.E.; Avorn, J.; Porsius, A.J.; de Boer, A. Reducing prescribing of highly anticholinergic antidepressants for elderly people: Randomised trial of group versus individual academic detailing. *BMJ* **2001**, *322*, 654–657. [CrossRef] [PubMed]
56. Fox, C.; Smith, T.; Maidment, I.; Chan, W.Y.; Bua, N.; Myint, P.K.; Boustani, M.; Kwok, C.S.; Glover, M.; Koopmans, I.; et al. Effect of medications with anti-cholinergic properties on cognitive function, delirium, physical function and mortality: A systematic review. *Age Ageing* **2014**, *43*, 604–615. [CrossRef] [PubMed]
57. Riordan, D.O.; Walsh, K.A.; Galvin, R.; Sinnott, C.; Kearney, P.M.; Byrne, S. The effect of pharmacist-led interventions in optimising prescribing in older adults in primary care: A systematic review. *SAGE Open Med.* **2016**, *4*, 2050312116652568. [CrossRef]
58. Øyane, N.M.F.; Finckenhagen, M.; Ruths, S.; Thue, G.; Lindahl, A.K. Improving drug prescription in general practice using a novel quality improvement model. *Scand. J. Prim. Health Care* **2021**, *39*, 174–183. [CrossRef]
59. van der Meer, H.G.; Wouters, H.; van Hulten, R.; Pras, N.; Taxis, K. Decreasing the load? Is a Multidisciplinary Multistep Medication Review in older people an effective intervention to reduce a patient's Drug Burden Index? Protocol of a randomised controlled trial. *BMJ Open* **2015**, *5*, e009213. [CrossRef]
60. Gurwitz, J.H.; Field, T.S.; Judge, J.; Rochon, P.; Harrold, L.R.; Cadoret, C.; Lee, M.; White, K.; LaPrino, J.; Erramuspe-Mainard, J.; et al. The incidence of adverse drug events in two large academic long-term care facilities. *Am. J. Med.* **2005**, *118*, 251–258. [CrossRef]
61. Martin, R.M.; Lunec, S.G.; Rink, E. UK postal survey of pharmacists working with general practices on prescribing issues: Characteristics, roles and working arrangements. *Int. J. Pharm. Pract.* **1998**, *6*, 133–139. [CrossRef]
62. Veggeland, T.; Dyb, S. The contribution of a clinical pharmacist to the improvement of medication at a geriatric hospital unit in Norway. *Pharm. Pract.* **2008**, *6*, 20–24. [CrossRef]
63. Romskaug, R.; Skovlund, E.; Straand, J.; Molden, E.; Kersten, H.; Pitkala, K.H.; Lundqvist, C.; Wyller, T.B. Effect of Clinical Geriatric Assessments and Collaborative Medication Reviews by Geriatrician and Family Physician for Improving Health-Related Quality of Life in Home-Dwelling Older Patients Receiving Polypharmacy: A Cluster Randomized Clinical Trial. *JAMA Intern. Med.* **2020**, *180*, 181–189. [CrossRef]
64. Gallagher, P.F.; O'Connor, M.N.; O'Mahony, D. Prevention of potentially inappropriate prescribing for elderly patients: A randomized controlled trial using STOPP/START criteria. *Clin. Pharmacol. Ther.* **2011**, *89*, 845–854. [CrossRef] [PubMed]
65. Clyne, B.; Smith, S.M.; Hughes, C.M.; Boland, F.; Bradley, M.C.; Cooper, J.A.; Fahey, T. Effectiveness of a Multifaceted Intervention for Potentially Inappropriate Prescribing in Older Patients in Primary Care: A Cluster-Randomized Controlled Trial (OPTI-SCRIPT Study). *Ann. Fam. Med.* **2015**, *13*, 545–553. [CrossRef] [PubMed]

66. Pasina, L.; Marengoni, A.; Ghibelli, S.; Suardi, F.; Djade, C.D.; Nobili, A.; Franchi, C.; Guerrini, G. A Multicomponent Intervention to Optimize Psychotropic Drug Prescription in Elderly Nursing Home Residents: An Italian Multicenter, Prospective, Pilot Study. *Drugs Aging* **2016**, *33*, 143–149. [CrossRef] [PubMed]
67. Jaam, M.; Naseralallah, L.M.; Hussain, T.A.; Pawluk, S.A. Pharmacist-led educational interventions provided to healthcare providers to reduce medication errors: A systematic review and meta-analysis. *PLoS ONE* **2021**, *16*, e0253588. [CrossRef]
68. García-Gollarte, F.; Baleriola-Júlvez, J.; Ferrero-López, I.; Cuenllas-Díaz, Á.; Cruz-Jentoft, A.J. An educational intervention on drug use in nursing homes improves health outcomes resource utilization and reduces inappropriate drug prescription. *J. Am. Med. Dir. Assoc.* **2014**, *15*, 885–891. [CrossRef]
69. Trivalle, C.; Cartier, T.; Verny, C.; Mathieu, A.M.; Davrinche, P.; Agostini, H.; Becquemont, L.; Demolis, P. Identifying and preventing adverse drug events in elderly hospitalised patients: A randomised trial of a program to reduce adverse drug effects. *J. Nutr. Health Aging* **2010**, *14*, 57–61. [CrossRef]
70. López-Álvarez, J.; Sevilla-Llewellyn-Jones, J.; Agüera-Ortiz, L. Anticholinergic Drugs in Geriatric Psychopharmacology. *Front Neurosci.* **2019**, *13*, 309. [CrossRef]
71. Kamarudin, G.; Penm, J.; Chaar, B.; Moles, R. Educational interventions to improve prescribing competency: A systematic review. *BMJ Open* **2013**, *3*, e003291. [CrossRef]
72. Picton, C.; Loughrey, C.; Webb, A. The need for a prescribing competency framework to address the burden of complex polypharmacy among multiple long-term conditions. *Clin. Med.* **2016**, *16*, 470–474. [CrossRef]
73. Salahudeen, M.S.; Duffull, S.B.; Nishtala, P.S. Anticholinergic burden quantified by anticholinergic risk scales and adverse outcomes in older people: A systematic review. *BMC Geriatr.* **2015**, *15*, 31. [CrossRef]

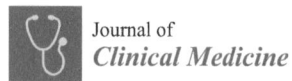

Article

Adherence to Medication in Older Adults with Type 2 Diabetes Living in Lubuskie Voivodeship in Poland: Association with Frailty Syndrome

Iwona Bonikowska [1,*], Katarzyna Szwamel [2] and Izabella Uchmanowicz [3]

[1] Institute of Health Sciences, University of Zielona Góra, 65-417 Zielona Gora, Poland
[2] Institute of Health Sciences, University of Opole, 45-060 Opole, Poland; katarzyna.szwamel@uni.opole.pl
[3] Department of Clinical Nursing, Wroclaw Medical University, 50-367 Wroclaw, Poland; izabella.uchmanowicz@umed.wroc.pl
* Correspondence: i.bonikowska@wlnz.uz.zgora.pl; Tel.: +48-602698252

Abstract: Purpose: Diabetic patients aged 65 years or older are more likely to be frail than non-diabetic older adults. Adherence to therapeutic recommendations in the elderly suffering from diabetes and co-existent frailty syndrome may prevent complications such as micro- or macroangiopathy, as well as significantly affect prevention and reversibility of frailty. The study aimed at assessing the impact of frailty syndrome (FS) on the level of adherence to medication in elderly patients with type 2 diabetes (DM2). Patients and Methods: The research was carried out among 175 DM2 patients (87; 49.71% women and 88; 50.29% men) whose average age amounted to 70.25 ± 6.7. Standardized research instruments included Tilburg frailty indicator (TFI) to assess FS and adherence in chronic disease scale questionnaire (ACDS) to measure adherence to medications. Results: The group of 101 (57.71%) patients displayed medium, 39 (22.29%)—low, and 35 (20.00%)—high adherence. As many as 140 of them (80.00%) were diagnosed with frailty syndrome. The median of the average result of TFI was significantly higher in the low adherence group ($p < 0.001$) (Mdn = 9, Q1–Q3; 7–10 pt.) than in the medium (Mdn = 6, Q1–Q3; 5–9 pt.) or high adherence (Mdn = 6.00, Q1–Q3; 4.5–8 pt.) ones. The independent predictors of the chance to be qualified to the non-adherence group included three indicators: TFI (OR 1.558, 95% CI 1.245–1.95), male gender (OR 2.954, 95% CI 1.044–8.353), and the number of all medications taken daily (each extra pill decreased the chance of being qualified to the non-adherence group by 15.3% (95% CI 0.728–0.954). Conclusion: Frailty syndrome in elderly DM2 patients influenced medical adherence in this group. The low adhesion group had higher overall TFI scores and separately higher scores in the physical and psychological domains compared to the medium and high adhesion groups.

Keywords: diabetes mellitus type 2; frailty syndrome; aged; treatment adherence and compliance

Citation: Bonikowska, I.; Szwamel, K.; Uchmanowicz, I. Adherence to Medication in Older Adults with Type 2 Diabetes Living in Lubuskie Voivodeship in Poland: Association with Frailty Syndrome. *J. Clin. Med.* 2022, 11, 1707. https://doi.org/10.3390/jcm11061707

Academic Editor: Francesco Mattace-Raso

Received: 27 December 2021
Accepted: 17 March 2022
Published: 19 March 2022

Publisher's Note: MDPI stays neutral with regard to jurisdictional claims in published maps and institutional affiliations.

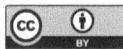

Copyright: © 2022 by the authors. Licensee MDPI, Basel, Switzerland. This article is an open access article distributed under the terms and conditions of the Creative Commons Attribution (CC BY) license (https://creativecommons.org/licenses/by/4.0/).

1. Introduction

Populations are aging and the prevalence of diabetes mellitus is increasing tremendously [1,2]. In 2019, it is estimated that 19.3% of people aged 65–99 years (135.6 million) lived with diabetes. It is projected that the number of people older than 65 years with diabetes will have reached 195.2 million by 2030 and 276.2 million by 2045 [2]. Diabetes mellitus type 2 (T2DM) is associated with complications including cardiovascular disease, retinopathy, renal failure, and peripheral vascular disease [3].

The risk of complications such as micro or macroangiopathy increases significantly after 10 years since diabetes is diagnosed and proper application of medical recommendations is crucial to prevent them [1,4]. Diabetes mellitus also leads to a significant deterioration in the quality of life due to premature disability, blindness, terminal chronic kidney disease, nontraumatic amputations, as well as frequent causes of hospitalization [5]. Recently, several data suggested that diabetes is accompanied not only by complications and disability but also frailty syndrome [4,6].

Frailty syndrome is a multidimensional clinical state that is common in older age [7]. The syndrome appears as a result of decreasing body physiological reserves and decreased the reply of the body to stressors' reaction connected with a deteriorating capacity of physiological systems and their deregulation. It leads to walking, balance, mobility as well as cognitive ability impairments. According to this concept developed by Fried et al., frailty is "a clinical syndrome in which three or more of the following criteria were present: unintentional weight loss (10 lbs in the past year), self-reported exhaustion, weakness (grip strength), slow walking speed and low physical activity" [8]. The current estimate of physical frailty prevalence among community-dwelling older Europeans is around 15% for adults aged 65 years and over [9].

Previous studies have shown that diabetic patients aged 65 years or older were more likely to be frail than nondiabetics [10,11]. The pathogenic linkage between DM and frailty potentially includes premature senescence of organ systems in a hyperglycemic status, chronic inflammation, increased oxidative stress, advanced glycation end-product accumulation, and insulin resistance [12]. Angulo et al., claim that the co-occurrence of diabetes and frailty in older people is not surprising since these two age-related conditions share common underlying pathophysiological mechanisms [13]. In patients with diabetes, death and cardiovascular diseases are attributed to classical risk factors such as hypertension, dyslipidemia, and smoking in approximately 60% of the patients and the contributing factor for the remaining 40% is frailty [14].

According to the recommendations, each person aged 65 and older should be given a chance to undergo a reliable screening test. After the diagnosis of frailty or prefrailty, further clinical assessment of the health condition should be carried out. All persons with frailty should receive social support as needed to address unmet needs and encourage adherence to a comprehensive care plan (strong recommendation) [15].

As it might be concluded, following therapeutic recommendations is especially important in the elderly suffering from diabetes as it might not only prevent such complications as micro and macroangiopathy but it is crucial for the prevention and reversibility of frailty [7,16]. Adherence to long-term therapy is defined as" the extent to which a person's behavior—taking medication, following a diet, and/or executing lifestyle changes, corresponds with agreed recommendations from a health care provider" [17]. It should be emphasized that about 50% of patients with chronic diseases do not have good adherence to their medication treatment plan [18]. The factors which contribute to non-adherence to therapeutic recommendations include patient-related factors (e.g., having negative beliefs and/or perceptions on medications, misconception about their medication), condition-related factors (co-morbidity, cognitive impairment, depression and anxiety, forgetfulness, alcohol consumption), socioeconomic-related factors (age > 60, lack of finances, poor health literacy) and therapy-related factors (e.g., the complexity of treatment regime and pill burden, the disappearance of symptoms, knowledge about DM and its medication) [19,20].

Medication non-adherence remains a significant barrier in achieving better health outcomes for patients with chronic diseases [21]. Following therapeutic recommendations among elderly DM patients might be even worse if frailty is co-existent. Diabetes and frailty are intricately linked; furthermore, diabetes is strongly associated with reduced mobility, activities of daily life, cognitive impairment, and dementia [22]. In recent years, researchers have repeatedly addressed the coexistence of frailty and diabetes in the elderly [23–26]. This problem was considered in the context of the impact of these diseases on the quality of life [5], cognitive and functional status [27–29], or on the results of clinical trials of these patients [29]. There are also studies in the literature focusing on the problem of non-adherence in various chronic diseases such as: COPD (chronic obstructive pulmonary disease [30], DM2 [31–33], chronic kidney disease [34], hypertension [35] or rheumatic heart disease [36], etc. There are also many studies, which show the level of adherence and effectiveness of interventions in patients with type 2 diabetes [37,38], although only some of these studies involve elderly patients. Previous studies showed that the coexistence of frailty syndrome has a negative impact on the adherence of older patients with hypertension [23] and with cardiovascular diseases [39]. However, the problem of adherence to medication in patients over 60 years of age with type 2 diabetes and coexisting frailty is rarely taken up. Analysis of our data allowed us to conclude that each score obtained on the TFI Scale increased the chance of qualifying for the non-adherence group by 55.8%. The relevant independent predictors of non-adherence qualification chance were three factors such as TFI score, male gender, and the number of all medications taken by a patient daily. We believe these results may be of great importance that should be shown and disseminated.

2. Materials and Methods

2.1. Study Design and Setting

The present study has a cross-sectional and observational design. The research was carried out between 2018 and 2019 after obtaining the consent of the Bioethics Committee at the Wroclaw Medical University (approval no. KB—207/2018) while maintaining the requirements of the Declaration of Helsinki of 1975 (amended in 2000) and Good Clinical Practice. The research was conducted among the patients of 5 primary health care centers located in Zielonogórskie District (Lubuskie Voivodeship, Poland).

2.2. Participants

To achieve an appropriate size for the study sample ($\alpha = 0.95$), invitation letters were sent to 365 persons randomized out of 39,197 patients with diagnoses of ICD-10 (E11–E11.9) in the age range of 60–89 years old living in the Lubuskie Voivodeship in 2017. Data regarding relevant inhabitants were obtained from Lubuskie Department of the National Health Fund from 2018 [40]. Invitations to the study were sent to the managers of all 30 primary health care centers located in Zielonogórskie District (Lubuskie Voivodeship). A positive response was obtained from five of them, therefore only patients from these centers were included in the study.

Doctors identified patients for the study according to the inclusion criteria. Then, the diabetes nurse interviewed the patient, presenting the purpose and method of the study and obtaining preliminary oral informed consent. Patients received a complete set of questionnaires and a written informed consent form to participate in the study.

The research inclusion criteria included: age ≥ 60, at least a year since diabetes was diagnosed, a written consent for the participation in the study and physical ability to fill in the questionnaire. The exclusion criteria included: neoplastic disease, chronic heart failure (NYHA IV), acute respiratory disease, ischemic heart disease (CCS-IV), end-stage renal disease or uremia, exacerbation of any diabetes complication making it impossible to complete the questionnaire (e.g., difficulties with reading the text of the questionnaire reported by the patient) and lack of a written consent for the participation in the study. Initially, 200 patients were accepted for the study but, eventually 175 T2DM patients were analyzed. The average age was 70.25 (SD = 6.7). The choice of the sample group is illustrated in Figure 1.

Before the examination, each patient was informed about its aim, method, and possibility of withdrawal at any stage of the research. The examinees were also assured full anonymity and the voluntary nature of the study. The aim and the procedures were explained during the selection phase and only those who voluntarily agreed were accepted. The patients filled in the questionnaire personally (paper-pen method) with a nurse specializing in diabetics present.

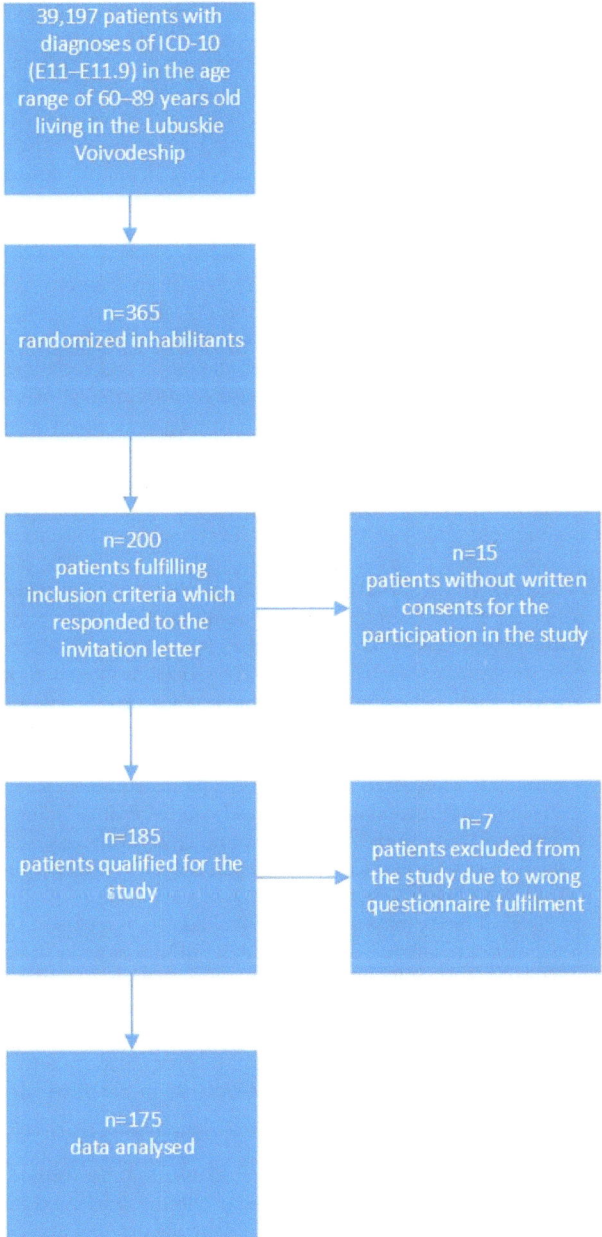

Figure 1. Sampling after considering research inclusion and exclusion criteria.

2.3. Research Tools

The questionnaire used in the research included basic socio-demographic data such as age, gender, education, place of residence, professional activity, marital status. Clinical data were collected from patients' medical files. Standardized research instruments also included adherence in chronic diseases scale—ACDS—and Tilburg frailty indicator (TFI).

Adherence in Chronic Diseases Scale—ACDS—allows to evaluate the adherence with medical recommendations by adult patients suffering from chronic diseases. The presumption of ACDS lies in the fact that only high adherence reflects good therapeutic plan realization in respect to pharmacology. The scale consists of 7 questions with 5 possible answers each. The questions reflect behaviors directly determining adherence (questions 1–5) and the situations and opinions indirectly affecting adherence (questions 6–7). The result of ACDS ranges from 0–28 points. The higher the result, the higher the adherence. The score might be interpreted in the following way: above 26 points—high adherence, between 21–26 points—medium adherence, below 21 points—low adherence [41].

Non-adherent patient—a patient who achieved between 0–20 points in ACDS.

Adherent patient—a patient whose score was medium (21–26 points) or high (27–28 points in ACDS).

Tilburg Frailty Indicator (TFI)—is an instrument created by Gobbens et al. [42]. It allows the assessing of frailty syndrome reliably and globally. The unquestionable asset of this test is the fact that it not only evaluates physical determinants as other similar tools do, but it has some insight into psychological and social determinants as well. TFI consists of two parts. TFI includes a tool for identifying factors that determine weakness. It has been validated in five languages, including the Polish version [43]. The first part A consists of 10 questions about the participant's socio-demographic characteristics. TFI includes a tool for identifying factors that determine weakness. Socio-demographic characteristics of age, sex, marital status and education, lifestyle, economic status, chronic diseases, stressful situations [44]. Part two B of the TFI comprises 15 self-reported questions, divided into three domains: physical, psychological, and social. The physical domain consists of eight questions related to physical health, unexplained weight loss, difficulty in walking, balance, hearing problems, vision problems, strength in hands, and physical tiredness (0–8 points). The psychological domain comprises four items related to cognition, depressive symptoms, anxiety, and coping (0–4 points). The social domain comprises three questions related to social relations, social support, and living alone (0–3 points). Eleven items of part two of the TFI have two response categories ("yes" and "no"), while the other items have three ("yes", "no," and "sometimes"). "Yes" or "sometimes" responses are scored 1 point each, while "no" responses are scored 0. The instrument's total score may range from 0 to 15: the higher the score, the higher one's frailty. Frailty is diagnosed when the total TFI score is ≥ 5 [40]. The TFI is valid and reproducible for the assessment of frailty syndrome among a Polish population. Cronbach's alpha reliability coefficients of the instrument ranged from 0.68 to 0.72 [45].

BMI (body mass index)—was calculated as a person's weight in kilograms divided by the square of height in meters. A high BMI can be an indicator of high body fatness. We classified BMI into following categories: normal body weight amounts for BMI 18.5–24.9 kg m^2, overweight ranges from BMI 25.0–29.9 kg m^2 and obesity is diagnosed if BMI > 30.0 kg m^2. BMI is a commonly applied indicator of obesity as it highly correlates with a percentage of fatty tissue in children and adults. The prognosis of a fatty tissue percentage is dependent on age (higher in older people), gender (higher in men), and race [46].

2.4. Statistical Analysis

The analysis of quantitative variables was performed by calculating the mean, standard deviation, median, quartiles, minimum, and maximum. The analysis of qualitative variables was performed by calculating the number and percentage of the occurrences of each value. Comparison of the values of qualitative variables in the groups was performed using the chi-square test (with Yates's correction for 2 × 2 tables) or the Fisher's exact test where low expected frequencies appeared in the tables. On the other hand, the comparison of the values of quantitative variables in the two groups was performed using the Mann-Whitney test. In turn, the comparison of the values of quantitative variables in the three groups was performed using the Kruskal-Wallis test. Post-hoc analysis with Dunn' test was performed to identify statistically significantly different groups after detecting statistically significant differences.

The multivariate analysis of the independent influence of many variables on the quantitative variable was performed using the logistic regression method. The results are presented in the form of values of the regression model parameters with a 95% confidence interval.

3. Results
3.1. Descriptive Data

The average age of the respondents amounted to 70.25 ± 6.70. The number of female to male patients was comparable—women (87; 49.71%) vs. men (88; 50.29%). Most of them were city residents (154; 88%), lived in a relationship (117; 66.86%) and completed secondary (80; 45.71%) or occupational education (44; 25.14%). The average duration of the diabetes treatment was 12.1 ± 8.52 years and the average number of medications taken was 8.07 ± 4.42. Most of the patients were on oral anti-diabetes medicines (106; 60.57%). The examinees were most frequently overweight (67; 38.29%) or of 1st-degree obesity (55; 31.43%). The most common co-existent diseases included hypertension (143; 81.71%) and kidney diseases (140; 80.00%). (Table 1).

Table 1. Socio-demographic and clinical characteristics of the sample group.

Variables		Total (*n* = 175)
Gender	Women	87 (49.71%)
	Men	88 (50.29%)
Age	M ± SD	70.25 ± 6.70
	median	69
	Q1–Q3	65–74
Marital status	Single	58 (33.14%)
	In relationship	117 (66.86%)
Place of residence	Village	21 (12.00%)
	City	154 (88.00%)
Education	Primary	19 (10.86%)
	Occupational	44 (25.14%)
	Secondary	80 (45.71%)
	High	32 (18.29%)
Diabetes duration [years]	M ± SD	12.1 ± 8.52
	median	10
	Q1–Q3	5–15
Number of all daily medications	M ± SD	8.07 ± 4.42
	median	7
	Q1–Q3	6–10
Number of anti-diabetes medications taken daily	M ± SD	1.81 ± 1.25
	median	2
	Q1–Q3	1–3
Diabetes treatment method	Oral anti-diabetes medications	106 (60.57%)
	Insulin	31 (17.71%)
	Oral anti-diabetes medications and insulin	33 (18.86%)
	non-pharmacological methods	5 (2.86%)
Body Mass Index (BMI)	normal body weight	19 (10.86%)
	overweight	67 (38.29%)
	1st degree obesity	55 (31.43%)
	2nd/3rd degree obesity	34 (19.43%)
Co-existent diseases: Hypertension	No	32 (18.29%)
	Yes	143 (81.71%)
Co-existent diseases: ischaemic heart disease	No	113 (64.57%)
	Yes	62 (35.43%)
Co-existent diseases: Rheumatic diseases	No	130 (74.29%)
	Yes	45 (25.71%)

Table 1. Cont.

Variables		Total (n = 175)
Co-existent diseases: Kidney's diseases	No	140 (80.00%)
	Yes	35 (20.00%)
Co-existent diseases: Respiratory system diseases	No	137 (78.29%)
	Yes	38 (21.71%)
Co-existent diseases: Locomotor system disorders	No	121 (69.14%)
	Yes	54 (30.86%)
Co-existent diseases: Diabetic foot syndrome	No	137 (78.29%)
	Yes	38 (21.71%)
Co-existent diseases: Eye diseases	No	103 (58.86%)
	Yes	72 (41.14%)

M—mean; SD—standard deviation, Q1—first quartile; Q3—third quartile; ACDS, adherence in chronic diseases scale.

3.2. The Prevalence of Frailty Syndrome and Level of Adherence to Medication in Type 2 Diabetes Elderly Patients

In the group of 175 patients, 101 (57.71%) displayed medium, 39 (22.29%) low, and 35 (20.00%)—high adherence. Frailty syndrome was diagnosed in as many as 140 out of 175 respondents (80.00%) (Table 2).

Table 2. Frailty syndrome occurrence and level of adherence to medication.

Instrument	Points	Interpretation	n	%
TFI	0–4	lack of frailty syndrome	35	20.00%
	5 and more	frailty syndrome	140	80.00%
ACDS	0–20	low adherence	39	22.29%
	21–26	medium adherence	101	57.71%
	27–28	high adherence	35	20.00%

TFI—Tilburg frailty indicator; ACDS—adherence in chronic diseases scale.

The average indicator of adherence to medication was 23.13 ± 3.72 and a TFI indicator amounted to 6.95 ± 2.75. The TFI in the physical domain was 3.68 ± 1.96, psychological domain 2.09 ± 0.93, and in the social domain 1.19 ± 0.75 on average (Table 3).

Table 3. Average distribution measures for standardized instruments.

Instrument	N	M	SD	Mdn	Min	Max	Q1	Q3
ACDS	175	23.13	3.72	24	13	28	21	26
TFI total score	175	6.95	2.75	7	0	13	5	9
TFI: physical domain	175	3.68	1.96	4	0	8	2	5
TFI: psychological domain	175	2.09	0.93	2	0	4	2	3
TFI: social domain	175	1.19	0.75	1	0	3	1	2

TFI, Tilburg frailty indicator; ACDS, adherence in chronic diseases scale; M, mean; SD, standard deviation; Mdn, median; Q1, first quartile; Q3, third quartile.

The respondents provided detailed answers to the questions contained in the TFI questionnaire concerning the following domains: physical, psychological, and social. A group of 63 respondents (36.00%) stated that they felt healthy in terms of their physical condition, 29 (16.57%) of the respondents lost more than 6 kg or more in the last 6 months or 3 kg in a month despite the lack of such intention. Our respondents experienced difficulties on a daily basis due to physical fatigue (121; 69.14%), difficulty walking (104; 59.43%), poor eyesight (100; 57.14%), lack of strength in the hands (70; 40.00%), poor hearing (55; 31.43%), difficulties in maintaining balance (53; 30.29%). The vast majority had problems with the psychological components of TFI—only 46 (26.29%) of the respondents had no problems with memory, 39 (22.29%) of the respondents did not experience a drop in mood over the last month, 18 (10.29%) of the respondents did not feel nervous over the last month and 43 (24.57%) were unable to cope well with the problems. In terms of the social components of TFI, the responses were as follows: a group of 145 (82.86%) of the respondents claimed that they received enough support from others, 143 (81.71%) indicated in the questionnaire that they missed the company of other people, and 35 (20.00%)—that they lived alone.

3.3. Socio-Demographic and Clinical Variables in Adherent and Non-Adherent Groups

Both adherent and non-adherent groups were similar in terms of age ($p = 0.053$), gender ($p = 0.493$), education ($p = 0.457$) marital status ($p = 0.078$) and place of residence ($p = 0.787$). They were also compliant as for analysed aspects of clinical condition (Table 4).

Table 4. Socio-demographic and clinical variables in adherent and non-adherent groups.

Variables		ACDS		p
		Adherent ($n = 136$)	Non-Adherent ($n = 39$)	
Age	M ± SD	69.64 ± 6.27	72.38 ± 7.72	U = 2113.5 $p = 0.053$
	Me	69	70	
	Q1–Q3	65–73	67.5–76	
Gender	Women	70 (51.47%)	17 (43.59%)	chi2 = 0.471 $p = 0.493$
	Men	66 (48.53%)	22 (56.41%)	
Marital status	Single	40 (29.41%)	18 (46.15%)	chi2 = 3.116 $p = 0.078$
	In relationship	96 (70.59%)	21 (53.85%)	
Education	Primary	14 (10.29%)	5 (12.82%)	$p = 0.457$
	Occupational	31 (22.79%)	13 (33.33%)	
	Secondary	64 (47.06%)	16 (41.03%)	
	High	27 (19.85%)	5 (12.82%)	
Place of residence	Village	16 (11.76%)	5 (12.82%)	$p = 0.787$
	City	120 (88.24%)	34 (87.18%)	
Diabetes duration [years]	M ± SD	11.88 ± 8.14	12.87 ± 9.81	U = 2576 $p = 0.786$
	Me	10	10	
	Q1–Q3	15–5	5–18.5	
Number of anti-diabetes medications taken daily	M ± SD	1.84 ± 1.3	1.69 ± 1.08	U = 2788.5 $p = 0.609$
	Me	2	2	
	Q1–Q3	1–3	1–2	
Number of all daily medications	M ± SD	8.11 ± 4.7	7.92 ± 3.32	U = 2524 $p = 0.645$
	Me	7	8	
	Q1–Q3	5–10.25	6–10	
Body Mass Index (BMI)	normal body weight	15 (11.03%)	4 (10.26%)	$p = 0.601$
	overweight	49 (36.03%)	18 (46.15%)	
	1st degree obesity	43 (31.62%)	12 (30.77%)	
	2nd/3rd degree obesity	29 (21.32%)	5 (12.82%)	

Table 4. Cont.

Variables		ACDS		p
		Adherent (n = 136)	Non-Adherent (n = 39)	
Co-existent diseases: Hypertension	No	26 (19.12%)	6 (15.38%)	chi2 = 0.088 p = 0.767
	Yes	110 (80.88%)	33 (84.62%)	
Co-existent diseases: ischaemic heart disease	No	90 (66.18%)	23 (58.97%)	chi2 = 0.408 p = 0.523
	Yes	46 (33.82%)	16 (41.03%)	
Co-existent diseases: Rheumatic diseases	No	103 (75.74%)	27 (69.23%)	chi2 = 0.374 p = 0.541
	Yes	33 (24.26%)	12 (30.77%)	
Co-existent diseases: Kidney's diseases	No	111 (81.62%)	29 (74.36%)	chi2 = 0.596 p = 0.44
	Yes	25 (18.38%)	10 (25.64%)	
Co-existent diseases: Respiratory system diseases	No	109 (80.15%)	28 (71.79%)	chi2 = 0.801 p = 0.371
	Yes	27 (19.85%)	11 (28.21%)	
Co-existent diseases: Locomotor system disorders	No	95 (69.85%)	26 (66.67%)	chi2 = 0.034 p = 0.855
	Yes	41 (30.15%)	13 (33.33%)	
Co-existent diseases: Diabetic foot syndrome	No	109 (80.15%)	28 (71.79%)	chi2 = 0.801 p = 0.371
	Yes	27 (19.85%)	11 (28.21%)	
Co-existent diseases: Eye diseases	No	81 (59.56%)	22 (56.41%)	chi2 = 0.028 p = 0.867
	Yes	55 (40.44%)	17 (43.59%)	
Diabetes treatment method	Oral anti-diabetes medications	81 (59.56%)	25 (64.10%)	p = 0.683
	Insulin	23 (16.91%)	8 (20.51%)	
	Oral anti-diabetes medications and insulin	27 (19.85%)	6 (15.38%)	
	non-pharmacological methods	5 (3.68%)	0 (0.00%)	

p—for quantitative variables the Mann-Whitney test, for qualitative variables chi-square test or Fisher's exact test, M—mean, SD—standard deviation, Me—median, Q1—first quartile, Q3—third quartile, ACDS—adherence in chronic diseases scale.

3.4. Frailty Syndrome vs. Adherence to Therapeutic Recommendations

The analysis of the correlation between adherence to medication and frailty syndrome revealed that the median of the overall score of TFI was significantly higher ($p < 0.001$) in the low adherence group (Mdn = 9, Q1–Q3; 7–10 pts) than in medium (Mdn = 6, Q1–Q3; 5–9 pts) or high (Me = 6.00, Q1–Q3; 4.5–8 pts) adherence groups. The median of the scores in the physical domain of TFI was also significantly higher in the low adherence group (Mdn = 5, Q1–Q3; 4–6 pts) than in the medium (Mdn = 4, Q1–Q3; 2–5 pts) or high adherence groups (Mdn = 3, Q1–Q3; 2–4.5 pts). A similar relevant correlation was observed in the psychological domain of TFI ($p = 0.034$). However, no essential correlations were noticed between average scores in the social domain of TFI and the level of adherence ($p = 0.339$) (Table 5).

Table 5. The correlation between adherence to medication and frailty syndrome.

Tilburg Frailty Indicator (TFI)		ACDS			p
		Low Adherence—A (n = 39)	Medium Adherence—B (n = 101)	High Adherence—C (n = 35)	
TFI total score	M ± SD Mdn Q1–Q3	8.62 ± 2.27 9 7–10	6.64 ± 2.69 6 5–9	6 ± 2.72 6 4.5–8	p < 0.001 * A > B, C
TFI: physical domain	M ± SD Mdn Q1–Q3	4.87 ± 1.64 5 4–6	3.43 ± 1.94 4 2–5	3.09 ± 1.82 3 2–4.5	p < 0.001 * A > B, C
TFI: psychological domain	M ± SD Mdn Q1–Q3	2.44 ± 0.99 2 2–3	2.02 ± 0.91 2 2–2	1.89 ± 0.83 2 1–2	p = 0.034 * A > B, C
TFI: social domain	M ± SD Mdn Q1–Q3	1.31 ± 0.92 1 1–2	1.2 ± 0.69 1 1–2	1.03 ± 0.66 1 1–1	p = 0.339

p—Kruskal-Wallis test and post-hoc analysis (Dunn's test), * statistically significant relationship (p < 0.05), TFI, Tilburg frailty indicator; M, mean; SD, standard deviation; Me, median; Q1, first quartile, Q3, third quartile.

3.5. Non-Adherence Predictors vs. Multifactorial Regression Model

The multifactorial logistic regression model showed that there were three factors significant as independent predictors of the chance to be qualified to the non-adherence group, namely, TFI, male gender, and the number of all medications taken daily by a patient. Each point scored at the TFI scale increased the chance of being qualified to the non-adherence group by 55.8% OR 1.558, (95% CI 1.245–1.95). Being male increased the chance by 2.954 times in comparison to being female, OR 2.954, (95% CI 1.044–8.353). The odds ratio for all the medications taken daily by a DM2 elderly patient was OR 0.847–each extra tablet/pill decreased the non-adherence group qualification chance by 15.3% (95% CI 0.728–0.954) (Table 6).

Table 6. Non-adherence predictors-multivariate logistic regression model.

Variables		OR	95% CI		p
Tilburg Frailty Indicator (total score)		1.558	1.245	1.95	<0.001 *
Age	(years)	1.062	0.98	1.152	0.144
Gender	Women Men	1 2.954	ref. 1.044	8.353	0.041 *
Marital status	Single In relationship	1 0.524	ref. 0.175	1.565	0.247
Education	Primary Occupational Secondary High	1 3.609 0.854 1.11	ref. 0.562 0.155 0.132	23.184 4.717 9.328	0.176 0.856 0.923
Place of residence	Village City	1 0.554	ref. 0.125	2.448	0.436
Body Mass Index (BMI)	normal body weight overweight 1st degree obesity 2nd/3rd degree obesity	1 1.839 1.747 0.728	ref. 0.374 0.347 0.121	9.048 8.786 4.375	0.454 0.499 0.728
Co-existent diseases: Hypertension	No Yes	1 3.111	ref. 0.76	12.729	0.114
Co-existent diseases: Ischemic heart disease	No Yes	1 1.271	ref. 0.476	3.399	0.632

Table 6. Cont.

Variables		OR	95% CI		p
Co-existent diseases: Rheumatic diseases	No	1	ref.		
	Yes	2.223	0.667	7.407	0.193
Co-existent diseases: Kidney's diseases	No	1	ref.		
	Yes	1.946	0.553	6.854	0.3
Co-existent diseases: Respiratory system diseases	No	1	ref.		
	Yes	1.119	0.361	3.471	0.846
Co-existent diseases: Locomotor system disorders	No	1	ref.		
	Yes	0.926	0.324	2.646	0.886
Co-existent diseases: Diabetic foot syndrome	No	1	ref.		
	Yes	0.384	0.106	1.391	0.145
Co-existent diseases: Eye diseases	No	1	ref.		
	Yes	1.149	0.402	3.285	0.796
Diabetes duration [years]	[years]	0.97	0.908	1.035	0.358
Diabetes treatment method	Oral anti-diabetes medications	1	ref.		
	Insulin	0.778	0.119	5.086	0.793
	Oral anti-diabetes medications and insulin	1.112	0.281	4.392	0.88
	non-pharmacological methods	0	0	Inf	0.991
Number of anti-diabetes medications taken daily		0.78	0.401	1.514	0.462
Number of all daily medications		0.847	0.728	0.984	0.03 *

p—multivariate logistic regression, * statistically significant relationship ($p < 0.05$), OR, odds ratio, ref.—reference category.

4. Discussion

Adherence to medical and dietary recommendations, undertaking physical activity and self-checks are crucially important to avoid severe and chronic complications in diabetes, however, they may all appear hard to fulfill in the elderly in terms of deteriorating mental and physical abilities [47]. One of the primary examinations carried out in Poland in the group of elderly DM2 patients is focused on assessing relevant predictors of adherence to medication and co-existent frailty syndrome.

The results of this research revealed that most of the elderly DM2 patients suffered from frailty syndrome as well. It was also proved that the level of adherence to medication was significantly determined by the existence of the syndrome. Eventually, it was observed that the low adherence group of patients achieved significantly higher overall TFI scores than the medium and high adherence groups. They had higher indicators of TFI in the physical and psychological domains of TFI as well. The relevant independent predictors of non-adherence qualification chance were three factors such as TFI score, male gender, and the number of all medications taken by a patient daily.

The results confirm the frequent co-existence of type 2 diabetes and frailty syndrome in patients aged over 60 as in 80% of the respondents diagnosed in the study. Such a high percentage of the coexistence of frailty syndrome in these patients is disturbing. The meta-analysis of the 32 studies by Kong et al. (2021) shows that the pooled prevalence of frailty and prefrailty in older adults with diabetes was 20.1% (95% CI = 16.0–24.2%) and 49.1% (95%CI = 45.1–53.1%), respectively, with significant heterogeneity across the studies [48]. The result obtained by us differs from the one presented in the meta-analysis; however, it is worth noting that Kong et al. did not take into account any of the Polish studies. Another study (Survey of Health, Aging, and Retirement in Europe, SHARE) showed that more than 50% of the European population aged 50 years and over were pre-frail or frail [49]. However, here the age threshold of the respondents was much lower compared to our study, and besides, the authors did not focus only on diabetic patients but on the general population. The available literature basically lacks research similar to ours conducted in Poland. However, this does not change the fact that the common prevalence of frailty syndrome surely calls for special attention to be paid to the adherence with therapeutic recommendations in this group of patients.

Diabetes and frailty are two conditions that frequently occur concurrently and are increasingly prevalent in older patient [50]. Yoon et al. (2019) claim that frailty syndrome appears to be the third category of complications in elderly diabetes patients along with common microvascular diseases and complications which lead to serious disabilities [6]. Diabetic patients are more likely to be frail than non-diabetic older adults [10,51]. In the study by Chhetri et al. (2017) ($n = 10, 039$, mean age of 70.51) the prevalence of frailty syndrome among diabetic patients was higher compared to non-diabetic older adults (19.32% vs. 11.92%). In this study diabetics were at 1.36 (95% CI = 1.18, 1.56) and 1.56 (95% CI = 1.32, 1.85) fold increase in risk of frailty compared to non-diabetic population for prevalence and incidence respectively [10]. The research by Ferri-Guerra et al. (2019) showed that in 763 DM patients (mean age 72.9 years) 50.5% were frail [52]. Other studies also confirmed that the prevalence of frailty in adults older than 65 years was three- to five-fold higher in patients with diabetes than that in the general population [51,53].

Patients with diabetes mellitus are at risk for developing frailty due to the complex interplay between different cardiometabolic factors [54]. A 2013 study by Bouillon et al. lists adiposity, low high-density lipoprotein (HDL)-cholesterol level, high blood pressure, and cigarette smoking as the risk factors of frailty syndrome occurrence [53]. García-Esquinas et al. (2015) explained the association between diabetes mellitus and frailty by unhealthy behaviors and obesity and to a greater extent by poor glucose control and altered serum lipid profile among diabetic individuals [55].

The self-report study is consistent with other studies because it focused on assessing the degree of adherence to treatment and its connotation with the weakness syndrome in elderly patients with type 2 diabetes. The results showed that the majority of respondents showed moderate and poor compliance. A high degree of compliance with the recommendations was noted only in every fifth respondent. An analysis of the correlation between drug use and the severity of the fragile syndrome also showed that the mean TFI overall score was significantly higher in the low adhesion group compared to the moderate and high adherence patients. Likewise, the numbers in the physical and psychological domains were relatively higher in the low adherence group.

Prevalence of non-adherence among DM2 patients ranged between 6.9% and 90.6%, which may be due to differences in study designs methodology and populations [56]. Following therapeutic recommendations forces patients to change their existing lifestyle, requires constant education, developing the ability to properly interpret changes in their health condition, and coping with new situations. Therefore, if the physical domain of frailty syndrome (physical health, unintended body weight loss, walking and balance problems, hearing and vision impairment, fatigue, and grip power decrease) is to be analyzed in the context of adherence, it is easily recognizable that the patients experienced serious issues in the field of physical health. Reports from 2005–2007 by other researchers also prove rapid pathological changes in diabetics. The research by health, aging, and body composition (Health ABC) showed that elderly type 2 diabetes patients lose the power in the knee extensor muscles much earlier than non-diabetics [57]. The English reported that elderly men with newly diagnosed diabetes revealed much weaker muscle strength and a higher probability of physical functions impairment than non-diabetic patients [58]. In the study by Bourdel-Marchasson et al. (2019) the sarcopenia symptoms were found more often in patients with frailty syndrome and were connected with a decreased volume of grey matter responsible for locomotor control [59]. Diabetes also influenced the grip strength in the study by Gundmi et al. 2018 [60]. Based on the results of the self-report, patients can conclude that the lower the adhesion to drugs, the higher the value in the physical domain of TFI. Motta et al. (2020) indicated that muscle strength is probably the most important factor that can be improved by exercise in patients with brittleness syndrome [61].

Therefore, while planning education among such patients suffering additionally from diabetes, we suggest taking advantage of this conclusion and the findings. They may serve as a strong motivator encouraging this age group to physical activity. As diabetes mellitus negatively affects muscle system functioning, such interventions, aimed at improving muscle functioning, should be implemented as soon as possible and patients should be informed about them. Due to the description of the sample group and current COVID-19 situation adjusting a proper method of adherence control may appear problematic. Telemedicine might be a good solution here. Telepharmacy increases adherence to therapeutic recommendations, especially when the system is enriched with the possibility of remote consultations between the patient and the pharmacist [62].

After the analysis of the self-reported results in the psychological domain of TFI, it might also be concluded that psychological components were at a higher level in the low adherence group in comparison to medium and high adherence groups. Earlier studies showed that DM2 patients are predestined to cognitive impairment and the changes affect adherence. For example, Tamura et al. (2018) showed that frailty and cognitive impairment are prevalent among patients with the cardiometabolic disease [63]. According to Munshi (2017), diabetes is a risk factor for the development of vascular as well as neurodegenerative dementia [64]. Considering what was mentioned above, patients with cognitive impairment may double medication doses or forget to take it, forget insulin injections and monitor blood glucose, as well as eat on time [19]. Apart from memory issues, half of the respondents in the study reported mood changes over the last month and the same number of them experienced nervousness. People with diabetes are two to three times more likely to develop depressive symptoms. Depressive symptoms are common in patients with uncontrolled type 2 diabetes who also have neuropathy and retinopathy. Hypertension, cardiovascular disease, and an unhealthy diet have been associated with depression [65,66].

In the other study of patients with DM2 (mean age 75.2 years old) carried out in Portugal, the group 22.3% had cognitive impairment, 16% had depression and 23.4% had anxiety. Those authors showed that higher anxiety and depression were associated with non-adherence to medication and to physical activity [19]. The analysis of the self-reported data in comparison to other studies confirms that planning proper management of diabetes mellitus in elderly patients should be based on the complex assessment of the patients in terms of frailty syndrome and its components (physical, psychological, and social). Frailty is the consequence of the interaction between the aging process and some chronic diseases and conditions that compromise functional systems [67].

Studies have shown that there are three factors of independent predictors of the chance of qualifying for non-adherence in the elderly, namely TFI score, male gender, and the number of medications taken daily by the patient. Self-report studies showed that each point obtained in the TFI scale increased the chance of qualifying a patient to the non-adherence group. Fragility negatively affected adherence by patients with other chronic diseases.

Another study from Poland shows that the coexistence of frailty syndrome has a negative impact on the adherence of older patients with hypertension [68]. In the study by Jankowska-Polańska et al. (2016), frail patients with hypertension had lower medication adherence in comparison to the non-frail subjects (6.60 ± 1.89 vs. 7.11 ± 1.42; $p = 0.028$) [69]. Frailty was associated with poor medication adherence in the study conducted among Chinese community-dwelling older patients with chronic diseases. In this study, authors concluded that medication necessity and medication concerns attenuated the total effect of frailty on medication adherence by 13.6% and 70.3% respectively [70]. The results above seem to confirm the opinion by Strain et al. (2021)—they are of the opinion that "frailty, rather than age, determines the prognosis for older adults with diabetes and should therefore be a key determinant of target setting and treatment choices when individualizing care" [71].

The self-reported study showed additionally that a significant predictor of non-adherence, except for TFI, was being male—it increased the chance of being qualified to the non-adherence group by 2954 times in comparison to being female. It was also found in the research of Horii et al. (2019) that being male was a significant predictor of adherence (OR 0.45, 95% CI 0.23–0.89, $p = 0.022$) [72]. It is worth mentioning that the impact of gender on adherence in DM2 patients was reported in existing studies heterogeneously. In the study by Demoz et al. (2020) predictors statistically associated with poor adherence were being female and the presence of at least one diabetic complication [73]. In the study by Aloudah et al. (2018) gender did not determine the level of adherence to oral hypoglycemic agents and lower adherence was associated with younger age, higher numbers of non-oral hypoglycemic agents, and higher HbA1c levels [74]. Gender did not influence adherence in the research by Aminde et al. (2019) either. In multivariable analysis, authors showed that an age above 60 years, alcohol consumption, and insulin-only therapy were associated with non-adherence [20].

The third aspect which affected adherence in the research was the number of medications taken by a patient daily. The odd ratio for all the medications taken daily was OR 0.847 and each extra tablet decreased the chance of being qualified to the non-adherence group by 15.3%. The method of DM treatment and the number of diabetic medications did not determine adherence.

Polypharmacy has previously been shown to be inversely associated with medication adherence in several studies of patients with DM2 [74,75] and in studies of patients with other chronic diseases [76,77]. The self-reported findings in correlation with the results by other researchers suggest reducing the number of medications to the most necessary ones to maintain optimal health conditions in over 60 years old with DM2, co-existent diseases, and frailty syndrome. It seems to be one of the non-adherence prophylaxis methods. The self-reported study also indicated the factors of non-adherence in over 60 years old DM2 patients. The similarities and differences between the results of the study and the results achieved by other researchers in terms of non-adherence predictors indicated a need for more personalized drug selection and therapeutic management to improve clinical outcomes in this group. It is important to notice that a lot of research cited in the discussion above is concentrated on adherence in respect to DM2, elderly age or frail patients with other chronic diseases. It stems from the deficits in literature on the topic of adherence, DM2, old age and frailty syndrome.

We suggest preceding the stage of planning proper diabetes management with a complex assessment of DM elderly patients for the occurrence of frailty syndrome and its components (physical, psychological, and social) with the use of a standardized instrument. We also suggest repeating the assessment in regular intervals or when needed to optimize health care. Moreover, there is a need for more personalized drug selection and therapeutic management to improve clinical outcomes in this group. The complex assessment of DM elderly patients for the occurrence of frailty syndrome and its components will allow members of the therapeutic team (doctors, nurses, social workers, nutritionists, rehabilitators) to jointly develop and implement individualized interventions aimed at the patient's needs to improve his adherence to medication. Rather, the focus should be on preventing non-adherence at an early stage of the disease by taking steps in the right order, i.e., (1) assessing the presence of the patient's weakness syndrome, (2) undertaking interventions aimed at the patient's physical, psychological, or social sphere depending on the assessment result, aimed at optimizing his adherence, (3) evaluating the medication adherence and glycemic control. However, checking the effectiveness of such a solution requires further research.

The first crucial limitation of the study derives from a small sample group analyzed and the limitation to one voivodship. The second is that only a questionnaire was used to assess adherence. The use of an analysis of pharmacy registers and medication use control in addition to the questionnaire would significantly increase the clinical value of the analysis however as Denicolò et al. (2021) notice there is no golden standard to assess adherence [56]. The third limitation referred to the ACDS questionnaire which only examined adherence in terms of pharmacotherapy, while in DM patients in the context of adherence, there are other elements equally essential such as regular physical activity, adherence with dietary recommendations, regular blood pressure, and glycemia measurements, etc.

5. Conclusions

Frailty syndrome was found in four-fifths of the DM2 elderly patients and it affected the adherence to medication in this group. The low adherence group achieved higher overall TFI scores and separately higher ones in physical and psychological domains in comparison to medium and high adherence groups. The independent predictors affecting non-adherence included three factors: a TFI score, male gender, and the number of all medications taken by a patient daily.

Author Contributions: I.B., K.S. and I.U.: Substantial contributions to conception and design, or acquisition of data, or analysis and interpretation of data. I.B., K.S. and I.U.: Manuscript draft or revising it critically for important intellectual content. I.B., K.S. and I.U.: Given final approval of the version to be published. Each author should have participated sufficiently in the work to take public responsibility for appropriate portions of the content. I.B., K.S. and I.U.: Agreed to be accountable for all aspects of the work in ensuring that questions related to the accuracy or integrity of any part of the work are appropriately investigated and resolved. All authors have read and agreed to the published version of the manuscript.

Funding: This research received no external funding.

Institutional Review Board Statement: The approval of the Bioethics Committee at the Medical University of Wrocław (approval number KB—207/2018) was obtained and the requirements of the Helsinki Declaration of 1975 (amended in 2000) and Good Clinical Practice were met.

Informed Consent Statement: Informed consent was obtained from all patients involved in the study.

Data Availability Statement: Data confirming the reported results can be found at the Department of Nursing of the University of Zielona Góra. Responsible person: Iwona Bonikowska.

Acknowledgments: We would like to thank you all the patients participating in the study.

Conflicts of Interest: The authors declare no conflict of interest.

References

1. Ogura, S.; Jakovljevic, M.M. Editorial: Global Population Aging—Health Care, Social and Economic Consequences. *Front. Public Health* **2018**, *6*, 335. [CrossRef] [PubMed]
2. Sinclair, A.; Saeedi, P.; Kaundal, A.; Karuranga, S.; Malanda, B.; Williams, R. Diabetes and global ageing among 65–99-year-old adults: Findings from the International Diabetes Federation Diabetes Atlas, 9th edition. *Diabetes Res. Clin. Pract.* **2020**, *162*, 108078. [CrossRef] [PubMed]
3. Goyal, R.; Jialal, I. *Diabetes Mellitus Type 2*; StatPearls Publishing: Treasure Island, FL, USA, 2022. Available online: https://www.ncbi.nlm.nih.gov/books/NBK513253/ (accessed on 16 March 2022).
4. Kao, C.C.; Hsieh, H.M.; Lee, D.Y.; Hsieh, K.P.; Sheu, S.J. Importance of medication adherence in treatment needed diabetic retinopathy. *Sci. Rep.* **2021**, *11*, 19100. [CrossRef] [PubMed]
5. Bello-Chavolla, O.Y.; Rojas-Martinez, R.; Aguilar-Salinas, C.A.; Hernández-Avila, M. Epidemiology of diabetes mellitus in Mexico. *Nutr. Rev.* **2017**, *75*, 4–12. [CrossRef] [PubMed]
6. Yoon, S.J.; Kim, K.I. Frailty and Disability in Diabetes. *Ann. Geriatr. Med. Res.* **2019**, *23*, 165–169. [CrossRef] [PubMed]
7. Bujnowska-Fedak, M.M.; Gwyther, H.; Szwamel, K.; D'Avanzo, B.; Holland, C.; Shaw, R.L.; Kurpas, D. A qualitative study examining everyday frailty management strategies adopted by Polish stakeholders. *Eur. J. Gen. Pract.* **2019**, *25*, 197–204. [CrossRef] [PubMed]
8. Fried, L.P.; Tangen, C.M.; Walston, J.; Newman, A.B.; Hirsch, C.; Gottdiener, J.; Seeman, T.; Tracy, R.; Kop, W.J.; Burke, G.; et al. Frailty in older adults: Evidence for a phenotype. *J. Gerontol. A Biol. Sci. Med. Sci.* **2001**, *56*, 146–156. [CrossRef] [PubMed]
9. O'Caoimh, R.; Galluzzo, L.; Rodríguez-Laso, Á.; Van der Heyden, J.; Ranhoff, A.H.; Lamprini-Koula, M.; Ciutan, M.; López-Samaniego, L.; Carcaillon-Bentata, L.; Kennelly, S.; et al. Prevalence of frailty at population level in European ADVANTAGE Joint Action Member States: A systematic review and meta-analysis. *Ann. Dell'istituto Super. Di Sanita* **2018**, *54*, 226–238.
10. Chhetri, J.K.; Zheng, Z.; Xu, X.; Ma, C.; Chan, P. The prevalence and incidence of frailty in Pre-diabetic and diabetic community-dwelling older population: Results from Beijing longitudinal study of aging II (BLSA-II). *BMC Geriatr.* **2017**, *17*, 47. [CrossRef] [PubMed]
11. MacKenzie, H.T.; Tugwell, B.; Rockwood, K.; Theou, O. Frailty and Diabetes in Older Hospitalized Adults: The Case for Routine Frailty Assessment. *Can. J. Diabetes* **2020**, *44*, 241–245. [CrossRef] [PubMed]

12. Chao, C.; Wang, J.; Chien, K.L.; COhort of GEriatric Nephrology in NTUH (COGENT) Study Group. Both pre-frailty and frailty increase healthcare utilization and adverse health outcomes in patients with type 2 diabetes mellitus. *Cardiovasc. Diabetol.* **2018**, *17*, 130. [CrossRef]
13. Angulo, J.; El Assar, M.; Álvarez-Bustos, A.; Rodríguez-Mañas, L. Physical activity and exercise: Strategies to manage frailty. *Redox. Biol.* **2020**, *35*, 101513. [CrossRef] [PubMed]
14. Ida, S.; Kaneko, R.; Imataka, K.; Murata, K. Relationship between frailty and mortality, hospitalization, and cardiovascular diseases in diabetes: A systematic review and meta-analysis. *Cardiovasc. Diabetol.* **2019**, *18*, 81. [CrossRef]
15. Dent, E.; Morley, J.E.; Cruz-Jentoft, A.J.; Woodhouse, L.; Rodríguez-Mañas, L.; Fried, L.P.; Woo, J.; Aprahamian, I.; Sanford, A.; Lundy, J.; et al. Physical Frailty: ICFSR International Clinical Practice Guidelines for Identification and Management. *Nutr. Health Aging* **2019**, *23*, 771–787. [CrossRef] [PubMed]
16. Lang, P.O.; Michel, J.P.; Zekry, D. Frailty syndrome: A transitional state in a dynamic process. *Gerontology* **2009**, *55*, 539–549. [CrossRef]
17. World Health Organization. Adherence to Long-Term Therapies: Evidence for Action. Available online: https://www.who.int/chp/knowledge/publications/adherence_full_report.pdf?ua=1 (accessed on 19 January 2021).
18. Fernandez-Lazaro, C.I.; García-González, J.M.; Adams, D.P.; Fernandez-Lazaro, D.; Mielgo-Ayuso, J.; Caballero-Garcia, A.; Racionero, F.M.; Córdova, A.; Miron-Canelo, J.A. Adherence to treatment and related factors among patients with chronic conditions in primary care: A cross-sectional study. *BMC Fam. Pract.* **2019**, *20*, 132. [CrossRef]
19. Mendes, R.; Martins, S.; Fernandes, L. Adherence to Medication, Physical Activity and Diet in Older Adults With Diabetes: Its Association With Cognition, Anxiety and Depression. *J. Clin. Med. Res.* **2019**, *11*, 583–592. [CrossRef] [PubMed]
20. Aminde, L.N.; Tindong, M.; Ngwasiri, C.A.; Aminde, J.A.; Njim, T.; Fondong, A.A.; Takah, N.F. Adherence to antidiabetic medication and factors associated with non-adherence among patients with type-2 diabetes mellitus in two regional hospitals in Cameroon. *BMC Endocr. Disord.* **2019**, *19*, 35. [CrossRef]
21. Hatah, E.; Rahim, N.; Makmor-Bakry, M.; Mohamed Shah, N.; Mohamad, N.; Ahmad, M.; Haron, N.H.; Hwe, C.S.; Wah, A.T.M.; Hassan, F.; et al. Adherence Development and validation of Malaysia Medication Assessment Tool (MyMAAT) for diabetic patients. *PLoS ONE* **2020**, *15*, e0241909. [CrossRef]
22. Tamura, Y.; Omura, T.; Toyoshima, K.; Araki, A. Nutrition Management in Older Adults with Diabetes: A Review on the Importance of Shifting Prevention Strategies from Metabolic Syndrome to Frailty. *Nutrients* **2020**, *12*, 3367. [CrossRef]
23. Pobrotyn, P.; Pasieczna, A.; Diakowska, D.; Uchmanowicz, B.; Mazur, G.; Banasik, M.; Kołtuniuk, A. Evaluation of Frailty Syndrome and Adherence to Recommendations in Elderly Patients with Hypertension. *J. Clin. Med.* **2021**, *10*, 3771. [CrossRef] [PubMed]
24. Uchmanowicz, I.; Nessler, J.; Gobbens, R.; Gackowski, A.; Kurpas, D.; Straburzyńska-Migaj, E.; Kałuzna-Oleksy, M.; Jankowska, E.A. Coexisting Frailty with Heart Failure. *Front. Physiol.* **2019**, *10*, 791. [CrossRef] [PubMed]
25. Bąk, E.; Młynarska, A.; Marcisz, C.; Bobiński, R.; Sternal, D.; Młynarski, R. The influence of frailty syndrome on quality of life in elderly patients with type 2 diabetes. *Qual. Life Res.* **2021**, *30*, 2487–2495. [CrossRef] [PubMed]
26. de Lima, B.F.; Gama, A.G.D.; da Nóbrega Dias, V.; da Silva, E.M.T.; da Costa Cavalcanti, F.A.; Gazzola, J.M. The frailty syndrome in older adults with type 2 diabetes mellitus and associated factors. *Rev. Bras. De Geriatr. E Gerontol.* **2020**, *23*, e190196. [CrossRef]
27. Mone, P.; Gambardella, J.; Lombardi, A.; Pansini, A.; De Gennaro, S.; Leo, A.L.; Famiglietti, M.; Marro, A.; Morgante, M.; Frullone, S.; et al. Correlation of physical and cognitive impairment in diabetic and hypertensive frail older adults. *Cardiovasc. Diabetol.* **2022**, *21*, 10. [CrossRef] [PubMed]
28. Thein, F.S.; Li, Y.; Nyunt, M.S.Z.; Gao, Q.; Wee, S.L.; Ng, T.P. Physical frailty and cognitive impairment is associated with diabetes and adversely impact functional status and mortality. *Postgrad. Med.* **2018**, *130*, 561–567. [CrossRef] [PubMed]
29. Casals, C.; Casals Sánchez, J.L.; Suárez Cadenas, E.; Aguilar-Trujillo, M.P.; Estébanez Carvajal, F.M.; Vázquez-Sánchez, M.Á. Fragilidad en el adulto mayor con diabetes mellitus tipo 2 y su relación con el control glucémico, perfil lipídico, tensión arterial, equilibrio, grado de discapacidad y estado nutricional [Frailty in older adults with type 2 diabetes mellitus and its relation with glucemic control, lipid profile, blood pressure, balance, disability grade and nutritional status]. *Nutr. Hosp.* **2018**, *35*, 820–826. [PubMed]
30. Dalon, F.; Van Ganse, E.; Correia Da Silva, C.; Nachbaur, G.; Saïl, L.; Belhassen, M. Revue générale sur l'adhésion aux traitements inhalés de la BPCO [Therapeutic adherence in chronic obstructive pulmonary disease: A literature review]. *Rev. Mal. Respir.* **2019**, *36*, 801–849. [CrossRef] [PubMed]
31. Rezaei, M.; Valiee, S.; Tahan, M.; Ebtekar, F.; Ghanei Gheshlagh, R. Barriers of medication adherence in patients with type-2 diabetes: A pilot qualitative study. *Diabetes Metab. Syndr. Obes.* **2019**, *1*, 589–599. [CrossRef] [PubMed]
32. Alshehri, K.A.; Altuwaylie, T.M.; Alqhtani, A.; Albawab, A.A.; Almalki, A.H. Type 2 Diabetic Patients Adherence Towards Their Medications. *Cureus* **2020**, *12*, e6932. [CrossRef] [PubMed]
33. Świątoniowska-Lonc, N.; Tański, W.; Polański, J.; Jankowska-Polańska, B.; Mazur, G. Psychosocial Determinants of Treatment Adherence in Patients with Type 2 Diabetes—A Review. *Diabetes Metab. Syndr. Obes.* **2021**, *16*, 2701–2715. [CrossRef] [PubMed]
34. Kefale, B.; Tadesse, Y.; Alebachew, M.; Engidawork, E. Management Practice, and Adherence and Its Contributing Factors among Patients with Chronic Kidney Disease at Tikur Anbessa Specialized Hospital: A Hospital Based Cross-Sectional Study. *Int. J. Nephrol.* **2018**, *29*, 2903139.

35. Algabbani, F.M.; Algabbani, A.M. Treatment adherence among patients with hypertension: Findings from a cross-sectional study. *Clin. Hypertens.* **2020**, *26*, 18. [CrossRef] [PubMed]
36. Mekonen, K.K.; Yismaw, M.B.; Abiye, A.A.; Tadesse, T.A. Adherence to Benzathine Penicillin G Secondary Prophylaxis and Its Determinants in Patients with Rheumatic Heart Disease at a Cardiac Center of an Ethiopian Tertiary Care Teaching Hospital. *Patient Prefer. Adherence* **2020**, *14*, 343–352. [CrossRef] [PubMed]
37. Enricho Nkhoma, D.; Jenya Soko, C.; Joseph Banda, K.; Greenfield, D.; Li, Y.J.; Iqbal, U. Impact of DSMES app interventions on medication adherence in type 2 diabetes mellitus: Systematic review and meta-analysis. *BMJ Health Care Inform.* **2021**, *28*, e100291. [CrossRef] [PubMed]
38. Tan, J.P.; Cheng, K.K.F.; Siah, R.C. A systematic review and meta-analysis on the effectiveness of education on medication adherence for patients with hypertension, hyperlipidaemia and diabetes. *J. Adv. Nurs.* **2019**, *75*, 2478–2494. [CrossRef] [PubMed]
39. Wleklik, M.; Denfeld, Q.; Lisiak, M.; Czapla, M.; Kałużna-Oleksy, M.; Uchmanowicz, I. Frailty Syndrome in Older Adults with Cardiovascular Diseases-What Do We Know and What Requires Further Research? *Int. J. Environ. Res. Public Health* **2022**, *19*, 2234. [CrossRef] [PubMed]
40. WSOZ-II.0123.28.2018; NFZ-Załącznik nr 1 Do Pisma Znak. National Health Fund: Warszawa, Poland, 2018.
41. Kubica, A.; Kosobucka, A.; Michalski, P.; Pietrzykowski, Ł.; Jurek, A.; Wawrzyniak, M.; Kasprzak, Ł. Skala adherence w chorobach przewlekłych—nowe narzędzie do badania realizacji planu terapeutycznego. *Folia Cardiol.* **2017**, *12*, 19.
42. Gobbens, R.J.; van Assen, M.A.; Luijkx, K.G.; Wijnen-Sponselee, M.T.; Schols, J.M. The Tilburg Frailty Indicator: Psychometric properties. *J. Am. Med. Dir. Assoc.* **2010**, *11*, 344–355. [CrossRef] [PubMed]
43. Uchmanowicz, I.; Jankowska-Polańska, B.; Uchmanowicz, B.; Kowalczuk, K.; Gobbens, R.J. Validity and Reliability of the Polish Version of the Tilburg Frailty Indicator (TFI). *J. Frailty Aging* **2016**, *5*, 27–32. [CrossRef] [PubMed]
44. Uchmanowicz, I.; Santiago, L.M. The Tilburg Frailty Indicator (TFI): New Evidence for Its Validity. *Clin. Interv. Aging* **2020**, *15*, 265–274.
45. Uchmanowicz, I.; Jankowska-Polańska, B.; Łoboz-Rudnicka, M.; Manulik, S.; Łoboz-Grudzień, K.; Gobbens, R.J. Cross-cultural adaptation and reliability testing of the Tilburg Frailty Indicator for optimizing care of Polish patients with frailty syndrome. *Clin. Interv. Aging* **2014**, *25*, 997–1001. [CrossRef] [PubMed]
46. Bray, G.A.; Gray, D.S. Obesity. Part I—Pathogenesis. *West. J. Med.* **1988**, *149*, 429–441. [CrossRef] [PubMed]
47. American Diabetes Association. Lifestyle Management: Standards of Medical Care in Diabetes. *Diabetes Care* **2018**, *41*, 38–50. [CrossRef] [PubMed]
48. Kong, L.N.; Lyu, Q.; Yao, H.Y.; Yang, L.; Chen, S.Z. The prevalence of frailty among community-dwelling older adults with diabetes: A meta-analysis. *Int. J. Nurs. Stud.* **2021**, *119*, 103952. [CrossRef] [PubMed]
49. Manfredi, G.; Midão, L.; Paúl, C.; Cena, C.; Duarte, M.; Costa, E. Prevalence of frailty status among the European elderly population: Findings from the Survey of Health, Aging and Retirement in Europe. *Geriatr. Gerontol. Int.* **2019**, *19*, 723–729. [CrossRef] [PubMed]
50. Cobo, A.; Vázquez, L.A.; Reviriego, J.; Rodríguez-Mañas, L. Impact of frailty in older patients with diabetes mellitus: An overview. *Endocrinol. Nutr.* **2016**, *63*, 291–303. [CrossRef] [PubMed]
51. Saum, K.U.; Dieffenbach, A.K.; Müller, H.; Holleczek, B.; Hauer, K.; Brenner, H. Frailty prevalence and 10-year survival in community-dwelling older adults: Results from the ESTHER cohort study. *Eur. J. Epidemiol.* **2014**, *29*, 171–179. [CrossRef] [PubMed]
52. Ferri-Guerra, J.; Aparicio-Ugarriza, R.; Salguero, D.; Baskaran, D.; Mohammed, Y.N.; Florez, H.; Ruiz, J.G. The Association of Frailty with Hospitalizations and Mortality among Community Dwelling Older Adults with Diabetes. *J. Frailty Aging* **2020**, *9*, 94–100. [CrossRef] [PubMed]
53. Bouillon, K.; Kivimäki, M.; Hamer, M.; Shipley, M.J.; Akbaraly, T.N.; Tabak, A.; Singh-Manoux, A.; Batty, G.D. Diabetes risk factors, diabetes risk algorithms, and the prediction of future frailty: The Whitehall II prospective cohort study. *J. Am. Med. Dir. Assoc.* **2013**, *14*, 851.e1–851.e6. [CrossRef] [PubMed]
54. Chao, C.T.; Wang, J.; Huang, J.W.; Chan, D.C.; Chien, K.L.; COhort of GEriatric Nephrology in NTUH (COGENT) Study Group. Hypoglycemic episodes are associated with an increased risk of incident frailty among new onset diabetic patients. *J. Diabetes Complicat.* **2020**, *34*, 107492. [CrossRef] [PubMed]
55. García-Esquinas, E.; Graciani, A.; Guallar-Castillón, P.; López-García, E.; Rodríguez-Mañas, L.; Rodríguez-Artalejo, F. Diabetes and risk of frailty and its potential mechanisms: A prospective cohort study of older adults. *J. Am. Med. Dir. Assoc.* **2015**, *16*, 748–754. [CrossRef] [PubMed]
56. Denicolò, S.; Perco, P.; Thöni, S.; Mayer, G. Non-adherence to antidiabetic and cardiovascular drugs in type 2 diabetes mellitus and its association with renal and cardiovascular outcomes: A narrative review. *J. Diabetes Complicat.* **2021**, *35*, 107931. [CrossRef] [PubMed]
57. Park, S.W.; Goodpaster, B.H.; Strotmeyer, E.S.; Kuller, L.H.; Broudeau, R.; Kammerer, C.; de Rekeneire, N.; Harris, T.B.; Schwartz, A.V.; Tylavsky, F.A.; et al. Accelerated loss of skeletal muscle strength in older adults with type 2 diabetes: The health, aging, and body composition study. *Diabetes Care* **2007**, *30*, 1507–1512. [CrossRef] [PubMed]
58. Sayer, A.A.; Dennison, E.M.; Syddall, H.E.; Gilbody, H.J.; Phillips, D.I.; Cooper, C. Type 2 diabetes, muscle strength, and impaired physical function: The tip of the iceberg? *Diabetes Care* **2005**, *28*, 2541–2542. [CrossRef] [PubMed]

59. Bourdel-Marchasson, I.; Catheline, G.; Regueme, S.; Danet-Lamasou, M.; Barse, E.; Ratsimbazafy, F.; Rodriguez-Manas, L.; Hood, K.; Sinclair, A.J. Frailty and Brain-Muscle Correlates in Older People with Type 2 Diabetes: A structural-MRI Explorative Study. *J. Nutr. Health Aging* **2019**, *23*, 637–640. [CrossRef] [PubMed]
60. Gundmi, S.; Maiya, A.G.; Bhat, A.K.; Ravishankar, N.; Hande, M.H.; Rajagopal, K.V. Hand dysfunction in type 2 diabetes mellitus: Systematic review with meta-analysis. *Ann. Phys. Rehabil. Med.* **2018**, *61*, 99–104. [CrossRef] [PubMed]
61. Motta, F.; Sica, A.; Selmi, C. Frailty in Rheumatic Diseases. *Front. Immunol.* **2020**, *29*, 576134. [CrossRef] [PubMed]
62. Le, T.; Toscani, M.; Colaizzi, J. Telepharmacy: A New Paradigm for Our Profession. *J. Pharm. Pract.* **2020**, *33*, 176–182. [CrossRef] [PubMed]
63. Tamura, Y.; Ishikawa, J.; Fujiwara, Y.; Tanaka, M.; Kanazawa, N.; Chiba, Y.; Iizuka, A.; Kaito, S.; Tanaka, J.; Sugie, M.; et al. Prevalence of frailty, cognitive impairment, and sarcopenia in outpatients with cardiometabolic disease in a frailty clinic. *BMC Geriatr.* **2018**, *18*, 264. [CrossRef] [PubMed]
64. Munshi, M.N. Cognitive dysfunction in older adults with diabetes: What a clinician needs to know. *Diabetes Care* **2017**, *40*, 461–467. [CrossRef] [PubMed]
65. Aljohani, W.; Algohani, L.; Alzahrani, A.; Bazuhair, M.; Bawakid, A.; Aljuid, L.; Al-Ahdal, A. Prevalence of Depression Among Patients With Type 2 Diabetes at King Abdullah Medical City. *Cureus* **2021**, *13*, e18457. [CrossRef] [PubMed]
66. Mathur, D.; Anand, A.; Srivastava, V.; Patil, S.S.; Singh, A.; Rajesh, S.K.; Nagendra, H.R.; Nagarathna, R. Depression in High-Risk Type 2 Diabetes Adults. *Ann. Neurosci.* **2020**, *27*, 204–213. [CrossRef] [PubMed]
67. Angulo, J.; El Assar, M.; Rodríguez-Mañas, L. Frailty and sarcopenia as the basis for the phenotypic manifestation of chronic diseases in older adults. *Mol. Asp. Med.* **2016**, *50*, 1–32. [CrossRef] [PubMed]
68. Uchmanowicz, B.; Chudiak, A.; Uchmanowicz, I.; Mazur, G. How May Coexisting Frailty Influence Adherence to Treatment in Elderly Hypertensive Patients? *Int. J. Hypertens.* **2019**, *2019*, 5245184. [CrossRef] [PubMed]
69. Jankowska-Polańska, B.; Dudek, K.; Szymanska-Chabowska, A.; Uchmanowicz, I. The influence of frailty syndrome on medication adherence among elderly patients with hypertension. *Clin. Interv. Aging* **2016**, *11*, 1781–1790. [CrossRef] [PubMed]
70. Qiao, X.; Tian, X.; Liu, N.; Dong, L.; Jin, Y.; Si, H.; Liu, X.; Wang, C. The association between frailty and medication adherence among community-dwelling older adults with chronic diseases: Medication beliefs acting as mediators. *Patient Educ. Couns.* **2020**, *103*, 2548–2554. [CrossRef] [PubMed]
71. Strain, W.D.; Down, S.; Brown, P.; Puttanna, A.; Sinclair, A. Diabetes and Frailty: An Expert Consensus Statement on the Management of Older Adults with Type 2 Diabetes. *Diabetes Ther.* **2021**, *12*, 1227–1247. [CrossRef] [PubMed]
72. Horii, T.; Momo, K.; Yasu, T.; Kabeya, Y.; Atsuda, K. Determination of factors affecting medication adherence in type 2 diabetes mellitus patients using a nationwide claim-based database in Japan. *PLoS ONE* **2019**, *14*, e0223431. [CrossRef] [PubMed]
73. Demoz, G.T.; Wahdey, S.; Bahrey, D.; Kahsay, H.; Woldu, G.; Niriayo, Y.L.; Collier, A. Predictors of poor adherence to antidiabetic therapy in patients with type 2 diabetes: A cross-sectional study insight from Ethiopia. *Diabetol. Metab. Syndr.* **2020**, *16*, 62. [CrossRef] [PubMed]
74. Aloudah, N.M.; Scott, N.W.; Aljadhey, H.S.; Araujo-Soares, V.; Alrubeaan, K.A.; Watson, M.C. Medication adherence among patients with Type 2 diabetes: A mixed methods study. *PLoS ONE* **2018**, *13*, e0207583. [CrossRef] [PubMed]
75. Priyanka, T.; Lekhanth, A.; Revanth, A.; Gopinath, C.; Babu, S.C. Effect of Polypharmacy on Medication Adherence in Patients with Type 2 Diabetes mellitus. *Indian J. Phar. Pract.* **2015**, *8*, 126–132. [CrossRef]
76. Akgol, J.; Erhan, E.; Ercument, O. Factors predicting treatment compliance among hypertensive patients in an urban area. *Med. Sci. Int. Med. J.* **2017**, *6*, 447–456. [CrossRef]
77. Awad, A.; Alhadab, A.; Albassam, A. Medication-Related Burden and Medication Adherence among Geriatric Patients in Kuwait: A Cross-Sectional Study. *Front. Pharmacol.* **2020**, *11*, 1296. [CrossRef] [PubMed]

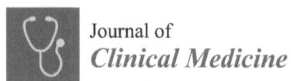

Article

The Multidimensional Prognostic Index Predicts Mortality in Older Outpatients with Cognitive Decline

Femke C. M. S. Overbeek [1], Jeannette A. Goudzwaard [1], Judy van Hemmen [2], Rozemarijn L. van Bruchem-Visser [1], Janne M. Papma [2], Harmke A. Polinder-Bos [1] and Francesco U. S. Mattace-Raso [1,*]

[1] Department of Geriatric Medicine, Erasmus MC University Medical Center, 3015 GD Rotterdam, The Netherlands; femkeoverbeek@hotmail.com (F.C.M.S.O.); j.goudzwaard@erasmusmc.nl (J.A.G.); r.l.visser@erasmusmc.nl (R.L.v.B.-V.); h.polinder-bos@erasmusmc.nl (H.A.P.-B.)

[2] Department of Neurology, Erasmus MC University Medical Center, 3015 GD Rotterdam, The Netherlands; j.vanhemmen@erasmusmc.nl (J.v.H.); j.papma@erasmusmc.nl (J.M.P.)

* Correspondence: f.mattaceraso@erasmusmc.nl; Tel.: +31-10-7035979

Abstract: Since the heterogeneity of the growing group of older outpatients with cognitive decline, it is challenging to evaluate survival rates in clinical shared decision making. The primary outcome was to determine whether the Multidimensional Prognostic Index (MPI) predicts mortality, whilst assessing the MPI distribution was considered secondary. This retrospective chart review included 311 outpatients aged ≥ 65 years and diagnosed with dementia or mild cognitive impairment (MCI). The MPI includes several domains of the comprehensive geriatric assessment (CGA). All characteristics and data to calculate the risk score and mortality data were extracted from administrative information in the database of the Alzheimer's Center and medical records. The study population (mean age 76.8 years, men = 51.4%) was divided as follows: 34.1% belonged to MPI category 1, 52.1% to MPI category 2 and 13.8% to MPI category 3. Patients with dementia have a higher mean MPI risk score than patients with MCI (0.47 vs. 0.32; $p < 0.001$). The HRs and corresponding 95% CIs for mortality in patients in MPI categories 2 and 3 were 1.67 (0.81–3.45) and 3.80 (1.56–9.24) compared with MPI category 1, respectively. This study shows that the MPI predicts mortality in outpatients with cognitive decline.

Keywords: dementia; Multidimensional Prognostic Index; cognitive decline; aging; mortality; frailty; geriatric assessment

1. Introduction

Cognitive decline is one of the most significant and common problems in older persons [1]. Dementia is an overall term for chronic and progressive neurodegenerative disorders with the loss of cognitive functioning [2]. Mild cognitive impairment (MCI) is a syndrome of having greater than expected cognitive decline for the person's age and education level, but in contrast to dementia, it does not significantly interfere with daily life activities [3]. Patients with MCI have an increased risk of developing dementia, and the conversion rate is almost 10% per year [4]. The prevalence rate of dementia in Europe in older persons aged over 65 is about 7%, and for MCI, this is four times greater [5,6]. The number of people living with dementia will double by 2050 [7]. Deaths from dementia are rising, making it the second leading cause of death in high-income countries [8]. Dementia appears to lead to higher mortality and is also associated with a loss of quality of life, higher healthcare costs, and, more often, institutionalization [9–11]. Nevertheless, it is still challenging for clinicians to inform their patients based on medical knowledge about the prognosis after being diagnosed with dementia or MCI.

The prognosis of older patients with cognitive decline is determined by their cognitive status and results from a combination of biological, functional, nutritional, environmental, psychological, and socioeconomic factors [12]. The comprehensive geriatric assessment (CGA) is the main tool to integrate information from all these domains and determine the prognosis [13]. In shared clinical decision-making, life expectancy and quality of life are important factors in evaluating diagnostic and therapeutic interventions [14]. Estimating the state of frailty and life expectancy of the patients is essential to point out the most appropriate decisions for treatment, prevention, institutionalization and care management [15]. Considering the heterogeneity of the group of patients with cognitive decline, it is challenging to evaluate survival rates.

The Multidimensional Prognostic Index (MPI) is derived from a standardized CGA. It uses a mathematic algorithm including information on eight domains relevant for assessing frail older persons (i.e., functional, cognitive and nutritional status, cohabitation status, comorbidities, polypharmacy and risk of pressure sores) using standardized and validated rating scales [13]. The MPI generates a numeric score between 0 and 1 that expresses the global risk index of multidimensional impairment. Therefore, the MPI can translate clinical outcomes of the CGA into a risk score that can predict negative outcomes. This tool has been developed and identified as well-calibrated to predict short and long-term mortality in several independent cohorts of hospitalized and community-dwelling older patients with acute and chronic diseases [1,13,14,16,17].

The present study aimed to investigate the distribution and the possible predictive value on mortality of the MPI within a population of outpatients with cognitive decline.

2. Materials and Methods

This study was a retrospective chart review study. All outpatients aged 65 years and older who were referred to the Alzheimer Center of the Erasmus MC University Medical Center, Rotterdam, from 1 January 2010 to 31 December 2020, and were primarily seen by a geriatrician were screened for inclusion in the study. Patients diagnosed with dementia or MCI after undergoing the standard workup were included. Exclusion criteria were a diagnosis of frontotemporal dementia (FTD), a psychiatric disorder and if data regarding calculating the MPI risk score was incomplete.

The present study was conducted according to the Declaration of Helsinki. In the Netherlands, ethical approval and patient consent are not required for a retrospective chart review study in which data collected during routine clinical care are extracted and analyzed anonymously. Two physicians were responsible for correctly extracting the information needed (ΓΟ, ΓMR).

All patients were included from the database of the Alzheimer's Center (n = 4461). The following data were already available: age, sex, Mini-Mental State Examination (MMSE) score and diagnosis. Information on mortality and the variables to calculate the MPI risk score were collected from the medical records. The MPI was determined based on information from eight different domains of the CGA [13]:

1. Cohabitation status was divided into three parts: living with family (with spouse and/or other relatives and/or a caregiver), institutionalized and alone;
2. Medication use was defined by the number of drugs used and was ranged into three groups: ≤ 3, from 4 to 6 and ≥ 7;
3. Functional status was evaluated by Katz's Activities of Daily Living (ADL) index [18];
4. Independence was defined by Lawton's Instrumental Activities of Daily Living (IADL) index [19];
5. Cognitive status was assessed with the Mini-Mental State Examination (MMSE). When appropriate, in case of a diverse cultural background and/or language barrier, the Rowland University Dementia Assessment Scale (RUDAS) was used [20,21];
6. Comorbidity was examined using the Cumulative Illness Rating Scale comorbidity index (CIRS-CI) [22];
7. The risk of developing pressure sores was evaluated through the Exton Smith Scale (ESS) [23];

8. Nutritional status was investigated with the Mini Nutritional Assessment short-form (MNA-SF) [24].

For each domain, a value is determined according to the conventional cutoff points derived from the literature (Table 1). Value 0 indicates no problem, 0.5 is a minor problem, and 1 is a severe problem. The sum of the calculated scores from the eight domains was divided by 8 to obtain the final MPI risk score ranging from 0 = no risk to 1 = highest risk. Additionally, the MPI was expressed as three categories of risk: MPI category 1 low risk (MPI risk score 0–0.33), MPI category 2 moderate risk (MPI risk score 0.34–0.66) and MPI category 3 high risk (MPI risk score 0.67–1) [13].

Table 1. MPI risk score is assigned to each domain based on the severity of the problem.

Assessment	No Problem (Value = 0)	Minor Problem (Value = 0.5)	Severe Problem (Value = 1)
CHS	Living with family	Institutionalized	Alone
Number of medications	0–3	4–6	≥ 7
ADL	6–5	4–3	2–0
IADL	8–6	5–4	3–0
MMSE (n = 289)	28–30	25–27	0–24
RUDAS (n = 22)	26–30	17–25	0–16
CIRS-CI	0	1–2	≥ 3
ESS	16–20	10–15	5–9
MNA-SF	≥ 12	8–11	0–7

Notes: Values are given in points. Abbreviations: MPI, Multidimensional Prognostic Index; CHS, cohabitation status; ADL, Activities of Daily Living; IADL, Instrumental Activities of Daily Living; MMSE, Mini-Mental State Examination; RUDAS, Rowland Universal Dementia Assessment Scale; CIRS-CI, Cumulative Illness Rating Scale Comorbidity Index; ESS, Exton Smith Scale; MNA-SF, Multi Nutritional Assessment Short Form.

The diagnosis of dementia was reached within the Alzheimer Center's team during weekly multidisciplinary consultation, according to the Diagnostic and Statistical Manual of Mental Disorders (DSM) 5th edition criteria [25].

Baseline characteristics were reported as frequencies for categorical variables and mean ± standard deviation (SD) for continuous variables. Comparisons across MPI categories were performed using a Chi-squared test for categorical variables and a one-way ANOVA test for continuous variables. For the comparisons between dementia and MCI, a Chi-squared test was used for categorical variables, and an independent samples T-test was used for continuous variables. To investigate the predictive role of MPI upon mortality, a Cox regression model was used to assess the hazard ratios (HR) and 95% confidence interval (95% CI). The model was adjusted for age and sex. Only 12 patients belonged to the MPI category 3, and we repeated the Cox regression analysis combining MPI categories 2 and 3 for further analysis. All statistical analyses were performed using SPSS Statistics 27. Two-sided p-values < 0.05 were considered statistically significant.

3. Results

The database included 4461 patients, of which 3802 were not included because of having visited another center, not being primarily seen by a geriatrician or age < 65 years. A total of 659 patients were screened for inclusion, and eventually, the study population included 311 patients (mean age 76.8 ± 6 years, 160 men (51.4%)) (Figure 1).

In total, 73% of patients had dementia, and 27% had MCI. In the dementia group, 45.4% were diagnosed with Alzheimer's disease, 16.7% with vascular dementia, 18.9% with mixed dementia (Alzheimer's and vascular dementia) and 18.9% with other forms of dementia (seven patients with Lewy body dementia, two with logopenic progressive aphasia, two with corticobasal degeneration and 32 remained undifferentiated). Table 2 shows the clinical characteristics of the patients included in the study. In total, 106 (34.1%) patients belonged to MPI category 1, 162 (52.1%) to MPI category 2 and 43 (13.8%) to MPI category 3. The majority (66.9%) of the patients lived together with family, 29.9% lived alone, and 3.2% were institutionalized. The daily number of drugs taken was high at 6.1 ± 3.9, and the comorbidity index (CIRS-CI) was rated at 3.2 ± 1.7. The patients had a moderate degree of dependence (ADL 5.3 ± 1.3; IADL 4.8 ± 2.4) but were cognitively impaired according to cognitive screening tests (MMSE 21.8 ± 5; RUDAS 18.8 ± 5.5). The cognitive status was scored using the MMSE in 289 patients (92.9%) and the RUDAS in 22 patients (7.1%). The risk of pressure ulcers was low (ESS score 17.5 ± 2.4), probably since the study population consisted of outpatients. With a mean MNA-SF of 11 ± 2.3, there was a moderate risk of malnutrition.

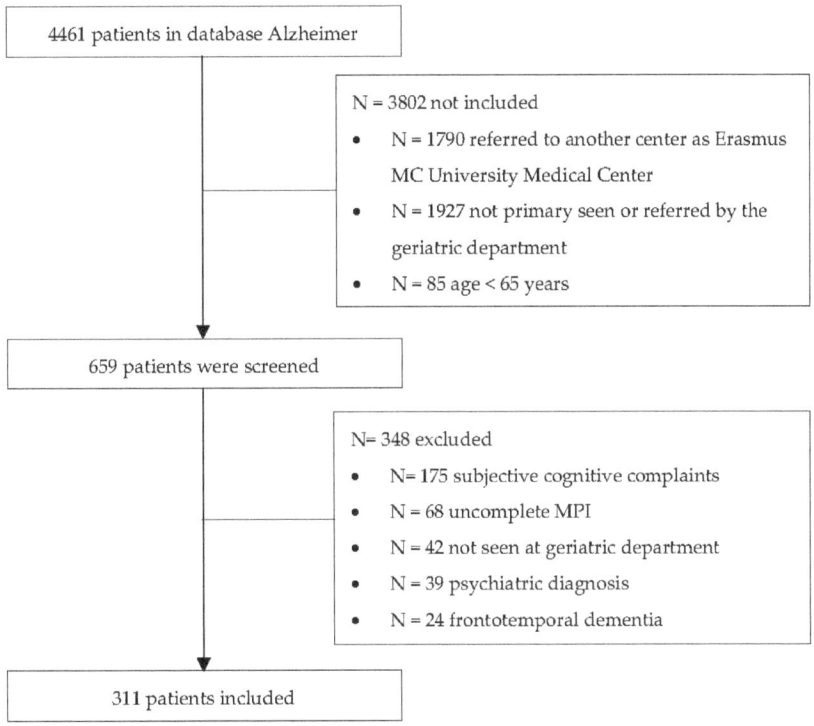

Figure 1. Flow chart of the study.

Table 3 presents the characteristics of the patients according to their MPI category. A higher MPI category is associated with a higher prevalence of dementia and a lower prevalence of MCI ($p < 0.001$ between MPI 1 and MPI 2/3; $p = 0.008$ between MPI 2 and MPI 3). Patients in MPI categories 2 and 3 were older ($p < 0.05$) than patients in MPI category 1. As expected, participants in higher MPI categories were more likely to use more medication, suffer from more comorbidities, be less independent in activities of daily living, have higher pressure sore risk and have a higher risk of malnutrition ($p < 0.001$ in all domains). The cognitive status of patients in MPI categories 2 and 3 was worse than in MPI category 1 ($p < 0.001$). There were fewer men in the dementia group than in the MCI group (45.4% vs. 67.9%, respectively; $p < 0.001$). The mean MPI risk score was higher in patients with dementia than with MCI (0.47 ± 0.18 vs. 0.32 ± 0.15; $p < 0.001$). Patients with dementia had worse ADL and IADL scores, cognitive status according to the MMSE or RUDAS, pressure sore risk and malnutrition risk ($p < 0.001$ in all domains) than patients with MCI. They were also more likely to use more medications than patients with MCI ($p = 0.035$).

Table 2. General characteristics (*n* = 311).

Men	160
Age (years)	76.8 ± 6
MCI	84
Dementia	227
Alzheimer's disease	103
Vascular dementia	38
Mixed dementia	43
Other	43
MPI-1	106
MPI-2	162
MPI-3	43
MPI risk score	0.43 ± 0.19
CHS	
With family	208
Institutionalized	10
Alone	93
Number of medications	6.1 ± 3.9
ADL	5.3 ± 1.3
IADL	4.8 ± 2.4

Notes: Values are given as n or mean ± SD. Abbreviations: SD, standard deviation; MCI, mild cognitive impairment; MPI, Multidimensional Prognostic Index; CHS, cohabitation status; ADL, activities of daily living; IADL, instrumental activities of daily living; MMSE, Mini-Mental State Examination; RUDAS, Rowland Universal Dementia Assessment Scale; CIRS-CI, Cumulative Illness Rating Scale Comorbidity Index; ESS, Exton Smith Scale; MNA-SF, Multi Nutritional Assessment Short Form.

Table 3. General characteristics according to MPI categories.

Variable	MPI 1 (*n* = 106)	MPI 2 (*n* = 162)	MPI 3 (*n* = 43)	*p*-Value
Men	56	88	16	* ns ** ns *** 0.046
Age (years)	75.6 ± 5.8	77.1 ± 5.7	78.3 ± 6.9	* 0.045 ** 0.012 *** ns
Dementia	58	127	42	* <0.001
MCI	48	35	1	** <0.001 *** 0.008
CHS				
With family	88	105	15	
Institutionalized	0	5	5	
Alone	18	52	23	
Number of medications	3.3 ± 3.1	7 ± 3.3	9.9 ± 3.3	<0.001
ADL	5.9 ± 0.4	5.5 ± 0.9	3.1 ± 1.6	<0.001
IADL	6.5 ± 1.7	4.4 ± 2.2	2 ± 1.6	<0.001
MMSE	24.5 ± 3.9	20.7 ± 5.1	19.1 ± 4.4	* <0.001 ** <0.001 *** ns
RUDAS	21.8 ± 5	18.3 ± 5.5	17.2 ± 6.1	ns
CIRS-CI	1.9 ± 1.3	3.6 ± 1.4	4.8 ± 1.4	<0.001

Notes: Values are given as n or mean ± SD. Abbreviations: SD, standard deviation; ns, not significant; MCI, mild cognitive impairment; MPI, Multidimensional Prognostic Index; CHS, cohabitation status; ADL, activities of daily living; IADL, instrumental activities of daily living; MMSE, Mini-Mental State Examination; RUDAS, Rowland Universal Dementia Assessment Scale; CIRS-CI, Cumulative Illness Rating Scale Comorbidity Index; ESS, Exton Smith Scale; MNA-SF, Multi Nutritional Assessment Short Form. * *p*-value between MPI 1 and MPI 2. ** *p*-value between MPI 1 and MPI 3. *** *p*-value between MPI 2 and MPI 3.

Seventy-one patients (22.8%) died during follow-up. After diagnosis, the average patient survival time was 2.5 years (from a minimum of 0.2 to a maximum of 10.4 years). Figure 2 shows the survival curve for the three MPI categories. The HRs and corresponding 95% CIs for mortality in patients in MPI category 2 and MPI category 3 were 1.67 (0.81–3.45) and 3.80 (1.56–9.24), respectively. When we combined patients in MPI categories 2 and 3, the HR for mortality was 3.98 (95% CI: 1.97—8.04, $p < 0.001$) compared to patients in MPI category 1.

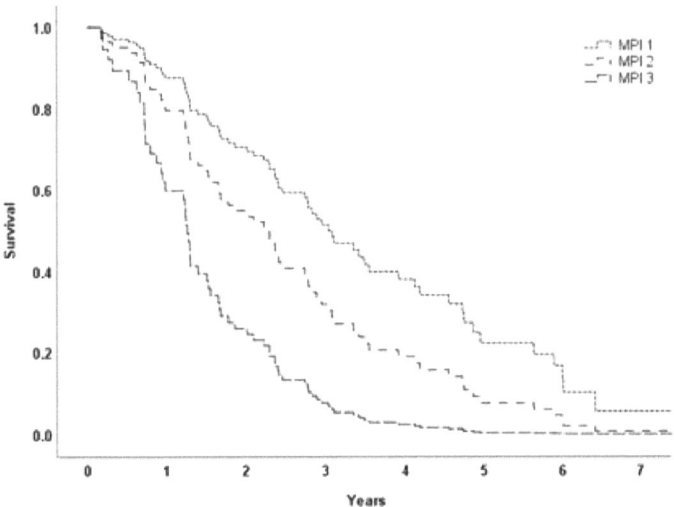

Figure 2. Cox regression survival curve stratified by MPI groups. Model adjusted for age and sex.

4. Discussion

In the present study, we found that older outpatients with cognitive decline and high MPI scores have an increased mortality risk. Patients with dementia had higher MPI scores than patients with MCI.

Several prognostic instruments have been investigated in older patients with cognitive decline. Nearly all instruments were validated in specific groups of patients such as institutionalized older patients with advanced dementia and Alzheimer's disease or investigated only the influence of single characteristics [26–29]. A systematic review of prognostic instruments based on literature confirmed the lack of prognostic indicators of 6-month mortality in older patients with advanced dementia [30]. A nationwide prospective cohort study in the Netherlands found an increased one- and five-year mortality risk in patients with dementia compared with the general population. Still, specific patient characteristics were not taken into account [31]. Recently, a nationwide registry-linkage study developed a survival time tool for older patients with dementia. This tool appeared to be very accurate in predicting the three-year survival [32].

A large prospective study found that the MPI had significantly better prognostic accuracy than three other frailty indices predicting short- and long-term mortality in different settings in hospitalized older patients [33]. A higher MPI risk score seemed, besides a higher risk of mortality, to be associated with other negative outcomes, such as institutionalization, rehospitalization and access to home care services [16,34]. As expected and in agreement with other recent studies, the MPI was also effective in predicting mortality in older patients with cognitive decline in this study [1,34]. The study of Pilotto et al. was based on hospitalized patients with dementia, and MCI was not considered. However, no study had explored whether the prevalence of dementia and MCI was higher or lower among the MPI categories [1].

The findings of our study should be interpreted with some limitations. First, the patients included were recruited within a single university medical center, and therefore we cannot extrapolate our findings to a general population. Second, we have used a modified version of the original MPI. Nevertheless, the different tools used in the present study were previously validated [22,35,36]. Third, transitions between the MPI categories over time can occur, potentially affecting the results. Information on education level was not available. Therefore, we cannot exclude that this might have biased the results.

This study has several strengths. First, a relatively large number of outpatients was included. Second, since the diagnosis is based on multidisciplinary consultation using biomarkers, diagnostic imaging and neuropsychological assessment, it is less likely that the diagnosis of dementia or MCI is missed or misdiagnosed. Third, including patients when only the RUDAS was available contributed to a culturally diverse background study population.

In conclusion, we found that a high MPI risk score was associated with an increased mortality rate in a group of older outpatients with cognitive decline. These findings need to be confirmed in larger and heterogeneous populations of patients with cognitive decline. If confirmed, the MPI would be a novel tool for risk stratification and medical decisions in this peculiar category of patients.

Author Contributions: Conceptualization, F.C.M.S.O. and F.U.S.M.-R.; methodology, F.C.M.S.O. and F.U.S.M.-R.; software, F.C.M.S.O. and F.U.S.M.-R.; validation, F.C.M.S.O. and F.U.S.M.-R.; formal analysis, F.C.M.S.O.; investigation, F.C.M.S.O., J.A.G., J.v.H., R.L.v.B.-V., J.M.P., H.A.P.-B. and F.U.S.M.-R.; data curation, J.v.H. and J.M.P.; writing—original draft preparation, F.C.M.S.O. and F.U.S.M.-R.; writing—review and editing, F.C.M.S.O., J.A.G., J.v.H., R.L.v.B.-V., J.M.P., H.A.P.-B. and F.U.S.M.-R.; visualization, F.C.M.S.O. and F.U.S.M.-R. supervision, F.U.S.M.-R. All authors have read and agreed to the published version of the manuscript.

Funding: This research received no external funding.

Institutional Review Board Statement: This study was conducted in accordance with the principles expressed in the Declaration of Helsinki. In The Netherlands, ethical approval and patient consent are not required for retrospective chart review studies in which data collected during routine clinical care are extracted and analyzed anonymously.

Informed Consent Statement: In The Netherlands, patient consent is not required for retrospective chart review studies in which data collected during routine clinical care are extracted and analyzed anonymously.

Data Availability Statement: Database of the Alzheimer Center of the Erasmus MC University Medical Center, Rotterdam.

Conflicts of Interest: The authors declare no conflict of interest.

References

1. Pilotto, A.; Sancarlo, D.; Panza, F.; Paris, F.; D'Onofrio, G.; Cascavilla, L.; Addante, F.; Seripa, D.; Solfrizzi, V.; Dallapiccola, B.; et al. The Multidimensional Prognostic Index (MPI), based on a comprehensive geriatric assessment predicts short- and long-term mortality in hospitalized older patients with dementia. *J. Alzheimer's Dis.* **2009**, *18*, 191–199. [CrossRef] [PubMed]
2. Gale, S.; Acar, D.; Daffner, K. Dementia. *Am. J. Med.* **2018**, *131*, 1161–1169. [CrossRef] [PubMed]
3. Gauthier, S.; Reisberg, B.; Zaudig, M.; Petersen, R.C.; Ritchie, K.; Broich, K.; Belleville, S.; Brodaty, H.; Bennett, D.; Chertkow, H.; et al. International Psychogeriatric Association Expert Conference on mild cognitive impairment. Mild cognitive impairment. *Lancet* **2006**, *367*, 1262–1270. [CrossRef]
4. Bruscoli, M.; Lovestone, S. Is MCI really just early dementia? A systematic review of conversion studies. *Int. Psychogeriatr.* **2004**, *16*, 129–140. [CrossRef] [PubMed]
5. Bacigalupo, I.; Mayer, F.; Lacorte, E.; Di Pucchio, A.; Marzolini, F.; Canevelli, M.; Di Fiandra, T.; Vanacore, N. A Systematic Review and Meta-Analysis on the Prevalence of Dementia in Europe: Estimates from the Highest-Quality Studies Adopting the DSM IV Diagnostic Criteria. *J. Alzheimer's Dis.* **2018**, *66*, 1471–1481. [CrossRef]
6. DeCarli, C. Mild cognitive impairment: Prevalence, prognosis, aetiology, and treatment. *Lancet Neurol.* **2003**, *2*, 15–21. [CrossRef]
7. Alzheimer Europe. Dementia in Europe Yearbook 2019. *Estimating the Prevalence of Dementia in Europa*. 2020. Available online: https://www.alzheimer-europe.org/Publications/Dementia-in-Europe-Yearbooks (accessed on 23 March 2021).
8. World Health Organization. The Top 10 Causes of Death. 2020. Available online: https://www.who.int/news-room/fact-sheets/detail/the-top-10-causes-of-death#:~{}:text=In%202019%2C%20Alzheimer\T1\textquoterights%20disease%20and,7th%20leading%20cause%20of%20death (accessed on 25 March 2021).
9. Jing, W.; Willis, R.; Feng, Z. Factors influencing quality of life of elderly people with dementia and care implications: A systematic review. *Arch. Gerontol. Geriatr.* **2016**, *66*, 23–41. [CrossRef]

10. Michalowsky, B.; Flessa, S.; Eichler, T.; Hertel, J.; Dreier, A.; Zwingmann, I.; Wucherer, D.; Rau, H.; Thyrian, J.R.; Hoffmann, W. Healthcare utilization and costs in primary care patients with dementia: Baseline results of the DelpHi-trial. *Eur. J. Health Econ.* **2018**, *19*, 87–102. [CrossRef]
11. Joling, K.J.; Janssen, O.; Francke, A.L.; Verheij, R.A.; Lissenberg-Witte, B.I.; Visser, P.J.; van Hout, H.P. Time from diagnosis to institutionalization and death in people with dementia. *Alzheimer's Dement.* **2020**, *16*, 662–671. [CrossRef]
12. Gill, T.M. The central role of prognosis in clinical decision making. *JAMA* **2012**, *307*, 199–200. [CrossRef]
13. Pilotto, A.; Ferrucci, L.; Franceschi, M.; D'Ambrosio, L.P.; Scarcelli, C.; Cascavilla, L.; Paris, F.; Placentino, G.; Seripa, D.; Dallapiccola, B.; et al. Development and validation of a multidimensional prognostic index for one-year mortality from comprehensive geriatric assessment in hospitalized older patients. *Rejuvenation Res.* **2008**, *11*, 151–161. [CrossRef] [PubMed]
14. Yourman, L.C.; Lee, S.J.; Schonberg, M.A.; Widera, E.W.; Smith, A.K. Prognostic indices for older adults: A systematic review. *JAMA* **2012**, *307*, 182–192. [CrossRef] [PubMed]
15. Reuben, D.B. Medical care for the final years of life: "When you're 83, it's not going to be 20 years". *JAMA* **2009**, *302*, 2686–2694. [CrossRef]
16. Pilotto, A.; Veronese, N.; Daragjati, J.; Cruz-Jentoft, A.J.; Polidori, M.C.; Mattace-Raso, F.; Paccalin, M.; Topinkova, E.; Siri, G.; Greco, A.; et al. Using the Multidimensional Prognostic Index to Predict Clinical Outcomes of Hospitalized Older Persons: A Prospective, Multicenter, International Study. *J. Gerontol. A Biol. Sci. Med. Sci.* **2019**, *74*, 1643–1649. [CrossRef] [PubMed]
17. Pilotto, A.; Gallina, P.; Fontana, A.; Sancarlo, D.; Bazzano, S.; Copetti, M.; Maggi, S.; Paroni, G.; Marcato, F.; Pellegrini, F.; et al. Development and validation of a Multidimensional Prognostic Index for mortality based on a standardized Multidimensional Assessment Schedule (MPI-SVaMA) in community-dwelling older subjects. *J. Am. Med. Dir. Assoc.* **2013**, *14*, 287–292. [CrossRef]
18. Katz, Z.; Ford, A.B.; Moskowitz, R.W.; Jackson, B.A.; Jaffe, M.W. Studies of Illness in the Aged. the Index of Adl: A Standardized Measure of Biological and Psychosocial Function. *JAMA* **1963**, *185*, 914–919. [CrossRef]
19. Lawton, M.P.; Brody, E.M. Assessment of older people: Self-maintaining and instrumental activities of daily living. *Gerontologist* **1969**, *9*, 179–186. [CrossRef]
20. Folstein, M.F.; Folstein, S.E.; McHugh, P.R. "Mini-mental state". A practical method for grading the cognitive state of patients for the clinician. *J. Psychiatr. Res.* **1975**, *12*, 189–198. [CrossRef]
21. Storey, J.E.; Rowland, J.T.J.; Conforti, D.A.; Dickson, H.G. The Rowland Universal Dementia Assessment Scale (RUDAS): A multicultural cognitive assessment scale. *Int. Psychogeriatr.* **2004**, *16*, 13–31. [CrossRef]
22. Bryant, K.; Sorich, M.J.; Woodman, R.J.; Mangoni, A.A. Validation and Adaptation of the Multidimensional Prognostic Index in an Older Australian Cohort. *J. Clin. Med.* **2019**, *8*, 1820. [CrossRef]
23. Bliss, M.R.; McLaren, R.; Exton-Smith, A.N. Mattresses for preventing pressure sores in geriatric patients. *Mon. Bull. Minist. Health Public Health Lab. Serv.* **1966**, *25*, 238–268. [PubMed]
24. Rubenstein, L.Z.; Harker, J.O.; Salvà, A.; Guigoz, Y.; Vellas, B. Screening for undernutrition in geriatric practice: Developing the short-form mini-nutritional assessment (MNA-SF). *J. Gerontol. A Biol. Sci. Med. Sci.* **2001**, *56*, M366–M372. [CrossRef] [PubMed]
25. American Psychiatric Association. *Diagnostic and Statistical Manual of Mental Disorders*, 5th ed.; American Psychiatric Association: Arlington, TX, USA, 2013.
26. Mitchell, S.L.; Miller, S.C.; Teno, J.M.; Davis, R.B.; Shaffer, M.L. The advanced dementia prognostic tool: A risk score to estimate survival in nursing home residents with advanced dementia. *J. Pain Symptom Manag.* **2010**, *40*, 639–651. [CrossRef] [PubMed]
27. Ruitenberg, A.; Kalmijn, S.; De Ridder, M.A.; Redekop, W.K.; van Harskamp, F.; Hofman, A.; Launer, L.J.; Breteler, M.M. Prognosis of Alzheimer's disease: The Rotterdam Study. *Neuroepidemiology* **2001**, *20*, 188–195. [CrossRef] [PubMed]
28. García-Ptacek, S.; Kåreholt, I.; Farahmand, B.; Cuadrado, M.L.; Religa, D.; Eriksdotter, M. Body-mass index and mortality in incident dementia: A cohort study on 11,398 patients from SveDem, the Swedish Dementia Registry. *J. Am. Med. Dir. Assoc.* **2014**, *15*, 447.e1–447.e7. [CrossRef] [PubMed]
29. Carcaillon, L.; Pérès, K.; Péré, J.J.; Helmer, C.; Orgogozo, J.M.; Dartigues, J.F. Fast cognitive decline at the time of dementia diagnosis: A major prognostic factor for survival in the community. *Dement. Geriatr. Cogn. Disord.* **2007**, *23*, 439–445. [CrossRef] [PubMed]
30. Brown, M.A.; Sampson, E.L.; Jones, L.; Barron, A.M. Prognostic indicators of 6-month mortality in elderly people with advanced dementia: A systematic review. *Palliat. Med.* **2013**, *27*, 389–400. [CrossRef]
31. van de Vorst, I.E.; Vaartjes, I.; Geerlings, M.I.; Bots, M.L.; Koek, H.L. Prognosis of patients with dementia: Results from a prospective nationwide registry linkage study in the Netherlands. *BMJ Open* **2015**, *5*, e008897. [CrossRef]
32. Haaksma, M.L.; Eriksdotter, M.; Rizzuto, D.; Leoutsakos, J.-M.S.; Rikkert, M.G.O.; Melis, R.J.; Garcia-Ptacek, S. Survival time tool to guide care planning in people with dementia. *Neurology* **2019**, *94*, e538–e548. [CrossRef]
33. Pilotto, A.; Rengo, F.; Marchionni, N.; Sancarlo, D.; Fontana, A.; Panza, F.; Ferrucci, L.; on behalf of the FIRI-SIGG Study Group. Comparing the prognostic accuracy for all-cause mortality of frailty instruments: A multicentre 1-year follow-up in hospitalized older patients. *PLoS ONE* **2012**, *7*, e29089. [CrossRef]
34. Gallucci, M.; Battistella, G.; Bergamelli, C.; Spagnolo, P.; Mazzuco, S.; Carlini, A.; Di Giorgi, E.; Boldrini, P.; Pilotto, A. Multidimensional prognostic index in a cognitive impairment outpatient setting: Mortality and hospitalizations. The Treviso Dementia (TREDEM) study. *J. Alzheimer's Dis.* **2014**, *42*, 1461–1468. [CrossRef] [PubMed]

35. Sancarlo, D.; D'Onofrio, G.; Franceschi, M.; Scarcelli, C.; Niro, V.; Addante, F.; Copetti, M.; Ferrucci, L.; Fontana, L.; Pilotto, A. Validation of a Modified-Multidimensional Prognostic Index (m-MPI) including the Mini Nutritional Assessment Short-Form (MNA-SF) for the prediction of one-year mortality in hospitalized elderly patients. *J. Nutr. Health Aging* **2010**, *15*, 169–173. [CrossRef] [PubMed]
36. Hooijer, C.; Dinkgreve, M.; Jonker, C.; Lindeboom, J.; Kay, D. Short screening tests for dementia in the elderly population. A comparison between AMTS, MMSE, MSQ and SPMSQ. *Int. J. Geriatr. Psychiatry* **1992**, *7*, 559–571. [CrossRef]

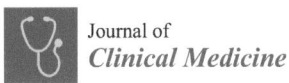

Article

Assessment of the Management of Patients with Chronic Pain Referred to a Specialized Pain Unit: A Cross-Sectional Multicenter Study (the DUO Project)

Víctor Mayoral Rojals [1], Ángeles Canós Verdecho [2], Begoña Soler López [3,*] and the Team DUO [†]

[1] Pain Unit, Hospital Universitari de Bellvitge, IDIBELL, L'Hospitalet de Llobregat, 08907 Barcelona, Spain; victormayoral@mac.com
[2] Pain Unit, Hospital Universitari i Politécnic La Fe, 46026 Valencia, Spain; canos_marver@gva.es
[3] Medical Department, E-C-BIO, S.L., Las Rozas, 28230 Madrid, Spain
* Correspondence: bsoler@ecbio.net
[†] Collaborators of the Team DUO is provided in the Supplementary section.

Abstract: A multicenter cross-sectional study was designed to assess the quality of treatment of 1190 patients with chronic pain at the time of referral to a specialized pain unit. A total of 119 physicians from 77 pain units throughout Spain collected 23 indicators of the quality of care from 10 consecutive clinical records of chronic pain patients (5 men, 5 women). Degenerative spinal diseases (38.6%) and lumbosciatic pain (29.8%) were the most common etiologies. At the time of referral to the pain unit, 9.8% of patients were not receiving any analgesic treatment. Treatment was modified in 88.1% of the patients by adding adjuvant drugs, adding opioids or increasing the doses of analgesic medications, and using analgesic techniques. Women had higher percentages of osteoarthritis, headache and fibromyalgia as the cause of pain, longer duration of pain and severe pain intensity, and a higher proportion of changes in the diagnosis of the underlying condition with which they had been referred to the pain unit. Improvements should be made in the patient management and referral protocols not only in the clinics prior to patient referral to the pain unit, but also in the pain units themselves.

Keywords: chronic pain; pain unit; quality indicators; analgesics; opioids; gender differences

1. Introduction

Chronic pain is one of the most common reasons for adults to seek medical care, particularly in primary care [1], and is associated with restrictions in daily life activities and mobility, reduced quality of life, anxiety and depression, and dependency on opioids [2,3]. The high prevalence of chronic pain and pain-related diseases as the leading cause of disability and disease burden globally has been confirmed in different studies, where 15–25% of adult population suffer chronic pain, reaching to the 50% in older than 65 [2,4–6]. Low back pain and recurrent tension-type headache are the conditions that cause most disability and dysfunction [7]. Additionally, the demand for pain care shows an increasing trend due to aging of the population and a high prevalence of chronic diseases [8,9].

Despite increased focus on the importance of pain control and effective analgesic medications, inadequate pain management has been widely reported with a large variability of undertreatment across studies and settings [10–12]. Barriers to the implementation of adequate pain control are multifactorial involving patient-related and biopsychosocial factors, disease-related factors, underestimation of pain intensity, lack of adequate training of healthcare providers, inadequate pain evaluation, and especially the complexity of the pathophysiological mechanisms of pain [13–16]. A multidisciplinary approach to pain management based on early multidimensional diagnosis of chronic pain and rapid initiation of evidence-based therapy according to an individual treatment plan is necessary to ensure the best outcomes [17,18].

Pain units were created to provide multidisciplinary pain assessment and care, involving a team of anesthetists, neurologists, psychiatrists, occupational therapists, nursing staff, and rehabilitation physicians [12]. In a meta-analysis of 65 studies, the effects of multidisciplinary treatments for chronic pain appeared to be stable over time and were not limited to improvements in pain but also extended to mood, interference with daily activities, and behavioral variables such as return to work or use of the health care system [19]. Multimodal pain management directed by pain specialists in pain clinics plays a pivotal role in the care of patients with chronic pain [20–26], but there is still little information on different aspects related to the profile of patients referred to these units, reason for referral, characteristics of pain management before referral, interventions and treatment prescribed by pain unit specialists, and outcomes attained. Although the use of the pain units is recommended worldwide, local rules for the referral of the patients could influence the characteristics of the patients for the first referral. Thus, in Spain, patients may be referred to the pain unit from primary health care or a specialist, mainly outpatients, when there is a problem diagnosing the underlying disease that generates the pain, and when the pain has not been controlled. Therefore, it is to be expected that the patient referred to the pain unit does not have the pain controlled, and this should be the main reason for his consultation [26]. This study aimed to evaluate the current practice of patients with chronic pain referred to pain units from a national perspective, and to provide useful information to assist stakeholders involved in pain care in their decision-making challenges.

2. Materials and Methods

2.1. Design

This was a multicenter, cross-sectional study conducted in pain units throughout Spain over a 5-month period (May–September 2020) and based on data collected from the medical records of patients with chronic pain (the DUO project). DUO is the Spanish acronym of "Dolor y Uso de Opiáceos" (Pain and Opioids Use). The primary objective of the study was to assess the clinical condition of patients with chronic pain at the time of referral to the pain unit, including the control of pain and details of treatment (medication and doses). The secondary objective was to assess the management of patients in the pain unit. The study protocol was approved by the Clinical Research Ethics Committee (CEIC) of Hospital Universitari de Bellvitge (code PR048/20, approval date 27 February 2020), and informed consent was waived because study data were collected from the electronic patients' medical records. All data were anonymized.

2.2. Participants

Patients of both genders aged 18 years or older were eligible provided that they presented with chronic pain, had been managed in the outpatient setting, and were referred to the pain unit for the first time. Chronic pain was defined according to the International Association for the Study of Pain (IASP) as either chronic primary or secondary pain in ≥ 1 anatomic region that is either persistent or recurs for >3 months and causes functional disability and emotional stress [24]. Chronic primary pain syndrome was also defined as pain that cannot be accounted for by any other chronic pain disorder.

2.3. Study Procedures

The scientific committee of the study was composed by two pain management specialists (V.M.R., A.C.V.) who developed the study questionnaire based on different recommendations of clinical practice guidelines for pain management [25,26]. The questionnaire included 35 questions, which were grouped into three sections: (a) indicators of the participating physician (4 items), (b) indicators of structure of the pain unit (8 items), and (c) indicators of the chronic pain process (23 items). The description of the study questionnaire is included in the Supplementary Material.

Study participants were staff physicians working in pain units throughout Spain. They were recruited by the contract research organization through formal e-mail invitations that included a brochure with full information about the project. The questionnaire was lodged in an internet microsite that could be accessed via a weblink, and only physicians who accepted to participate in the study were provided with access to the questionnaire platform URL and the user's password. Participation in the study was anonymous and voluntary. To complete the section of process indicators, participating physicians collected data of 10 consecutive patients (5 men and 5 women) with chronic pain who were referred to the pain unit during the study period.

2.4. Statistical Analysis

A sample size of 120 pain units was necessary to describe the process indicators selected for the study with an estimated precision of ±6% in the confidence intervals (CI) of the proportions, with a 94% statistical power for a two-tailed alpha error of 0.05. Categorical variables are expressed as frequencies and percentages, and continuous variables as mean and 95% CI. The chi-square test or the Fisher's exact test was used for the comparison of categorical variables, and the Student's *t*-test for quantitative variables. In relation to process indicators, differences between men and women were analyzed using the Student's *t*-test or the Mann–Whitney *U* test for the comparison of the mean values and 95% CI for valid cases (number of patients in which the value of the variable was available) and the mean percentages and 95% CI of compliance with the indicator for valid cases in each pain unit. Statistical significance was set at $p < 0.05$. The SPSS version 27.0 statistical package (IBM SPSS, Chicago, IL, USA) was used for the analysis of data.

3. Results

3.1. Characteristics of Participants

A total of 119 physicians from pain units completed the study questionnaire and provided pooled data of 1190 patients with chronic pain. Pain units were located in 16 out of total 17 regions of Spain. There were 57 men and 62 women, with a mean age of 46.2 years and mean years of professional experience of 12.5. Most physicians were specialists in anesthesiology (86.6%) and worked in public hospitals (89.9%) (Table 1).

Table 1. Characteristics of 119 participants.

Variables	Number (%)	Mean (95% CI)
Participating physicians		
Gender		
Male	57 (47.9)	
Female	62 (52.1)	
Age of the participating physician		46.2 (44.5–48.0)
Years of professional experience in the field of pain		12.5 (10.8–14.1)
Current clinical specialty		
Anesthesiology	103 (86.6)	
Primary care	5 (4.2)	
Physical medicine and rehabilitation	10 (8.4)	
Neurosurgery	1 (0.8)	
Structure indicators		
Type of center to which the unit belongs		
Public hospital/center	107 (89.9)	
Mixed center	12 (10.1)	
What level does your pain unit correspond to?		
Level I	10 (8.4)	
Level I	58 (47.1)	
Level III	53 (44.5)	

Table 1. *Cont.*

Variables	Number (%)	Mean (95% CI)
Number of patients seen in the unit in one month		462.6 (402.8–522.4)
Number of new patients referred to the unit in one month		103.8 (89.8–117.8)
Does the unit have a pain assessment protocol?		
No	25 (21.2)	
Yes	93 (78.8)	
Does the unit use validated chronic pain assessment scales?		
No	5 (4.2)	
Yes	114 (95.8)	
Is health-related quality of life of patients with chronic pain evaluated using validated scales?		
No	59 (49.6)	
Yes	60 (50.4)	
Is mental health of patients with chronic pain evaluated using validated scales?		
No	85 (71.4)	
Yes	34 (28.6)	

CI: confidence interval; Level I: monographic unit; Level II: multidisciplinary pain treatment unit; Level III: multidisciplinary pain center or unit for the study and treatment of pain.

3.2. Structure Indicators

The mean number of new patients referred to the pain unit in one month was 104, accounting for 26.2% of new consultations. Pain assessment protocols were available in 78.8% of the pain units, and validated scales for the assessment of chronic pain were used in 95.8% of the cases. Validated scales for assessing quality of life and mental health were used in 50.4% and 28.6% of cases, respectively (Table 1).

3.3. Process Indicators

Details of process indicators are shown in Tables 2 and 3. Around 45% of patients were referred to the pain unit from orthopaedic surgery and traumatology; men as compared with women were more frequently referred from neurology/neurosurgery (11.7% vs. 7.6%, $p = 0.02$) and oncology (4.2% vs. 2.4%, $p = 0.03$) services, whereas a higher percentage of women were referred from rheumatology services (9.3% vs. 4.7%, $p = 0.001$). Women were also older than men (61.9 vs. 59.1 years, $p = 0.001$). Regarding the employment status, more men were in the active category, whereas more women were housewives. Leading causes of chronic pain were degenerative spinal diseases and lumbosciatic pain. Lumbosciatic pain was significantly more common in men ($p = 0.001$), whereas osteoarthritis ($p = 0.001$), headache ($p = 0.033$) and fibromyalgia ($p < 0.0001$) were significantly more frequent in women. Women also showed a significantly longer duration of chronic pain (32.7 months) than men (26.8 months) ($p = 0.007$). In relation to the type of pain, significant gender differences included somatic pain ($p = 0.001$) and primary pain ($p = 0.045$) more frequent in women, and neuropathic pain more frequent in men ($p = 0.008$). The intensity of pain assessed on a 0–10 scale at the time of pain unit consultation was 6.9 (95% CI 6.7–7.2) in women and 6.6 (95% CI 6.3–6.8) in men ($p = 0.041$). Moreover, severe pain was reported by a higher percentage of women ($p = 0.033$) and mild pain by a higher percentage of men ($p = 0.033$).

More than 80% of patients had impaired functionality due to chronic pain and more than 50% sleep disturbances caused by the pain condition. Breakthrough pain was present in 27% of patients. Differences between men and women in these variables were not observed.

Table 2. Process indicators in 1190 patients with chronic pain referred to the pain unit.

Variables	Total % (95% CI)	Gender		p Value
		Men % (95% CI)	Women % (95% CI)	
Specialty from which the patient is referred				
Orthopaedic surgery and traumatology	44.7 (40.6–48.9)	43.5 (38.6–48.3)	45.8 (41.0–50.6)	
Neurology/neurosurgery	9.7 (7.3–12.0)	11.7 (8.5–14.9)	7.6 (5.1–10.1)	0.02
Rheumatology	7.0 (5.3–8.7)	4.7 (2.8–6.5)	9.3 (6.8–11.9)	0.001
Primary care	14.3 (11.3–17.3)	13.8 (10.6–17.0)	14.9 (11.3–18.5)	
Oncology	3.3 (2.1–4.5)	4.2 (2.7–5.8)	2.4 (1.1–3.7)	0.03
Physical medicine and rehabilitation	13.0 (10.0–15.9)	12.7 (9.4–16.1)	13.2 (9.5–16.9)	
Internal medicine	1.4 (0.7–2.2)	1.7 (0.7–2.7)	1.2 (0.3–2.1)	
Others	7.0 (5.2–8.8)	7.7 (5.1–10.3)	6.4 (4.4–8.5)	
Patient age, years, mean (95% CI)	60.5 (59.6–61.4)	59.1 (57.7–60.3)	61.9 (60.6–63.1)	0.001
Patient employment status				
Active	36.8 (33.4–40.1)	43.9 (39.6–48.3)	29.6 (25.7–33.5)	<0.0001
Unemployed	11.7 (9.1–14.3)	12.1 (9.0–15.1)	11.4 (8.1–14.6)	
Pensioner	42.6 (39.0–46.2)	42.8 (38.6–47.0)	42.4 (37.3–47.5)	
Housewives	8.6 (6.7–10.5)	0.7 (0.0–1.3)	16.4 (12.8–20.1)	<0.0001
Student	0.3 (0.0–0.5)	0.5 (−0.1–1.1)	0 (0.0–0.0)	
Main cause of chronic pain				
Degenerative spinal diseases	38.6 (34.4–42.8)	36.8 (32.1–41.5)	40.5 (35.2–45.9)	
Lumbosciatic pain	29.8 (26.3–33.2)	34.5 (29.9–39.0)	25.1 (20.8–29.4)	0.001
Trauma	3.1 (1.8–4.5)	3.9 (1.8–5.9)	3.9 (1.9–5.9)	
Complex regional syndrome	4.1 (2.6–5.6)	3.7 (2.1–5.3)	4.6 (2.3–6.8)	
Osteoarthritis extremities	9.0 (6.9–11.1)	6.7 (4.6–8.8)	11.2 (8.3–14.1)	0.001
Peripheral neuropathy	5.6 (4.0–7.3)	6.6 (4.3–8.8)	4.8 (2.9–6.6)	
Visceral	1.4 (0.7–2.2)	1.9 (0.8–2.9)	0.9 (0.1–1.6)	
Neoplastic	3.6 (2.4–4.8)	4.4 (2.8–6.0)	2.7 (1.3–4.1)	
Headache	0.8 (0.3–1.4)	0.3 (−0.1–0.8)	1.2 (0.3–2.1)	0.033
Fibromyalgia	4.0 (2.6–5.4)	0.5 (−0.1–1.1)	7.6 (5.1–10.2)	<0.0001
Herpes zoster	1.7 (1.0–2.4)	2.0 (0.9–3.1)	1.4 (0.4–2.3)	
Other	5.6 (3.5–7.6)	4.4 (2.8–6.0)	2.7 (1.3–4.1)	
Duration of pain, months, mean (95% CI)	29.7 (26.7–32.6)	26.9 (23.1–30.6)	32.7 (28.2–37.2)	0.007
Type of pain				
Somatic	23.2 (19.3–27.2)	19.5 (15.5–23.5)	27.2 (22.3–32.1)	0.001
Visceral	1.4 (0.7–2.1)	1.2 (0.3–2.1)	1.7 (0.7–2.7)	
Neuropathic	24.0 (20.6–27.4)	27.0 (22.9–31.2)	21.1 (17.1–25.2)	0.008
Mixed	50.2 (45.5–54.9)	52.0 (46.9–57.0)	47.9 (42.4–53.5)	
Primary	1.5 (0.5–2.6)	0.5 (−0.1–1.1)	2.6 (0.6–4.5)	0.045
Pain intensity measurement with a validated scale before referral	39.9 (31.8–47.9)	40.4 (32.1–48.8)	38.6 (30.3–46.9)	
Pain intensity (0–10) at pain unit consultation, mean (95% CI)	6.8 (6.6–6.9)	6.6 (6.4–6.8)	6.9 (6.7–7.2)	0.041
Current pain intensity (0–10 points)				
Mild (0–4)	13.1 (9.8–16.5)	15.3 (11.1–19.5)	11.1 (7.6–14.7)	0.033
Moderate (5–7)	55.5 (51.6–59.4)	56.6 (51.9–61.4)	54.7 (49.9–59.4)	
Severe (8–10)	32.5 (28.1–36.8)	29.0 (24.1–33.8)	35.6 (30.6–40.6)	0.033
Impaired functionality due to chronic pain	82.6 (78.0–87.2)	81.5 (76.6–86.4)	84.3 (79.6–89.0)	
Sleep disturbance due to chronic pain	58.7 (53.3–64.0)	56.9 (51.1–62.7)	61.7 (56.0–67.5)	
Assessment of sleep disturbance using validated scales	16.3 (10.2–22.3)	16.0 (9.7–22.2)	16.0 (9.9–22.1)	
Presence of breakthrough pain	26.6 (20.7–32.4)	26.7 (20.5–32.9)	26.2 (20.1–32.3)	

Table 2. Cont.

Variables	Total % (95% CI)	Gender		p Value
		Men % (95% CI)	Women % (95% CI)	
Analgesic step of the patient on visiting the pain unit				
No treatment	9.8 (7.5–12.2)	10.6 (7.8–13.4)	9.1 (6.1–12.1)	
First step: non-opioid analgesic	24.1 (20.1–28.1)	25.0 (20.1–30.0)	23.3 (18.8–27.7)	
First step: non-opioid analgesic + adjuvant	13.7 (11.5–16.0)	15.9 (12.4–19.5)	11.7 (8.7–14.7)	
Second step: weak opioid	10.8 (8.0–13.6)	9.3 (6.2–12.3)	11.6 (8.0–15.2)	
Second step: weak opioid + adjuvant	10.3 (7.9–12.7)	10.3 (7.4–13.2)	10.6 (7.4–13.8)	
Second step: weak opioid + non-opioid analgesic	8.8 (6.7–10.9)	8.0 (5.0–11.0)	9.6 (6.8–12.4)	
Second step: weak opioid + non-opioid analgesic + adjuvant	8.1 (6.0–10.2)	8.2 (5.7–10.8)	8.0 (5.3–10.8)	
Third step: strong opioid	5.5 (3.8–7.3)	5.6 (3.3–7.9)	5.7 (3.6–7.8)	
Third step: strong opioid + adjuvant	6.6 (4.7–8.5)	7.3 (4.7–9.9)	6.0 (3.7–8.2)	
Third step: strong opioid + non-opioid analgesic	4.4 (2.9–5.8)	3.4 (1.6–5.1)	5.3 (3.3–7.3)	
Third step: strong opioid + non-opioid analgesic + adjuvant	6.7 (4.5–8.9)	6.6 (4.1–9.1)	6.8 (4.1–9.6)	
Interventional techniques, drug administration via spinal route, peripheral nerve block, sympathetic or neurolytic block, electrical stimulation techniques, neurosurgery	2.2 (0.9–3.5)	2.5 (0.8–4.2)	1.8 (0.4–3.2)	
Instructions for the use of rescue analgesics	45.5 (38.4–52.5)	44.5 (37.2–51.8)	45.9 (38.4–53.3)	

CI: confidence interval.

Table 3. Pain treatment in 1190 patients with chronic pain referred to the pain unit.

Variables	Total % (95% CI)	Gender		p Value
		Men % (95% CI)	Women % (95% CI)	
Drug treatment on admission to the pain unit				
None	8.4 (5.9–11.0)	9.1 (6.2–11.9)	7.7 (4.8–10.7)	
Non-steroidal anti-inflammatory agents	37.6 (30.9–44.3)	42.6 (33.3–51.9)	34.8 (27.5–42.0)	0.049
Metamizole	24.5 (20.4–28.6)	22.0 (17.3–26.7)	28.2 (22.2–34.2)	0.042
Paracetamol	54.5 (47.8–61.1)	53.2 (45.1–61.4)	56.5 (49.2–63.9)	
Codeine	1.3 (0.4–2.2)	0.7 (−0.4–1.7)	1.8 (0.4–3.3)	
Tramadol	40.0 (34.8–45.1)	40.0 (33.4–46.7)	40.5 (34.6–46.3)	
Buprenorphine	2.5 (1.2–3.7)	2.4 (1.0–3.7)	2.8 (0.7–4.8)	
Fentanyl	9.4 (6.6–12.3)	8.3 (5.1–11.6)	10.6 (7.2–14.0)	
Hydromorphone	0.2 (−0.1–0.4)	0.2 (−0.2–0.5)	0.2 (−0.2–0.5)	
Morphine	1.6 (0.2–3.1)	1.4 (0.1–2.7)	2.0 (0.1–3.9)	
Oxycodone	0.4 (0.0–0.8)	0.5 (−0.2–1.2)	0.3 (−0.1–0.8)	
Oxycodone/naloxone	5.4 (2.8–8.1)	5.5 (3.1–7.9)	5.5 (1.7–9.2)	
Tapentadol	11.6 (8.6–14.6)	10.5 (7.1–14.0)	12.9 (8.7–17.0)	
Lidocaine	1.2 (0.4–2.0)	0.8 (0.0–1.6)	1.5 (0.3–2.6)	
Capsaicin	1.8 (0.6–3.0)	0.8 (0.1–1.6)	3.0 (0.2–5.7)	
Amitriptyline	7.4 (5.3–9.5)	6.2 (3.8–8.5)	8.5 (5.6–11.3)	
Duloxetine	1.8 (0.6–3.0)	1.0 (0.0–2.0)	2.8 (0.2–5.5)	
Venlafaxine	26.6 (22.8–30.5)	27.2 (22.1–32.4)	26.0 (21.0–30.9)	

Table 3. Cont.

Variables	Total % (95% CI)	Gender		p Value
		Men % (95% CI)	Women % (95% CI)	
Pregabalin	10.7 (8.3–13.1)	12.0 (8.6–15.3)	10.2 (5.9–14.4)	
Gabapentin	2.8 (1.4–4.2)	2.8 (1.1–4.4)	2.8 (1.1–4.4)	
Corticosteroids	6.5 (4.4–8.7)	7.3 (4.7–9.9)	5.6 (2.9–8.2)	
Mean drug doses on admission to the pain unit				
Metamizole (mg)	1369.1 (1223.7–1514.5)	1413.1 (1192.2–1634.0)	1329.5 (1133.0–1526.0)	
Paracetamol (mg)	1886.7 (1766.9–2006.6)	1821.0 (1645.6–1996.5)	1962.9 (1797.7–2128.1)	
Codeine (mg)	55.0 (16.0–94.0)	90.0	49.6 (5.4–93.9)	
Tramadol (mg)	139.7 (129.9–149.6)	138.7 (124.0–153.3)	140.8 (127.4–154.2)	
Buprenorphine (µg)	40.4 (32.1–48.7)	37.9 (27.2–48.6)	43.4 (28.3–58.6)	
Fentanyl (µg)	87.2 (56.5–117.8)	109.7 (52.2–167.3)	71.9 (37.8–106.0)	
Hydromorphone (mg)	8.0	-	8.0	
Morphine (mg)	35.0 (19.0–51.0)	39.0 (12.0–66.0)	32.0 (7.0–57.0)	
Oxycodone (mg)	29.0 (6.0–53.0)	24.0 (−15.0–63.0)	38.0 (−8.0–83.0)	
Oxycodone/naloxone (mg)	29.0 (22.0–36.0)	29.0 (19.0–39.0)	28.0 (17.0–40.0)	
Tapentadol (mg)	130.0 (112.0–148.0)	137.0 (105.0–170.0)	124.0 (104.0–143.0)	
Amitriptyline (mg)	24.7 (19.5–29.8)	29.1 (17.1–41.0)	22.0 (18.0–25.0)	
Duloxetine (mg)	60.0 (53.0–68.0)	53.0 (43.0–62.0)	67.0 (56.0–78.0)	
Venlafaxine (mg)	109.0 (67.0–151.0)	139.0 (10.0–267.0)	99.0 (49.0–149.0)	
Pregabalin (mg)	165.1 (148.5–181.8)	180.9 (155.7–206.1)	147.0 (126.1–167.9)	
Gabapentin (mg)	847.0 (735.0–959.0)	876.0 (737.0–1014.0)	805.0 (608.0–1002.0)	
Actions taken at the pain unit regarding drug treatment				
No action, previous treatment maintained	11.9 (8.8–15.1)	13.3 (9.7–16.8)	10.6 (7.1–14.1)	
First step dose modification	10.4 (5.8–14.9)	10.5 (6.1–14.9)	11.2 (4.8–17.6)	
Second step dose modification	14.6 (10.3–18.8)	14.3 (10.0–18.5)	13.8 (9.0–18.7)	
Third step dose modification	10.4 (6.9–13.8)	8.4 (5.2–11.6)	12.4 (6.7–18.1)	
Change of the first step non-opioid analgesic	7.7 (3.5–11.8)	6.1 (2.8–9.4)	10.0 (2.6–17.3)	
Moved from the first to the second step	16.8 (12.4–21.3)	17.6 (12.8–22.4)	16.9 (10.7–23.2)	
Change-rotation of second step opioid	4.7 (1.4–8.1)	4.3 (1.5–7.1)	6.0 (0.5–11.5)	
Change weak to strong opioid (2nd to 3rd step)	16.2 (11.2–21.2)	14.9 (10.6–19.2)	18.6 (11.0–26.2)	
Change-rotation of third step opioid	6.7 (3.1–10.3)	7.2 (4.3–10.1)	7.2 (0.3–14.1)	
Change of adjuvant	7.8 (4.3–11.4)	6.4 (3.4–9.4)	10.2 (4.4–16.0)	
Addition of one or more non-opioid analgesics	7.5 (5.0–10.1)	7.8 (4.8–10.9)	7.4 (4.5–10.3)	
Addition of one or more adjuvants	28.1 (23.3–33.0)	28.0 (22.5–33.5)	28.3 (22.6–34.0)	
Start of interventional techniques, drug administration via spinal route, peripheral nerve block, sympathetic or neurolytic block, electrical stimulation techniques or neurosurgery	60.4 (44.6–76.3)	60.0 (48.1–71.9)	53.0 (44.1–61.9)	
Reasons for treatment changes				
Lack of efficacy	60.2 (55.2–65.1)	62.1 (56.6–67.6)	58.4 (64.1)	
Side effects	9.1 (6.7–11.4)	7.8 (5.3–10.3)	10.3 (7.3–13.4)	
Insufficient dose	24.2 (19.6–28.7)	23.6 (18.8–28.4)	25.1 (19.8–30.4)	
Others	10.6 (7.5–13.8)	13.6 (6.5–20.8)	9.8 (6.5–13.2)	
Patient follow-up				
Refer the patient for a second consultation appointment at the pain unit	90.3 (87.9–92.8)	90.8 (87.8–93.7)	89.8 (86.8–92.9)	
Refer the patient to the service from which he/she was referred	2.8 (1.5–4.1)	2.2 (1.0–3.4)	3.4 (1.5–5.3)	

Table 3. Cont.

Variables	Total % (95% CI)	Gender		p Value
		Men % (95% CI)	Women % (95% CI)	
Refer the patient to a different specialist from which he/she came from	2.6 (1.4–3.8)	2.4 (0.9–3.9)	2.9 (1.4–4.3)	
Refer the patient to primary care	4.6 (2.9–6.4)	5.2 (3.1–7.3)	4.1 (2.1–6.0)	
Modification of the previous diagnosis	17.3 (13.1–21.5)	14.8 (10.6–19.0)	19.0 (14.4–23.6)	0.043
Exclusion of addictive disorders in opioid-treated patients	57.6 (49.7–65.4)	60.6 (52.4–68.8)	55.2 (47.0–63.5)	
Information that opioids may affect driving ability	59.3 (51.5–67.0)	61.6 (53.5–69.8)	57.9 (49.5–66.4)	

CI: confidence interval.

Figure 1 summarizes treatment according to the analgesic ladder steps on referral to the pain unit and modification of treatment recommended in the pain unit. A total of 9.8% of the patients with chronic pain were not receiving any treatment at the time of referral to the pain unit. The remaining 90.2% were receiving some analgesic treatment, with 37.8% of patients treated according to the first ladder step (mainly non-opioid analgesics only), 38% to the second ladder step (weak opioids with or without adjuvant drugs in 21% of cases), and 23% to the third step (strong opioids alone in only 5.5% of cases) (Table 2). Other therapeutic interventions, such as peripheral nerve block, electrical stimulation techniques, analgesia through the spinal route, sympathetic/neurolytic block were only used in 2% of patients. On the other hand, only 44% of patients had received instructions for use of rescue analgesia. Gender-related differences in the distribution of patients according to the analgesic ladder were not observed.

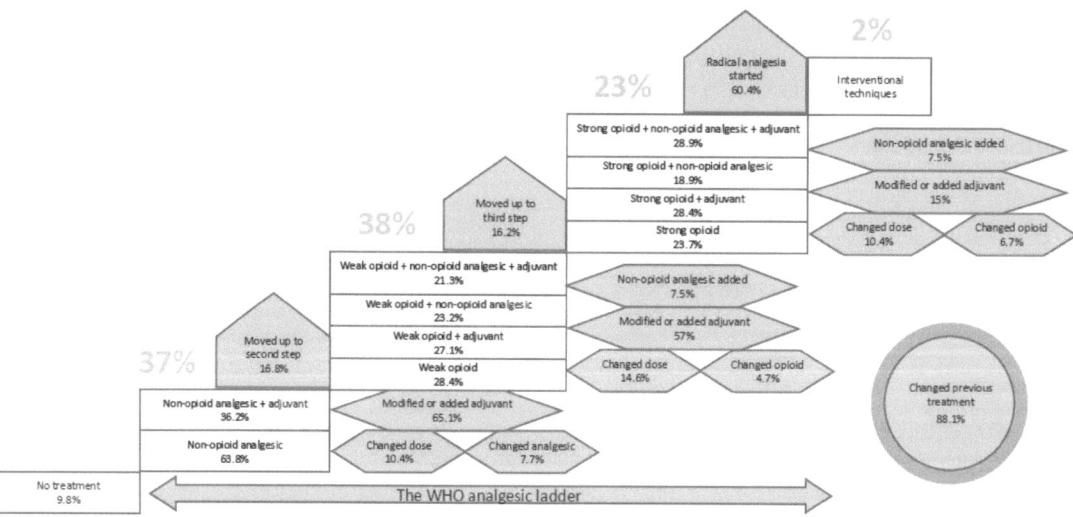

Figure 1. Treatment details according to the steps of the analgesic ladder in first-time referral to the pain unit (white boxes) and actions taken at the pain unit regarding modification of treatment (grey boxes).

Paracetamol, non-steroidal anti-inflammatory drugs (NSAIDs), tramadol, metamizole and venlafaxine were the most commonly used medications (Table 3). Metamizole was use by a significantly higher percentage of women as compared with men (28.2% vs. 22%, $p = 0.042$), whereas NSAIDs were more commonly used in men (42.6% vs. 34.7%, $p = 0.049$). On admission to the pain unit, drug treatment was changed in 88.1% of patients, with lack of efficacy being the main reason for change in about 60% of patients. Addition of one or more adjuvant drugs, modification of doses of second step analgesics, change from the first to the second step, and change from weak to strong opioid were the actions more frequently recommended, with similar percentages in men and women (Table 3). However, the previous diagnosis was modified in 19% of women and in 14.8% in men ($p = 0.043$).

Finally, after the first consultation in the pain unit, 90.3% of patients were appointed for a second visit in the pain unit, 4.6% were referred to the primary care setting, 2.8% to the same service or specialty than the one they came from, and 2.6% to a different specialty.

4. Discussion

This study aimed to gather knowledge on the clinical profile of patients with chronic pain at the time of referral to a specialized pain unit, usually because of poor control of pain. The nationwide perspective of the project is supported by the participation of 119 physicians from 77 pain units out of the 123 accredited units in the Spanish public healthcare system [27]. Additionally, the physicians who completed the survey had a mean experience in the pain field of 12 years excluding their training period, and most of them were specialists in anesthesiology. Seventy-nine percent of pain units had a written protocol for pain assessment, although it would be desirable for all units to implement a protocolized evaluation of pain. There was a reduced percentage of units in which health-related quality of life and mental health of patients with chronic pain were evaluated on a routine basis, a relevant aspect that should be improved because of the deleterious effect of chronic pain on daily functioning and the risk of triggering anxiety, depression, and other mental health issues [28]. Perhaps one of the barriers of the pain therapy centers is that they have limited time and insufficient resources to test and follow patients' quality of life.

Patients were referred to the pain units from different settings, especially from orthopaedic surgery and traumatology (45%), followed by primary care (14%) and physical medicine and rehabilitation (13%), which is consistent with common causes of pain, including degenerative spinal diseases, lumbosciatic pain, and arthrosis. In a previous study of 269 patients referred to 12 outpatient hospital pain clinics in Catalonia, Spain, 50% of patients were referred by specialists in orthopaedic surgery and traumatology and 20% by primary care [21]. Despite that fact that most patients suffered from moderate-severe pain with impaired functionality in more than 80% of cases and sleep disturbance in almost 60%, pain had not been measured using a validated instrument in 40% of patients prior to referral to the pain unit. The impact of pain on the quality of sleep was only evaluated in 16% of patients. Moreover, chronic pain was long-lasting with a mean duration of more than 2 years. These findings indicate that there is still large room for improvement in the management of chronic pain before referral to pain specialists. However, differences in the duration of pain according to types and causes of pain or referral services were not analyzed. Some differences found between men and women could be expected as women showed a higher proportion of arthrosis, headache and fibromyalgia, as well as pain intensity, which agrees with data from a Norwegian population-based study in which women reported significantly higher pain intensity scores than men [29].

Data reported in other studies regarding undertreatment of chronic pain [12,21,30,31] were also found in the present study, including around 10% of patients who had not received any pain therapy and the fact that drug treatment was modified in 88.1% of patients on the first visit to the pain clinic. The proportion of patients receiving drugs of the first and second step of the WHO analgesic ladder was similar (38%), and 23% of patients were treated with strong opioids (third step). It should be noted that 45.4% of patients received adjuvant drugs, particularly over the first and second steps. The most commonly prescribed analgesic medication was paracetamol (in more than half of the patients) followed by tramadol, NSAIDs, and metamizole. However, paracetamol has been shown to be ineffective in the treatment of low back pain and provides minimal short-term benefits in patients with osteoarthritis [32]. The use of adjuvant agents together with the main drugs is allowed on all analgesic ladders [33]. Adjuvant drugs improve the analgesic response and are particularly useful for some types of pain, such as neuropathic pain. These drugs include antidepressants, anxiolytics, steroids, muscle relaxants, capsaicin or local anesthetics. The analgesic effect is probably produced via enhancement of transmitter concentrations in pain-modulating pathways [34]. Interestingly, venlafaxine was the most common adjuvant drug used by patients at the time of referral to the pain unit (26.6%), but duloxetine, which has significant analgesic effects for managing chronic pain associated with fibromyalgia and peripheral neuropathic pain [35], was used by 1.8% of the patients only.

The main action taken in the pain unit was a change of treatment in 88.1% of the patients to achieve a better control of pain because of lack of efficacy or insufficient doses of previous medications. In patients in the second and third steps, a non-opioid analgesic was added. Moreover, 17% of patients in the first analgesic step moved to the second step, and 16% of those in the second step moved to the third step. Interventional procedures for analgesia are measures mainly adopted by pain specialists and were indicated in 60% of the patients. In none of the actions taken at the pain unit, significant differences between men and women were found, except for modifying the previous diagnosis, which occurred more frequently in women than in men, although changes related to individual diagnosis were not evaluated. On the other hand, some of the differences found in our study between men and women in relation to higher pain intensity, longer duration of pain, and chronic conditions, such as headache, back pain, and fibromyalgia, have been reported in other studies also [29,36].

Pooled data collection prevented individual patient comparisons. Data were recorded during the first visit to the pain clinic and, although pain conditions continued to be managed by pain specialists in subsequent visits, the course of patients was not evaluated. Despite these limitations, the sample of pain units accounted for 63% of all pain units available in the public healthcare system of the country, supporting the representativeness of the sample.

5. Conclusions

The present findings indicate that improvements should be made in the patient management and referral protocols, with reinforcement of the importance of using validated instruments to assess the intensity of pain and the impacts of chronic pain on quality of life and mental health. Gender-related differences require attention, especially in relation to higher pain intensity and causes of chronic pain in women. Efforts should be made to provide an integrated multidisciplinary care of patients with chronic pain with the objective of optimizing drug treatment and improving adequate long-lasting control of pain.

Supplementary Materials: The following supporting information can be downloaded at: https://www.mdpi.com/article/10.3390/jcm11133586/s1, Study questionnaire. The Team DUO (members by alphabetical order): Carolina Abellán Aracil, Aranjuez, Madrid; Alejandro Alcina Navarro, Madrid; Ignacio Javier Alejandro Alejandro, Las Palmas; Lucía Ángel Redondo, Sevilla; Mónica Araujo Vázquez, Pontevedra; Martín Zacarías Arcas Molina, Albacete; Enrique Bárez Hernández, Araba/Álava; Dolores Bedmar Cruz, Madrid; Moncef Belaouchi Belaouchi, Valencia; Ara Bermejo Marín, Valencia; José David Bravo Corrales, Ciudad Real; Carlos Burguera Baldoví, Valencia; José Enrique Calderón Seoane, Cádiz; Noelia Calvo García, Bizkaia; Elena Cano Serrano, Granada; Luz Cánovas Martínez, Ourense; Miguel Ángel Caramés Álvarez, Las Palmas; Martín Carpintero Porrero, Asturias; Félix Cebeiro Balda, Navarra; Joan Coma Coma, Barcelona; José de la Cueva Aguilera Cádiz; Juan Carlos de la Pinta García, Madrid; Marta del Valle Hoyos, Málaga; Eva María Díaz Ibáñez, Murcia; Clara Díaz-Alejo Marchante, Alicante; Enrique Domínguez Suárez, Lugo; Francisco Duca Rezzulini, Barcelona; Cristina Embid Román, Alicante; Sara Estévez Sarmiento, Las Palmas; Gustavo Fabregat Cid, Valencia; Jaime Fandiño Vaquero, Pontevedra; Mariano Fernández Baena, Málaga; Alfredo Fernández Esplá, Madrid; María del Rosario Fernández Fernández, Asturias; Montserrat Fernández García, Barcelona; Ana Fernández López, Madrid; Urides Armando Fernández Orraca, Barcelona; Lourdes Ferreira Laso, La Rioja; Julia M. Ferreras Zamora, Barcelona; Jordi Folch Ibáñez, Barcelona; Cristina Garcés San José, Zaragoza; Juan Carlos García Collada, Cuenca; María Jesús García Menéndez, Asturias; José Antonio Girón Mombiela, Zaragoza; José Luis Gómez Palonés, Castellón;

María Cristina Gómez Vega, Bizkaia; Juana González Fernández, Granada; Eduardo González García, Valladolid; Raquel González Jiménez, Madrid; José Manuel González Mesa, Málaga; Marcos González Cabano, A Coruña; Agustín Guerri Cebollada, Valencia; Jordi Guitart Vela, Barcelona; Mª Anunciación Gutiérrez Gómez, Burgos; Zeina Hachoue Saliba, Madrid; María José Hernandez Cádiz, Valencia; María Inmaculada Herrador Montiel, Córdoba; Carla Iglesias Morales, Toledo; Rosa Ma Izquierdo Aguirre, Valencia; Paula Jiménez Vázquez, Sevilla; Ma Rocío López Díez, Ourense; Josep López Garrido, Barcelona; María López Gómez, Toledo; Mónica López-Tafall Cáceres, Araba/Álava; José Leonardo Mansilla Moret, IIIes Balears; Jenaro Mañero Rey, Barcelona; César Margarit Ferri, Alicante; Diana Mariñansky Mlynarzewicz, Girona; Mercedes Martínez García, Madrid; Javier Mata Estévez, IIIes Balears; Mónica Mayo Moldes, Pontevedra; Javier Medel Rebollo, Barcelona; Ana Belén Mencías Hurtado, Santa Cruz de Tenerife; Juan Manuel Mercado Escribá, Castellón; Bartolomé Mir Darder, IIIes Balears; Rosse Mery Molina Sánchez, Barcelona; María del Mar Monerris Tabasco, Barcelona; Onel Morales Torres, Girona; Rafael Morales Valero, Córdoba; Manuel Muñoz Martínez, Madrid; María Navarro Martínez, Burgos; Minerva Navarro Rivero, Las Palmas; María Luz Padilla Del Rey, Murcia; Ángela Catalina Palacios Córdoba, Granada; Ernesto Pastor Martínez, Valencia; María Amparo Pérez Díaz, A Coruña; Arelis Pérez Fernández, Albacete; Guillermo Petinal Algás, Pontevedra; Mauricio Polanco García, Barcelona; Patricia Puiggròs Hernández, IIIes Balears; Miriam Puyo Olmo, Barcelona; Montserrat Reche García, Valencia; Ma Carmen Ribera Montés, Alicante; Paloma Ricós Bugeda, Barcelona; María Belén Rodríguez Campoó, Madrid; Isabel Rodríguez Fernández, Cáceres; Iria Rodríguez Rodríguez, A Coruña; María Cristina Rodríguez Roca, Madrid; Elena Rojo Rodríguez, Madrid; María Blanca Rondeau Marco, Murcia; Alberto Sánchez Campos, Bizkaia; Esperanza Sánchez Navarro, Madrid; Calixto Andrés Sánchez Pérez, Alicante; Roger Sánchez Toll, Valencia; José Antonio Sánchez Tirado, Zaragoza; Yolanda Sastre Peris, Alicante; Ancor Serrano Afonso, Barcelona; Anna Server Salvà, Barcelona; Carlos Solano Perea, Cádiz; Ana Suárez Cobian, Madrid; Alberto Taborga Echevarría, Cantabria; Humberto Víctor Torres Lamberti, Asturias; Ma Isabel Vargas Domingo, Barcelona; Alberto Vela de Toro, Granada; Rafael Vergel Eleuterio, Murcia; Vicente Luis Villanueva Pérez, Valencia; Francisco Villegas Estévez, Castellón; and Marta Yus López, Madrid, Spain.

Author Contributions: Conceptualization, V.M.R., Á.C.V. and B.S.L.; Data curation, B.S.L.; Supervision, V.M.R. and Á.C.V.; Validation, B.S.L.; Writing—original draft, B.S.L.; Writing—review & editing, V.M.R. and Á.C.V. All authors have read and agreed to the published version of the manuscript.

Funding: This research was supported by Neuraxpharm Spain, S.L.

Institutional Review Board Statement: The study was conducted in accordance with the Declaration of Helsinki and approved by the Clinical Research Ethics Committee of Hospital Universitari de Bellvitge (protocol code PR048/20, approval date 27 February 2020).

Informed Consent Statement: Patient consent was waived because study data were collected from the electronic patients' medical records.

Data Availability Statement: Data of the study are available from the corresponding author upon request.

Acknowledgments: The authors thank Marta Pulido for editing the manuscript and editorial assistance.

Conflicts of Interest: V. Mayoral Rojals and A. Canós Verdecho received fees for the coordination of the DUO project and B. Soler López was contracted by Neuraxpharm Spain, S.L., for the design, monitoring, and statistical analysis.

References

1. Smith, B.H.; Torrance, N. Management of chronic pain in primary care. *Curr. Opin. Support. Palliat. Care* **2011**, *5*, 137–142. [CrossRef]
2. Breivik, H.; Collett, B.; Ventafridda, V.; Cohen, R.; Gallacher, D. Survey of chronic pain in Europe: Prevalence, impact on daily life, and treatment. *Eur. J. Pain* **2006**, *10*, 287–333. [CrossRef] [PubMed]
3. van Hecke, O.; Torrance, N.; Smith, B.H. Chronic pain epidemiology and its clinical relevance. *Br. J. Anaesth.* **2013**, *111*, 13–18. [CrossRef] [PubMed]
4. Cohen, S.P.; Vase, L.; Hooten, W.M. Chronic pain: An update on burden, best practices, and new advances. *Lancet* **2021**, *397*, 2082–2097. [CrossRef]

5. GBD 2017 Disease and Injury Incidence and Prevalence Collaborators. Global, regional, and national incidence, prevalence, and years lived with disability for 354 diseases and injuries for 195 countries and territories, 1990–2017. A systematic analysis for the Global Burden of Disease Study 2017. *Lancet* **2018**, *392*, 1789–1858. [CrossRef]
6. Mills, S.E.E.; Nicolson, K.P.; Smith, B.H. Chronic pain: A review of its epidemiology and associated factors in population-based studies. *Br. J. Anaesth.* **2019**, *123*, e273–e283. [CrossRef]
7. Miró, J.; Paredes, S.; Rull, M.; Queral, R.; Miralles, R.; Nieto, R.; Huguet, A.; Baos, J. Pain in older adults: A prevalence study in the Mediterranean region of Catalonia. *Eur. J. Pain* **2007**, *11*, 83–92. [CrossRef]
8. Zimmer, Z.; Zajacova, A. Persistent, consistent, and extensive: The trend of increasing pain prevalence in older Americans. *J. Gerontol. B Psychol. Sci. Soc. Sci.* **2020**, *75*, 436–447. [CrossRef]
9. Zimmer, Z.; Zajacova, A.; Grol-Prokopczyk, H. Trends in pain prevalence among adults aged 50 and older across Europe, 2004 to 2015. *J. Aging Health* **2020**, *32*, 1419–1432. [CrossRef]
10. Deandrea, S.; Montanari, M.; Moja, L.; Apolone, G. Prevalence of undertreatment in cancer pain. A review of published literature. *Ann. Oncol.* **2008**, *19*, 1985–1991. [CrossRef]
11. Sinatra, R. Causes and consequences of inadequate management of acute pain. *Pain Med.* **2010**, *11*, 859–1871.
12. Dubois, M.Y.; Gallagher, R.M.; Lippe, P.M. Pain medicine position paper. *Pain Med.* **2009**, *10*, 972–1000. [CrossRef] [PubMed]
13. Kwon, J.H.; Hui, D.; Chisholm, G.; Hong, W.T.; Nguyen, L.; Bruera, E. Experience of barriers to pain management in patients receiving outpatient palliative care. *J. Palliat. Med.* **2013**, *16*, 908–914. [CrossRef] [PubMed]
14. Carr, E. Barriers to effective pain management. *J. Perioper. Pract.* **2007**, *17*, 200–208. [CrossRef]
15. Kwon, J.H. Overcoming barriers in cancer pain management. *J. Clin. Oncol.* **2014**, *32*, 1727–1733. [CrossRef]
16. Majedi, H.; Dehghani, S.S.; Soleyman-Jahi, S.; Tafakhori, A.; Emami, S.A.; Mireskandari, M.; Hosseini, S.M. Assessment of factors predicting inadequate pain management in chronic pain patients. *Anesth. Pain Med.* **2019**, *9*, e97229. [CrossRef]
17. Pergolizzi, J.; Ahlbeck, K.; Aldington, D.; Alon, E.; Coluzzi, F.; Dahan, A.; Huygen, F.; Kocot-Kępska, M.; Mangas, A.C.; Mavrocordatos, P.; et al. The development of chronic pain: Physiological CHANGE necessitates a multidisciplinary approach to treatment. *Curr. Med. Res. Opin.* **2013**, *29*, 1127–1135. [CrossRef]
18. Scascighini, L.; Toma, V.; Dober-Spielmann, S.; Sprott, H. Multidisciplinary treatment for chronic pain: A systematic review of interventions and outcomes. *Rheumatology* **2008**, *47*, 670–678. [CrossRef]
19. Flor, H.; Fydrich, T.; Turk, D.C. Efficacy of multidisciplinary pain treatment centers: A meta-analytic review. *Pain* **1992**, *49*, 221–230. [CrossRef]
20. Patwardhan, A.; Matika, R.; Gordon, J.; Singer, B.; Salloum, M.; Ibrahim, M. Exploring the role of chronic pain clinics: Potential for opioid reduction. *Pain Physician* **2018**, *21*, E603–E610.
21. Videla, S.; Català, E.; Ribera, M.V.; Montes, A.; Samper, D.; Fuentes, J.; Busquets, C.; Pain Units of Hospitals in Catalonia Group. Characteristics and outcomes of chronic pain patients referred to hospital pain clinics: A prospective observational study. *Minerva Anestesiol.* **2017**, *83*, 12–22. [CrossRef] [PubMed]
22. Lakha, S.F.; Yegneswaran, B.; Furlan, J.C.; Legnini, V.; Nicholson, K.; Mailis-Gagnon, A. Referring patients with chronic noncancer pain to pain clinics: Survey of Ontario family physicians. *Can. Fam. Physician* **2011**, *57*, e106–e112. [PubMed]
23. Fogelman, Y.; Carmeli, E.; Minerbi, A.; Harash, B.; Vulfsons, S. Specialized pain clinics in primary care: Common diagnoses, referral patterns and clinical outcomes—Novel pain management model. *Adv. Exp. Med. Biol.* **2018**, *1047*, 89–98. [PubMed]
24. Treede, R.D.; Rief, W.; Barke, A.; Aziz, Q.; Bennett, M.I.; Benoliel, R.; Cohen, M.; Evers, S.; Finnerup, N.B.; First, M.B.; et al. Chronic pain as a symptom or a disease: The IASP Classification of Chronic Pain for the International Classification of Diseases (ICD-11). *Pain* **2019**, *160*, 19–27. [CrossRef] [PubMed]
25. Tejedor Fernández, M.; Gálvez Mateos, R. Programa de Seguridad del Paciente en las Unidades de Tratamiento del Dolor. Informes de Evaluación de Tecnologías Sanitarias. AETSA 2009/II. Available online: https://www.aetsa.org/download/publicaciones/antiguas/AETSA_2009-11.pdf (accessed on 14 November 2021).
26. Unidad de Tratamiento del Dolor. Estándares y Recomendaciones de Calidad y Seguridad. Informes, Estudios e Investigación 2011. Ministerio de Sanidad, Política Social e Igualdad. Available online: https://www.mscbs.gob.es/organizacion/sns/planCalidadSNS/docs/EERR/Unidad_de_tratamiento_del_dolor.pdf (accessed on 14 November 2021).
27. González-Escalada, J.R.; Camba, A.; Sánchez, I. Censo de las unidades del dolor en España. Análisis de la estructura organizativa, dotación, cartera de servicios e indicadores de calidad y buenas prácticas. *Rev. Soc. Esp. Dolor* **2014**, *21*, 149–161. [CrossRef]
28. Kawai, K.; Kawai, A.T.; Wollan, P.; Yawn, B.P. Adverse impacts of chronic pain on health-related quality of life, work productivity, depression and anxiety in a community-based study. *Fam. Pract.* **2017**, *34*, 656–661. [CrossRef]
29. Rustøen, T.; Wahl, A.K.; Hanestad, B.R.; Lerdal, A.; Paul, S.; Miaskowski, C. Gender differences in chronic pain—Findings from a population-based study of Norwegian adults. *Pain Manag. Nurs.* **2004**, *5*, 105–117. [CrossRef]
30. Zorba Paster, R. Chronic pain management issues in the primary care setting and the utility of long-acting opioids. *Expert Opin. Pharm.* **2010**, *11*, 1823–1833. [CrossRef]
31. García, C.A.; Santos Garcia, J.B.; Rosario Berenguel Cook, M.D.; Colimon, F.; Flores Cantisani, J.A.; Guerrero, C.; Núñez, M.D.R.G.; Castro, J.J.H.; Kraychete, D.C.; Lara-Solares, A.; et al. Undertreatment of pain and low use of opioids in Latin America. *Pain Manag.* **2018**, *8*, 181–196. [CrossRef]

32. Machado, G.C.; Maher, C.G.; Ferreira, P.H.; Pinheiro, M.B.; Lin, C.W.C.; Day, R.O.; McLachlan, A.; Ferreira, M.L. Efficacy and safety of paracetamol for spinal pain and osteoarthritis: Systematic review and meta-analysis of randomised placebo controlled trials. *BMJ* **2015**, *350*, h1225. [CrossRef]
33. World Health Organization. *Cancer Pain Relief: With a Guide to Opioid Availability*, 2nd ed.; World Health Organization: Geneva, Switzerland, 1996. Available online: https://apps.who.int/iris/handle/10665/37896 (accessed on 18 November 2021).
34. Knotkova, H.; Pappagallo, M. Adjuvant analgesics. *Med. Clin. N. Am.* **2007**, *91*, 113–124. [CrossRef] [PubMed]
35. Bellingham, G.A.; Peng, P.W. Duloxetine: A review of its pharmacology and use in chronic pain management. *Reg. Anesth. Pain Med.* **2010**, *35*, 294–303. [CrossRef] [PubMed]
36. Munce, S.E.; Stewart, D.E. Gender differences in depression and chronic pain conditions in a national epidemiologic survey. *Psychosomatics* **2007**, *48*, 394–399. [CrossRef] [PubMed]

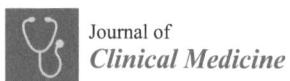

Article

Prevalence and Clinical Conditions Related to Sarcopaenia among Older Persons Living in the Community

Encarnación Blanco-Reina [1,*], Ricardo Ocaña-Riola [2], Gabriel Ariza-Zafra [3], María Rosa García-Merino [4], Lorena Aguilar-Cano [5], Jenifer Valdellós [4], Claudia Torres-Blanco [6] and Inmaculada Bellido-Estévez [1]

1. Pharmacology and Therapeutics Department, Instituto de Investigación Biomédica de Málaga-IBIMA, School of Medicine, University of Málaga, 29016 Málaga, Spain; ibellido@uma.es
2. Escuela Andaluza de Salud Pública, 18011 Granada, Spain; ricardo.ocana.easp@juntadeandalucia.es
3. Geriatrics Department, Complejo Hospitalario Universitario, 02006 Albacete, Spain; gariza@sescam.jccm.es
4. Health District of Málaga-Guadalhorce, 29009 Málaga, Spain; rosaballet@yahoo.es (M.R.G.-M.); jenny_dok7@hotmail.com (J.V.)
5. Physical Medicine and Rehabilitation Department, Hospital Regional Universitario, 29010 Málaga, Spain; loagca2011@hotmail.com
6. Pharmacology and Therapeutics Department, School of Medicine, University of Málaga, 29016 Málaga, Spain; claudiatblanco4@gmail.com
* Correspondence: eblanco@uma.es; Tel.: +34-952-136-648

Abstract: (1) Background: In health care and in society at large, sarcopaenia is a disorder of major importance that can lead to disability and other negative health-related events. Our study aim is to determine the prevalence of sarcopaenia among older people attended in primary care and to analyse the factors associated with this age-related clinical condition; (2) Methods: A multicentre cross-sectional study was conducted of 333 community-dwelling Spanish adults aged 65 years or more. Sociodemographic, clinical, functional, anthropometric, and pharmacological data were collected. Sarcopaenia was defined following European Working Group on Sarcopaenia in Older People (EWGSOP) criteria; (3) Results: Sarcopaenia was present in 20.4% of the study sample, and to a severe degree in 6%. The intensity of the association between sarcopaenia and frailty was weak-moderate (Cramer V = 0.45). According to the multinomial logistic regression model performed, sarcopaenia was positively associated with age and with the presence of psychopathology (OR = 2.72; 95% CI = 1.30–5.70) and was inversely correlated with body mass index (OR = 0.73; 95% CI = 0.67–0.80); (4) Conclusions: Sarcopaenia commonly affects community-dwelling older persons and may be associated with age, body mass index, and psychopathology. The latter factor may be modifiable or treatable and is therefore a possible target for intervention.

Keywords: sarcopaenia; older adults; primary care; psychopathology; frailty; body mass index

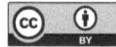

1. Introduction

In recent years, there has been growing interest in identifying age-related conditions that can lead to disability. In this context, special attention has been paid to the study of sarcopaenia, a condition that is closely related to physical function impairment. The term sarcopaenia was originally proposed in 1989 to describe age-related decrease in muscle mass [1,2]. Subsequently, various operational definitions and diagnostic criteria have been proposed. It has been suggested that defining sarcopaenia only in terms of muscle mass is of very limited value, for several reasons. Firstly, the association between this criterion alone and adverse health outcomes is weak. Moreover, muscle strength does not depend exclusively on muscle mass, and the relationship between them is not linear [3,4]. In response to these observations, a functional dimension has been added to the term. In 2010, the European Working Group on Sarcopaenia in Older People (EWGSOP) provided a working definition for sarcopaenia [5], proposing that it be diagnosed using the twin criteria of low muscle mass and low muscle function (either low strength and/or low physical performance). This operational definition represented an important change and is currently in wide use, worldwide. More recently, however, in order to reflect the growing body of new scientific and clinical evidence regarding this question, the EWGSOP recommendations have been updated (as EWGSOP2) [6], and the broad description of sarcopaenia is that it is a muscle disease (or failure) rooted in adverse muscle changes that accrue over a lifetime. In fact, sarcopaenia is already formally recognised as a muscle disease, with a specific ICD-10-MC diagnosis code, which represents an important step forward towards a generally accepted classification [7,8].

Progressive muscle loss in the elderly is due in part to physiological age-related changes, such as the loss of motoneuron units, decreased hormone status, and increased insulin sensitivity, which in turn lead to increased proteolysis, decreased muscle protein synthesis, and increased fat infiltration of the muscle [9]. Other factors that may contribute to the development of sarcopaenia include immobility, inflammation, an inactive lifestyle, and malnutrition. We believe it important to seek a better understanding of this geriatric syndrome due to its prevalence, its association with negative health-related events, the existence of certain potentially reversible factors, and because it is, at least initially, a treatable condition. In this respect, physical exercise to gain muscle resistance and a focused nutritional intervention are of fundamental importance.

Widely varying accounts have been given of the prevalence of sarcopaenia [10–14]. In part, this is because it depends on the characteristics of the population under study (such as age, gender, comorbidity, and race) and on the healthcare setting considered, but the value obtained is also subject to the methodology used to assess muscle mass and even to the definition made of sarcopaenia [11]. Even when focusing exclusively on community-dwelling older people, the heterogeneity of the samples analysed, the criteria used, and the cut-off points selected combine to affect the prevalence obtained, reported values of which range from 6% to 59.8% [11], or from 9.9% to 40.4% according to other sources [12–14]. In any case, the global rate of sarcopaenia is undoubtedly rising across the world, and the impact is especially high among the elderly population in nursing homes and those who are hospitalised or in rehabilitation units [11].

Sarcopaenia has a major impact on society and its healthcare systems, imposing severe personal, social, and economic burdens [15]. Among other consequences, it increases the risk of falls and fractures [16,17], impairs patients' ability to perform activities of daily living [18], provokes mobility disorders [19], limits independence [20], decreases the quality of life [21], and can even lead to death [22,23].

In view of these considerations, a heightened awareness of the dangers of sarcopaenia should become a part of clinical routine, with special regard to community-dwelling older persons. Primary care is the most common health contact point for most of the older population. Moreover, attention is usually comprehensive and personalised, making this healthcare environment very suitable for the identification, management, and study of sarcopaenia. However, the assessment and treatment of sarcopaenia at the outpatient level is still uncommon. Accordingly, this complex syndrome is probably underdiagnosed [24]. In view of its relationship with disability and other negative health-related events, and the need to continue characterising its prevalence in different settings, the present study was designed to address these questions. The progression of sarcopaenia depends on various factors, and their joint effects are directly relevant to the possibilities of prevention and treatment [25]. The main aim of the present study is to determine the prevalence of sarcopaenia among older adults living in the community in Spain, where life expectancy rates are among the highest in the world [26], and to analyse related factors, some of which are potentially modifiable through specific interventions and preventive actions.

2. Materials and Methods

This multicentre cross-sectional study was carried out within a primary healthcare context.

2.1. Reference Population and Study Sample

The study sample was composed of persons aged 65 years or more, living in the community, attended at primary care centres in Malaga (Spain). All participants were registered in the database of the Spanish NHS, were treated in an outpatient setting (i.e., not institutionalised), and provided signed informed consent to take part in the study. As exclusion criteria, none had implanted metal devices (pacemakers or osteoarticular prostheses, because they might cause interference with electric bioimpedanciometry measurements), had suffered the complete or partial amputation of a limb, or had an advanced or terminal illness. The patients were recruited at nine primary healthcare centres, using stratified random sampling designed to obtain a representative sample. The study population was allocated in proportion to the size of each healthcare centre. Based on a published prevalence of sarcopaenia in primary care of 22% [27,28] and assuming a margin of error of less than 4.5% and a 95% confidence interval, we calculated that the minimum sample size required for this study would be 325 persons.

2.2. Data Collection and Global Assessment

The participants were interviewed using a structured questionnaire, and various physical tests were conducted to assess the presence and degree of sarcopaenia. Further data were obtained from medication packaging and digital medical records. A complete set of sociodemographic, clinical, functional, and pharmacological data were collected from all participants. The clinical data included all diseases recorded, possible comorbidities, and Charlson's comorbidity index (CCI) [29]. Information was also obtained about the medication prescribed (indication, dosage, and duration of any treatment received during the last three months or more). Polypharmacy was defined as the chronic prescription of five or more drugs.

Cognitive function was evaluated using Pfeiffer's short portable mental state questionnaire (SPMSQ) [30], and mood status was determined using Yesavage's geriatric depression scale (GDS-15) [31]. The patients' independence in performing instrumental activities of daily living (IADL) was assessed using the Lawton scale [32]. The body mass index (BMI) was calculated, and nutritional screening was performed using the Spanish version (Nestlé Nutrition Institute) of the Mini Nutritional Assessment-Short Form [33]. The different BMI categories (underweight, normal, overweight, and obesity) were operationalised following the World Health Organization cut-off values.

Frailty was assessed according to the phenotype proposed by Fried et al. [34], which consists of the following criteria: (a) unintentional weight loss of 4.5 kg or more in the previous year; (b) self-reported exhaustion, identified by two questions on the Center for Epidemiological Studies Depression (CES-D) scale; (c) weakness, defined by low handgrip strength and measured in kg in the dominant hand using a dynamometer (highest of three consecutive measurements), adjusted for gender and BMI (grip strength was classified as low when the force exerted was below the first quintile of the distribution); (d) slow walking speed (lowest quintile of gait speed), assessed by the walking time (in seconds) over a distance of 4.57 m, adjusted for gender and height; and (e) low physical activity, measured by the weighted score of kilocalories expended per week, obtained from the Minnesota Leisure Time Activity Questionnaire and adjusted for gender. Participants were classified as non-frail (robust) if they met none of the criteria, pre-frail if they met one or two criteria, and frail if three or more criteria were met.

2.3. Assessment of Sarcopaenia

The main study outcome was sarcopaenia, which was defined following EWGSOP criteria [5]. According to these criteria, diagnosis of sarcopaenia required the documentation of low muscle mass plus the documentation of either low muscle strength or low physical performance.

2.3.1. Muscle Mass

Muscle mass was measured by bioelectrical impedance analysis (BIA). The BIA resistance (measurement range 150–1200 Ohms) was determined using a Tanita BC-418 body composition analyser (Tanita Corporation, Tokyo, Japan) with an 8-electrode method and an operating frequency of 50 kHz. Muscle mass was calculated using Janssen's bioelectrical impedance analysis equation [35]. Absolute skeletal muscle mass was converted to skeletal muscle index (SMI) by dividing the limb skeletal muscle mass (kg) by the square of the height (m^2). Low muscle mass was defined as the SMI of two standard deviations (SDs) or more below the normal sex-specific mean for young persons. Using the cut-off points indicated in the EWGSOP consensus, low muscle mass was classified as SMI < 8.87 kg/m^2 in men and <6.42 kg/m^2 in women.

2.3.2. Muscle Strength

Muscle strength was assessed by grip strength, measured using a Jamar hydraulic grip hand dynamometer SP-5030J1 (Lafayette Instrument Company, Lafayette, IN, USA). Patients were instructed to perform a maximal isometric contraction, and the highest value of three consecutive measurements was recorded. BMI-adjusted values were used as cut-off points to classify low muscle strength (following EWGSOP recommendations for men/women) [5].

2.3.3. Physical Performance

Usual walking speed (m/s) on a 4-metre course was used as an objective measure of physical performance. The time elapsed from the start to the finish point was recorded by an investigator with a digital chronometer, and the best time of two attempts was recorded. A cut-off point of 0.8 m/s or less in gait speed was used to define low physical performance [5].

Sarcopaenia was diagnosed as follows: low muscle mass alone was defined as pre-sarcopaenia; the joint presence of low muscle mass and low muscle strength or low performance was defined as sarcopaenia; and the presence of all three criteria was considered as severe sarcopaenia.

All data were measured and collected by primary care clinicians, who were active members of the research team.

2.4. Statistical Analysis

Exploratory data analysis and frequency tables were used to describe the study variables. Taking into account the four possible categories of the main variable according to the EWGSOP conceptual stages of sarcopaenia (pre-sarcopaenia, sarcopaenia, severe sarcopaenia, and no sarcopaenia), a multinomial logistic regression model was used to study the relationship between the independent variables and the outcome variable, sarcopaenia [36]. All independent variables were included in the regression model. The influence of various factors on the states of pre-sarcopaenia, sarcopaenia, and severe sarcopaenia was examined, taking non-sarcopaenic patients as a benchmark. Odds ratios (OR) and 95% confidence intervals (CI) were calculated for each covariate included in the model. A 5% significance level was assumed to indicate statistical significance. All statistical data analyses were performed using SPSS version 24.0 (IBM SPSS Statistics, Armonk, NY, USA).

2.5. Ethical Considerations

This study was conducted in accordance with the Declaration of Helsinki. The Málaga Clinical Research Ethics Committee approved the study (PI-0234-14), and informed consent was obtained from all patients prior to their inclusion.

3. Results

3.1. Characteristics of the Study Population

The study population consisted of 333 community-dwelling Spanish adults aged 65 years or more. Their mean age was 72.81 years (standard deviation 5.1, range 65–91), and slightly more than half were female. Only 19.5% lived alone; the rest lived with a partner, family member(s), or caretaker (professional or otherwise). The average CCI score was 1.30 (standard deviation 1.4, range 0–7), and 33.3% of the patients had a score > 2. Each patient presented an average of 7.4 diagnoses (standard deviation 3.4, range 0–20) and was consuming 6.5 drugs (standard deviation 4.0; range 0–21), with a polymedication prevalence of 65.8%. The most prevalent chronic conditions were bone and joint disorders (mainly osteoarthritis of the knee, hip, hand, and shoulder) (76.9%), hypertension (68.2%), and dyslipidaemia (51.7%). Some form of psychopathology (mainly anxiety and/or depression) was present in 37.8% of the patients, and 42.6% suffered insomnia. The mean score on the Lawton scale was 6.7 (standard deviation 1.7, range 0–8) with half of the sample being independently capable of performing IADL. Regarding anthropometric and nutritional characteristics, the mean BMI was 30.3 kg/m^2 (standard deviation 4.9, range 18.9–52.3). Only 14.7% of the patients had a normal weight; 39.6% presented overweight and 45.6% obesity. Among the participants with obesity, more than half (56.6%) were class I (30–34.9 kg/m^2), 34.9% were class II (35–39.9 kg/m^2), and 8.5% were obesity class III or severe (>40 kg/m^2). Nevertheless, according to the MNA, 95.5% of the participants had a good nutritional status and only 3.3% were at risk of malnutrition or were malnourished (1.2%). The sociodemographic, functional, cognitive, and clinical characteristics of the study participants are summarised in Table 1.

Table 1. Characteristics of the study population (n = 333).

Quantitative Variables	Mean	Standard Deviation
Age (years)	72.8	5.1
Lawton (IADL)	6.7	1.7
BMI (kg/m^2)	30.3	4.9
Number of comorbidities	7.4	3.4
Number of drugs per patient	6.5	4
Qualitative Variables	**Subjects (n)**	**Percentage (%)**
Gender		
Male	138	41.4
Female	195	58.6
Lawton (IADL)		
0–1	4	1.2
2 3	19	5.7
4–5	44	13.2
6–7	95	28.5
8	171	51.4
SPMSQ (Pfeiffer)		
0–2 errors	305	91.6
3–4 errors	21	6.3
5 errors and over	7	2.1
GDS-15		
0–5	255	76.6
6–9	56	16.8
10 and over	22	6.6
BMI categories		
Underweight	0	0

Table 1. *Cont.*

Qualitative Variables	Subjects (*n*)	Percentage (%)
Normal	49	14.7
Overweight	132	39.6
Obese	152	45.6
Nutritional status		
Normal	318	95.5
Malnutrition risk	11	3.3
Malnourished	4	1.2
Charlson Comorbidity Index		
0–1	219	65.8
2	53	15.9
3 or more	61	18.3
Specific comorbidities		
Bone and joint disorders	256	76.9
Hypertension	227	68.2
Dyslipidaemia	172	51.7
Insomnia	142	42.6
Psychopathology	126	37.8
Diabetes mellitus	89	26.8
Heart disease	81	24.3
Respiratory disease	125	21.5
Osteoporosis	57	17.1
Polymedication	219	65.8
Frailty states		
Robust (non-frail)	72	21.6
Pre-frail	190	57.1
Frail	71	21.3
Fried criterion		
Unintentional weight loss	22	6.6
Exhaustion	68	20.4
Weakness	209	62.8
Slow walking speed	59	17.7
Low physical activity	164	49,2

IADL: Instrumental activities of daily living; BMI: Body mass index (0.0–18.5: underweight; 18.5–24.9: normal; 25.0–29.9: overweight; 30 and over: obese); SPMSQ: Short Portable Mental Status Questionnaire (0–2 errors: normal mental functioning; 3–4 errors: mild cognitive impairment; 5 errors and over: moderate-severe cognitive impairment); GDS-15: Geriatric Depression Scale (0–5: no depression; 6–9: suggestive of depression, 10 and over: almost always depression).

Frailty was present in 21.3% of participants; 57.1% were pre-frail and 21.6% were non-frail. The most prevalent Fried phenotype criterion observed in the sample was weakness (62.8%), followed by low physical activity (49.2%) and exhaustion (20.4%).

3.2. Assessment of Sarcopaenia and Related Factors

According to the EWGSOP algorithm, 20.4% of the community-dwelling older adults in the sample had sarcopaenia, and 6% had severe sarcopaenia. Slightly more than half (57.7%) of the participants did not meet any criteria for sarcopaenia and 15.9% were considered pre-sarcopaenic (low muscle mass alone) (Table 2). The mean SMI was 7.6 kg/m^2 (standard deviation 1.4; range 4.8–12.0). For the female participants, the mean SMI was 6.7 kg/m^2 (standard deviation 0.8; range 4.8–9.2), and for the men, it was 9.0 kg/m^2 (standard deviation 0.9; range 5.8–12.0). Therefore, sarcopaenia was present, overall, in 26.4% of this elderly population. The condition was more common in women (29.2%) than in men (22.5%), and among the non-obese than the obese (37% vs. 13.8%, respectively; $p < 0.001$). The coincidence of obesity and sarcopaenia was present in 6.3% of the sample. In this respect, too, the mean BMI was higher in non-sarcopaenic than in sarcopaenic patients (31.3 kg/m^2 versus 27.6 kg/m^2, respectively; $p < 0.001$).

Table 2. Sarcopaenia categories and criteria according to EWGSOP (n = 333).

	Subjects (n)	Percentage (%)
Sarcopaenia categories		
No sarcopaenia	192	57.7
Pre-sarcopaenia	53	15.9
Sarcopaenia	68	20.4
Severe sarcopaenia	20	6
Criteria		
Low muscle mass	141	42.3
Low muscle strength	209	62.8
Slow walking speed	59	17.7

Categories: No sarcopaenia: 0 criteria present; Pre-sarcopaenia: low muscle mass alone; Sarcopaenia (2 criteria present): low muscle mass + low muscle strength or low performance; Severe sarcopaenia: 3 criteria present.

Regarding the combination of sarcopaenia and frailty, 7.8% of participants were both frail and sarcopaenic, while 13.5% were frail-only. None were sarcopaenic-only. Therefore, there were no patients who were sarcopaenic and robust at the same time, and all sarcopaenic individuals were either in a state of pre-frailty (70.5%) or one of frailty (29.5%). The prevalence of frailty among those with sarcopaenia was 40.2%; among those with frailty, the prevalence of sarcopaenia was 36.6%. The intensity of the association between sarcopaenia and frailty was weak-moderate (Cramer V = 0.45).

A multinomial logistic regression analysis was performed to further examine the influence of the independent variables on the EWGSOP sarcopaenia categories (Table 3). The two factors that were most consistently associated with the presence of sarcopaenia were BMI and the diagnosis of a psychopathology. In fact, the odds of presenting sarcopaenia and severe sarcopaenia decreased by 27% and 25% for each additional point (kg/m^2) of BMI (OR = 0.73, 95% CI = 0.67–0.80; OR = 0.75, 95% CI = 0.66–0.86), respectively. However, these odds rose sharply for persons with a psychopathology, for all states of sarcopaenia. Thus, the OR of patients with vs. without a psychopathology were 2.56 (95% CI = 1.06–6.19) for pre-sarcopaenia, 2.72 (95% CI = 1.30–5.70) for sarcopaenia, and 7.89 (95% CI = 2.25–27.59) for severe sarcopaenia, with all other covariates being equal. No relevant association was found between sarcopaenia and the other prevalent pathologies considered or with the number of medications consumed. In this population sample, gender did not behave as a predictor variable; however, age was related to severe sarcopaenia. Thus, for each additional year of life, the odds of presenting severe sarcopaenia increased by 10% (OR = 1.11, 95% CI = 1.01–1.22).

Table 3. Factors related to sarcopaenia. Multinomial logistic regression for pre-sarcopaenia, sarcopaenia, and severe sarcopaenia states (with respect to non-sarcopenic).

Independent Variable	Pre-Sarcopaenia OR (95% CI)	Sarcopaenia OR (95% CI)	Severe Sarcopaenia OR (95% CI)
Age	0.94 (0.87–1.02)	0.98 (0.92–1.04)	1.11 (1.01–1.22) *
Number of comorbidities	0.79 (0.65–0.97) *	0.92 (0.78–1.08)	1.04 (0.82–1.33)
Number of medicines	1.08 (0.95–1.24)	0.98 (0.87–1.10)	1.03 (0.85–1.24)
BMI	0.74 (0.67–0.83) ***	0.73 (0.67–0.0.80) ***	0.75 (0.66–0.86) ***
Gender			
Male	0.51 (0.22–1.18)	0.64 (0.31–1.31)	0.46 (0.11–1.84)
Female	1	1	1
Diabetes mellitus			
Yes	1.12 (0.45–2.76)	0.76 (0.33–1.74)	2.58 (0.79–8.41)
No	1	1	1

Table 3. Cont.

Independent Variable	Pre-Sarcopaenia OR (95% CI)	Sarcopaenia OR (95% CI)	Severe Sarcopaenia OR (95% CI)
Heart disease			
Yes	1.04 (0.34–3.09)	1.09 (0.43–2.75)	0.44 (0.89–2.24)
No	1	1	1
Bone and joint disorder			
Yes	0.38 (0.16–0.89) *	0.73 (0.32–1.65)	1.59 (0.16–15.09)
No	1	1	1
Osteoporosis			
Yes	0.87 (0.31–2.45)	0.28 (0.10–0.79) *	1.10 (0.34–3.58)
No	1	1	1
Psychopathology			
Yes	2.56 (1.06– 6.19) *	2.72 (1.30–5.70) **	7.89 (2.25–27.59) ***
No	1	1	1
Low physical activity			
Yes	0.31 (0.13–0.72) *	0.95 (0.48–1.85)	1.90 (0.59–6.09)
No	1	1	1

OR: odds ratio; BMI: Body mass index (kg/m^2). * $p < 0.05$; ** $p < 0.01$; *** $p < 0.001$.

4. Discussion

The results of the present study show that sarcopaenia (assessed using the EWGSOP algorithm) is present in about a quarter of community-dwelling older patients (sarcopaenia in 20.4% and severe sarcopaenia in 6%). These prevalence data are slightly higher than those reported by similar studies conducted in Spain [27] or elsewhere [28] and are close to the upper limit of the expected range in this health setting. Systematic reviews of studies also carried out on elderly outpatient populations, using the same diagnostic criteria, have reported prevalences ranging from 9.9–40.4% [13], 1–33 % [10], and 10–27% [37]. This considerable heterogeneity between the studies may reflect differences in the diagnostic criteria used, in the cut-off points chosen, and in the characteristics of the target population. In our study, the EWGSOP algorithm was used because it was the working definition most commonly employed when the study began, and thus provided the best comparability with previous work in this area. Moreover, the EWGSOP operational definition offered cut-off points for muscle strength that corresponded to those of the weakness item in the Fried criteria. Very recent studies have shown that the EWGSOP2 diagnostic criteria detect lower prevalences than EWGSOP [38], i.e., the 2010 original version presents greater sensitivity [39].

According to our findings, sarcopaenia is positively associated with age and with the presence of one or more psychopathologies, and inversely correlated with BMI. In our study population, the prevalence of sarcopaenia was higher in women than in men, but a statistically significant association with gender was not confirmed in the multivariate regression model. Although some studies have observed a higher prevalence in the female population [40], most systematic reviews report that more men than women are affected by sarcopaenia [11,14]. There is no clear explanation in this regard, nor has this conclusion been definitively established. It has been suggested that the cut-off value threshold could influence the question [41], or that reduced functional status in men is more closely related to the loss of muscle mass, while in women this decline would be more associated with osteoarthritis, osteoporosis, or depression [42]. We did find a significant relationship with age, such that for each additional year of life, the odds of presenting severe sarcopenia increased by 10%. This is a biologically plausible result that is consistent with previous findings [40,43,44].

Regarding comorbidities, the clinical condition that was associated with all states of sarcopaenia was the diagnosis of psychopathology (mainly anxiety and depression), which doubled the odds of a patient presenting pre-sarcopaenia or sarcopaenia and multiplied them by seven for severe sarcopaenia. Sarcopaenia has most frequently been associated with other chronic conditions such as chronic lung disease, neurological disease, and neoplasia. However, some evidence of a relationship with depression has also been observed, but this association appears to be weaker and is less commonly reported [45–47]. An association has also been reported between mental pathology and frailty [48,49]. It has been observed that persons with a psychopathology tend to be less physically active, to have a less active social life, and to consume a less healthy diet, and that any or all of these factors could be related to a loss of strength and muscle mass.

Our findings show that after adjusting for potential confounders, BMI is closely associated with sarcopaenia. Thus, the odds of a patient presenting sarcopaenia and severe sarcopaenia decrease by 27% and 25% for each additional point (kg/m^2) of BMI, respectively. In consequence, we found the prevalence of sarcopaenia among those with obesity to be significantly lower than among the non-obese population (13.8% vs. 37%, respectively). This inverse relationship between BMI and sarcopaenia is consistent with other studies [43,44]. However, although BMI has been considered an approximate marker of nutritional status, sarcopaenia sometimes coexists with obesity. In our study sample, the prevalence of sarcopaenic obesity was 6.3%, an intermediate figure according to data from a recent systematic review and meta-analysis (2–9%) [37]. It seems that adipose inflammation leads to intra-abdominal fat redistribution and fat infiltration in the muscle. Accordingly, synergy between the loss of muscle mass and this fat infiltration could trigger the pathogenesis of sarcopaenic obesity [50]. In any case, the nutritional status of our community-dwelling older persons was very good (only 1.2% malnutrition), but the presence of obesity was high compared to previous reports. Thus, a study of older adults in 21 European countries reported only 20.9% obesity compared to 45.6% in our sample population [51]. Among other causes, this high prevalence could be due to a certain north-south gradient. According to a national study conducted in Spain, obesity is higher in the south (where Malaga is located) than in the rest of the country [52].

The coexistence of frailty and sarcopaenia was observed in 7.8% of the patients in our study. This rate is lower than that found in another multicentre study conducted in Spain, but the latter focused on hospitalised patients with a higher disease burden, which would explain the discrepancy (18%) [43]. In a recent cohort study of community-dwelling older adults in Australia, more similar to ours, only 2.8% of participants were both frail and sarcopaenic. Among these participants, with either condition, the risk of mortality was over three times higher [53]. The prevalence of frailty among those with sarcopaenia was 40.2%, and that of sarcopaenia among frail patients was 36.6%, results very similar to those found by Reijinierse et al. (42.1% and 36.4%, respectively) who concluded that outpatients with sarcopaenia were more likely to be frail than frail outpatients to be sarcopaenic [54]. Therefore, although sarcopaenia and frailty are related processes and indeed there is some overlap between the criteria that define them, the combined prevalence is low, which reflects the fact that they are different constructs and represent different types of pathophysiology. Sarcopaenia consists of impaired function and muscle mass, while frailty is a broader, multifactorial process that reduces homeostatic reserves. This slight degree of concordance corroborates the conclusions of previous research, in which the two diagnoses did not always coincide according to all definitions applied [54]. In addition, our results show that the intensity of the association between sarcopaenia and frailty was only weak-moderate (Cramer V = 0.45), a low intercorrelation previously reported by the Toledo Study of Healthy Aging (Cramer V = 0.16) [27]. Therefore, it is important to diagnose these conditions separately in order to perform the most appropriate intervention. In accordance with Thompson et al., we believe that individuals identified as frail would benefit from an assessment for sarcopaenia, and vice versa, as a joint assessment is more predictive of mortality than one of either condition alone [53].

It seems well established that progressive resistance training and an adequate protein intake help build muscle mass. In this respect, too, certain dietary interventions (mainly concerning amino acids, vitamin D, antioxidants, and other supplements) are currently being considered [55]. However, although sarcopaenia is currently a topic of great interest, some authors have drawn attention to the possible adverse effects of overdiagnosis and of classifying this phenomenon as a disease. Indeed, it has not been shown that diagnosing sarcopaenia reduces morbidity and mortality, or that the specific treatment for this condition produces better results than the general recommendations of appropriate physical exercise and diet. Moreover, the diagnostic criteria applied tend to be varied and even arbitrary [56]. In view of these considerations, we believe that while sarcopaenia screening studies are positive, encouraging awareness of this condition, revealing its impact and underlining the necessity to adopt an appropriate lifestyle and diet, nevertheless unnecessary labelling should be avoided, and more and better evidence should be obtained about sarcopaenia and its impact on the elderly population.

The study we describe has various strengths. It is based on the analysis of data obtained from a representative sample of healthcare centres and on the global assessment of the participants. The data considered are sufficient in quantity and quality, having been collected directly via personal interviews, anthropometric tests, and medical records. Moreover, in our opinion, the outpatient setting is ideal for assessing conditions such as frailty and sarcopaenia because it is where large numbers of elderly patients are attended and where certain interventions are best performed. Among other strong points of our analysis, the EWGSOP diagnostic criteria were rigorously applied, and the cut-off points used to classify low muscle mass coincide with those of many other studies [40,41,44,57,58]. This parameter was assessed using BIA, as in most studies in the field, due to its accessibility, ease of use, and portability within the health centre. Although DXA is a more precise method, its use in clinical routine is limited by cost considerations and the need for more specialised equipment and personnel. In addition, data suggest there is a good correlation between BIA and DXA [59]. Among the limitations of the study are its cross-sectional design, which means that causal relationships cannot be established, and the fact that it was carried out in a single region and country, which reduces its external validity. However, we believe that the sample considered is representative of a large proportion of community-dwelling older adults, and that the findings found provide a good reflection of circumstances in similar socio-sanitary environments. Another possible limitation of the study is not having considered among the exclusion criteria possible cachexia status, such as cancer and COPD, which are circumstances that can also cause muscle loss.

5. Conclusions

According to the EWGSOP criteria, sarcopaenia is a common condition among community-dwelling older persons and may be associated with factors such as age, body mass index, and the presence of one or more psychopathologies. The latter predictive factor may be modifiable or treatable, and thus constitutes a possible area of intervention. Therefore, more attention should be paid to certain signs (or symptoms) to better detect anxiety and depression in the elderly, as these processes tend to be underdiagnosed and appropriate remedial measures would promote healthy aging. Sarcopaenia and frailty are related but separate conditions and require specific approaches.

Author Contributions: Conceptualization, E.B.-R. and G.A.-Z.; methodology, E.B.-R. and R.O.-R.; formal analysis, E.B.-R. and R.O.-R.; investigation, E.B.-R., R.O.-R., G.A.-Z., L.A.-C., M.R.G.-M., J.V., C.T.-B. and I.B.-E.; resources, E.B.-R. and I.B.-E.; data curation: L.A.-C., M.R.G.-M., J.V., and C.T.-B.; writing-original draft preparation, E.B.-R., R.O.-R. and G.A.-Z.; writing—review and editing, E.B.-R., R.O.-R., G.A.-Z. and I.B.-E.; visualization, E.B.-R., R.O.-R. and I.B.-E.; supervision, E.B.-R.; project administration, E.B.-R.; funding acquisition: E.B.-R. All authors have read and agreed to the published version of the manuscript.

Funding: This research was funded by the Fundación Pública Andaluza Progreso y Salud, Con-sejería de Salud, Junta de Andalucía, through the Programme Proyectos de Investigación Biomé-dica (Grant number PI 0234/14). The APC was funded by the University of Málaga. The funders had no role in the design of the study; in the collection, analyses, or interpretation of data; in the writing of the manuscript; or in the decision to publish the results.

Institutional Review Board Statement: The study was conducted according to the guidelines of the Declaration of Helsinki and approved by the Málaga Clinical Research Ethics Committee (protocol EBR-MED-2013-01, PI-0234-14; approval date, 25 July 2013).

Informed Consent Statement: Informed consent was obtained from all subjects involved in the study.

Data Availability Statement: The data that support the findings of this study are not publicly available due to being used for further investigational objectives and because the data contain information that could compromise the privacy of research participants. However, specific information can be obtained from the corresponding author upon reasonable request (E.B.-R.).

Acknowledgments: The authors wish to thank the Primary Care Management Team (Health District of Málaga-Guadalhorce) for providing access to the health centres and patient lists.

Conflicts of Interest: The authors declare no conflict of interest.

References

1. Rosenberg, I.H. Summary comments: Epidemiological and methodological problems in determining nutritional status of older people. *Am. J. Clin. Nutr.* **1989**, *50*, 1231–1233. [CrossRef]
2. Rosenberg, I.H. Sarcopenia: Origins and clinical relevance. *J. Nutr.* **1997**, *127*, 990S–991S. [CrossRef] [PubMed]
3. Goodpaster, B.H.; Park, S.W.; Harris, T.B.; Kritchevsky, S.B.; Nevitt, M.; Schwartz, A.V.; Simonsick, E.M.; Tylavsky, F.A.; Visser, M.; Newman, A.B. The loss of skeletal muscle strength, mass, and quality in older adults: The health aging and body composition study. *J. Gerontol. A Biol. Sci. Med. Sci.* **2006**, *61*, 1059–1064. [CrossRef] [PubMed]
4. Janssen, I.; Baumgartner, R.; Ross, R.; Rosenberg, I.H.; Roubenoff, R. Skeletal muscle cutpoints associated with elevated physical disability risk in older men and women. *Am. J. Epidemiol.* **2004**, *159*, 413–421. [CrossRef]
5. Cruz-Jentoft, A.J.; Baeyens, J.P.; Bauer, J.M.; Boirie, Y.; Cederholm, T.; Landi, F.; Martin, F.C.; Michel, J.-P.; Rolland, Y.; Schneider, S.M.; et al. Sarcopenia: European consensus on definition and diagnosis: Report of the European Working Group on Sarcopenia in Older People. *Age Ageing* **2010**, *39*, 412–423. [CrossRef] [PubMed]
6. Cruz-Jentoft, A.J.; Bahat, G.; Bauer, J.; Boirie, Y.; Bruyere, O.; Cederholm, T.; Cooper, C.; Landi, F.; Rolland, Y.; Sayer, A.A.; et al. Sarcopenia: Revised European consensus on definition and diagnosis. *Age Ageing* **2019**, *48*, 16–31. [CrossRef]
7. Anker, S.D.; Morley, J.E.; von Haehling, S. Welcome to the ICD-10 code for sarcopenia. *J. Cachexia Sarcopenia Muscle* **2016**, *7*, 512–514. [CrossRef]
8. 2022 ICD-10-CM Diagnosis Code M62.84. Sarcopenia. Available online: https://www.icd10data.com/ICD10CM/Codes/M00-M99/M60-M63/M62-/M62.84 (accessed on 30 May 2022).
9. International Working Group on Sarcopenia. Sarcopenia: An undiagnosed condition in older adults. Current consensus definition: Prevalence, etiology, and consequences. *J. Am. Med. Dir. Assoc.* **2011**, *12*, 249–256. [CrossRef]
10. Cruz-Jentoft, A.J.; Landi, F.; Schneider, S.M.; Zúñiga, C.; Arai, H.; Boirie, Y.; Chen, L.-K.; Fielding, R.A.; Martin, F.C.; Michel, J.-E.; et al. Prevalence of and interventions for sarcopenia in ageing adults: A systematic review. Report of the International Sarcopenia Initiative (EWGSOP and IWGS). *Age Ageing* **2014**, *43*, 748–759. [CrossRef]
11. Lardiés-Sánchez, B.; Sanz-Paris, A.; Boj-Carceller, D.; Cruz-Jentoft, A.J. Systematic review: Prevalence of sarcopenia in ageing people using bioelectrical impedance analysis to assess muscle mass. *Eur. Geriatr. Med.* **2016**, *7*, 256–261. [CrossRef]
12. Shafiee, G.; Keshtkar, A.; Soltani, A.; Ahadi, Z.; Larijani, B.; Heshmat, R. Prevalence of sarcopenia in the world: A systematic review and meta-analysis of general population studies. *J. Diabetes Metab. Disord.* **2017**, *16*, 21. [CrossRef] [PubMed]
13. Mayhew, A.J.; Amog, K.; Phillips, S.; Parise, G.; McNicholas, P.D.; de Souza, R.J.; Thabane, L.; Raina, P. The prevalence of sarcopenia in community-dwelling older adults, an exploration of differences between studies and within definitions: A systematic review and meta-analyses. *Age Ageing* **2019**, *48*, 48–56. [CrossRef] [PubMed]
14. Papadopoulou, S.K.; Tsintavis, P.; Potsaki, P.; Papandreou, D. Differences in the Prevalence of Sarcopenia in Community-Dwelling, Nursing Home and Hospitalized Individuals. A Systematic Review and Meta-Analysis. *J. Nutr. Health Aging* **2020**, *24*, 83–90. [CrossRef]
15. Mijnarends, D.M.; Luiking, Y.C.; Halfens, R.J.G.; Evers, S.M.A.A.; Lenaerts, E.L.A.; Verlaan, S.; Wallace, M.; Schols, J.M.G.A.; Meijers, J.M.M. Muscle, health and costs: A glance at their relationship. *J. Nutr. Health Aging* **2018**, *22*, 766–773. [CrossRef] [PubMed]
16. Bischoff-Ferrari, H.A.; Orav, J.E.; Kanis, J.A.; Rizzoli, R.; Schlögl, M.; Staehelin, H.B.; Willett, W.C.; Dawson-Hughes, B. Comparative performance of current definitions of sarcopenia against the prospective incidence of falls among community-dwelling seniors age 65 and older. *Osteoporos Int.* **2015**, *26*, 2793–2802. [CrossRef]
17. Schaap, L.A.; van Schoor, N.M.; Lips, P.; Visser, M. Associations of sarcopenia definitions, and their components, with the incidence of recurrent falling and fractures: The longitudinal aging study Amsterdam. *J. Gerontol. A Biol. Sci. Med. Sci.* **2018**, *73*, 1199–1204. [CrossRef]
18. Malmstrom, T.K.; Miller, D.K.; Simonsick, E.M.; Ferrucci, L.; Morley, J.E. SARC-F: A symptom score to predict persons with sarcopenia at risk for poor functional outcomes. *J. Cachexia Sarcopenia Muscle* **2016**, *7*, 28–36. [CrossRef]

19. Morley, J.E.; Abbatecola, A.M.; Argiles, J.M.; Baracos, V.; Bauer, J.; Bhasin, S.; Cederholm, T.; Coats, A.J.S.; Cummings, S.R.; Evans, W.J.; et al. Sarcopenia with limited mobility: An international consensus. *J. Am. Med. Dir. Assoc.* **2011**, *12*, 403–409. [CrossRef]
20. Dos Santos, L.; Cyrino, E.S.; Antunes, M.; Santos, D.A.; Sardinha, L.B. Sarcopenia and physical independence in older adults: The independent and synergic role of muscle mass and muscle function. *J. Cachexia Sarcopenia Muscle* **2017**, *8*, 245–250. [CrossRef]
21. Beaudart, C.; Biver, E.; Reginster, J.Y.; Rizzoli, R.; Rolland, Y.; Bautmans, I.; Petermans, J.; Gillain, S.; Buckinx, F.; Dardenne, N.; et al. Validation of the SarQoL(R), a specific health-related quality of life questionnaire for Sarcopenia. *J. Cachexia Sarcopenia Muscle* **2017**, *8*, 238–244. [CrossRef]
22. De Buyser, S.L.; Petrovic, M.; Taes, Y.E.; Toye, K.R.C.; Kaufman, J.M.; Lapauw, B.; Goemaere, S. Validation of the FNIH sarcopenia criteria and SOF frailty index as predictors of long-term mortality in ambulatory older men. *Age Ageing* **2016**, *45*, 602–608. [CrossRef] [PubMed]
23. Liu, P.; Hao, Q.; Hai, S.; Wang, H.; Cao, L.; Dong, B. Sarcopenia as a predictor of all-cause mortality among community-dwelling older people: A systematic review and meta-analysis. *Maturitas* **2017**, *103*, 16–22. [CrossRef] [PubMed]
24. Montero-Errasquín, B.; Cruz-Jentoft, A.J. The value of sarcopenia in the prevention of disability. *Med. Clin.* **2019**, *153*, 243–244. [CrossRef] [PubMed]
25. Dent, E.; Morley, J.E.; Cruz-Jentoft, A.J.; Arai, H.; Kritchevsky, S.B.; Guralnik, J.; Bauer, J.M.; Pahor, M.; Clark, B.C.; Cesari, M.; et al. International Clinical Practice Guidelines for Sarcopenia (ICFSR): Screening diagnosis and management. *J. Nutr. Health Aging* **2018**, *22*, 1148–1161. [CrossRef]
26. Foreman, K.J.; Marquez, N.; Dolgert, A.; Fukutaki, K.; Fullman, N.; McGaughey, M. Forecasting life expectancy, years of life lost, and all-cause and cause-specific mortality for 250 causes of death: Reference and alternative scenarios for 2016-40 for 195 countries and territories. *Lancet* **2018**, *392*, 2052–2090. [CrossRef]
27. Davies, B.; García, F.; Ara, I.; Artalejo, F.R.; Rodriguez-Mañas, L.; Walter, S. Relationship Between Sarcopenia and Frailty in the Toledo Study of Healthy Aging: A Population Based Cross-Sectional Study. *J. Am. Med. Dir. Assoc.* **2018**, *19*, 282–286. [CrossRef]
28. Yamada, M.; Nishiguchi, S.; Fukutani, N.; Tanigawa, T.; Yukutake, T.; Kayama, H.; Aoyama, T.; Arai, H. Prevalence of sarcopenia in community-dwelling Japanese older adults. *J. Am. Med. Dir. Assoc.* **2013**, *14*, 911–915. [CrossRef]
29. Charlson, M.E.; Pompei, P.; Ales, K.L.; MacKenzie, C.R. A new method of classifying prognostic comorbidity in longitudinal studies: Development and validation. *J. Chronic. Dis.* **1987**, *40*, 373–383. [CrossRef]
30. Pfeiffer, E. A short portable mental status questionnaire for the assessment of organic brain deficit in elderly patients. *J. Am. Geriatr. Soc.* **1975**, *23*, 433–441. [CrossRef]
31. Sheikh, J.I.; Yesavage, J.A. Geriatric Depression Scale (GDS): Recent evidence and development of a shorter version. *Clin. Geront.* **1986**, *5*, 165–173.
32. Lawton, M.P.; Brody, E.M. Assessment of older people: Self-maintaining and instrumental activities of daily living. *Gerontologist* **1969**, *9*, 179–186. [CrossRef] [PubMed]
33. Kaiser, M.J.; Bauer, J.M.; Ramsch, C.; Uter, W.; Guigoz, Y.; Cederholm, T.; Sieber, C.C. MNA-International Group. Validation of the Mini Nutritional Assessment short-form (MNA-SF): A practical tool for identification of nutritional status. *J. Nutr. Health Aging* **2009**, *13*, 782–788. [CrossRef] [PubMed]
34. Fried, L.P.; Tangen, C.M.; Walston, J.; Newman, A.B.; Hirsch, C.; Gottdiener, J.; Seeman, T.; Tracy, R.; Kop, W.J.; Burke, G.; et al. Frailty in older adults: Evidence for a phenotype. *J. Gerontol. A Biol. Sci. Med. Sci.* **2001**, *56*, M146–M156. [CrossRef] [PubMed]
35. Janssen, I.; Heymsfield, S.B.; Baumgartner, R.N.; Ross, R. Estimation of skeletal muscle mass by bioelectrical impedance analysis. *J. Appl. Physiol.* **2000**, *89*, 465–471. [CrossRef]
36. Hosmer, D.W.; Lemeshow, S.; Sturdivant, R.X. *Applied Logistic Regression*, 3rd ed.; John Wiley & Sons: Hoboken, NJ, USA, 2013.
37. Petermann-Rocha, F.; Balntzi, V.; Gray, S.R.; Lara, J.; Ho, F.K.; Pell, J.P.; Celis-Morales, C. Global prevalence of sarcopenia and severe sarcopenia: A systematic review and meta-analysis. *J. Cachexia Sarcopenia Muscle* **2022**, *13*, 86–99. [CrossRef]
38. Fernandes, L.V.; Paiva, A.E.G.; Silva, A.C.B.; de Castro, I.C.; Santiago, A.F.; de Oliveira, E.P.; Porto, L.C.J. Prevalence of sarcopenia according to EWGSOP1 and EWGSOP2 in older adults and their associations with unfavorable health outcomes: A systematic review. *Aging Clin. Exp. Res.* **2022**, *34*, 505–514. [CrossRef]
39. Vágnerová, T.; Michálková, H.; Dvořáčková, O.; Topinková, E. Comparison between EWGSOP1 and EWGSOP2 criteria and modelling of diagnostic algorithm for sarcopenic obesity in over 70 years old patients. *Eur. Geriatr. Med.* **2022**, *13*, 641–648. [CrossRef]
40. Volpato, S.; Bianchi, L.; Cherubini, A.; Landi, F.; Maggio, M.; Savino, E.; Bandinelli, S.; Ceda, G.P.; Guralnik, J.M.; Ferrucci, L. Prevalence and clinical correlates of sarcopenia in community-dwelling older people: Application of the EWGSOP definition and diagnostic algorithm. *J. Gerontol. A Biol. Sci. Med. Sci.* **2014**, *69*, 438–446. [CrossRef]
41. Smoliner, C.; Sieber, C.C.; Wirth, R. Prevalence of sarcopenia in geriatric hospitalized patients. *J. Am. Med. Dir. Assoc.* **2014**, *15*, 267–272. [CrossRef]
42. Kim, I. Age and gender differences in the relation of chronic diseases to activity of daily living (ADL) disability for elderly South Koreans: Based on representative dataH. *J. Prev. Med. Public Health* **2011**, *4*, 32–40. [CrossRef]
43. Bernabeu-Wittel, M.; González-Molina, A.; Fernández-Ojeda, R.; Díez-Manglano, J.; Salgado, F.; Soto-Martín, M.; Muniesa, M.; Ollero-Baturone, M.; Gómez-Salgado, J. Impact of Sarcopenia and Frailty in a Multicenter Cohort of Polypathological Patients. *J. Clin. Med.* **2019**, *8*, 535. [CrossRef] [PubMed]

44. Bianchi, L.; Abete, P.; Bellelli, G.; Bo, M.; Cherubini, A.; Corica, F.; Di, B.M.; Maggio, M.; Manca, G.M.; Rizzo, M.R.; et al. GLISTEN Group Investigators. Prevalence and Clinical Correlates of Sarcopenia, Identified According to the EWGSOP Definition and Diagnostic Algorithm, in Hospitalized Older People: The GLISTEN Study. *J. Gerontol. A Biol. Sci. Med. Sci.* **2017**, *72*, 1575–1581. [CrossRef]
45. Kirk, B.; Zanker, J.; Bani Hassan, E.; Bird, S.; Brennan-Olsen, S.; Duque, G. Sarcopenia Definitions and Outcomes Consortium (SDOC) Criteria are Strongly Associated With Malnutrition, Depression, Falls, and Fractures in High-Risk Older Persons. *J. Am. Med. Dir. Assoc.* **2021**, *22*, 741–745. [CrossRef] [PubMed]
46. Pilati, I.; Slee, A.; Frost, R. Sarcopenic Obesity and Depression: A Systematic Review. *J. Frailty Aging* **2022**, *11*, 51–58. [CrossRef] [PubMed]
47. Fábrega-Cuadros, R.; Cruz-Díaz, D.; Martínez-Amat, A.; Aibar-Almazán, A.; Redecillas-Peiró, M.T.; Hita-Contreras, F. Associations of sleep and depression with obesity and sarcopenia in middle-aged and older adults. *Maturitas* **2020**, *142*, 1–7. [CrossRef]
48. Kume, Y.; Takahashi, T.; Itakura, Y.; Lee, S.; Makizako, H.; Ono, T. Polypharmacy and Lack of Joy Are Related to Physical Frailty among Northern Japanese Community-Dwellers from the ORANGE Cohort Study. *Gerontology* **2021**, *67*, 184–193. [CrossRef]
49. Blanco-Reina, E.; Aguilar-Cano, L.; García-Merino, M.R.; Ocaña-Riola, R.; Valdellós, J.; Bellido-Estévez, I.; Ariza-Zafra, G. Assessing Prevalence and Factors Related to Frailty in Community-Dwelling Older Adults: A Multinomial Logistic Analysis. *J. Clin. Med.* **2021**, *10*, 3576. [CrossRef]
50. Li, C.W.; Yu, K.; Shyh-Chang, N.; Jiang, Z.; Liu, T.; Ma, S.; Luo, L.; Guang, L.; Liang, K.; Ma, W.; et al. Pathogenesis of sarcopenia and the relationship with fat mass: Descriptive review. *J. Cachexia Sarcopenia Muscle* **2022**, *13*, 781–794. [CrossRef]
51. Marconcin, P.; Ihle, A.; Werneck, A.O.; Gouveia, E.R.; Ferrari, G.; Peralta, M.; Marques, A. The Association of Healthy Lifestyle Behaviors with Overweight and Obesity among Older Adults from 21 Countries. *Nutrients* **2021**, *13*, 315. [CrossRef]
52. Pérez-Rodrigo, C.; Gianzo Citores, M.; Hervás Bárbara, G.; Aranceta-Bartrina, J. Prevalence of obesity and abdominal obesity in Spanish population aged 65 years and over: ENPE study. *Med. Clin.* **2022**, *58*, 49–57. [CrossRef]
53. Thompson, M.Q.; Yu, S.; Tucker, G.R.; Adams, R.J.; Cesari, M.; Theou, O.; Visvanathan, R. Frailty and sarcopenia in combination are more predictive of mortality than either condition alone. *Maturitas* **2021**, *144*, 102–107. [CrossRef] [PubMed]
54. Reijnierse, E.M.; Trappenburg, M.C.; Blauw, G.J.; Verlaan, S.; de van der Schueren, M.A.; Meskers, C.G.; Maier, A.B. Common Ground? The Concordance of Sarcopenia and Frailty Definitions. *J. Am. Med. Dir. Assoc.* **2016**, *17*, e7–e12. [CrossRef] [PubMed]
55. Cruz-Jentoft, A.J.; Dawson Hughes, B.; Scott, D.; Sanders, K.M.; Rizzoli, R. Nutritional strategies for maintaining muscle mass and strength from middle age to later life: A narrative review. *Maturitas* **2020**, *132*, 57–64. [CrossRef] [PubMed]
56. Haase, C.B.; Brodersen, J.B.; Bülow, J. Sarcopenia: Early prevention or overdiagnosis? *BMJ* **2022**, *376*, e052592. [CrossRef]
57. Landi, F.; Liperoti, R.; Fusco, D.; Mastropaolo, S.; Quattrociocchi, D.; Proia, A.; Tosato, M.; Bernabei, R.; Onder, G. Sarcopenia and mortality among older nursing home residents. *J. Am. Med. Dir. Assoc.* **2012**, *13*, 121–126. [CrossRef]
58. Legrand, D.; Vaes, B.; Matheï, C.; Swine, C.; Degryse, J.M. The prevalence of sarcopenia in very old individuals according to the European consensus definition: Insights from the BELFRAIL study. *Age Ageing* **2013**, *42*, 727–734. [CrossRef]
59. Reiss, J.; Iglseder, B.; Kreutzer, M.; Weilbuchner, I.; Treschnitzer, W.; Kässmann, H.; Pirich, C.; Reiter, R. Case finding for sarcopenia in geriatric inpatients: Performance of bioimpedance analysis in comparison to dual X-ray absorptiometry. *BMC Geriatr.* **2016**, *16*, 52. [CrossRef]

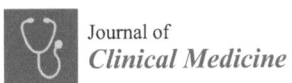

Article

Inflammaging and Blood Pressure Profiles in Late Life: The Screening for CKD among Older People across Europe (SCOPE) Study

Lisanne Tap [1,*], Andrea Corsonello [2], Mirko Di Rosa [2], Paolo Fabbietti [2], Francesc Formiga [3], Rafael Moreno-González [3], Johan Ärnlöv [4,5], Axel C. Carlsson [5,6], Harmke A. Polinder-Bos [1], Regina E. Roller-Wirnsberger [7], Gerhard H. Wirnsberger [7], Tomasz Kostka [8], Agnieszka Guligowska [8], Rada Artzi-Medvedik [9], Ilan Yehoshua [10], Christian Weingart [11], Cornel C. Sieber [11], Pedro Gil [12], Sara Lainez Martinez [12], Fabrizia Lattanzio [2] and Francesco U. S. Mattace-Raso [1,†] on behalf of the SCOPE Investigators

1. Department of Internal Medicine, Section of Geriatric Medicine, Erasmus MC, University Medical Center Rotterdam, 3015 GD Rotterdam, The Netherlands
2. Italian National Research Center on Aging (INRCA), 60124 Ancona, Italy
3. Geriatric Unit, Internal Medicine Department, Bellvitge University Hospital-IDIBELL-L'Hospitalet de Llobregat, 08907 Barcelona, Spain
4. School of Health and Social Studies, Dalarna University, 791 31 Falun, Sweden
5. Division of Family Medicine and Primary Care, Department of Neurobiology, Care Sciences and Society (NVS), Karolinska Institutet, 171 77 Stockholm, Sweden
6. Academic Primary Health Care Centre, Stockholm Region, 113 65 Stockholm, Sweden
7. Department of Internal Medicine, Medical University of Graz, 8036 Graz, Austria
8. Department of Geriatrics, Healthy Ageing Research Centre, Medical University of Lodz, 90-549 Lodz, Poland
9. Department of Nursing, The Recanati School for Community Health Professions, Faculty of Health Sciences, Ben-Gurion University of the Negev, Beer Sheva 84105, Israel
10. Maccabi Healthcare Services, Southern Region, Tel Aviv 69978, Israel
11. Department of General Internal Medicine and Geriatrics, Krankenhaus Barmherzige Brüder Regensburg and Institute for Biomedicine of Aging, Friedrich-Alexander-Universität Erlangen-Nürnberg, 93049 Regensburg, Germany
12. Department of Geriatric Medicine, Hospital Clinico San Carlos, 28040 Madrid, Spain
* Correspondence: l.tap@erasmusmc.nl; Tel.: +31-10-7035979
† SCOPE Investigators are listed in acknowledgments.

Abstract: The neutrophil-to-lymphocyte ratio (NLR) is a marker for systemic inflammation. Since inflammation plays a relevant role in vascular aging, the aim of this study was to investigate whether NLR is associated with blood pressure profiles in older adults. This study was performed within the framework of the SCOPE study including 2461 outpatients aged 75 years and over. Mean blood pressure values, namely systolic blood pressure (SBP), diastolic blood pressure (DBP) and pulse pressure (PP) were investigated across tertiles of NLR. Change in blood pressure levels in 2 years of follow-up were compared across categories of baseline NLR. Data of 2397 individuals were used, of which 1854 individuals had hypertension. Mean values of blood pressure did not differ across categories of baseline NLR in individuals without hypertension. Individuals with hypertension with a high-range NLR had lower SBP and PP when compared to those in low-range NLR (mean difference SBP −2.94 mmHg, p = 0.032 and PP −2.55 mmHg, p = 0.030). Mean change in blood pressure in 2 years did only slightly differ in non-clinically relevant ranges, when compared across tertiles of baseline NLR. NLR as a marker of inflammaging was not associated with unfavorable blood pressure profiles in older individuals with or without hypertension.

Keywords: inflammation; neutrophil-to-lymphocyte ratio; hypertension; blood pressure; vascular aging; older adults

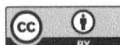

Citation: Tap, L.; Corsonello, A.; Di Rosa, M.; Fabbietti, P.; Formiga, F.; Moreno-González, R.; Ärnlöv, J.; Carlsson, A.C.; Polinder-Bos, H.A.; Roller-Wirnsberger, R.E.; et al. Inflammaging and Blood Pressure Profiles in Late Life: The Screening for CKD among Older People across Europe (SCOPE) Study. *J. Clin. Med.* 2022, 11, 7311. https://doi.org/10.3390/jcm11247311

Academic Editor: Antonio Gonzalez-Perez

Received: 13 November 2022
Accepted: 6 December 2022
Published: 9 December 2022

Publisher's Note: MDPI stays neutral with regard to jurisdictional claims in published maps and institutional affiliations.

Copyright: © 2022 by the authors. Licensee MDPI, Basel, Switzerland. This article is an open access article distributed under the terms and conditions of the Creative Commons Attribution (CC BY) license (https://creativecommons.org/licenses/by/4.0/).

1. Introduction

Hypertension is very common in older adults and viewed as an accelerated form of vascular aging [1,2]. Vascular aging is characterized by breaks in elastic fibers and accumulation of collagen in the arterial wall, resulting in a decline of elastic properties and thus an increase in arterial stiffness [3]. Increased arterial stiffness is also associated with subsequent development of hypertension and related blood pressure alterations, such as a decline in diastolic blood pressure (DBP) and an increase in systolic blood pressure (SBP) and pulse pressure (PP) [4]. Besides age and cardiovascular risk factors, systemic inflammation also plays a relevant role in the rate of vascular aging [5]. However, whether 'inflammaging' is associated with vascular aging at older age is not completely clear.

Immunosenescence refers to the significant changes of the immune system with aging [6]. It results in remodeling of specific cell types, higher levels of pro-inflammatory cytokines and seems to induce a permanent low-grade state of chronic inflammation [7]. A variety of biochemical and hematological markers can be measured to assess this systemic inflammation [8]. For instance, the role of C-reactive protein has been widely observed in observational studies in several chronic conditions [9–11]. Interestingly, more recent literature indicates that the ratio of blood cells subtypes have a significant prognostic value for cardiovascular diseases [12,13]. The neutrophil-to-lymphocyte ratio (NLR), derived directly from the differential white blood cell count, is a relatively novel marker reflecting the balance between two aspects of the immune system: acute and chronic inflammation (neutrophil count) and adaptive immunity (lymphocyte count) [14]. During (chronic) illness and various pathological states, this balance shifts due to systemic inflammation and oxidative stress. The NLR has proven its prognostic value in several diseases, such as cardiovascular diseases [15,16], infections [17] and several types of cancer [18], in which higher NLR values represent higher rates of inflammation. NLR is an inexpensive, 'easy to obtain' and highly available measurement, making it a very accessible tool in clinical practice.

The aim of this study was to explore whether NLR as marker of inflammation is associated with blood pressure profiles in older adults aged 75 years and over with and without hypertension.

2. Materials and Methods

The present study was performed within the framework of the Screening for Chronic Kidney Disease among Older People across Europe (SCOPE) study. The SCOPE study (European Grant Agreement no. 436849), is a multicenter 2-year prospective cohort study involving patients older than 75 years attending outpatient services in participating institutions in Austria, Germany, Israel, Italy, the Netherlands, Poland and Spain. Methods of the SCOPE study have been extensively described elsewhere [19]. Participants were requested to sign a written informed consent before entering the study. The study protocol was approved by ethics committees at all participating institutions, and complies with the Declaration of Helsinki and Good Clinical Practice Guidelines.

2.1. Inflammation

Blood samples were obtained during baseline visit to assess clinical laboratory tests including the differentiated white blood cell count. The NLR was calculated by dividing the absolute neutrophil count by the absolute lymphocyte count. No specific normal values or cut-off point of NLR in older adults exist and most researchers have explored NLR in categories in their own population. The authors decide to categorize participants in groups of low-range, mid-range and high range values of NLR using tertiles stratified for the presence of hypertension.

2.2. Blood Pressure Profiles

Blood pressure measurements were conducted during baseline visit and also every following visit after 1 and 2 years of follow-up using an oscillometric device with a brachial cuff in resting position. SBP and DBP were measured and documented in millimetres of mercury (mmHg). PP, also expressed in mmHg, was calculated as the difference between SBP and DBP. PP is a marker of age-related vascular stiffness in which higher values of PP indicate greater stiffness (i.e., less elasticity) [20]. Since blood pressure was also measured during follow-up, change in blood pressure values (SBP, DBP and PP) was calculated and documented as change in mmHg. Hypertension was registered when present in medical history and/or when antihypertensive medication was used for this indication.

2.3. Other Variables

Demographic data and socioeconomic status were documented. Information on alcohol use, smoking status, medical history and use of medication was collected, including the use and type of antihypertensive medication. Additionally, the cumulative illness rating scale for geriatrics (CIRS-G) was calculated [21]. During the study visit, a comprehensive geriatric assessment (CGA) was performed including information on other domains, such as information on cognition and functional status [22].

2.4. Statistical Analysis

Descriptive statistics were expressed as percentage for categorical variables and mean and standard deviation (SD) or median and interquartile ranges (IQR) for continuous variables, depending on normal or non-normal distribution. First, characteristics were compared between participants with and without hypertension using the Chi square test for categorical variables and T-test or Mann–Whitney U test for continuous variables, depending on normal or non-normal distribution. Second, cross-sectional analyses were conducted in which mean values of SBP, DBP and PP were compared across tertiles of NLR using analysis of variance (ANOVA) stratified for the presence of hypertension. Multivariate analyses were also conducted with adjustment for covariates age, sex, BMI, diabetes mellitus, CIRS-G and the use of antihypertensive medication. Third, mean change of SBP, DBP and PP in two years of follow-up were compared across tertiles of NLR stratified for the presence of hypertension using ANOVA. In multivariate analyses, these tests were adjusted for baseline value of SBP, DBP or PP and previous identified covariates. Individuals who were lost to follow-up, died or with missing data were excluded from related analyses (Figure 1). A *p*-value of <0.05 was considered statistically significant.

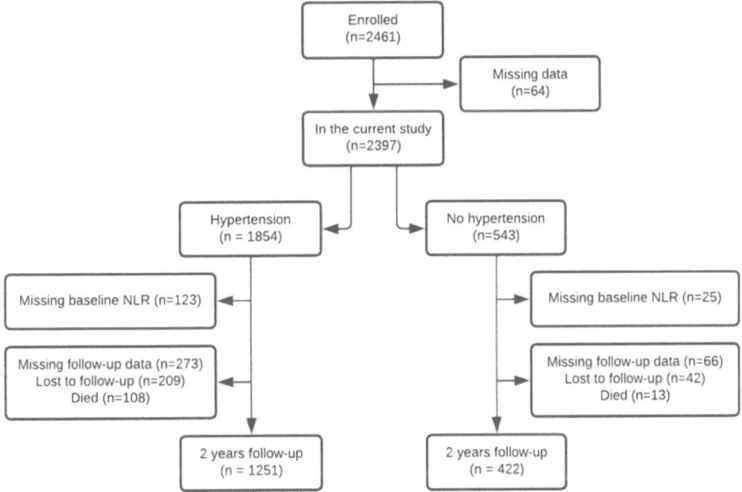

Figure 1. Flowchart on in- and exclusion of individuals within the current study.

3. Results

In total, 2461 participants were enrolled in the SCOPE study and 2397 participants were included in the analyses as result of missing data on 64 participants. The complete flowchart on the included and excluded individuals is shown in Figure 1. A total of 1854 individuals (77.3%) had a medical history of hypertension and/or used anti-hypertensive medication for this indication and 543 participants (22.7%) had no hypertension. Overall baseline characteristics stratified for the presence of hypertension are presented in Table 1.

Table 1. Overall sample description in individuals with and without hypertension.

Variable	Hypertension (n = 1854)	No Hypertension (n = 543)	p-Value
Age, years	80 [77–83]	79 [77–82]	<0.001
Women	1034 (55.8%)	307 (56.5%)	NS
Living alone	456 (24.6%)	119 (21.9%)	NS
BMI, kg/m^2	27.7 [25.1–30.8]	25.8 [23.4–28.6]	<0.001
Alcohol consumption	449 (24.2%)	161 (29.7%)	0.009
Current Smoker	73 (3.9%)	30 (5.5%)	NS
Former Smoker	698 (37.6%)	201 (37%)	NS
ADL dependent	475 (25.6%)	99 (18.2%)	0.001
iADL dependent	822 (44.3%)	156 (28.7%)	<0.001
CKD	1306 (70.4%)	274 (50.5%)	<0.001
eGFR-BIS, mL/min	52.9 [41.4–62.0]	59.9 [52.5–66.7]	<0.001
TIA	175 (9.4%)	35 (6.4%)	0.030
Stroke	126 (6.8%)	13 (2.4%)	<0.001
Cancer	328 (17.7%)	87 (16%)	NS
COPD	239 (12.9%)	48 (8.8%)	0.011
CHF	360 (19.4%)	38 (7%)	<0.001
Diabetes Mellitus	541 (29.2%)	64 (11.8%)	<0.001
Atrial fibrillation	319 (17.2%)	44 (8.1%)	<0.001
Vascular disease	259 (14%)	43 (7.9%)	<0.001
SBP, mmHg	140 [130–152]	132 [120–147]	<0.001
DBP, mmHg	79 [70–85]	78 [70–83]	NS
PP, mmHg	62 [52–73]	55 [48–67]	<0.001
CIRS-G, total score	9 [6–12]	5 [3–8]	<0.001
CIRS-G, severity index	1.5 [1.3–1.8]	1.4 [1.0–1.7]	<0.001
Neutrophils, 10^9/L	4.0 [3.2–5.1]	3.5 [2.8–4.4]	<0.001
Lymphocytes, 10^9/L	1.7 [1.3–2.1]	1.6 [1.3–2.1]	NS
NLR [1]	2.4 [1.8–3.3]	2.1 [1.6–2.8]	<0.001
Antihypertensives	1795 (94.9%)	139 (25.6%)	<0.001
Calcium channel blockers	606 (32.7%)	16 (3.0%)	<0.001
ACE-inhibitors/ARB	1344 (72.5%)	50 (9.2%)	<0.001
Diuretics	866 (46.7%)	40 (7.4%)	<0.001
Beta-blockers	915 (49.4%)	92 (16.9%)	<0.001

Values are expressed as number (percentage) or median [IQR]. p-values are based on chi-squared test for categorical variables and Mann–Whitney U test for continuous variables; [1] Data available on 1731 individuals with hypertension and 518 without hypertension. Abbreviations: BMI, Body Mass Index; (i) ADL, (instrumental) Activities of Daily Living; CKD; chronic kidney disease, eGFR-BIS, estimated Glomerular Filtration Rate-Berlin Initiative Study; TIA, transient ischemic attack; COPD, chronic obstructive pulmonary disease; CHF, chronic heart failure; SBP, systolic blood pressure; DBP, diastolic blood pressure; PP, Pulse Pressure; CIRS-G, Cumulative Illness Rating Scale for Geriatrics; NLR; neutrophils-to-lymphocyte ratio; ACE, angiotensin-converting enzyme; ARBs, angiotensin receptor blockers.

Individuals with hypertension were older (80 vs. 79 years, $p < 0.001$), had higher BMI (27.7 vs. 25.8 kg/m^2, $p < 0.001$), SBP (140 vs. 132 mmHg, $p < 0.001$) and PP (62 vs. 55 mmHg, $p = 0.001$) than individuals without hypertension. Additionally, the prevalence of comorbidities was higher in individuals with hypertension, than in those without hypertension, such as the prevalence of chronic kidney disease (70.4% vs. 50.5%, $p < 0.001$), stroke (6.8% vs. 2.4%, $p < 0.001$) and diabetes mellitus (29.2% vs. 11.8%, $p < 0.001$), resulting in higher comorbidity score (CIRS-G 9 vs. 5, $p < 0.001$). The amount of neutrophils was higher in individuals with hypertension than in those without hypertension (4.0 vs. 3.5 × 10^9/L, $p < 0.001$), whereas lymphocytes count did not differ between groups (1.7 vs. 1.6 × 10^9/L), resulting in higher values of NLR in individuals with hypertension (2.4 vs. 2.1, $p < 0.001$). Individuals with hypertension more often used anti-hypertensive medication than individuals without hypertension (94.9% vs. 24.6%, $p < 0.001$). Most frequently, individuals with hypertension used ACE-inhibitors/ARBs (72.5%). They also used beta-blockers (49.4%), diuretics (46.7%) or calcium channel blockers (32.7%).

3.1. Individuals with Hypertension

The low-range NLR tertile contained individuals with a value up to 1.95 and the high-range NLR started from 3.01. Mean values of blood pressure across tertiles of NLR are presented in Figure 2A–C.

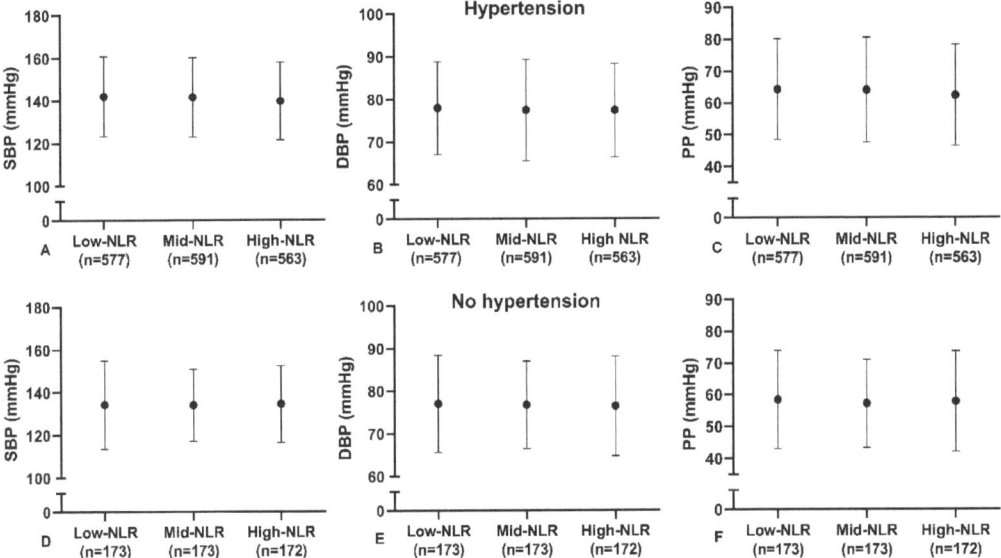

Figure 2. Mean values of blood pressure across tertiles of NLR in individuals with hypertension (**A–C**) and no hypertension (**D–F**). Dots represent mean values, bars represent standard deviation. Figure **A** and **D**, systolic blood pressure (SBP) in mmHg; Figure **B** and **E**, diastolic blood pressure (DBP) in mmHg; Figure **C** and **F** pulse pressure (PP) in mmHg.

Mean values of SBP were 142.0 ± 18.8 mmHg, 141.5 ± 18.7 mmHg and 139.7 ± 18.3 mmHg from lowest to highest tertile of NLR, respectively. Individuals in the high-range NLR had slightly lower SBP when compared to low-range NLR (mean difference −2.94 mmHg, 95% CI −5.70; −0.18 mmHg, $p = 0.032$). Mean values of DBP were 77.9 ± 10.9 mmHg, 77.4 ± 11.9 mmHg and 77.3 ± 11.0 mmHg, respectively, with no differences across categories. Mean values of PP were 64.3 ± 15.9 mmHg, 64.1 ± 16.5 mmHg and 62.4 ± 16.0 mmHg, respectively. Individuals in the high-range NLR had lower PP when compared to low-range NLR (mean difference −2.55 mmHg, 95% CI −4.93; −0.18 mmHg, $p = 0.030$).

Mean change of blood pressure levels were compared across tertiles of baseline NLR and presented in Table 2.

Mean changes from lowest to highest tertile of baseline NLR were 2.8 ± 20.8 mmHg, 0.7 ± 21.3 mmHg and 1.4 ± 21.4 mmHg for SBP, 0.4 ± 33.8 mmHg, 0.4 ± 12.2 mmHg and 0.6 ± 12.3 mmHg for DBP and 0.9 ± 17.4 mmHg, 1.1 ± 18.7 mmHg and 0.9 ± 18.2 mmHg for PP (respectively).

Mean change in blood pressure values in 2 years did only slightly differ in non-clinically relevant ranges.

Table 2. Mean change of blood pressure values across tertiles of NLR in individuals with and without hypertension.

Hypertension (n = 1251)	Low NLR (n = 432)	Mid NLR (n = 429)	High NLR (n = 390)
ΔSBP, mmHg	2.8 ± 20.8	0.7 ± 21.3	1.4 ± 21.4
ΔDBP, mmHg	0.4 ± 33.8	0.4 ± 12.2	0.6 ± 12.3
ΔPP, mmHg	0.9 ± 17.4	1.1 ± 18.7	0.9 ± 18.2
No Hypertension (n = 422)	Low NLR (n = 152)	Low NLR (n = 145)	Low NLR (n = 125)
ΔSBP, mmHg	0.6 ± 19.0	0.6 ± 19.3	2.9 ± 21.1
ΔDBP, mmHg	1.3 ± 11.9	1.1 ± 11.7	1.7 ± 11.8
ΔPP, mmHg	0.1 ± 15.8	1.8 ± 14.4	1.2 ± 17.4

Values are expressed as mean (±SD); Δ = delta/change; p-values are based on one-way ANOVA comparison. Abbreviations: SBP, systolic blood pressure; DBP, diastolic blood pressure; NLR; neutrophil-to-lymphocyte ratio.

3.2. Individuals without Hypertension

The low-range NLR tertile contained individuals with a value up to 1.77, whereas the high-range NLR started from 2.53. Mean values of blood pressure across tertiles of NLR are presented in Figure 2D–F. Mean values of SBP were 134.2 ± 20.8 mmHg, 133.9 ± 16.9 mmHg and 134.3 ± 18.1 mmHg from lowest to highest tertile of NLR, respectively. Mean values of DBP were 77.0 ± 11.4 mmHg, 76.7 ± 10.3 mmHg and 76.4 ± 11.7 mmHg from lowest to highest tertile of NLR, respectively. Mean values of PP were 58.4 ± 15.5 mmHg, 57.2 ± 13.9 mmHg and 57.9 ± 15.9 mmHg from lowest to highest tertile of NLR, respectively. There were no differences in blood pressure levels across categories.

Mean change of blood pressure levels in individuals without hypertension are also presented in Table 2. Mean changes from lowest to highest tertile of baseline NLR were 0.6 ± 19.0 mmHg, 0.6 ± 19.3 mmHg and 2.9 ± 21.1 mmHg for SBP, 1.3 ± 11.9 mmHg, 1.1 ± 11.7 mmHg and 1.7 ± 11.8 mmHg for DBP and 0.1 ± 15.8 mmHg, 1.8 ± 14.4 mmHg and 1.2 ± 17.4 mmHg for PP (respectively). There was no difference in changes of blood pressure levels across categories.

4. Discussion

NLR as a marker of inflammaging, was not associated with unfavorable blood pressure profiles in individuals with and without hypertension aged 75 years and over. Mean changes in blood pressure levels during a follow up of 2 years were close to zero and no differences could be observed in changes of blood pressure levels, when comparing individuals with low-range, mid-range or high-range NLR.

The role of oxidative stress and inflammation in vascular aging and development of hypertension is well established [5]. During aging of the immune system, specific cell types will remodel and a permanent state of chronic inflammation is induced [23]. Several studies found that higher levels of C-reactive protein and pro-inflammatory cytokines are associated with increased arterial stiffness [24,25]. Chronic inflammation can affect blood vessel structures and this effect is most likely due to the role of inflammatory state in endothelial dysfunction, by inhibiting endothelium-dependent vasodilatation. In middle-aged adults, a cross-sectional study investigated the possible association between NLR and 24 h blood pressure measurements in patients with newly diagnosed hypertension [26]. Results showed that patients with no antihypertensive therapy in the upper two quartiles of NLR had the highest systolic and diastolic blood pressure. Additionally, a significant association between NLR and high blood pressure load was found. Interestingly, the quartiles of NLR were comparable with the tertiles used in our study, namely first < 1.55, second 1.55–1.92, third 1.92–2.48 and fourth > 2.48. Since this study involves a specific group of untreated patients with hypertension with a mean age of 49 years, the main results could not be compared to our older adults, who commonly have a history of decades with hypertension. Another cross-sectional study performed in England investigated the relation between NLR and 24 h blood pressure measurements in 508 individuals between the age of 18–80 years who underwent the blood pressure measurement for the diagnosis or evaluation of hypertension [27]. A positive association between NLR and arterial stiffness was found. Moreover, increasing NLR was an independent predictor of cardiovascular outcomes. Included patients had a mean age of 58.8 ± 14.0 and this study did not focus on blood pressure profiles and NLR, and therefore these results in younger patients could not be completely compared to our findings.

As far as we are concerned, no studies have investigated the possible association between NLR and blood pressure profiles in old age. We had hypothesized that a higher rate of inflammation would be associated with unfavorable blood pressure levels, however, the findings could not confirm our hypothesis. We took into account also the potential of anti-inflammatory effects of the different type of antihypertensive medication on this association [28–30], however adjusting for this potential confounder did not change our results. A potential explanation for our findings could be due to a ceiling effect. There is an association between inflammation and blood pressure levels at younger age, however, in our population of individuals aged 75 years and over, a ceiling effect might explain our findings. Additionally, it is possible that seriously ill patients with unfavorable inflammation and blood pressure profiles or the highest rate of comorbidities, were not included in this study, due to death or no willingness to participate due to health-related issues. Additionally, death during follow-up could have affected our results. Eventually, the annual change in blood pressure levels in our population might be too small to be investigated during a follow-up of 2 years. A study conducted in the USA which included older adults of 75 years and over found a mean annual change in SBP of <1 mmHg in men and circa 2 mmHg in women and a mean annual change in DBP of circa 1.2 mmHg in both sexes [31]. We found quite an opposite result as than what we expected in individuals with hypertension, namely the group with the highest NLR had the lowest SBP and PP. A possible explanation for this finding could lay in the fact that theoretically, patients with hypertension and high NLR represent a group with the least favorable health status. Consequently, those older adults might be the ones with most frequent hospital visits and better health-care surveillance leading to better blood pressure control.

Some limitations of the present study deserve consideration. First, we decided to analyse blood pressure levels across tertiles of NLR, instead of a continuous number which could have affected the results. This decision was based on the fact that no normal values for older adults exist and since it is not known whether or not every step of higher or lower NLR is as relevant. Second, blood pressure values were documented from one measurement per visit, while 24 h blood pressure measurement could have provided another view on blood pressure profiles. Third, we did not took into account changes in medication during follow-up which could have affected the mean levels of blood pressure of time. Fourth, as stated previously, we cannot exclude that the length of follow-up might be too short to investigate a possible relation between inflammation and blood pressure profiles. Fifth, survival bias could have led to a ceiling effect in which individuals with the most unfavorable profiles were not included or could not be followed up. The present study also has strengths. We have studied a large real-world population of older adults in 7 different countries, with no strict inclusion criteria, therefore our findings may apply for a large population of older adults across Europe. Moreover, all data were obtained systematically in participating centers, which makes these results very reliable. Furthermore, NLR is a novel and interesting marker to investigate, so the present study contributes in this relatively new field of research. Additionally, multiple blood pressure values were included, among which SBP, DBP and PP. Since blood pressure profiles can change with aging those three included measurements were able to reflect different angles of vascular aging.

5. Conclusions

In conclusion, in older adults with higher rates of inflammation, we expected to find unfavorable blood pressure profiles reflecting elevated arterial stiffness and higher rate of vascular aging. However, this association was not found. The search for contributing factors to accelerated vascular aging even at higher age is still highly relevant in order to recognize individuals at risk for cardiovascular outcomes and optimize possible treatment strategies.

Author Contributions: L.T. and F.U.S.M.-R.: participated in study protocol design, data collection, leading statistical analysis, manuscript drafting and revision. A.C. and F.L.: conceived the study, coordinated study protocol and data collection, participated in statistical analysis and manuscript revision. M.D.R., P.F. and H.A.P.-B.: participated in statistical analysis and manuscript revision. F.F., R.M.-G., J.Ä., A.C.C., R.E.R.-W., G.H.W., T.K., A.G., R.A.-M., I.Y., C.W., C.C.S., P.G. and S.L.M.: participated in study protocol and data collection, participated in manuscript revision. All authors have read and agreed to the published version of the manuscript.

Funding: The SCOPE project was granted by the European Union Horizon 2020 program, under the Grant Agreement n°634869.

Institutional Review Board Statement: The study was conducted in accordance with the Declaration of Helsinki, and approved by Ethics Committees in participating institutions as follows: Italian National Research Center on Aging (INRCA), Italy, #2015 0522 IN, 27 January 2016; University of Lodz, Poland, #RNN/314/15/KE, 17 November 2015; Medizinische Universität Graz, Austria, #28–314 ex 15/16, 5 August 2016; Erasmus MC University Medical Center Rotterdam, The Netherlands, #MEC-2016-036 #NL56039.078.15, v.4, 7 March 2016; Hospital Clínico San Carlos, Madrid, Spain, # 15/532-E_BC, 16 September 2016; Bellvitge University Hospital Barcelona, Spain, #PR204/15, 29 January 2016; Friedrich-Alexander University Erlangen-Nürnberg, Germany, #340_15B, 21 January 2016; Helsinki committee in Maccabi Healthcare services, Bait Ba-lev, Bat Yam, Israel, #45/2016, 24 July 2016.

Informed Consent Statement: Informed consent was obtained from all subjects involved in the study.

Data Availability Statement: Data will be available for SCOPE consortium on request from the principal investigator, Fabrizia Lattanzio, Italian National Research Center on Aging (IRCCS INRCA), Ancona, Fermo and Cosenza, Italy. f.lattanzio@inrca.it.

Acknowledgments: SCOPE study investigators, Coordinating center: Fabrizia Lattanzio, Italian National Research Center on Aging (INRCA), Ancona, Italy–Principal Investigator. Andrea Corsonello, Silvia Bustacchini, Silvia Bolognini, Paola D'Ascoli, Raffaella Moresi, Giuseppina Di Stefano, Cinzia Giammarchi, Anna Rita Bonfigli, Roberta Galeazzi, Federica Lenci, Stefano Della Bella, Enrico Bordoni, Mauro Provinciali, Robertina Giacconi, Cinzia Giuli, Demetrio Postacchini, Sabrina Garasto, Annalisa Cozza–Italian National Research Center on Aging (INRCA), Ancona, Fermo and Cosenza, Italy–Coordinating staff. Romano Firmani, Moreno Nacciariti, Mirko Di Rosa, Paolo Fabbietti–Technical and statistical support; Participating centers: Department of Internal Medicine, Medical University of Graz, Austria: Gerhard Hubert Wirnsberger, Regina Elisabeth Roller-Wirnsberger, Carolin Herzog, Sonja Lindner; Section of Geriatric Medicine, Department of Internal Medicine, Erasmus MC, University Medical Center Rotterdam, The Netherlands: Francesco Mattace-Raso, Lisanne Tap, Gijsbertus Ziere, Jeannette Goudzwaard, Harmke Polinder-Bos; Department of Geriatrics, Healthy Ageing Research Centre, Medical University of Lodz, Poland: Tomasz Kostka, Agnieszka Guligowska, Łukasz Kroc, Bartłomiej K Sołtysik, Małgorzata Pigłowska, Agnieszka Wójcik, Zuzanna Chrząstek, Natalia Sosowska, Anna Telążka, Joanna Kostka, Elizaveta Fife, Katarzyna Smyj, Kinga Zel; The Recanati School for Community Health Professions at the faculty of Health Sciences at Ben-Gurion University of the Negev, Israel: Rada Artzi-Medvedik, Yehudit Melzer, Mark Clarfield, Itshak Melzer; and Maccabi Healthcare services southern region, Israel: Rada Artzi-Medvedik, Ilan Yehoshua, Yehudit Melzer; Geriatric Unit, Internal Medicine Department and Nephrology Department, Hospital Universitari de Bellvitge, Institut d'Investigació Biomèdica de Bellvitge-IDIBELL, L'Hospitalet de Llobregat, Barcelona, Spain: Francesc Formiga, Rafael Moreno-González, Xavier Corbella, Yurema Martínez, Carolina Polo, Josep Maria Cruzado; Department of Geriatric Medicine, Hospital Clínico San Carlos, Madrid: Pedro Gil Gregorio, Sara Laínez Martínez, Mónica González Alonso, Jose A. Herrero Calvo, Fernando Tornero Molina, Lara Guardado Fuentes, Pamela Carrillo García, María Mombiedro Pérez; Department of General Internal Medicine and Geriatrics, Krankenhaus Barmherzige Brüder Regensburg and Institute for Biomedicine of Aging, Friedrich-Alexander-Universität Erlangen-Nürnberg, Germany: Alexandra Renz, Susanne Muck, Stephan Theobaldy, Andreas Bekmann, Revekka Kaltsa, Sabine Britting, Robert Kob, Christian Weingart, Ellen Freiberger, Cornel Sieber; Department of Medical Sciences, Uppsala University, Sweden: Johan Ärnlöv, Axel Carlsson, Tobias Feldreich; Scientific advisory board (SAB): Roberto Bernabei, Catholic University of Sacred Heart, Rome, Italy; Christophe Bula, University of Lausanne, Switzerland; Hermann Haller, Hannover Medical School, Hannover, Germany; Carmine Zoccali, CNR-IBIM Clinical Epidemiology and Pathophysiology of Renal Diseases and Hypertension, Reggio Calabria, Italy; Data and Ethics Management Board (DEMB): Kitty Jager, University of Amsterdam, The Netherlands; Wim Van Biesen, University Hospital of Ghent, Belgium. Paul E. Stevens, East Kent Hospitals University NHS Foundation Trust, Canterbury, United Kingdom.

Conflicts of Interest: The authors declare no conflict of interest. The funder had no role in the design of the study; in the collection, analyses, or interpretation of data; in the writing of the manuscript; or in the decision to publish the results.

References

1. Harvey, A.; Montezano, A.C.; Touyz, R.M. Vascular biology of ageing-Implications in hypertension. *J. Mol. Cell. Cardiol.* **2015**, *83*, 112–121. [CrossRef] [PubMed]
2. Muli, S.; Meisinger, C.; Heier, M.; Thorand, B.; Peters, A.; Amann, U. Prevalence, awareness, treatment, and control of hypertension in older people: Results from the population-based KORA-age 1 study. *BMC Public Health* **2020**, *20*, 1049. [CrossRef] [PubMed]
3. Laurent, S.; Boutouyrie, P.; Lacolley, P. Structural and genetic bases of arterial stiffness. *Hypertension* **2005**, *45*, 1050–1055. [CrossRef]
4. Mitchell, G.F. Arterial stiffness and hypertension: Chicken or egg? *Hypertension* **2014**, *64*, 210–214. [CrossRef] [PubMed]
5. Guzik, T.J.; Touyz, R.M. Oxidative stress, inflammation, and vascular aging in hypertension. *Hypertension* **2017**, *70*, 660–667. [CrossRef] [PubMed]
6. Aw, D.; Silvia, A.B.; Palmer, D.B. Immunosenescence: Emerging challenges for an aging population. *Immunology* **2007**, *120*, 435–446. [CrossRef]
7. Fulop, T.; Larbi, A.; Dupuis, G.; Le Page, A.; Frost, E.H.; Cohen, A.A.; Witkowski, J.M.; Franceschi, C. Immunosenescence and Inflamm-Aging As Two Sides of the Same Coin: Friends or Foes? *Front. Immunol.* **2017**, *8*, 1960. [CrossRef]
8. Germolec, D.R.; Frawley, R.P.; Evans, E. Markers of inflammation. *Methods Mol. Biol.* **2010**, *598*, 53–73. [CrossRef]
9. Lee, S.; Choe, J.W.; Kim, H.K.; Sung, J. High-sensitivity C-reactive protein and cancer. *J. Epidemiol.* **2011**, *21*, 161–168. [CrossRef]
10. Yasue, H.; Hirai, N.; Mizuno, Y.; Harada, E.; Itoh, T.; Yoshimura, M.; Kugiyama, K.; Ogawa, H. Low-grade inflammation, thrombogenicity, and atherogenic lipid profile in cigarette smokers. *Circ. J.* **2006**, *70*, 8–13. [CrossRef]
11. Folsom, A.R.; Aleksic, N.; Catellier, D.; Juneja, H.S.; Wu, K.K. C-reactive protein and incident coronary heart disease in the Atherosclerosis Risk In Communities (ARIC) study. *Am. Heart J.* **2002**, *144*, 233–238. [CrossRef] [PubMed]
12. Agarwal, R.; Aurora, R.G.; Siswanto, B.B.; Muliawan, H.S. The prognostic value of neutrophil-to-lymphocyte ratio across all stages of coronary artery disease. *Coron. Artery Dis.* **2022**, *33*, 137–143. [CrossRef] [PubMed]
13. Özpelit, E.; Akdeniz, B.; Özpelit, M.E.; Tas, S.; Bozkurt, S.; Tertemiz, K.C.; Sevinç, C.; Badak, Ö. Prognostic value of neutrophil-to-lymphocyte ratio in pulmonary arterial hypertension. *J. Int. Med. Res.* **2015**, *43*, 661–671. [CrossRef] [PubMed]
14. Imtiaz, F.; Shafique, K.; Mirza, S.S.; Ayoob, Z.; Vart, P.; Rao, S. Neutrophil lymphocyte ratio as a measure of systemic inflammation in prevalent chronic diseases in Asian population. *Int. Arch. Med.* **2012**, *5*, 2. [CrossRef]
15. Angkananard, T.; Anothaisintawee, T.; McEvoy, M.; Attia, J.; Thakkinstian, A. Neutrophil Lymphocyte Ratio and Cardiovascular Disease Risk: A Systematic Review and Meta-Analysis. *BioMed Res. Int.* **2018**, *2018*, 2703518. [CrossRef] [PubMed]
16. Verma, S.; Husain, M.; Madsen, C.; Leiter, L.A.; Rajan, S.; Vilsboll, T.; Rasmussen, S.; Libby, P. Neutrophil-to-lymphocyte ratio predicts cardiovascular events in patients with type 2 diabetes: Post hoc analysis of SUSTAIN 6 and PIONEER 6. *Eur. Heart J.* **2021**, *42* (Suppl. S1), ehab724.2479. [CrossRef]
17. Cataudella, E.; Giraffa, C.M.; Di Marca, S.; Pulvirenti, A.; Alaimo, S.; Pisano, M.; Terranova, V.; Corriere, T.; Ronsisvalle, M.L.; Di Quattro, R.; et al. Neutrophil-to-lymphocyte ratio: An emerging marker predicting prognosis in elderly adults with community-acquired pneumonia. *J. Am. Geriatr. Soc.* **2017**, *65*, 1796–1801. [CrossRef]
18. Templeton, A.J.; McNamara, M.G.; Šeruga, B.; Vera-Badillo, F.E.; Aneja, P.; Ocaña, A.; Leibowitz-Amit, R.; Sonpavde, G.; Knox, J.J.; Tran, B.; et al. Prognostic role of neutrophil-to-lymphocyte ratio in solid tumors: A systematic review and meta-analysis. *J. Natl. Cancer Inst.* **2014**, *106*, dju124. [CrossRef]
19. Corsonello, A.; Tap, L.; Roller-Wirnsberger, R.; Wirnsberger, G.; Zoccali, C.; Kostka, T.; Guligowska, A.; Mattace-Raso, F.; Gil, P.; Fuentes, L.G.; et al. Design and methodology of the screening for CKD among older patients across Europe (SCOPE) study: A multicenter cohort observational study. *BMC Nephrol.* **2018**, *19*, 260. [CrossRef]
20. Safar, M.E.; Nilsson, P.M.; Blacher, J.; Mimran, A. Pulse pressure, arterial stiffness, and end-organ damage. *Curr. Hypertens. Rep.* **2012**, *14*, 339–344. [CrossRef]
21. Conwell, Y.; Forbes, N.T.; Cox, C.; Caine, E.D. Validation of a measure of physical illness burden at autopsy: The Cumulative Illness Rating Scale. *J. Am. Geriatr. Soc.* **1993**, *41*, 38–41. [CrossRef] [PubMed]

22. Ellis, G.; Whitehead, M.A.; O'Neill, D.; Langhorne, P.; Robinson, D. Comprehensive geriatric assessment for older adults admitted to hospital. *Cochrane Database Syst. Rev.* **2011**, *7*, CD006211. [CrossRef]
23. Franceschi, C.; Bonafè, M.; Valensin, S.; Olivieri, F.; De Luca, M.; Ottaviani, E.; De Benedictis, G. Inflamm-aging. An evolutionary perspective on immunosenescence. *Ann. N. Y. Acad. Sci.* **2000**, *908*, 244–254. [CrossRef] [PubMed]
24. Mattace-Raso, F.U.; van der Cammen, T.J.; van der Meer, I.M.; Schalekamp, M.A.; Asmar, R.; Hofman, A.; Witteman, J.C. C-reactive protein and arterial stiffness in older adults: The Rotterdam Study. *Atherosclerosis* **2004**, *176*, 111–116. [CrossRef]
25. Mahmud, A.; Feely, J. Arterial stiffness is related to systemic inflammation in essential hypertension. *Hypertension* **2005**, *46*, 1118–1122. [CrossRef]
26. Çimen, T.; Sunman, H.; Efe, T.H.; Erat, M.; Şahan, H.F.; Algül, E.; Guliyev, I.; Akyel, A.; Doğan, M.; Açıkel, S.; et al. The relationship between 24-hour ambulatory blood pressure load and neutrophil-to-lymphocyte ratio. *Rev. Port. Cardiol.* **2017**, *36*, 97–105. [CrossRef]
27. Boos, C.J.; Toon, L.T.; Almahdi, H. The relationship between ambulatory arterial stiffness, inflammation, blood pressure dipping and cardiovascular outcomes. *BMC Cardiovasc. Disord.* **2021**, *21*, 139. [CrossRef]
28. Montecucco, F.; Pende, A.; Mach, F. The Renin-Angiotensin System Modulates Inflammatory Processes in Atherosclerosis: Evidence from Basic Research and Clinical Studies. *Mediat. Inflamm.* **2009**, *2009*, 752406. [CrossRef]
29. Ohtsuka, T.; Hamada, M.; Hiasa, G.; Sasaki, O.; Suzuki, M.; Hara, Y.; Shigematsu, Y.; Hiwada, K. Effect of beta-blockers on circulating levels of inflammatory and anti-inflammatory cytokines in patients with dilated cardiomyopathy. *J. Am. Coll. Cardiol.* **2001**, *37*, 412–417. [CrossRef]
30. Riku, D.; Tim, B.; David, R.V.W.; Edward, F.P. L-Type Calcium Channel Blockers Exert an Antiinflammatory Effect by Suppressing Expression of Plasminogen Receptors on Macrophages. *Circ. Res.* **2009**, *105*, 167–175. [CrossRef]
31. Langer, R.D.; Criqui, M.H.; Barrett-Connor, E.L.; Klauber, M.R.; Ganiats, T.G. Blood pressure change and survival after age 75. *Hypertension* **1993**, *22*, 551–559. [CrossRef] [PubMed]

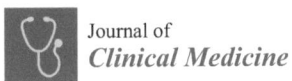

Article

The Effect of Age on Non-Invasive Hemodynamics in Chronic Heart Failure Patients on Left-Ventricular Assist Device Support: A Pilot Study

Else-Marie van de Vreede [1,†], Floor van den Berg [1,†], Parsa Jahangiri [2], Kadir Caliskan [2] and Francesco Mattace-Raso [1,*]

[1] Department of Geriatric Medicine, Erasmus MC University Medical Center, 3015 GD Rotterdam, The Netherlands
[2] Department of Cardiology, Erasmus MC University Medical Center, 3015 GD Rotterdam, The Netherlands
* Correspondence: f.mattaceraso@erasmusmc.nl; Tel.: +31-10-7035979
† These authors contributed equally to this work.

Abstract: Background: Implantation of continuous flow left ventricular assist devices (LVAD's) has been increasingly used in patients with advanced heart failure (HF). Little is known about the non-invasive hemodynamics and the relationship with adverse events in this specific group of patients. We aimed to identify any differences in non-invasive hemodynamics in patients with an LVAD in different age categories and to investigate if there is an association with major adverse events. Methods: In this observational cross-sectional study, HF patients with a continuous flow LVAD were included. Non-invasive hemodynamic parameters were measured with a validated, automated oscillometric blood pressure monitor. The occurrences of adverse events were registered by reviewing the medical records of the patients. An independent-samples T-test and Chi-square test were used to compare different groups of patients. Results: Forty-seven patients were included; of these, only 12 (25.6%) had a successful measurement. Heart rate, heart rate-adjusted augmentation index, and pulse wave velocity were higher in the ≥55 years of age LVAD group compared to the <55 years of age LVAD group (all $p < 0.05$). Stroke volume was significantly lower in the ≥55 years of age LVAD group compared to the <55 years of age LVAD group ($p = 0.015$). Patients with adverse events such as cardiovascular events, GI-bleeding, or admission to a hospital had lower central pulse pressure (cPP) than patients without any adverse event. Conclusion: Older LVAD patients have a significantly higher heart rate, heart rate-adjusted augmentation index, and pulse wave velocity and a significantly lower stroke volume compared to participants aged < 55 years. The pulsatile component of blood pressure was decreased in patients with adverse events.

Keywords: aging; non-invasive hemodynamics; blood pressure; heart failure; continuous flow; LVAD; non-pulsatility; adverse events

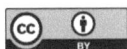

1. Introduction

Implantation of a left-ventricular assist device (LVAD) has been increasingly used in advanced heart failure (HF) patients that are refractory to optimal medical therapy. It can be used as a bridge-to-heart transplantation therapy, or as destination therapy [1]. Bridge-to-heart transplantation therapy reduces mortality and improves patients' overall condition [2]. Patients undergoing destination therapy are, by definition, ineligible for transplantation, mostly due to increased age or other comorbidities [3]. Heart failure remains a potentially fatal disease despite advances in therapy [4]. If evolved therapies for advanced heart failure patients give no result, LVAD implantation can be used. The small pool of donor hearts and the growing group of heart failure patients in need of a transplant causes an increase in LVAD destination therapy [1].

LVADs improves clinical outcomes in HF patients by improving hemodynamics, but with a non-physiological non-pulsatile, continuous-flow hemodynamics [5]. Little is known about the hemodynamics patterns in patients implanted with an LVAD. Because of the improvement of continuous-flow LVADs (CF-LVADs) in durability, the cumulative effects of these changed hemodynamics have become an important area of interest [6]. Despite improvements in survival, CF-LVADs are associated with complications such as long-term end-organ dysfunction, gastro-intestinal (GI) bleeding, hospitalization, and cardiovascular events. Both low arterial pulsatility and increased aortic stiffness may increase the risk of those adverse events [7–9].

Clarification of hemodynamic parameters in LVAD patients may help to optimize these parameters and improve clinical outcomes. While there is no conclusive evidence to suggest that this will occur, we hypothesize that LVAD patients will have a specific blood pressure profile that differs from patients without an LVAD. Therefore, we will investigate non-invasive hemodynamic parameters in patients with an LVAD. The purpose of this study is to identify any differences in non-invasive hemodynamics between patients with an LVAD within different age categories and whether specific hemodynamic patterns are associated with any adverse event.

2. Materials and Methods

2.1. Patient Selection

We included outpatients with HF with an LVAD who were followed by the department of Cardiology at the Erasmus MC University Medical Center, Rotterdam, in the period of December 2021 until March 2022. Patients were asked to participate in the study if they were >18 years when they were implanted with an LVAD. Written informed consent was obtained from all participants before we started the measurements. The study protocol (MEC-2015-405) was approved by the medical-ethical board of Erasmus MC University Medical Center, Rotterdam.

2.2. Variables

Demographic data used: age, sex, weight, length, BMI (kg/m^2), etiology of HF, indication for LVAD, and device type; medications were assessed by reviewing the medical records of the patients. Renal function (assessed by eGFR–creatinine based), bilirubin, NT-proBNP, and hemoglobin were measured during laboratory control.

2.3. Hemodynamic Data

LVAD device values and blood pressure values were collected by reviewing the electronic medical records of the patients. Non-invasive hemodynamic data were collected through measurements with a Mobil-O-Graph The Mobil O Graph (IEM, Rheinland, Germany) is a previously validated, automated oscillometric blood pressure monitor [10,11]. Besides brachial blood pressure readings, the monitor provides an estimation of the aortic pulse wave velocity (aPWV) through analysis of brachial pulse wave morphology. The measurements were performed in a quiet examination room, with the patient seated with both legs uncrossed on the floor, after two minutes rest. The brachial cuff was applied to the right upper arm on the right spot of the brachial artery and inflated two times to perform a complete measurement.

Other hemodynamic parameters obtained during the same measurement, using inbuilt algorithms, included mean arterial pressure (MAP), heart rate (HR), pulse pressure (PP), stroke volume (SV), cardiac output (CO), peripheral vascular resistance (SVR), cardiac index (CIx), augmentation pressure, and augmentation index (AIx). The collected data were uploaded into HMS Client Server 5.1 software, Rheinland, Germany.

2.4. Adverse Events Registration

We retrospectively reviewed the electronic medical records of patients who were selected in the study to register if there were adverse events in people on the waiting list or after LVAD implantation. We focused on three major complications. Adverse events were defined as cardiovascular events such as myocardial infarct or CVA, gastro-intestinal bleeding, and admission to a hospital.

2.5. Statistical Analysis

Statistical analyses were performed using IBM SPSS Statistics 28, Chicago, IL, USA, version for Windows. All patients with a successful or failed measurement were analyzed for baseline characteristics and LVAD device values. For further analyses, patients without a successful measurement were excluded. Normally distributed data are presented as median and interquartile range (IQR) for continuous variables and frequency (%) for categorical variables. Characteristics were compared between the group patients with and without complications, using the T-test for continuous variables. The Chi-square test was used to compare percentages. To investigate the possible role of aging patients, patients were divided into age categories < 55 years and ≥55 years. A two-tailed *p*-value of ≤0.05 was considered statistically significant.

3. Results

Figure 1 shows the flowchart of the inclusion of patients. In total, 47 patients were asked to participate in the study. All 47 patients underwent a blood pressure measurement with the Mobil-O-Graph. Thirty-five patients were excluded from analyses of the non-invasive hemodynamics because we were not able to perform a successful measurement in these patients. We included 12 patients for analyses of the non-invasive hemodynamics.

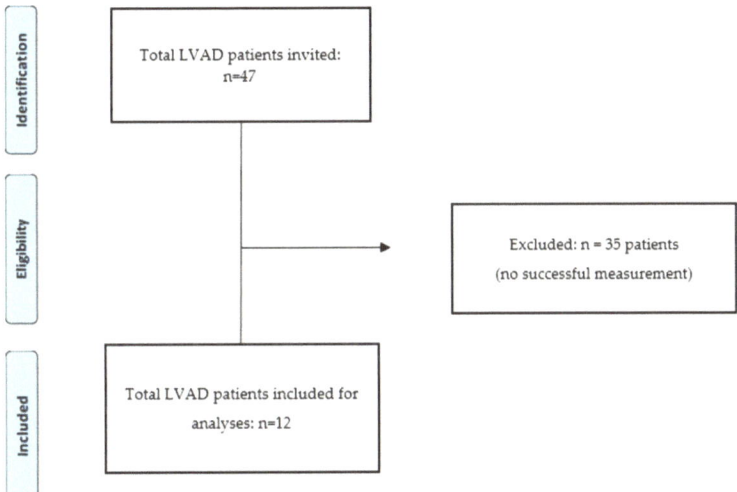

Figure 1. Flowchart inclusion of patients.

Table 1 shows the baseline characteristics for patients with HF with an LVAD with a successful blood pressure measurement, compared with patients with a non-successful measurement. In 25.6%, we were able to perform a successful measurement in HF with an LVAD. There was no statistically significant difference in age, sex, weight, BMI, time since LVAD implantation, or etiology of HF between groups. In both groups, most of the patients were men. Only one patient had an LVAD device type HM-II; all other patients had a device type HM-III. There was also no statistically significant difference between the blood pressure values measured by the LVAD nurse practitioner. The LVAD parameters flow and PI were significant different between groups. In patients with a failed measurement, we found a higher flow ($p = 0.014$) and a lower PI ($p = 0.002$). The mean NT-proBNP in patients with a failed measurement was higher; however, this difference was barely statistically significant ($p = 0.057$).

Table 1. Baseline characteristics of HF with an LVAD with successful or failed measurement.

Characteristics	Successful Measurement (12)	Failed Measurement (35)	p-Value
Age, years, IQR	57 (34–66)	60 (53–64)	ns
Sex, men, n (%)	10 (83.3)	30 (85.7)	ns
Weight, kg	80 (78–96)	88.2 (77.6–101.2)	ns
BMI, kg/m^2	26.6 (25.3–30)	27.8 (25.3–30.0]	ns
Time on LVAD, months	19.5 (3–30)	23 (13–41]	ns
Etiology of HF, ischemic, % (n)	58.3 (7)	57.1 (20)	ns
Smoking, %	2 (16.7)	2 (5.7)	ns
Diabetes, %	2 (16.7)	5 (14.3)	ns
Hypertension, %	2 (16.7)	6 (17.1)	ns
LVAD device type, HM-3, % (n)	11 (91.7)	35 (100)	ns
SBP, mmHg	108 (104–116)	102 (99–112)	ns
MAP, mmHg	93 (84–96)	85 (82–90)	ns
DBP, mmHg	83 (75–87)	79 (73–84)	ns
PP, mmHg	23 (17–28)	26 (23–30)	ns
LVAD parameters			
• RPM, r/min	5300 (5200–5400)	5400 (5300–5500)	ns
• Flow, L/min	4.4 (4.1–4.5)	4.6 (4.3–4.9)	0.014
• PI	4.4 (3.9–5.7)	3.6 (2.9–4.40)	0.002
• Pulse Power, Watt	3.8 (3.8–4)	4.0 (3.8–4.2)	ns
eGFR, ml/min/1.73 m^2	69 (63–90)	60.0 (43–77)	ns
Hb, mmol/L	8.7 (7.7–9)	8.6 (7.8–9.3)	ns
Bilirubin, μmol/L	9.0 (8–16)	11.0 (8–17)	ns
NT-proBNP, pmol/L	152 (99–213)	190 (138–390)	0.057

Abbreviations: LVAD, left ventricular assist device; BMI, body mass index; HF, heart failure; HM-II, Heartmate II; HM-III, Heartmate III; SBP, systolic blood pressure; MAP, mean arterial pressure; DBP, diastolic blood pressure; PP, pulse pressure; RPM, revolutions per minute; PI, pulsatility index; eGFR, estimated glomerular filtration rate; Hb, hemoglobin; NT-proBNP, N-terminal pro-brain natriuretic peptide.

Table 2 shows the baseline characteristics of patients with an LVAD in the different age categories, <55 years and ≥55 years. The <55 years group included four patients, the group with patients ≥ 55 years included seven patients.

Figure 2 shows the mean levels and distribution of the non-invasive hemodynamic parameters in the age categories < 55 years and ≥55 years. Heart rate, heart rate-adjusted augmentation index, and pulse wave velocity were statistically significant higher in the ≥55 years of age LVAD group compared to the <55 years of age LVAD group (all $p < 0.05$). Stroke volume was significantly lower in the ≥55 years of age LVAD group compared to the <55 years of age LVAD group ($p = 0.015$).

In Table 3, the baseline characteristics of patients with HF with an LVAD are presented. We included 12 patients with HF with an LVAD, of which seven patients had no adverse event and five patients had adverse event. Adverse events include hospitalization (for cardiac causes), GI-bleeding, and a cardiovascular event. There was no statistically significant difference in any of the baseline characteristics between the two groups. Patients with any adverse event did have a longer median time since LVAD implantation (13.5 versus 28.3 months). Only one patient had an LVAD device type HM-II, all other patients had an LVAD device type HM-III. The LVAD parameters, such as RPM, flow, PI, and pulse power, were measured by the LVAD technician on the same day our measurement was performed. This also applies for the blood pressure values and the lab results. There were no missing data for any of the patients.

Table 2. Baseline characteristics of HF with an LVAD in different age categories.

Characteristics	Age < 55 Years (n = 4)	Age ≥ 55 Years (n = 6)	p-Value
Age, years, IQR	33 (24.5–49)	62 (57–72)	<0.001
Sex, men, n (%)	4 (100)	6 (75)	ns
Weight, kg	81.7 (77.9–112.6)	80 (78–96)	ns
BMI, kg/m^2	25.7 (29.4–25.2)	27.9 (25.7–29.9)	ns
Time since LVAD, months	29 (14.3–66.3)	6.0 (2–25)	ns
Etiology of HF, ischemic, n (%)	0	7 (87.5)	0.004
Smoking, %	0	2 (25)	ns
Diabetes, %	1 (25)	1 (12.5)	ns
Hypertension, %	0	2 (25) 25% (2)	ns
LVAD device type, HM-III, % (n)	1 (25)	0	ns
SBP, mmHg	108.5 (98.3–117.3)	108 (104–116)	ns
MAP, mmHg	90 (78.8–96)	93 (87–95)	ns
DBP, mmHg	79.5 (69.8–88.5)	83 (80–87)	ns
PP, mmHg	25 (21.3–33.3)	23 (15–28)	ns
LVAD parameters			
• RPM, r/min	5250 (5200–7350)	5300 (5250–5250)	ns
• Flow, L/min	4.4 (4.1–4.5)	4.4 (4.2–4.5)	ns
• PI	5.1 (4.5–6.4)	4.1 (3.9–4.6)	ns
• Pulse Power, Watt	4.0 (3.8–4.8)	3.8 (3.8–4.0)	ns
eGFR, m/min/1.73 m^2	75.7 (67.5–86)	63 (54–83.5)	ns
Hb, mmol/L	9.0 (8.6–9.3)	8.4 (7.7–8.9)	ns
Bilirubin, μmol/L	16 (7.5–29)	9 (8.5–10.5)	ns
NT-proBNP, pmol/L	117.5 (39.5–201)	152 (120–215)	ns

Abbreviations: LVAD, left ventricular assist device; BMI, body mass index; HF, heart failure; HM-II, Heartmate II; HM-III, Heartmate III; SBP, systolic blood pressure; MAP, mean arterial pressure; DBP, diastolic blood pressure; PP, pulse pressure; RPM, revolutions per minute; PI, pulsatility index; eGFR, estimated glomerular filtration rate; Hb, hemoglobin; NT-proBNP, N-terminal pro-brain natriuretic peptide.

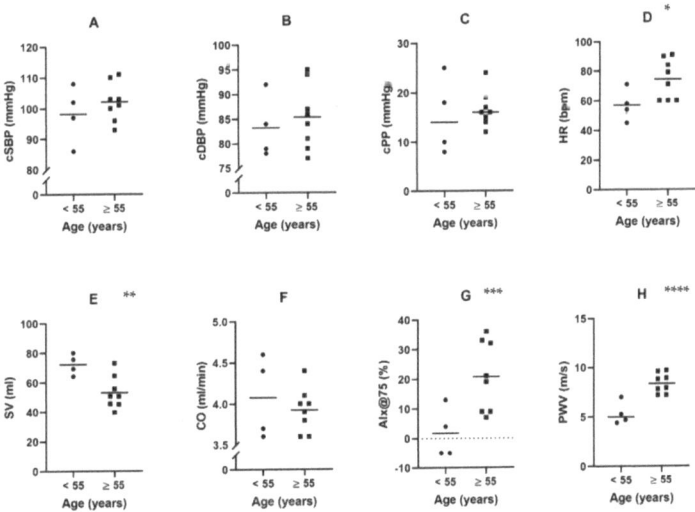

Figure 2. Distribution of non-invasive hemodynamics in HF with an LVAD within different age categories (**A–H**). Abbreviations: cSBP, central systolic blood pressure; cDBP, central diastolic blood pressure; cPP, central pulse pressure; HR, heart rate; SV, stroke volume; CO, cardiac output; AIx, augmentation index; PWV, pulse wave velocity. Note: bars represent mean values, dots represent individual patients. * $p = 0.034$; ** $p = 0.015$; *** $p = 0.013$; **** $p = 0.001$.

Table 3. Baseline characteristics of patients with an LVAD with and without any adverse event.

Characteristics	LVAD without Adverse Event (7)	LVAD with Any Adverse Event (5)	p-Value
Age, years	57.5 (29.5–63)	55 (44–72)	ns
Sex, men, n (%)	5 (71.4)	5 (100)	ns
Weight, kg	78.5 (77.5–86.6)	96 (79.5–110.1)	ns
BMI, kg/m²	25.8 (24.7–28.1)	30 (25.9–30.4)	ns
Time since LVAD, months	13.5 (1.75–28)	28.3 (7.5–53)	ns
Etiology of HF, ischemic, % (n)	57.1 (4)	60 (3)	ns
Smoking, %	2 (28.6)	0	ns
Diabetes, %	0	2 (40)	ns
Hypertension, %	2 (28.6)	0	ns
LVAD device type, HM-III, % (n)	6 (100)	4 (80)	ns
SBP, mmHg	112 (102–118.3)	107 (102–113)	ns
MAP, mmHg	93.5 (84.5–97.8)	91 (777–95.5)	ns
DBP, mmHg	82.5 (77–89.3)	83 (65.5–88)	ns
PP, mmHg	20 (14.8–29.8)	24 (21.5–32.5)	ns
LVAD parameters			
• RPM, r/min	5300 (5175–5300)	5400 (5200–5400)	ns
• Flow, L/min	4.3 (3.9–4.4)	4.5 (4.3–4.5)	ns
• PI	4.2 (3.7–7.6)	4.4 (4.2–5.3)	ns
• Pulse Power, Watt	3.8 (3.7–4.0)	3.9 (3.8–4.7)	ns
eGFR, mL/min/1.73 m²	73 (58.5–84)	66 (54–90)	ns
Hb, mmol/L	8 (7.7–9.5)	9 (8.6–9)	ns
Bilirubin, μmol/L	9 (6.8–12.8)	12 (8–25)	ns
NT-proBNP, pmol/L	162 (90.2–256.5)	152 (66–212)	ns

Abbreviations: LVAD, left ventricular assist device; BMI, body mass index; HF, heart failure; HM-II, Heartmate II; HM-III, Heartmate III; SBP, systolic blood pressure; MAP, mean arterial pressure; DBP, diastolic blood pressure; PP, pulse pressure; RPM, revolutions per minute; PI, pulsatility index; eGFR, estimated glomerular filtration rate; Hb, hemoglobin; NT-proBNP, N-terminal pro-brain natriuretic peptide.

In Figure 3, the mean values and the distribution of the non-invasive hemodynamic parameters are shown in different groups, with and without complications. Only the central pulse pressure (cPP) was statistically significant different between the two groups. Patients without adverse events had a median cPP of 18.5 IQR 14.3–24.3, patients with adverse events had a median cPP of 14 IQR 9–16, $p = 0.044$. There was no statistically significant difference between the mean values of the other hemodynamics.

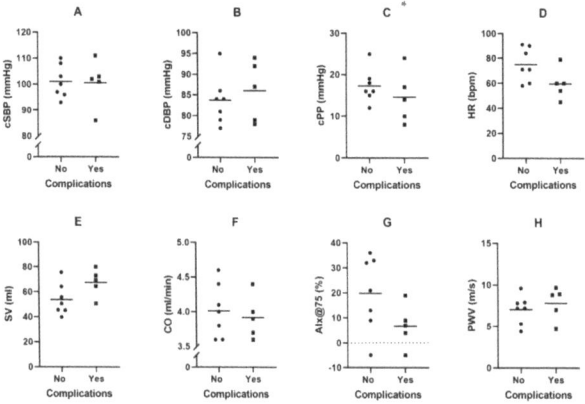

Figure 3. Distribution of non-invasive hemodynamics in HF with an LVAD with and without adverse events (**A–H**). Abbreviations: cSBP, central systolic blood pressure; cDBP, central diastolic blood pressure; cPP, central pulse pressure; HR, heart rate; SV, stroke volume; CO, cardiac output; AIx, augmentation index; PWV, pulse wave velocity. Note: bars represent mean values, dots represent individual patients. * $p = 0.044$.

4. Discussion

In this cross-sectional study, we found that older LVAD patients had higher aortic stiffness, augmentation index, and heart rate but lower stroke volume compared to participants aged < 55 years. The pulsatile component of blood pressure was decreased in patients with previous adverse events.

LVAD patients have a reduced arterial pulse pressure [12], which makes it difficult to measure the blood pressure with an automated oscillometric blood pressure monitor. Nonetheless, previous studies validated blood pressure measurements with the Mobil-O-Graph in LVAD patients using an A-line comparison. Even though this methodology was previously validated [10,13] with a success rate of 91% [13] and 82% [10], we were able to obtain the measurements in only 25.6% of the LVAD patients.

Castagna et al. found that a lower HeartMate II speed was associated with a higher success rate ($p < 0.05$) [10]. In our study, we also compared the RPM speed between the successful and failed measurement group. We found no significant difference, but our study group consisted of only one HeartMate II against 46 HeartMate III implants, which could make this comparison questionable. Furthermore, they found that no other measured parameters were associated with measurement success. Meanwhile, we did find that LVAD flow, LVAD Pulse Index (PI), and NT-proBNP were associated with measurement success. Lower values of the PI indicate lower filling pressures and lower contractility of the left ventricle. With lower values of the PI, the LVAD is providing greater support and the flow pulse coming from the left ventricle is lower [14]. This is a possible explanation why it is harder to measure the blood pressure in patients with a lower PI.

A previous study by Schofield et al. [15] investigated a limited number of hemodynamic parameters in LVAD patients and is the only study who investigated this subject. Because of the limited existing literature about hemodynamics in LVAD patients, we compared our study findings to the literature regarding the association between hemodynamics and age in healthy individuals. First of all, Houghton et al. [16] found that stroke volume under resting conditions in healthy individuals reduces with increasing age. Our study also found a significantly lower stroke volume in LVAD patients $\geq$ 55 years compared to LVAD patients < 55 years. The same study of Houghton et al. [16] also investigated the association between aging and heart rate and found that there was no significant difference between heart rate in younger and older participants. Surprisingly, in our LVAD patients we did find a significant increase in heart rate with increasing age. PWV is a marker for arterial stiffness, which is an indicator for vascular aging. It can predict cardiovascular events according to several studies [17–19]. According to Styczynski et al. [20], there is an age-related increase in PWV. In our study we also found that LVAD patients $\geq$ 55 years had a significantly higher PWV than LVAD patients < 55 years. Thus, an increased age is associated with a higher PWV, which could function as a predictor for cardiovascular events. Notable is that the augmentation index is not significantly different in LVAD patients divided in different age categories in our study. Augmentation index is an indirect measure of arterial stiffness and is calculated with the augmentation pressure and pulse pressure. According to Fantin et al. [21], the AIx increases with age up to 55 years and tend to plateau thereafter. Because our age categories are divided into < 55 years and $\geq$ 55 years, this could explain why there is no significant difference due to the plateauing of the AIx increase. An associated hemodynamic parameter is the heart rate-adjusted augmentation index. To confound for the influence of heart rate, the augmentation index is calculated as it would be at 75 beats per minute. Beckmann et al. [22] found that the AIx@75 significantly increases with age. In our study, the AIx@75 also significantly increased between age categories <55 years and $\geq$55 years.

All non-invasive hemodynamic parameters were not significantly different between men and women. This outcome is difficult to judge because our study population only consisted of two women and nine men. Because of the small study group and imbalance, it is injudicious to conclude that there is truly no significant difference between men and women for all non-invasive hemodynamic parameters.

The non-invasive hemodynamic parameters measured in the previous studies discussed above were investigated in participants without an LVAD and should therefore be taken into consideration. What is interesting to see is that some non-invasive hemodynamic parameters show the same difference in age categories in patients with and without an LVAD. This may highlight that, on some levels, the blood pressure profile of heart failure patients with and without an LVAD is very similar. However, there are also some differences between our study and the existing literature, such as heart rate, which indicates that LVAD patients do have a different blood pressure profile.

As a result of a small pool of heart donors and the large growing group of heart failure patients in need of a transplant, destination therapy with an LVAD, which mainly consist of older patients > 60 years, is growing and accounts for progressively more implants than before [23]. Technological improvements in pump design and surgical techniques have made the efficiency of LVAD support longer [24]. As a result of the fast development in LVAD technology and the longer efficiency of LVAD support, understanding hemodynamics in LVAD patients has become more clinically relevant. In patients with HF with an LVAD, we found that a decrease in cPP in patients was associated with adverse events. This is consistent with findings in earlier studies that showed that adverse events in patients with an LVAD may be partly a result of chronic exposure to a low pulsatility. Patients with CF-LVADs with a low PP can have elevated levels of sympathetic nerve activity (SNA) [25], which, by causing high BP levels, predisposes to adverse events [26]. Furthermore, it has been suggested that higher levels of increased sympathetic tone can cause smooth muscle relaxation. This can lead to arteriovenous dilatation and ultimately arteriovenous malformation, which causes GI-bleeding [27]. Crow et al. retrospectively compared patients with pulsatile versus non-pulsatile LVADs and they found higher rates of GI-bleeding in patients with a non-pulsatile flow [28]. CF-LVADs give a continuous blood flow with minimal pulsatility that decreases the cyclical stretch of the arterial wall, leading to increased aortic stiffness [29]. It is reported that the aortic stiffness increases immediately after LVAD implantation, with attenuation of this increase in the first year [29]. Higher aortic stiffness is associated with significantly higher rates of common complications of CF-LVAD therapy [8].

Limitations: The findings of our study must be interpreted cautiously because of the relatively small group of patients included. While measuring, we were only able to successfully measure in a small percentage of our patients. The difficulty of measuring LVAD patients is most likely due to different flow. LVAD patients have a constant flow, while patients without an LVAD have a pulsatile flow. Application of non-invasive haemodynamic assessment based on an oscillometric blood pressure monitor might not be feasible in LVAD patients. This means that the LVAD represents an obstacle to carrying out valuable pulse wave analysis. We assessed patients at different times after LVAD implantation of since they were diagnosed with HF. Especially in patients with an LVAD, it is possible that in the early phase after LVAD implantation they were not completely stabilized and recovered from the device implantation. Because of the cross-sectional design, we did not perform serial assessments; therefore, we cannot rule out the possibility that the non-invasive hemodynamics may change over time. One strength of our explorative study is the examination of a relatively novel and increasing population with an increasing relevance in the future. Second, measurements with the Mobil-O-Graph only take a few minutes and could easily be applied in daily practice. Before this can be applied, research is necessary regarding the clinical relevance of the measured non-invasive hemodynamics.

5. Conclusions

In this cross-sectional study, we found that LVAD patients aged 55 years and older had higher levels of aortic stiffness, augmentation index, and heartrate and a lower stroke volume when compared with younger patients. The pulsatile component of blood pressure is decreased in patients with adverse events.

Considering the explorative character of this study, future research is necessary to investigate whether the non-invasive hemodynamics can predict the occurrence of adverse events in patients with HF with an LVAD.

Author Contributions: Conceptualization, F.M.-R.; Methodology, K.C.; Formal analysis, E.-M.v.d.V. and F.v.d.B.; Investigation, E.-M.v.d.V., F.v.d.B., P.J. and F.M.-R.; Data curation, E.-M.v.d.V. and F.v.d.B.; Writing—original draft, E.-M.v.d.V., F.v.d.B. and P.J.; Writing—review & editing, K.C. and F.M.-R.; Supervision, K.C. and F.M.-R.; Project administration, F.M.-R. All authors have read and agreed to the published version of the manuscript.

Funding: This research received no external funding.

Institutional Review Board Statement: This study was conducted in accordance with the principles expressed in the Declaration of Helsinki. The medical-ethical board of Erasmus MC University Medical Center, Rotterdam approved the study (MEC-2015-405).

Informed Consent Statement: Informed consent was given by all participants.

Data Availability Statement: Database of the Geriatric Medicine Division of the Erasmus MC University Medical Center, Rotterdam.

Acknowledgments: The authors would like to thank Wave Medical BV, Heerenveen, the Netherlands, for logistic support for performing this study (Mobil-O-Graph device).

Conflicts of Interest: The authors have no conflict of interest.

References

1. Patel, S.; Nicholson, L.; Cassidy, C.J.; Wong, K.Y. Left ventricular assist device: A bridge to transplant or destination therapy? *Postgrad. Med. J.* **2016**, *92*, 271–281. [CrossRef] [PubMed]
2. Frazier, O.H.; Rose, E.A.; Oz, M.C.; Dembitsky, W.; McCarthy, P.; Radovancevic, B.; Poirier, V.L.; Dasse, K.A.; HeartMate LVAS Investigators. Multicenter clinical evaluation of the HeartMate vented electric left ventricular assist system in patients awaiting heart transplantation. *J. Thorac. Cardiovasc. Surg.* **2001**, *122*, 1186–1195. [CrossRef] [PubMed]
3. Slaughter, M.S.; Singh, R. The role of ventricular assist devices in advanced heart failure. *Rev. Esp. Cardiol. Engl. Ed.* **2012**, *65*, 982–985. [CrossRef] [PubMed]
4. Bleumink, G.S.; Knetsch, A.M.; Sturkenboom, M.C.; Straus, S.M.; Hofman, A.; Deckers, J.W.; Witteman, J.C.; Stricker, B.H. Quantifying the heart failure epidemic: Prevalence, incidence rate, lifetime risk and prognosis of heart failure The Rotterdam Study. *Eur. Heart J.* **2004**, *25*, 1614–1619. [CrossRef] [PubMed]
5. Rose, E.A.; Gelijns, A.C.; Moskowitz, A.J.; Heitjan, D.F.; Stevenson, L.W.; Dembitsky, W.; Long, J.W.; Ascheim, D.D.; Tierney, A.R.; Levitan, R.G.; et al. Long-term use of a left ventricular assist device for end-stage heart failure. *N. Engl. J. Med.* **2001**, *345*, 1435–1443. [CrossRef] [PubMed]
6. Slaughter, M.S.; Rogers, J.G.; Milano, C.A.; Russell, S.D.; Conte, J.V.; Feldman, D.; Sun, B.; Tatooles, A.J.; Delgado, R.M., III; Long, J.W.; et al. Advanced heart failure treated with continuous-flow left ventricular assist device. *N. Engl. J. Med.* **2009**, *361*, 2241–2251. [CrossRef]
7. Kirklin, J.K.; Naftel, D.C.; Kormos, R.L.; Pagani, F.D.; Myers, S.L.; Stevenson, L.W.; Givertz, M.M.; Young, J.B. Quantifying the effect of cardiorenal syndrome on mortality after left ventricular assist device implant. *J. Heart Lung Transpl.* **2013**, *32*, 1205–1213. [CrossRef]
8. Rosenblum, H.; Pinsino, A.; Zuver, A.; Javaid, A.; Mondellini, G.; Ji, R.; Cockcroft, J.R.; Yuzefpolskaya, M.; Garan, A.R.; Shames, S.; et al. Increased Aortic Stiffness Is Associated with Higher Rates of Stroke, Gastrointestinal Bleeding and Pump Thrombosis in Patients With a Continuous Flow Left Ventricular Assist Device. *J. Card. Fail.* **2021**, *27*, 696–699. [CrossRef]
9. Imamura, T.; Nguyen, A.; Kim, G.; Raikhelkar, J.; Sarswat, N.; Kalantari, S.; Smith, B.; Juricek, C.; Rodgers, D.; Ota, T.; et al. Optimal haemodynamics during left ventricular assist device support are associated with reduced haemocompatibility-related adverse events. *Eur. J. Heart Fail.* **2019**, *21*, 655–662. [CrossRef]
10. Castagna, F.; McDonnell, B.J.; Stöhr, E.J.; Yuzefpolskaya, M.; Trinh, P.N.; Topkara, V.K.; Garan, A.R.; Flannery, M.A.; Takeda, K.; Takayama, H.; et al. Non-invasive measurement of peripheral, central and 24-hour blood pressure in patients with continuous-flow left ventricular assist device. *J. Heart Lung Transpl.* **2017**, *36*, 694–697. [CrossRef]
11. Hametner, B.; Wassertheurer, S.; Kropf, J.; Mayer, C.; Eber, B.; Weber, T. Oscillometric estimation of aortic pulse wave velocity: Comparison with intra-aortic catheter measurements. *Blood Press. Monit.* **2013**, *18*, 173–176. [CrossRef] [PubMed]
12. Bennett, M.K.; Roberts, C.A.; Dordunoo, D.; Shah, A.; Russell, S.D. Ideal methodology to assess systemic blood pressure in patients with continuous-flow left ventricular assist devices. *J. Heart Lung Transpl.* **2010**, *29*, 593–594. [CrossRef] [PubMed]

13. Castagna, F.; McDonnell, B.; Yuzefpolskaya, M.; Topkara, V.; Garan, A.; Willey, J.; Trinh, P.; Wong, K.; Cagliostro, B.; Flannery, M.; et al. Validity and Reliability of a Next Generation Non-Invasive Blood Pressure Monitor in Patients with Continuous-Flow Left Ventricular Assist Device. *J. Heart Lung Transpl.* **2016**, *35*, S326–S327. [CrossRef]
14. Barić, D. Why pulsatility still matters: A review of current knowledge. *Croat. Med. J.* **2014**, *55*, 609–620. [CrossRef]
15. Schofield, R.S.; Pierce, G.L.; Nichols, W.W.; Klodell, C.T.; Aranda, J.M.; Pauly, D.F.; Hill, J.A.; Braith, R.W. Arterial-wave reflections are increased in heart failure patients with a left-ventricular assist device. *Am. J. Hypertens.* **2007**, *20*, 622–628. [CrossRef]
16. Houghton, D.; Jones, T.W.; Cassidy, S.; Siervo, M.; MacGowan, G.A.; Trenell, M.I.; Jakovljevic, D.G. The effect of age on the relationship between cardiac and vascular function. *Mech. Ageing Dev.* **2016**, *153*, 1–6. [CrossRef]
17. Mattace-Raso, F.; van der Cammen, T.J.; Hofman, A.; van Popele, N.M.; Bos, M.L.; Schalekamp, M.A.; Asmar, R.; Reneman, R.S.; Hoeks, A.P.; Breteler, M.M.; et al. Arterial stiffness and risk of coronary heart disease and stroke: The Rotterdam study. *Circulation* **2006**, *113*, 657–663. [CrossRef]
18. Sutton-Tyrrell, K.; Najjar, S.S.; Boudreau, R.; Venkitachalam, L.; Kupelian, V.; Simonsick, E.M.; Havlik, R.; Lakatta, E.G.; Spurgeon, H.; Kritchevsky, S.; et al. Elevated aortic pulse wave velocity, a marker of arterial stiffness, predicts cardiovascular events in well-functioning older adults. *Circulation* **2005**, *111*, 3384–3390. [CrossRef]
19. Mitchell, G.F.; Hwang, S.-J.; Vasan, R.S.; Larson, M.G.; Levy, D.; Benjamin, E.J.; Pencina, M.J.; Hamburg, N.M.; Vita, J.A. Arterial stiffness and cardiovascular events: The Framingham Heart Study. *Circulation* **2010**, *121*, 505–511. [CrossRef]
20. Styczynski, G.; Cienszkowska, K.; Ludwiczak, M.; Szmigielski, C. Age-related values of aortic pulse wave velocity in healthy subjects measured by Doppler echocardiography. *J. Hum. Hypertens.* **2021**, *35*, 1081–1087. [CrossRef]
21. Fantin, F.; Mattocks, A.; Bulpitt, C.J.; Banya, W.; Rajkumar, C. Is augmentation index a good measure of vascular stiffness in the elderly? *Age Ageing* **2007**, *36*, 43–48. [CrossRef] [PubMed]
22. Beckmann, M.; Jacomella, V.; Kohler, M.; Lachat, M.; Salem, A.; Amann-Vesti, B.; Husmann, M. Risk Stratification of Patients with Peripheral Arterial Disease and Abdominal Aortic Aneurysm Using Aortic Augmentation Index. *PLoS ONE* **2015**, *10*, e0139887. [CrossRef] [PubMed]
23. Kirklin, J.K.; Naftel, D.C.; Pagani, F.D.; Kormos, R.L.; Stevenson, L.W.; Blume, E.D.; Miller, M.A.; Baldwin, J.T.; Young, J.B. Sixth INTERMACS annual report: A 10,000-patient database. *J. Heart Lung Transpl.* **2014**, *33*, 555–564. [CrossRef] [PubMed]
24. Shaffer, A.; Cogswell, R.; John, R. Future developments in left ventricular assist device therapy. *J. Thorac. Cardiovasc. Surg.* **2021**, *162*, 605–611. [CrossRef] [PubMed]
25. Markham, D.W.; Fu, Q.; Palmer, M.D.; Drazner, M.H.; Meyer, D.M.; Bethea, B.T.; Hastings, J.L.; Fujimoto, N.; Shibata, S.; Levine, B.D. Sympathetic neural and hemodynamic responses to upright tilt in patients with pulsatile and nonpulsatile left ventricular assist devices. *Circ. Heart Fail.* **2013**, *6*, 293–299. [CrossRef]
26. Pinsino, A.; Castagna, F.; Zuver, A.M.; Royzman, E.A.; Nasiri, M.; Stöhr, E.J.; Cagliostro, B.; McDonnell, B.; Cockcroft, J.R.; Garan, A.R.; et al. Prognostic implications of serial outpatient blood pressure measurements in patients with an axial continuous-flow left ventricular assist device. *J. Heart Lung Transpl.* **2019**, *38*, 396–405. [CrossRef]
27. Cappell, M.S.; Lebwohl, O. Cessation of recurrent bleeding from gastrointestinal angiodysplasias after aortic valve replacement. *Ann. Intern. Med.* **1986**, *105*, 54–57. [CrossRef]
28. Crow, S.; John, R.; Boyle, A.; Shumway, S.; Liao, K.; Colvin-Adams, M.; Toninato, C.; Missov, E.; Pritzker, M.; Martin, C.; et al. Gastrointestinal bleeding rates in recipients of nonpulsatile and pulsatile left ventricular assist devices. *J. Thorac. Cardiovasc. Surg.* **2009**, *137*, 208–215. [CrossRef]
29. Patel, A.C.; Dodson, R.B.; Cornwell, W.K.; Hunter, K.S.; Cleveland, J.C.; Brieke, A.; Lindenfeld, J.; Ambardekar, A.V. Dynamic Changes in Aortic Vascular Stiffness in Patients Bridged to Transplant with Continuous-Flow Left Ventricular Assist Devices. *JACC Heart Fail.* **2017**, *5*, 449–459. [CrossRef]

Disclaimer/Publisher's Note: The statements, opinions and data contained in all publications are solely those of the individual author(s) and contributor(s) and not of MDPI and/or the editor(s). MDPI and/or the editor(s) disclaim responsibility for any injury to people or property resulting from any ideas, methods, instructions or products referred to in the content.

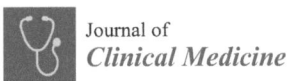

Article

Better Handgrip Strength Is Related to the Lower Prevalence of Pain and Anxiety in Community-Dwelling Older Adults

Natalia Sosowska [1], Agnieszka Guligowska [1], Bartłomiej Sołtysik [1], Ewa Borowiak [2], Tomasz Kostka [1] and Joanna Kostka [3],*

[1] Department of Geriatrics, Healthy Ageing Research Centre, Medical University of Lodz, 90-419 Lodz, Poland; natalia.sosowska@umed.lodz.pl (N.S.); agnieszka.guligowska@umed.lodz.pl (A.G.); bartlomiej.soltysik@umed.lodz.pl (B.S.); tomasz.kostka@umed.lodz.pl (T.K.)

[2] Department of Conservative Nursing, Medical University of Lodz, 90-419 Lodz, Poland; ewa.borowiak@umed.lodz.pl

[3] Department of Gerontology, Medical University of Lodz, 90-419 Lodz, Poland

* Correspondence: joanna.kostka@umed.lodz.pl

Abstract: Although handgrip strength (HGS) may be treated as a biomarker of many health problems, there is little evidence on the potential role of HGS in the prevention of pain or anxiety in older adults. We investigated the relationship of HGS to the presence of pain and anxiety among community-dwelling older adults. The study was performed in 2038 outpatients, aged 60 to 106 years. The Jamar hand-held hydraulic dynamometer was used to measure HGS. The prevalence of pain and anxiety was assessed with the Euroqol 5D questionnaire. Symptoms of depression were recorded with 15-item Geriatric Depression Scale (GDS). In the multivariate logistic regression model taking into account age, sex, BMI and concomitant diseases, the significant influence of HGS on the presence of pain (odds ratio [OR] = 0.988) in the entire study population and among men (OR = 0.983) was found. HGS was a significant independent predictor for the presence of anxiety in the entire study population (OR = 0.987), in women (OR = 0.985) and in men (OR = 0.988). In the fully adjusted model with included GDS, 1 kg higher HGS was still associated with 1.2% and 1.3% lower probability of the presence of pain and anxiety, respectively. We conclude that low HGS is associated with the presence of pain and anxiety among older adults, independent of age, sex, depression symptoms and concomitant chronic diseases. Future research should assess whether improvement of HGS would alleviate psychological dysfunction in older adults.

Keywords: pain; anxiety; elderly; handgrip; quality of life

1. Introduction

Chronic pain is common among older adults and is associated with suffering, falls and disability. It is a risk factor for premature death and accelerated cognitive decline. It also causes social isolation and generates greater costs and burden on health systems [1]. Drug treatment is only partially effective and is associated with adverse effects [2]. As the number of older adults in the population increases, anxiety is also becoming a common problem, resulting in increased burden on healthcare, contributing to high social and individual costs. Late detection of this disorder is associated with uncharacteristic symptoms, multimorbidity and the ageing process itself [3]. Therefore, more research should be implemented to improve the diagnosis of pain and anxiety in the elderly and explore their relationship with other factors, which may contribute to better prevention, influence the way these complaints are approached and improve the quality of treatment.

One of the potential simple measures related to pain and anxiety may be handgrip strength (HGS) [4,5]. Because of greater muscle mass, males are on average stronger than females [6]. HGS may be treated as a biomarker, as it can be used to determine overall strength, upper limb function, sarcopenia, frailty syndrome, bone mineral density, fractures, falls, malnutrition, cognitive impairment, depression, sleep problems, diabetes, multimorbidity and quality of life at the same time [4,7–10]. Monitoring and sustaining HGS can act as a preventive measure of mortality and the appearance of diseases, functional decline and hospitalization problems [11–14]. Routine use of HGS can be as a single measurement or as part of several investigations to identify older adults who may present with poor health [4].

In the available literature, there are some data on the impact of HGS on pain or anxiety in specific populations of patients [15–19]. Nevertheless, there is a paucity of data on the potential role of sustaining HGS in the prevention of feelings of pain or anxiety in older adults, especially in larger populations of seniors. Therefore, in this work, we investigated the relationship of HGS to the presence of pain and anxiety among community-dwelling older adults.

2. Materials and Methods

The study was performed in 2038 outpatients of the Geriatric Clinic of the Medical University of Lodz, Poland, aged 60 to 106 years who volunteered to participate in the study. The inclusion criteria were age 60 years and over, living in the community, in-person contact that allows them to understand the instructions logically and written consent to participate in the study. We excluded patients who were not able or refused to perform the necessary tests and who had recently undergone hand surgery or treated for inflammation at this location.

The study was approved by the Bioethics Committee of the Medical University of Lodz and complies with the Declaration of Helsinki and Good Clinical Practice Guidelines.

2.1. Euroqol 5D Quality of Life Assessment Questionnaire

The Euroqol 5D questionnaire is a widely used and validated generic instrument [20,21]. The test is divided into two parts. The first consists of five statements relating to mobility, self-care, usual activities, pain/discomfort and anxiety/depression. One can choose from 'no problems', 'moderate problems' and 'extreme problems'. The second part is a visual analogue scale or Euroqol-VAS and is a 'thermometer' where 100 indicates 'best imaginable health state' and 0 indicates 'worst imaginable health state'. The patient assesses his or her health status using both parts. For the purposes of this study, part of the Euroqol 5D questionnaire was used, namely that concerned with the prevalence of pain and anxiety among the study group [21].

2.2. The Geriatric Depression Scale (GDS)

The GDS was created for the assessment of depression among older people [22]. It is composed of simple answers (Yes/No). The shorter version of the test consists of 15 questions selected from the longer version. Each question is scored as 0 or 1 point. A score of 0–4 is indicative of normal; 5–8 of mild depression; 9–11 of moderate depression; and 12–15 of severe depression. The GDS is a fairly sensitive and specific test [22].

2.3. Handgrip Strength

The Jamar hand-held hydraulic dynamometer (Sammons Preston, Rolyon, Bolingbrook, IL, USA) was used to measure muscle strength (HGS) according to the standardized protocol [23]. The patient repeated tests 3 times with each hand. The best score was used for analysis.

2.4. Statistical Methods

Statistical analysis was performed using Statistica (13) software (StatSoft, Kraków, Poland).

The quantitative values are presented as means with standard deviations and qualitative variables as numbers and percentages. One-way analysis of variance (ANOVA) and the Chi^2 test were used to compare the two groups. The logistic regression model was established to predict the probability of presence of pain and anxiety as dependent variables using the stepwise regression method, with the age, sex, body mass index (BMI), the presence of diseases, GDS score and HGS as independent variables.

A multivariate logistic regression model was constructed by employing the forward–backward stepwise selection procedure. The first model was without the GDS variable and the second was with the GDS variable.

An analysis of the comparison of the presence of pain in the group of men with HGS < 27 and with HGS ≥ 27 kg and in the group of women with HGS < 16 and with HGS ≥ 16 kg was also performed. Those cut-off points have been proposed by the European Working Group on Sarcopenia [24].

For all statistical analyses, values of $p < 0.05$ were considered significant.

3. Results

3.1. Demographic and Clinical Data

Seventy-seven percent of the participants reported pain and sixty-five percent reported anxiety. The characteristics of the patients according to the prevalence of pain and anxiety have been presented in Tables 1–6.

Table 1. Characteristics of pain prevalence among study patients.

	Pain		
Variable	Yes (n = 1570)	No (n = 468)	p-Value
Age [years]	74.53 ± 8.47	72.16 ± 8.13	≤0.001 [a]
Men [n (%)]	405 (25.8)	169 (36.1)	≤0.001 [b]
BMI [kg/m^2]	27.46 ± 4.80	26.94 ± 4.42	≤0.05 [a]
Diabetes [n (%)]	313 (19.9)	74 (15.8)	≤0.05 [b]
Respiratory diseases [n (%)]	201 (12.8)	50 (10.7)	ns [b]
Musculoskeletal disorders [n (%)]	326 (20.8)	102 (21.8)	ns [b]
Chronic heart failure [n (%)]	626 (39.9)	103 (22)	≤0.001 [b]
Myocardial infarction [n (%)]	159 (10.1)	30 (6.4)	≤0.05 [b]
Hypertension [n (%)]	1072 (68.3)	267 (57)	≤0.001 [b]
Stroke [n (%)]	193 (12.3)	36 (7.7)	≤0.01 [b]
Cancer [n (%)]	131 (8.3)	34 (7.3)	ns [b]
GDS	5.03 ± 3.76	3.05 ± 2.93	≤0.001 [a]
HGS [kg]	30.11 ± 14.23	34.21 ± 14.94	≤0.001 [a]

The quantitative values are presented as mean ± SD and as number and percentage. [a] Analysis of variance (ANOVA) test; [b] Chi^2 test. Abbreviations: BMI—body mass index, GDS—Geriatric Depression Scale, HGS—handgrip strength.

Table 2. Characteristics of anxiety prevalence among study patients.

	Anxiety		
Variable	Yes (n = 1330)	No (n = 708)	p-Value
Age [years]	74.48 ± 8.41	73.06 ± 8.45	≤0.001 [a]
Men [n (%)]	303 (22.8)	271 (38.3)	≤0.001 [b]
BMI [kg/m^2]	27.35 ± 4.87	27.32 ± 4.42	ns [a]
Diabetes [n (%)]	269 (20.2)	118 (16.7)	ns [b]
Respiratory diseases [n (%)]	171 (12.8)	80 (11.3)	ns [b]
Musculoskeletal disorders [n (%)]	280 (21)	148 (20.9)	ns [b]
Chronic heart failure [n (%)]	544 (40.9)	185 (26.1)	≤0.001 [b]
Myocardial infarction [n (%)]	134 (10.1)	55 (7.8)	ns [b]
Hypertension [n (%)]	902 (67.8)	437 (61.7)	≤0.01 [b]
Stroke [n (%)]	172 (12.9)	57 (8)	≤0.001 [b]
Cancer [n (%)]	111 (8.3)	54 (7.6)	ns [b]
GDS	5.6 ± 3.71	2.65 ± 2.73	≤0.001 [a]
HGS [kg]	29.21 ± 13.7	34.52 ± 15.32	≤0.001 [a]

The quantitative values are presented as mean ± SD and as number and percentage. [a] Analysis of variance (ANOVA) test; [b] Chi^2 test. Abbreviations: BMI—body mass index, GDS—Geriatric Depression Scale, HGS—handgrip strength, ns—not significant.

Table 3. Characteristics of pain prevalence among women.

	Pain among Women		
Variable	Yes (*n* = 1165)	No (*n* = 299)	*p*-Value
Age [years]	75.29 ± 8.45	72.92 ± 8.27	≤0.001 [a]
BMI [kg/m^2]	27.51 ± 4.94	26.63 ± 4.52	≤0.01 [a]
Diabetes [*n* (%)]	226 (19.4)	37 (12.37)	≤0.01 [b]
Respiratory diseases [*n* (%)]	127 (10.9)	36 (12.04)	ns [b]
Musculoskeletal disorders [*n* (%)]	241 (20.7)	79 (26.42)	≤0.05 [b]
Chronic heart failure [*n* (%)]	482 (41.4)	75 (25.08)	≤0.001 [b]
Myocardial infarction [*n* (%)]	98 (8.4)	18 (6.02)	ns [b]
Hypertension [*n* (%)]	793 (68.1)	184 (61.54)	≤0.05 [b]
Stroke [*n* (%)]	138 (11.8)	23 (7.69)	≤0.05 [b]
Cancer [*n* (%)]	101 (8.7)	24 (8.03)	ns [b]
GDS	5.20 ± 3.77	3.33 ± 3.09	≤0.001 [a]
HGS [kg]	25.31 ± 10.69	27.28 ± 11.41	≤0.01 [a]

The quantitative values are presented as mean ± SD and as number and percentage. [a] Analysis of variance (ANOVA) test; [b] Chi^2 test. Abbreviations: BMI—body mass index, GDS—Geriatric Depression Scale, HGS—handgrip strength, ns—not significant.

Table 4. Characteristics of pain prevalence among men.

	Pain among Men		
Variable	Yes (*n* = 405)	No (*n* = 169)	*p*-Value
Age [years]	72.34 ± 8.14	70.82 ± 7.71	≤0.05 [a]
BMI [kg/m^2]	27.29 ± 4.38	27.49 ± 4.2	ns [a]
Diabetes [*n* (%)]	87 (21.5)	37 (21.89)	ns [b]
Respiratory diseases [*n* (%)]	74 (18.3)	14 (8.28)	≤0.01 [b]
Musculoskeletal disorders [*n* (%)]	85 (21)	23 (13.61)	≤0.05 [b]
Chronic heart failure [*n* (%)]	144 (35.6)	28 (16.57)	≤0.001 [b]
Myocardial infarction [*n* (%)]	61 (15.1)	12 (7.1)	≤0.01 [b]
Hypertension [*n* (%)]	279 (68.9)	83 (49.11)	≤0.001 [b]
Stroke [*n* (%)]	55 (13.6)	13 (7.69)	≤0.05 [b]
Cancer [*n* (%)]	30 (7.4)	10 (5.92)	ns [b]
GDS	4.54 ± 3.7	2.56 ± 2.56	≤0.001 [a]
HGS [kg]	43.91 ± 14.17	46.45 ± 12.37	≤0.05 [a]

The quantitative values are presented as mean ± SD and as number and percentage. [a] Analysis of variance (ANOVA) test; [b] Chi^2 test. Abbreviations: BMI—body mass index, GDS—Geriatric Depression Scale, HGS—handgrip strength, ns—not significant.

Table 5. Characteristics of anxiety prevalence among women.

	Anxiety among Women		
Variable	Yes (*n* = 1027)	No (*n* = 437)	*p*-Value
Age [years]	75.17 ± 8.46	73.96 ± 8.42	≤0.05 [a]
BMI [kg/m^2]	27.43 ± 4.98	27.11 ± 4.6	ns [a]
Diabetes [*n* (%)]	201 (19.6)	62 (14.19)	≤0.05 [b]
Respiratory diseases [*n* (%)]	115 (11.2)	48 (10.98)	ns [b]
Musculoskeletal disorders [*n* (%)]	219 (21.3)	101 (23.11)	ns [b]
Chronic heart failure [*n* (%)]	433 (42.2)	124 (28.38)	≤0.001 [b]
Myocardial infarction [*n* (%)]	86 (8.4)	30 (6.86)	ns [b]
Hypertension [*n* (%)]	700 (68.2)	277 (63.39)	ns [b]
Stroke [*n* (%)]	128 (12.5)	33 (7.55)	≤0.01 [b]
Cancer [*n* (%)]	92 (9)	33 (7.55)	ns [b]
GDS	5.66 ± 3.7	2.82 ± 2.91	≤0.001 [a]
HGS [kg]	25.06 ± 10.32	27.26 ± 11.91	≤0.001 [a]

The quantitative values are presented as mean ± SD and as number and percentage. [a] Analysis of variance (ANOVA) test; [b] Chi^2 test. Abbreviations: BMI—body mass index, GDS—Geriatric Depression Scale, HGS—handgrip strength, ns—not significant.

Table 6. Characteristics of anxiety prevalence among men.

	Anxiety among Men		
Variable	Yes ($n = 1027$)	No ($n = 437$)	p-Value
Age [years]	72.16 ± 7.81	71.59 ± 8.29	ns [a]
BMI [kg/m^2]	27.08 ± 4.48	27.65 ± 4.13	ns [a]
Diabetes [n (%)]	68 (22.4)	56 (20.66)	ns [b]
Respiratory diseases [n (%)]	56 (18.5)	32 (11.81)	≤0.05 [b]
Musculoskeletal disorders [n (%)]	61 (20.1)	47 (17.34)	ns [b]
Chronic heart failure [n (%)]	111 (36.6)	61 (22.51)	≤0.001 [b]
Myocardial infarction [n (%)]	48 (15.8)	25 (9.23)	≤0.05 [b]
Hypertension [n (%)]	202 (66.7)	160 (59.04)	ns [b]
Stroke [n (%)]	44 (14.5)	24 (8.86)	≤0.05 [b]
Cancer [n (%)]	19 (6.3)	21 (7.75)	ns [b]
GDS	5.39 ± 3.75	2.36 ± 2.39	≤0.001 [a]
HGS [kg]	43.26 ± 14.38	46.22 ± 12.75	≤0.01 [a]

The quantitative values are presented as mean ± SD and as number and percentage. [a] Analysis of variance (ANOVA) test; [b] Chi^2 test. Abbreviations: BMI—body mass index, GDS—Geriatric Depression Scale, HGS—handgrip strength, ns—not significant.

Subjects with pain were older, more often women, had higher BMI, higher prevalence of diabetes, heart failure, myocardial infarction, hypertension and stroke (Table 1). Subjects with anxiety were older, more often women, had higher prevalence of heart failure, hypertension and stroke (Table 2). Both pain and anxiety sufferers were characterized by higher GDS score and lower HGS as compared to the subjects without these problems (Tables 1 and 2). Those associations were generally similar when assessed separately in women and men, especially with consistent differences for GDS and HGS (Tables 3–6). The presence of chronic diseases was generally related to higher prevalence of pain and anxiety.

Of interest is an inverse association between the presence of musculoskeletal disorders and the manifestation of pain in women. A similar trend was observed for anxiety in women. Different associations of musculoskeletal disorders with the manifestation of pain in both sexes was confirmed with statistically significant interaction ($p = 0.0028$) between musculoskeletal disorders and sex with the manifestation of pain as a dependent variable.

3.2. Multivariate Regression Models

In the first multivariate logistic regression model (without the GDS), several independent predictors of pain and anxiety were identified. Statistically significant effects of female sex on the presence of pain and anxiety; higher age and BMI on the presence of pain, especially among women; chronic heart failure on the presence of pain and anxiety among both men and women; stroke on the presence of anxiety, especially among women; hypertension on the presence of pain, especially among men; and respiratory diseases and musculoskeletal disorders on the presence of pain were found.

Particular attention was directed to the effects of HGS on the presence of pain and anxiety in a multivariate design. Significant influence of HGS on the presence of pain (odds ratio [OR] = 0.988, 95% confidence interval [CI] = 0.980–0.995; $p = 0.002$) (forward regression) in the entire study population was found, in addition to presence of pain among men (OR = 0.983, 95% CI = 0.969–0.998; $p = 0.022$). HGS was a significant independent predictor for the presence of anxiety in the entire study population (OR = 0.987, 95% CI = 0.979–0.995; $p = 0.001$), in addition to presence of anxiety among women (OR = 0.985, 95% CI = 0.975–0.996; $p = 0.005$) and among men (OR = 0.988, 95% CI = 0.975–1.000; $p = 0.047$). Except for the regression with pain in the entire population, all other results were the same for the forward and backward designs.

In the second multivariate logistic regression model, GDS was also included as an independent variable. GDS was selected as the most powerful ($p < 0.001$ for all analyses) independent predictor of pain or anxiety both in the entire study population and separately in women and men. Together with GDS, there were found statistically significant effects for being female on the presence of pain and anxiety; higher age on the presence of anxiety and pain, especially among women; higher BMI on the presence of pain, especially among women; chronic heart failure in all groups except anxiety among men; and hypertension on the presence of pain, especially among men.

HGS was a significant independent predictor for the presence of pain in the entire study population (OR = 0.988, 95% CI = 0.980–0.995; p = 0.001) (forward regression), and also for the presence of anxiety in the entire study population (OR = 0.987, 95% CI = 0.977–0.996; p = 0.007) (backward regression) and presence of anxiety among women (OR = 0.988, 95% CI = 0.976–1.000; p = 0.049) (backward regression).

The main findings on the effects of HGS on the presence of pain and anxiety from the multivariate regression models have been shown in Table 7. Independent of other co-determinants, the contribution of HGS to the lower prevalence of pain and anxiety varied from 1.2% to 1.7% per 1 kg increase as a measure of HGS.

Table 7. Independent of other co-determinants, the contribution of HGS (increase in HGS per 1 kg) to the lower prevalence of pain and anxiety among study patients.

	Multivariate Logistic Regression Model without GDS			Multivariate Logistic Regression Model with GDS		
	Study Population	Women	Men	Study Population	Women	Men
Pain	↓1.2%	-	↓1.7%	↓1.2%	-	-
Anxiety	↓1.5%	↓1.3%	↓1.2%	↓1.3%	↓1.2%	-

GDS—Geriatric Depression Scale, HGS—handgrip strength.

3.3. Comparison to Sarcopenia HGS Cut-Off Points

Male and female groups with and without pain were compared according to sarcopenia HGS cut-off points proposed by the European Working Group on Sarcopenia (Figure 1). The prevalence of pain tended to be higher (p = 0.0858 for men and p = 0.0674 for women) in subjects fulfilling the HGS criteria for sarcopenia. Those associations were even more visible for anxiety (Figure 2). The prevalence of anxiety was higher (p < 0.001 for men and p = 0.0013 for women) in subjects fulfilling the HGS criteria for sarcopenia.

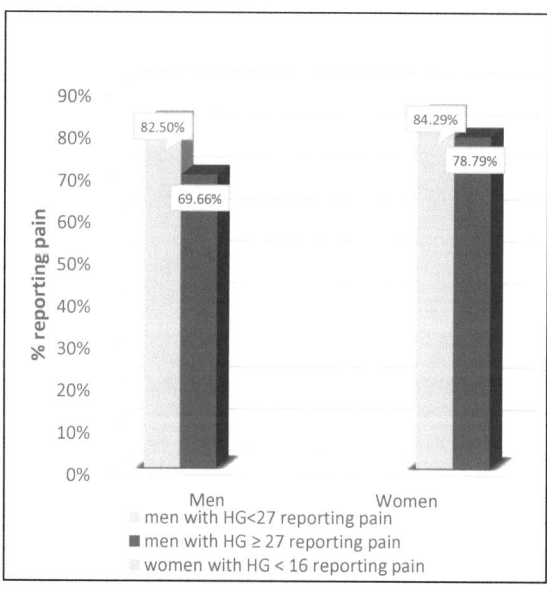

Figure 1. Comparison of the presence of pain by sex with a specific HGS cut-off points: in men with HGS < 27 (n = 40) and ≥ 27 kg (n = 534) and in women with HGS < 16 (n = 210) and HGS ≥ 16 kg (n = 1254). Chi^2 score for men: p = 0.0858; Chi^2 score for women: p = 0.0674.

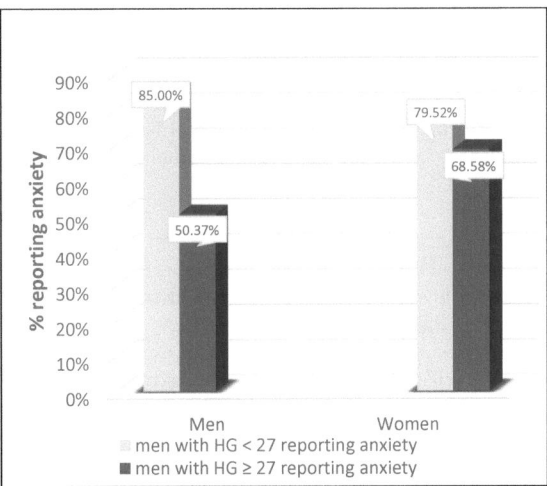

Figure 2. Comparison of the presence of anxiety by sex with specific HGS cut-off points: in men with HGS < 27 (n = 40) and ≥ 27 kg (n = 534) and in women with HGS < 16 (n = 210) and HGS ≥ 16 kg (n = 1254). Chi^2 score for men: p < 0.001; Chi^2 score for women: p = 0.0013.

4. Discussion

This study analyzed the relationship between handgrip strength (HGS) and the presence of pain and anxiety among older adults. The data on this subject available in the literature are not consistent. Our study shows that both pain and anxiety are very common in the study population and that HGS influences the presence of pain and anxiety among older adults independent of age, sex and concomitant chronic diseases. This relationship is generally similar in males and females, but the co-contribution of concomitant disorders may differ between the two sexes.

The prevalence of pain and anxiety increases with age [2,3]. Both pain and anxiety are associated with decreased functioning, poor mental health and have a negative impact on quality of life for older people [3,25,26]. Chronic pain and anxiety also increase health care costs [3,26]. HGS is a simple, quick and reliable method of assessing maximum voluntary compressive force. This measurement is useful for assessing qualitative and functional aspects of muscle strength, but also for evaluating nutritional status and general health. In addition, HGS is associated with many chronic diseases [27].

Recent data have shown that HGS can be an independent predictor of quality of life in a variety of disease settings, from arthritis to chronic liver disease and depression [28]. Lower HGS was significantly associated with prevalence of pain, anxiety and poor quality of life in cancer survivors [28,29]. Pain intensity and HGS were dysfunctions affecting upper limb disability in women with bilateral idiopathic carpal tunnel syndrome [15], and carpal tunnel syndrome patients with low levels of education showed reduced HGS and more catastrophic thinking [16]. The results of the study by Daliri et al. [17] show that anxiety correlates with pain and lower HGS in patients with cervical radiculopathy. Furthermore, this correlation is almost similar in patients with carpal tunnel syndrome. Disability in patients with carpal tunnel syndrome as well as cervical radiculopathy is associated with anxiety, depression and catastrophic thinking. The authors suggest that further research should determine whether psychological distress causes more disability or the reverse [17]. In a cross-sectional study of 439 women with fibromyalgia, lower physical performance assessed through the Senior Fitness Test battery and HGS test was associated with higher levels of anxiety [30]. In women with early rheumatoid arthritis HGS was found to be significantly reduced in those with widespread pain as compared to women without widespread pain [31]. The effects of preoperative pain, anxiety and depression on arm, shoulder and hand disability; quality of life; HGS strength and range of motion in the first year after salvage wrist surgery were studied [18]. Negative effects of pain and anxiety on patient-reported outcomes were found. Preoperative pain or tendency to anxiety had a strong negative effect on postoperative disability. Anxiety also resulted in lower postoperative quality of life, while pain had a negative effect on HGS [18]. In contrast, severe fatigue in people with rheumatoid arthritis was associated more with self-rated health, pain and anxiety/depression rather than with physical capacity tests (lower limb function, HGS and aerobic capacity) [32].

Similar to with specific diseases, several general population studies indicated an association between HGS and mental health. Korean men and women with low HGS had poor mobility and pain or discomfort on the Euroqol-5D scale [33]. In middle-aged Japanese women, low grip strength and insomnia were independently associated with pain symptoms. The authors suggested that treating insomnia in these women may offset muscle and joint pain and thus improve HGS, or treating pain may reduce insomnia in addition to improving HGS [34]. In 3952 subjects aged ≥50 years, a one-standard-deviation increase in HGS was associated with 12.1% lower odds of prevalent Generalized Anxiety Disorder (GAD), and middle- and high-strength tertiles were associated with 27.3% and 23.1% lower odds, respectively [35]. In a 7-year prospective cohort study of 152,978 UK Biobank participants, an exercise test and dynamometer were used to measure cardiorespiratory fitness and HGS, respectively [36]. Patient Health Questionnaire-9 and Generalised Anxiety Disorder-7 scales estimated the incidence of common mental disorders at follow-up. Low and medium HGS were associated with 1.381 and 1.116 higher odds of common mental disorder compared to high HGS. Individuals in the lowest group for both cardiorespiratory fitness and HGS had 1.981 higher odds of depression and 1.599 higher odds of anxiety, compared to a high level of fitness group [36]. In another analysis from the UK Biobank prospective cohort study, of the 162,167 participants included, 5462 (3.4%) developed depression and 6614 (4.1%) anxiety, over a median follow-up period of 10.0 years. In the fully adjusted model, a 5 kg lower HGS rating was associated with a 7% and 8% higher risk of depression and anxiety, respectively. The authors recommend that future research should assess if resistance training aimed at increasing HGS can prevent the occurrence of mental health conditions [37].

Relatively few studies assessed the relationship of HGS to the prevalence of pain or anxiety in older populations. Imai et al. assessed the frailty and chronic pain of 107 older adults. The prevalence of chronic pain with pre-frailty was high, and chronic pain and pre-frailty were strongly related [26]. A recent meta-analysis demonstrated a relationship between low muscle strength and intensified depressive symptoms in older populations [38]. In contrast, in 173 institutionalized older individuals, there were no differences in HGS values between the groups with and without chronic pain [39].

Our data show that both pain and anxiety are very common in the older population, especially in women. Presence of symptoms of depression (GDS) was selected as the most powerful independent predictor of pain or anxiety, both in the entire study population and separately in women and men. Higher HGS was related to the lower presence of pain and anxiety among older adults independent of age, GDS and concomitant chronic diseases. In the fully adjusted model, a HGS rating higher than 1kg was associated with 1.2% and 1.3% lower probability of the presence of pain and anxiety, respectively. These data seem comparable to the analysis from the UK Biobank prospective cohort [37]. The association of HGS to the prevalence of pain and anxiety was apparently similar in males and females. Nevertheless, the co-contribution of concomitant disorders may differ between the two sexes. While the presence of chronic diseases was generally related to higher prevalence of pain and anxiety, an inverse association of the presence of musculoskeletal disorders to the manifestation of pain, with a similar trend for anxiety, was observed in women. This phenomenon may be explained by the fact that women with musculoskeletal disorders were almost three years younger ($p < 0.001$) as compared to women without those diseases. Therefore, it seems that younger women are more prone to suffer from musculoskeletal diseases, while with age this problem becomes less troublesome.

Our study has some limitations. Its cross-sectional character excludes any firm causality statements. In addition, the study was conducted in a central European population, and results may be different in other cultures. Nevertheless, the key strengths of this study are the careful recruitment procedures and the large study population.

5. Conclusions

A significant relationship between low HGS and the presence of pain and anxiety in the study population was found. Maintenance of high HGS may be considered an important protective factor against feelings of pain and anxiety, independent of age, depression and concomitant diseases. Future research should prospectively assess reciprocal associations between HGS and pain or anxiety and whether improvement of HGS would alleviate psychological dysfunction in older adults. It seems that this would also be helpful for the geriatric healthcare system.

Author Contributions: Conceptualization, N.S., T.K. and J.K.; Methodology, T.K., J.K. and E.B.; Formal analysis, J.K. and T.K.; Investigation, A.G., B.S., E.B., T.K. and J.K.; Resources, T.K.; data curation, N.S., J.K. and T.K.; Writing—original draft preparation, N.S., J.K. and T.K.; Writing—review and editing, N.S., A.G., B.S., E.B., T.K. and J.K.; Visualization, N.S.; Supervision, T.K. and J.K.; Project administration, T.K.; Funding acquisition, J.K. All authors have read and agreed to the published version of the manuscript.

Funding: The authors were supported by grants founded by the Medical University of Lodz, Poland (503/6-077-01/503-61-001-19-00 and 503/6-127-06/503-61-001-19-00).

Institutional Review Board Statement: The study was conducted in accordance with the Declaration of Helsinki and approved by the Committee on the Ethics of Research of Human Experimentation at the Medical University of Lodz, Poland (RNN/647/14/KB, 23 September 2014).

Informed Consent Statement: Informed consent was obtained from all individual participants included in the study.

Data Availability Statement: Data will be available on request from the corresponding author.

Conflicts of Interest: The authors declare no conflict of interest.

References

1. Ogliari, G.; Ryg, J.; Andersen-Ranberg, K.; Scheel-Hincke, L.L.; Collins, J.T.; Cowley, A.; Di Lorito, C.; Howe, L.; Robinson, K.R.; Booth, V.; et al. Association of pain and risk of falls in community-dwelling adults: A prospective study in the Survey of Health, Ageing and Retirement in Europe (SHARE). *Eur. Geriatr. Med.* **2022**, *13*, 1441–1454. [CrossRef] [PubMed]
2. Domenichiello, A.F.; Ramsden, C.E. The silent epidemic of chronic pain in older adults. *Prog. Neuropsychopharmacol. Biol. Psychiatry* **2019**, *93*, 284–290. [CrossRef]
3. Balsamo, M.; Cataldi, F.; Carlucci, L.; Fairfield, B. Assessment of anxiety in older adults: A review of self-report measures. *Clin. Interv. Aging* **2018**, *13*, 573–593. [CrossRef] [PubMed]
4. Bohannon, R.W. Grip Strength: An Indispensable Biomarker for Older Adults. *Clin. Interv. Aging* **2019**, *14*, 1681–1691. [CrossRef] [PubMed]
5. Noh, H.M.; Park, Y.S. Handgrip strength, dynapenia, and mental health in older Koreans. *Sci. Rep.* **2020**, *10*, 4004. [CrossRef]
6. Perna, F.M.; Coa, K.; Troiano, R.P.; Lawman, H.G.; Wang, C.-Y.; Li, Y.; Moser, R.P.; Ciccolo, J.T.; Comstock, B.A.; Kraemer, W.J. Muscular Grip Strength Estimates of the U.S. Population from the National Health and Nutrition Examination Survey 2011–2012. *J. Strength Cond. Res.* **2016**, *30*, 867–874. [CrossRef]
7. Jacob, M.E.; O'Donnell, A.; Samra, J.; Gonzales, M.M.; Satizabal, C.; Pase, M.P.; Murabito, J.M.; Beiser, A.; Seshadri, S. Grip Strength, Gait Speed and Plasma Markers of Neurodegeneration in Asymptomatic Middle-aged and Older Adults. *J. Frailty Aging* **2022**, *11*, 291–298. [CrossRef] [PubMed]
8. Nakamura, K.; Kawasaki, A.; Suzuki, N.; Hosoi, S.; Fujita, T.; Hachisu, S.; Nakano, H.; Naraba, H.; Mochizuki, M.; Takahashi, Y. Grip Strength Correlates with Mental Health and Quality of Life after Critical Care: A Retrospective Study in a Post-Intensive Care Syndrome Clinic. *J. Clin. Med.* **2021**, *10*, 3044. [CrossRef] [PubMed]
9. Tajika, T.; Kuboi, T.; Oya, N.; Endo, F.; Shitara, H.; Ichinose, T.; Sasaki, T.; Hamano, N.; Chikuda, H. Association Between Upper-Extremity Health Condition and Depressive Status in an Elderly General Population. *Inquiry* **2021**, *58*, 469580211059952. [CrossRef]

10. Esteban-Cornejo, I.; Ho, F.K.; Petermann-Rocha, F.; Lyall, D.M.; Martinez-Gomez, D.; Cabanas-Sánchez, V.; Ortega, F.B.; Hillman, C.H.; Gill, J.M.R.; Quinn, T.J.; et al. Handgrip strength and all-cause dementia incidence and mortality: Findings from the UK Biobank prospective cohort study. *J. Cachexia Sarcopenia Muscle* **2022**, *13*, 1514–1525. [CrossRef]
11. Milman, R.; Zikrin, E.; Shacham, D.; Freud, T.; Press, Y. Handgrip Strength as a Predictor of Successful Rehabilitation After Hip Fracture in Patients 65 Years of Age and Above. *Clin. Interv. Aging* **2022**, *17*, 1307–1317. [CrossRef] [PubMed]
12. Kawamoto, R.; Kikuchi, A.; Akase, T.; Ninomiya, D.; Kumagi, T. Thigh circumference and handgrip strength are significantly associated with all-cause mortality: Findings from a study on Japanese community-dwelling persons. *Eur. Geriatr. Med.* **2021**, *12*, 1191–1200. [CrossRef] [PubMed]
13. Nagaoka, S.; Yoshimura, Y.; Eto, T.; Kumagi, M. Low handgrip strength is associated with reduced functional recovery and longer hospital stay in patients with osteoporotic vertebral compression fractures: A prospective cohort study. *Eur. Geriatr. Med.* **2021**, *12*, 767–775. [CrossRef] [PubMed]
14. Ko, S.H.; Park, S.J.; Kim, N.Y.; Jeon, W.; Shin, D.A.; Kim, S.H. Influence of Preoperative Handgrip Strength on Length of Stay after Lumbar Fusion Surgery. *J. Clin. Med.* **2022**, *11*, 3928. [CrossRef] [PubMed]
15. Yoshida, A.; Kurimoto, S.; Iwatsuki, K.; Saeki, M.; Nishizuka, T.; Nakano, T.; Yoneda, H.; Onishi, T.; Yamamoto, M.; Tatebe, M.; et al. Upper extremity disability is associated with pain intensity and grip strength in women with bilateral idiopathic carpal tunnel syndrome. *NeuroRehabilitation* **2019**, *44*, 199–205. [CrossRef] [PubMed]
16. Núñez-Cortés, R.; Cruz-Montecinos, C.; Antúnez-Riveros, M.A.; Pérez-Alenda, S. Does the educational level of women influence hand grip and pinch strength in carpal tunnel syndrome? *Med. Hypotheses* **2020**, *135*, 109474. [CrossRef]
17. Mahla Daliri, B.O.; Khorasani, H.M.; Olia, N.D.B.; Azhari, A.; Shakeri, M.; Moradi, A. Association of psychological factors with limb disability in patients with cervical radiculopathy: Comparison with carpal tunnel syndrome. *BMC Musculoskelet. Disord.* **2022**, *23*, 667. [CrossRef]
18. Swärd, E.M.; Brodda-Jansen, G.; Schriever, T.U.; Andersson-Franko, M.; Wilcke, M.K. The impact of psychological factors on outcome after salvage surgery for wrist osteoarthritis. *J. Hand Surg. Eur. Vol.* **2022**, *47*, 805–811. [CrossRef]
19. Kim, H.J.; Ban, M.G.; Yoon, K.B.; Jeon, W.; Kim, S.H. Neuropathic-like Pain Symptoms and Their Association with Muscle Strength in Patients with Chronic Musculoskeletal Pain. *J. Clin. Med.* **2022**, *11*, 5471. [CrossRef]
20. Kind, P.; Dolan, P.; Gudex, C.; Williams, A. Variations in population health status: Results from a United Kingdom national questionnaire survey. *Bmj* **1998**, *316*, 736–741. [CrossRef]
21. EQ-5D. Available online: https://euroqol.org/ (accessed on 27 May 2023).
22. Yesavage, J.A.; Brink, T.L.; Rose, T.L.; Lum, O.; Huang, V.; Adey, M.; Leirer, V.O. Development and validation of a geriatric depression screening scale: A preliminary report. *J. Psychiatr. Res.* **1982**, *17*, 37–49. [CrossRef] [PubMed]
23. Rantanen, T.; Guralnik, J.M.; Foley, D.; Masaki, K.; Leveille, S.; Curb, J.D.; White, L. Midlife hand grip strength as a predictor of old age disability. *JAMA* **1999**, *281*, 558–560. [CrossRef] [PubMed]
24. Cruz-Jentoft, A.J.; Bahat, G.; Bauer, J.; Boirie, Y.; Bruyère, O.; Cederholm, T.; Cooper, C.; Landi, F.; Rolland, Y.; Sayer, A.A.; et al. Sarcopenia: Revised European consensus on definition and diagnosis. *Age Ageing* **2019**, *48*, 16–31. [CrossRef] [PubMed]
25. Sit, R.W.S.; Choi, S.Y.K.; Wang, B.; Chan, D.C.C.; Zhang, D.; Yip, B.H.K.; Wong, S.Y.S. Neuromuscular exercise for chronic musculoskeletal pain in older people: A randomised controlled trial in primary care in Hong Kong. *Br. J. Gen. Pract.* **2021**, *71*, e226–e236. [CrossRef]
26. Imai, R.; Imaoka, M.; Nakao, H.; Hida, M.; Tazaki, F.; Omizu, T.; Ishigaki, T.; Nakamura, M. Association between chronic pain and pre-frailty in Japanese community-dwelling older adults: A cross-sectional study. *PLoS ONE* **2020**, *15*, e0236111. [CrossRef]
27. Shah, S.A.; Safian, N.; Mohammad, Z.; Nurumal, S.R.; Wan Ibadullah, W.A.H.; Mansor, J.; Ahmad, S.; Hassan, M.R.; Shobugawa, Y. Factors Associated with Handgrip Strength Among Older Adults in Malaysia. *J. Multidiscip. Healthc.* **2022**, *15*, 1023–1034. [CrossRef] [PubMed]
28. Paek, J.; Choi, Y.J. Association between hand grip strength and impaired health-related quality of life in Korean cancer survivors: A cross-sectional study. *BMJ Open* **2019**, *9*, e030938. [CrossRef]
29. Kim, H.; Yoo, S.; Kim, H.; Park, S.G.; Son, M. Cancer Survivors with Low Hand Grip Strength Have Decreased Quality of Life Compared with Healthy Controls: The Korea National Health and Nutrition Examination Survey 2014-2017. *Korean J. Fam. Med.* **2021**, *42*, 204–211. [CrossRef]
30. Córdoba-Torrecilla, S.; Aparicio, V.A.; Soriano-Maldonado, A.; Estévez-López, F.; Segura-Jiménez, V.; Álvarez-Gallardo, I.; Femia, P.; Delgado-Fernández, M. Physical fitness is associated with anxiety levels in women with fibromyalgia: The al-Ándalus project. *Qual. Life Res.* **2016**, *25*, 1053–1058. [CrossRef]
31. Bilberg, A.; Bremell, T.; Bjersing, J.; Mannerkorpi, K. High prevalence of widespread pain in women with early rheumatoid arthritis. *Scand. J. Rheumatol.* **2018**, *47*, 447–454. [CrossRef]
32. Demmelmaier, I.; Pettersson, S.; Nordgren, B.; Dufour, A.B.; Opava, C.H. Associations between fatigue and physical capacity in people moderately affected by rheumatoid arthritis. *Rheumatol. Int.* **2018**, *38*, 2147–2155. [CrossRef] [PubMed]
33. Kang, S.Y.; Lim, J.; Park, H.S. Relationship between low handgrip strength and quality of life in Korean men and women. *Qual. Life Res.* **2018**, *27*, 2571–2580. [CrossRef] [PubMed]
34. Terauchi, M.; Odai, T.; Hirose, A.; Kato, K.; Akiyoshi, M.; Miyasaka, N. Muscle and joint pains in middle-aged women are associated with insomnia and low grip strength: A cross-sectional study. *J. Psychosom. Obstet. Gynaecol.* **2020**, *41*, 15–21. [CrossRef] [PubMed]

35. Gordon, B.R.; McDowell, C.P.; Lyons, M.; Herring, M.P. Associations between grip strength and generalized anxiety disorder in older adults: Results from the Irish longitudinal study on ageing. *J. Affect Disord.* **2019**, *255*, 136–141. [CrossRef]
36. Kandola, A.A.; Osborn, D.P.J.; Stubbs, B.; Choi, K.W.; Hayes, J.F. Individual and combined associations between cardiorespiratory fitness and grip strength with common mental disorders: A prospective cohort study in the UK Biobank. *BMC Med.* **2020**, *18*, 303. [CrossRef]
37. Cabanas-Sánchez, V.; Esteban-Cornejo, I.; Parra-Soto, S.; Petermann-Rocha, F.; Gray, S.R.; Rodríguez-Artalejo, F.; Ho, F.K.; Pell, J.P.; Martínez-Gómez, D.; Celis-Morales, C. Muscle strength and incidence of depression and anxiety: Findings from the UK Biobank prospective cohort study. *J. Cachexia Sarcopenia Muscle* **2022**, *13*, 1983–1994. [CrossRef]
38. Zasadzka, E.; Pieczyńska, A.; Trzmiel, T.; Kleka, P.; Pawlaczyk, M. Correlation between Handgrip Strength and Depression in Older Adults-A Systematic Review and a Meta-Analysis. *Int. J. Environ. Res. Public Health* **2021**, *18*, 4823. [CrossRef]
39. Ribeiro, D.d.S.; Garbin, K.; Jorge, M.S.G.; Doring, M.; Portella, M.R.; Wibelinger, L.M. Prevalence of chronic pain and analysis of handgrip strength in institutionalized elderly. *BrJP* **2019**, *2*, 242–246. [CrossRef]

Disclaimer/Publisher's Note: The statements, opinions and data contained in all publications are solely those of the individual author(s) and contributor(s) and not of MDPI and/or the editor(s). MDPI and/or the editor(s) disclaim responsibility for any injury to people or property resulting from any ideas, methods, instructions or products referred to in the content.

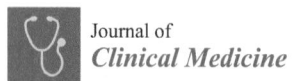

Article

Quality of Life and Kidney Function in Older Adults: Prospective Data of the SCOPE Study

Rada Artzi-Medvedik [1,2], Robert Kob [3], Mirko Di Rosa [4], Fabrizia Lattanzio [4], Andrea Corsonello [4], Ilan Yehoshua [2], Regina E. Roller-Wirnsberger [5], Gerhard H. Wirnsberger [5], Francesco U. S. Mattace-Raso [6], Lisanne Tap [6], Pedro G. Gil [7], Francesc Formiga [8], Rafael Moreno-González [8], Tomasz Kostka [9], Agnieszka Guligowska [9], Johan Ärnlöv [10,11], Axel C. Carlsson [11,12], Ellen Freiberger [3,*] and Itshak Melzer [13,*] on behalf of the SCOPE Investigators

[1] Department of Nursing, The Recanati School for Community Health Professions at the Faculty of Health Sciences, Ben-Gurion University of the Negev, Beer-Sheva 8443944, Israel; rada.artzi@gmail.com
[2] Maccabi Health Services, Southern District, Omer 8496500, Israel
[3] Department of Internal Medicine-Geriatrics, Institute for Biomedicine of Aging (IBA), Friedrich-Alexander-Universität Erlangen-Nürnberg, 90408 Nürnberg, Germany
[4] Italian National Research Center on Aging (IRCCS INRCA), 60124 Ancona, Italy
[5] Department of Internal Medicine, Medical University of Graz, 8036 Graz, Austria
[6] Department of Internal Medicine, Section of Geriatric Medicine, Erasmus MC, University Medical Center Rotterdam, P.O. Box 2040, 3000 CA Rotterdam, The Netherlands
[7] Department of Geriatric Medicine, Hospital Clinico San Carlos, 28040 Madrid, Spain
[8] Geriatric Unit, Internal Medicine Department, Bellvitge University Hospital—IDIBELL—L'Hospitalet de Llobregat, 08907 Barcelona, Spain
[9] Department of Geriatrics, Healthy Ageing Research Centre, Medical University of Lodz, 90-647 Lodz, Poland
[10] School of Health and Social Studies, Dalarna University, 79188 Falun, Sweden
[11] Division of Family Medicine and Primary Care, Department of Neurobiology, Care Sciences and Society (NVS), Karolinska Institutet, 17177 Huddinge, Sweden
[12] Academic Primary Health Care Centre, Stockholm Region, 10405 Stockholm, Sweden
[13] Department of Physical Therapy, The Recanati School for Community Health Professions at the Faculty of Health Sciences, Ben-Gurion University of the Negev, Beer-Sheva 8443944, Israel
* Correspondence: ellen.freiberger@fau.de (E.F.); itzikm@bgu.ac.il (I.M.)

Abstract: A longitudinal alteration in health-related quality of life (HRQoL) over a two-year period and its association with early-stage chronic kidney disease (CKD) progression was investigated among 1748 older adults (>75 years). HRQoL was measured by the Euro-Quality of Life Visual Analog Scale (EQ-VAS) at baseline and at one and two years after recruitment. A full comprehensive geriatric assessment was performed, including sociodemographic and clinical characteristics, the Geriatric Depression Scale-Short Form (GDS-SF), Short Physical Performance Battery (SPPB), and estimated glomerular filtration rate (eGFR). The association between EQ-VAS decline and covariates was investigated by multivariable analyses. A total of 41% of the participants showed EQ-VAS decline, and 16.3% showed kidney function decline over the two-year follow-up period. Participants with EQ-VAS decline showed an increase in GDS-SF scores and a greater decline in SPPB scores. The logistic regression analyses showed no contribution of a decrease in kidney function on EQ-VAS decline in the early stages of CKD. However, older adults with a greater GDS-SF score were more likely to present EQ-VAS decline over time, whereas an increase in the SPPB scores was associated with less EQ-VAS decline. This finding should be considered in clinical practice and when HRQoL is used to evaluate health interventions among older adults.

Keywords: quality of life; chronic kidney disease; older adults; prospective studies; cohort studies; disease progression

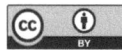

1. Introduction

The increase in the prevalence of chronic kidney disease (CKD) among older adults is related to a broad range of health concerns, including impaired physical, cognitive, and mental function [1–3], malnutrition [4], sarcopenia [5], and frailty [6,7]. These health-related problems among older adults increase the use of healthcare resources and challenge healthcare systems [8,9] more than other diseases [10–12]. This contributes to reducing the health-related quality of life (HRQoL) of community-dwelling older adults even in the early stages of CKD [13]. HRQoL was suggested to be a significant outcome, and its repeated evaluations are recommended to assess the quality of care in patients with end-stage renal disease (ESRD) [14].

HRQoL is a subjective perception of individuals or groups of their physical and mental health [15]. Not surprisingly, patients with severe CKD and ESRD show lower HRQoL scores [16–20]. Reduced HRQoL in patients with ESRD is associated with lower survival and higher hospitalization rates [16–18]. A previous cross-sectional study showed that even in early CKD stages in community-dwelling older adults, HRQoL was significantly lower compared to healthy older adults, and that the impact of CKD on HRQoL is multifactorial and partly mediated by physical performance and depressive symptoms [13]. This finding is consistent with other cross-sectional studies that have shown lower HRQoL even in the early stages (e.g., 3a and 3b) of CKD [21–24]. Longitudinal data on the association between CKD progression and HRQoL decline among older adults are rare, especially in the early stages of CKD, because this topic is less investigated. Yet, a few studies have shown that morbidity and mortality outcomes are associated with low HRQoL in patients with CKD [25–28]. In these studies, physical performance, psychological state, and HRQoL were significantly associated with increased risks of ESRD and mortality among CKD patients.

The SCOPE study represents a valuable opportunity to investigate the associations between decreased HRQoL and decline in kidney function over a two-year follow-up period in non-end-stage renal disease participants [29]. Because HRQoL is not directly affected by core symptoms of CKD, but by the deterioration in physical and psychological function [13], the aims of the present study were to investigate the association between alterations in HRQoL over a two-year period and the progression of early-stage CKD among older adults. Thus, four research questions were formulated to be addressed in the present analyses: (1) Are changes in physical functioning and depressive symptoms over a two-year period associated with decreased HRQoL? (2) Is baseline HRQoL associated with CKD progression over a two-year period? (3) Are there changes in HRQoL over a two-year period in community-dwelling older adults? (4) Is CKD progression over a two-year period associated with decreased HRQoL? The findings of this analysis will help to deepen the understanding of the impact of negative aspects of CKD on HRQoL among older adults in the early stages of the disease and to better evaluate HRQoL, not only as a consequence of the disease but also as a broad reflection of well-being among the older population.

2. Materials and Methods

2.1. Study Design and Participants

The present analysis was performed within the framework of the "Screening for Chronic Kidney Disease among Older People across Europe" (SCOPE) project, a multicenter 2-year prospective cohort study involving people older than 75 years attending outpatient services in participating institutions in Austria, Germany, Israel, Italy, the Netherlands, Poland, and Spain (clinical trial number NCT02691546, registered on 25th February 2016 at clinicaltrials.gov). Methods of the SCOPE study have been described in detail elsewhere [29]. A full comprehensive geriatric assessment (CGA) was performed at the baseline (T0), at one year (12-month follow-up visit, T1), and 2 years (24-month follow-up visit, T2) after the recruitment. Overall, 2461 participants were initially enrolled in the study, but only 1748 provided complete HRQoL data at all three time points and were included in this analysis (Figure 1). A comparison between 1748 older adults whom we included vs. 713 who were excluded from the analysis due to incomplete HRQoL data can be found in Supplementary Table S1.

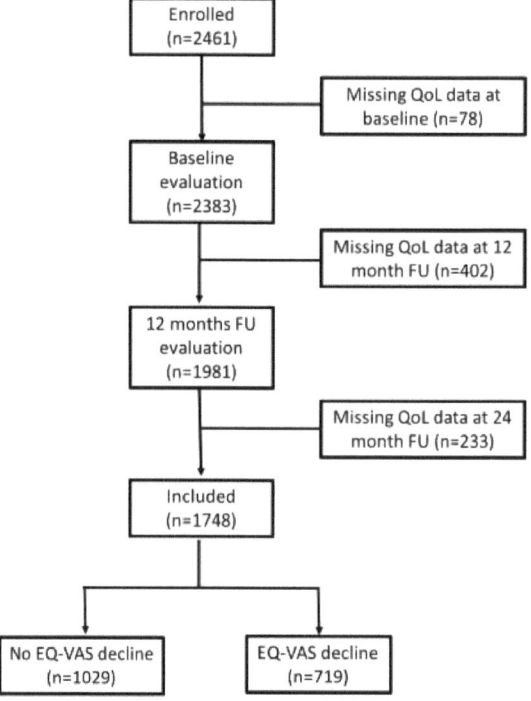

Figure 1. Flowchart on in- and exclusion of individuals within the current analysis.

2.2. Study Protocol and Instruments

During face-to-face interviews, demographic and clinical variables were collected as follows: sex, age, education, marital status; blood pressure, body mass index (BMI, kg/m^2); Mini-Mental State Examination (MMSE) [30]; history of medical conditions (e.g., diabetes mellitus, hypertension, stroke, hip fracture, chronic obstructive pulmonary disease (COPD), osteoporosis, Parkinson's disease, anemia); the presence of lower urinary tract symptoms (LUTS) [31]; and history of falls during the last year. Overall comorbidity was assessed by the Cumulative Illness Rating Scale for Geriatrics (CIRS-G) [32] and by the number of prescribed medications taken by the participants during the past month (four or less or more than five). A 15-item Geriatric Depression Scale-Short Form (GDS-SF) [33] was used for the evaluation of self-reported symptoms of depression. Short Physical Performance Battery (SPPB) [34] and a hand grip strength test [35] were used for physical performance evaluation. Further, blood and urine laboratory tests were performed at T0, T1, and T2 and included hemoglobin, albumin, serum creatinine, urinary protein-to-creatinine ratio, and estimated glomerular filtration rate (eGFR).

2.3. HRQoL Assessment

HRQoL was assessed by the Euro-Quality of Life Visual Analogue Scale (EQ-VAS) and the Euro-Quality of Life 5 Dimensions (EQ-5D) [36]. The EQ-VAS asks participants to indicate their overall health on a visual analog scale, ranging from "worst possible" (score = 0) to "best possible" health (score = 100). Higher scores on this scale represent better subjective HRQoL. The EQ-5D is used to evaluate the HRQoL measure with one question on five different dimensions, which include mobility, self-care, usual activities, pain/discomfort, and anxiety/depression. The answers given to EQ-5D are scored from

1: "I have no problems ..." for perfect health status, to 5: "I am unable to ..." for bad health status. The 5-digit numbers for the five dimensions are combined and describe the patient's total self-rated health status. This means that the higher the EQ-5D score on this scale, the worse HRQoL is. The EQ-VAS scores were the explanatory variable in this study. Similar to our previous cross-sectional study [13], we defined three categories of HRQoL: low as an EQ-VAS score of 0–50; intermediate as an EQ-VAS score of 51–75; and high as EQ-VAS score of 76–100.

2.4. HRQoL Decline Outcome

The HRQoL decline over the two-year follow-up period was defined as a downgrading of at least one category according to the EQ-VAS score (i.e., from high to intermediate or low; or from intermediate to low). Based on the above, the participants were divided into two groups: (1) the EQ-VAS decline group; and (2) the no EQ-VAS decline group. We also calculated the variation in EQ-VAS from T0 to T2 as the difference in the EQ-VAS score = Δ EQ-VAS.

2.5. Kidney Function Evaluation

In this analysis, eGFR was calculated using the Berlin Initiative Study (BIS) Equations (1) and (2) [37]:

$$\text{Women: eGFR} = (3736 \times (\text{Scr}) - 0.87 \times (\text{age}) - 0.95) \times 0.82 \qquad (1)$$

$$\text{Men: eGFR} = 3736 \times (\text{Scr}) - 0.87 \times (\text{age}) - 0.95, \qquad (2)$$

Serum creatinine was measured by Isotope Dilution Mass Spectrometry (IDMS) traceable methods. According to K/DOQI clinical practice guidelines [14], CKD is divided into 5 stages, from stage 1 with normal renal filtration rate (eGFR $\geq$ 90 mL/min/1.73 m^2) to stage 5, including kidney failure or end-stage renal disease (eGFR < 15 mL/min/1.73 m^2). For the purpose of our analysis, CKD stages 1 and 2 were combined, defined as non-CKD patients (eGFR $\geq$ 60 mL/min/1.73 m^2), stages 3a + 3b defined as moderate CKD (GFR, 30–59.9 mL/min/1.73 m^2), stage 4 defined as severe CKD (GFR, 15–29.9 mL/min/1.73 m^2), and stage 5 defined as ESRD (GFR < 14.9 mL/min/1.73 m^2). CKD was defined as eGFR < 59.9 mL/min/1.73 m^2.

2.6. CKD Progression Outcome

CKD progression was defined as a worsening of at least one CKD stage at least once during the two-year follow-up period (i.e., a decline from CKD stages 3a + b to stages 4 or lower). Based on the above, we divided the participants into two groups: (1) CKD progression group; and (2) no CKD progression group. In addition, Δ eGFR was calculated as the difference in the eGFR from T0 to T2.

2.7. Physical and Mental Functions Decline Outcomes

Worsening of self-reported symptoms of depression was indicated by the positive difference in the GDS-SF score from T0 to T2 (Δ GDS-SF). Deterioration in physical functioning was assessed as the difference from T0 to T2 in the following indicators: overall SPPB score; balance score; gait speed test; chair stand test; and hand grip strength test. Negative Δ SPPB scores and Δ handgrip strength are related to declining/worsening physical function.

2.8. Statistical Analysis

Continuous variables were reported as a mean and standard deviation; comparisons between groups (EQ-VAS decline vs. no EQ-VAS decline) were performed by Student's t-test or Mann–Whitney U test on the basis of their distribution (assessed using Shapiro–Wilk test). Categorical variables were expressed as absolute frequencies and percentages, and statistical differences were analyzed by Chi-square test. We first computed descriptive statistics for the subject's characteristics at baseline and the changes over a 2-year period, i.e., from baseline (T0) to T2 (Δ). Associations between ΔEQ-VAS and variation variables (i.e., ΔeGFR, ΔSPPB—overall and subscales, and ΔGDS-SF) were assessed with Spearman rank correlation with Bonferroni-adjusted significance level and graphically represented with scatterplot diagrams. Possible interactions of co-morbidities with ΔeGFR as a factor of quality-of=life decline were also tested. Finally, three multivariable logistic models (unadjusted, age- and sex-adjusted, and fully adjusted) for each variation variable were performed to estimate their relation to EQ-VAS decline. Odds ratios (OR) and 95% confidence intervals (CI) were reported for each potential determinant. Fully adjusted models included age, gender, educational level, EQ-VAS at baseline, MMSE at baseline, BMI at baseline, GDS-SF at baseline, grip strength at baseline, and more than five prescribed medications at baseline. The variance inflation factors (VIFs) and tolerance were additionally measured in the multivariable logistic regression analysis to investigate the degree of multicollinearity among covariates: VIF >10 and tolerance <0.25 were used to define the presence of high multicollinearity (Miles J. Tolerance and variance inflation factor. First published in 29 September 2014, Wiley StatsRef Stat Ref Online, (Hoboken, New Jersey, USA); 2014. https://doi.org/10.1002/9781118445112.stat06593).

Data were analyzed using STATA version 15.1 Statistical Software Package for Windows (Stata Corp, College Station, TX, USA). Statistical significance was set a priori at $p < 0.05$.

3. Results

3.1. Participants' Characteristics

In our cohort of 1748 older adults, 1029 (58.7%) were found with no EQ-VAS decline, and 719 (41.3%) had EQ-VAS decline (Table 1). Compared to the no EQ-VAS decline group, the older adults in the EQ-VAS decline group were more frequently females, had a higher educational level, higher BMI, lower MMSE; were taking more than five prescribed medications per day; had higher GDS-SF, higher EQ-5D, higher EQ-VAS, and lower grip strength. Interestingly, Δ GDS-SF increased in the EQ-VAS decline group vs. the no EQ-VAS decline group (+0.1 vs. −0.2, $p = 0.046$). Compared to the no EQ-VAS decline group, the EQ-VAS decline group showed a significantly higher decline in Δ SPPB balance and Δ SPPB gait speed (−0.1 vs. −0.2, $p = 0.029$ and −0.1 vs. −0.3, $p = 0.034$, respectively). No influence of Δ eGFR was found on EQ-VAS decline.

Table 1. Sociodemographic, clinical, physical, and emotional characteristics at baseline and their change over a two-year follow-up period (i.e., Δ) of: (1) older adults with no EQ-VAS decline and (2) older adults with EQ-VAS decline.

	Total	No EQ-VAS Decline	EQ-VAS Decline	p-Value
	N − 1748	N = 1029	N = 719	
Baseline Assessment				
Sex, *female* n(%)	969(55.4%)	547(53.2%)	422(58.7%)	0.022
Age, mean ± SD	79.9 ± 3.9	79.9 ± 3.9	80.0 ± 3.9	0.631
Education (years), mean ± SD	11.5 ± 4.9	11.3 ± 5.0	11.7 ± 4.9	0.026
Marital status, *widow* n(%)	553(31.6%)	312(30.3%)	241(33.5%)	0.157
BMI, mean ± SD	27.7 ± 4.3	27.4 ± 4.2	28.0 ± 4.4	0.011
MMSE, mean ± SD	28.1 ± 2.5	28.2 ± 2.5	27.9 ± 2.6	0.001
Diabetes mellitus, n(%)	398(22.8%)	227(22.1%)	171(23.8%)	0.398
Hypertension, n(%)	1314(75.2%)	770(74.8%)	544(75.7%)	0.692
Stroke, n(%)	94(5.4%)	61(5.9%)	33(4.6%)	0.222
Hip fracture, n(%)	74(4.2%)	50(4.9%)	24(3.3%)	0.120
COPD, n(%)	203(11.6%)	110(10.7%)	93(12.9%)	0.149
Osteoporosis, n(%)	534(30.5%)	317(30.8%)	217(30.2%)	0.780
Parkinson's disease, n(%)	26(1.5%)	16(1.6%)	10(1.4%)	0.780
Anemia, n(%)	296(16.9%)	169(16.4%)	127(17.7%)	0.299
LUTS, n(%)	493(28.2%)	273(26.5%)	220(30.6%)	0.116

Table 1. Cont.

	Total	No EQ-VAS Decline	EQ-VAS Decline	p-Value
	N = 1748	N = 1029	N = 719	
Falls history, n(%)	521(29.8%)	313(30.4%)	208(28.9%)	0.503
CKD, n(%)	1111(63.6%)	664(64.5%)	447(62.2%)	0.154
eGFR (mL/min/1.73 m^2), mean ± SD	54.6 ± 14.1	54.6 ± 14.1	54.7 ± 14.1	0.605
CIRS-G score, mean ± SD	8.3 ± 4.5	8.2 ± 4.5	8.3 ± 4.4	0.624
5+ prescribed medications, n(%)	1123(64.2%)	631(61.3%)	492(68.4%)	0.004
GDS-SF score, mean ± SD	2.5 ± 2.6	2.4 ± 2.7	2.8 ± 2.4	0.000
EQ-5D, mean ± SD	7.9 ± 3.0	7.8 ± 3.1	8.0 ± 2.8	0.003
EQ-VAS, mean ± SD	72.0 ± 17.2	70.3 ± 18.4	74.5 ± 15.0	0.000
SPPB score, mean ± SD	9.0 ± 2.8	9.0 ± 2.8	9.1 ± 2.6	0.836
Balance test, mean ± SD	3.3 ± 1.1	3.2 ± 1.1	3.3 ± 1.0	0.141
Gait speed test, mean ± SD	3.3 ± 1.0	3.3 ± 1.0	3.3 ± 0.9	0.671
Chair stand test, mean ± SD	2.7 ± 1.2	2.7 ± 1.2	2.6 ± 1.2	0.227
Grip strength test, mean ± SD	25.1 ± 10.1	25.7 ± 10.2	24.1 ± 9.7	0.002
After a two-year follow-up period				
CKD progression, n(%)	284(16.3%)	166(16.1%)	118(16.4%)	0.190
Δ eGFR (mL/min/1.73 m^2), mean ± SD	−0.1 ± 18.2	7.8 ± 14.4	−11.4 ± 17.0	0.360
Δ GDS-SF score, mean ± SD	−0.1 ± 2.5	−0.2 ± 2.5	+0.1 ± 2.4	0.046
Δ SPPB score, mean ± SD	−0.6 ± 2.3	−0.5 ± 2.2	−0.8 ± 2.4	0.075
Δ Balance, mean ± SD	−0.1 ± 1.2	−0.1 ± 1.2	−0.2 ± 1.2	0.029
Δ Gait speed, mean ± SD	−0.2 ± 1.0	−0.1 ± 0.9	−0.3 ± 1.0	0.034
Δ Chair stand, mean ± SD	−0.1 ± 1.1	−0.1 ± 1.1	−0.1 ± 1.2	0.512
Δ Grip strength, mean ± SD	−1.1 ± 5.5	−1.0 ± 4.9	−1.2 ± 6.2	0.837

Abbreviations: EQ-VAS, Euro-Quality of Life Visual Analog Scale; BMI, body mass index; MMSE, Mini-Mental State Examination; COPD, chronic obstructive pulmonary disease; LUTS, lower urinary tract symptoms; CKD, chronic kidney disease; eGFR, estimated glomerular filtration rate; CIRS-G, Cumulative Illness Rating Scale for Geriatrics; GDS-SF, Geriatric Depression Scale-Short Form; EQ-5D, Euro-Quality of Life 5 Dimensions; SPPB, short physical performance battery. Note: Negative value of Δ eGFR, Δ SPPB, Δ balance, and/or Δ gait indicates a progression of CKD and physical performance, respectively, and a positive value of Δ GDS-SF indicates a progression in self-reported depressive symptoms.

3.2. Associations between Δ EQ-VAS, Δ eGFR, and Other Health-Related Variables

The association between Δ EQ-VAS score during the two-year follow-up was assessed using Spearman rank correlation with Δ eGFR, Δ SPPB score, Δ hand grip strength, and Δ GDS-SF score, as shown in Figure 2A–D. Figure 2A clearly shows no associations between Δ EQ-VAS and Δ eGFR (Rs = 0.026, p = 0.366). However, an increase in GDS-SF score (i.e., Δ GDS-SF) was negatively associated with Δ EQ-VAS (Rs = 0.109, p < 0.001, Figure 2B), suggesting that increased depressive symptoms during the two-year follow-up had a significant association with HRQoL decline among older adults. Further, changes in physical performance over time, i.e., Δ SPPB score and Δ SPPB balance score, have a low yet significantly positive association with Δ EQ-VAS (Rs = 0.096, p = 0.001 and Rs = 0. 0.097, p = 0.001, respectively, Figure 2C,D), suggesting that reduced balance during the 2-year follow-up had a significant effect on HRQoL decline among older adults. In addition, we found no association between Δ EQ-VAS and hand grip strength. Spearman's rank correlation coefficients remained statistically significant once Bonferroni correction was applied. There was no association between co-morbidities (e.g., diabetes mellitus, hypertension, stroke, hip fracture, COPD, osteoporosis, Parkinson's disease, anemia, LUTS, and falls history at baseline) and decline in eGFR.

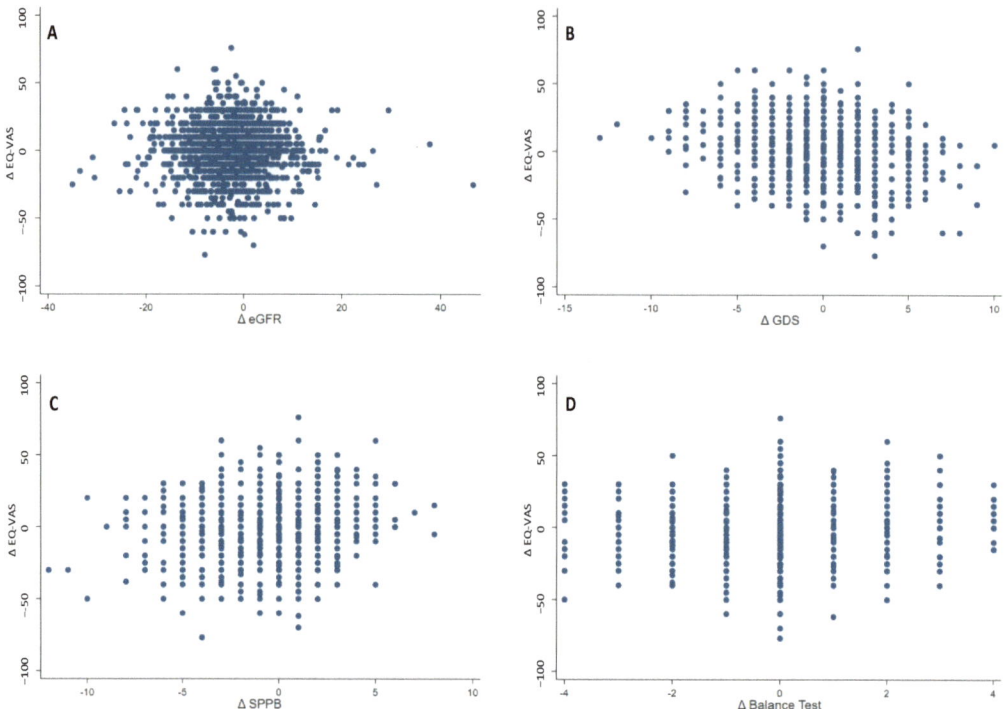

Figure 2. Scatterplot and linear fitted values of the difference in the EQ-VAS score from T0 to T2 (Δ EQ-VAS) and (**A**) Δ eGFR; (**B**) Δ GDS; (**C**) Δ SPPB scores; and (**D**) Δ SPPB balance scores, i.e., the difference from T0 to T2.

According to the logistic regression analyses (Table 2), there is no contribution of a decrease in kidney function in the early stages of CKD (i.e., Δ eGFR) on EQ-VAS decline. We found that older adults who had more depressive symptoms over the two-year period (i.e., positive Δ GDS) were more likely to report having EQ-VAS decline also after adjusting for age and sex; the EQ-VAS decline was similar (OR = 1.06, 95%CI = 1.02–1.11). When adjusting for educational level, EQ-VAS at baseline, MMSE at baseline, BMI at baseline, GDS-SF at baseline, grip strength at baseline, and more than five prescribed medications at baseline contributed to a somewhat higher EQ-VAS decline (OR = 1.14, 95%CI = 1.09–1.20). Interestingly, an increase in the overall SPPB score during the two-year follow-up period was associated with less EQ-VAS decline by 5% (OR = 0.95, 95%CI = 0.91–0.99). These results were similar after adjusting for age, sex, educational level, EQ-VAS at baseline, MMSE at baseline, BMI at baseline, GDS-SF at baseline, grip strength at baseline, and more than five prescribed medications at baseline. The potential "protection effect" was even higher for Δ SPPB balance and Δ SPPB gait (OR = 0.92, 95%CI = 0.85–0.99 and OR = 0.89, 95%CI = 0.81–0.99, respectively). Adjusting for age and sex (model 2) and for educational level, EQ-VAS at baseline and MMSE at baseline (model 3) did not change the ORs. In addition, Δ SPPB chair stand and Δ hand grip revealed no association with EQ-VAS decline. As for the validity of the analyses, for Models 2 and 3, the mean VIF was <10, ranging from 1.31 and 1.41, and tolerance was >0.25 for each independent variable, confirming that no collinearity issue existed.

Table 2. Determinants of EQ-VAS decline, OR (95%CI).

Independent Variable	Δ eGFR	Δ GDS-SF	Δ SPPB Total Score	Δ SPPB Balance	Δ SPPB Gait	Δ Sit to Stand	Δ Hand Grip
Model 1. Only independent variable	1.01 (0.99–1.02)	1.06 (1.02–1.10)	0.95 (0.91–0.99)	0.92 (0.85–0.99)	0.89 (0.81–0.99)	1.03 (0.93–1.13)	0.99 (0.97–1.01)
Model 2. Model 1 adjusted for age and sex	1.01 (0.99–1.02)	1.06 (1.02–1.11)	0.94 (0.91–0.99)	0.92 (0.85–0.99)	0.89 (0.80–0.98)	1.02 (0.92–1.12)	0.99 (0.97–1.01)
Model 3. Model 2 adjusted for educational level, EQ-VAS at baseline, MMSE at baseline, BMI at baseline, GDS-SF at baseline, grip strength at baseline, more than five prescribed medications at baseline	1.01 (0.99–1.02)	1.14 (1.09–1.20)	0.95 (0.91–0.99)	0.92 (0.84–1.00)	0.88 (0.78–0.98)	1.03 (0.93–1.14)	0.98 (0.96–1.01)

Abbreviations: EQ-VAS, Euro-Quality of Life Visual Analog Scale; OR, odds ratio; BMI, body mass index; MMSE, Mini-Mental State Examination; eGFR, estimated glomerular filtration rate; GDS-SF, Geriatric Depression Scale-Short Form; SPPB, short physical performance battery.

4. Discussion

In the present study, we found that 16.3% of older adults showed a decline in kidney function over the two-year follow-up period. A similar percentage of decline was found in a study conducted in the UK (18% of the participants showed a decline in kidney function within five years), whereas the risk of ESRD was very low (0.2%) [38]. However, we found a considerable decrement in HRQoL over the two-year period, whereas approximately 41% (n = 719) reported an EQ-VAS decline. Our study provides evidence that HRQoL decline among older adults is not associated with early stages of kidney function decline over a two-year period. Previous studies found that only patients with CKD on dialysis or with ESRD have a significantly lower HRQoL [39,40]. In patients with pre-dialysis chronic renal failure, the decline in HRQoL has been shown to be faster than that in the general population and was associated with an increase in serum creatinine and a decrease in hematocrit levels [25]. It has also been reported that the physical and psychological domains and HRQoL scores were significantly associated with increased risk of ESRD and mortality among CKD patients [28]. Low HRQoL across numerous subscales was independently associated with a higher risk of cardiovascular events and mortality in CKD patients, but not with CKD progression [27]. In an earlier study, an increased risk of CKD progression and mortality was associated with a lower physical health component of the SF-36 score [26]. The physical function in the above studies [26–28] was evaluated using an indirect measure of physical function, i.e., the physical component score of SF-12 and SF-36; thus, it was hard to compare to our cohort, in which physical function was measured using SPPB. In an earlier study [2], reduced renal function was associated with poorer physical performance (SPPB total score < 5) among older hospitalized patients with CKD, which suggests that these older hospitalized adults were more frail than in our cohort of community-dwelling independent older adults. Additionally, Tsai et al. [28] reported that 41.3% of their cohort suffered from depression compared with 14% in our cohort [13], suggesting that their cohort was less resilient. These previous findings combined with our results suggest that HRQoL decline among patients with CKD is associated with ESRD or dialysis, but not at the early stages of CKD progression.

Although earlier studies provide important findings, they are limited in scope, since they did not include older adults in the early CKD stages, which most patients with CKD belong to. More broadly, the association between HRQoL and longitudinal outcomes of physical and psychological domains among older adults in early CKD stages has not been examined. A significant body of research has investigated the possible association between HRQoL and the physical function of patients with ESRD or following kidney transplant, but these factors are not well-explored in those with less severe CKD [41]. This highlights the significance of our finding. Among the possible interpretations of our results, it is worth noting that changes in physical function and depressive symptoms over time have the strongest impact on the decline in EQ-VAS among community-dwelling elderly adults. The multivariate regression analyses showed that the decline in physical functioning and the increase in depressive symptoms over time were independently associated with HRQoL decline. Changes in physical performance over time, i.e., Δ SPPB, have a low yet significantly positive association with Δ EQ-VAS over time; these results may suggest that balance and gait function may 'protect' older adults from a decline in HRQoL. Another explanation might be that a better HRQoL leads to better physical function among older adults. Since our results are based on a cross-sectional study design that permits us to determine associations between variables and not causal relationships, the answer to this question should be investigated separately in a later prospective study. Most of the time, HRQoL has been interpreted as an accompanying outcome of one's disease. However, our findings suggest that HRQoL is an important person-centered measurement, since changes in HRQoL seem to be an indicator of changes in physical and mental health status. Thus, it can be used for general population surveys, clinical research, and health policy evaluation. HRQoL also provides insight into treatment methods, since the improvement in both physical and mental function may improve HRQoL, and this may play an important role in clinical decisions and policy making. The exact mechanism underlying the association between HRQoL and the progression of CKD is abstract and difficult to explore. The decline in EQ-VAS that was found in our study is associated with reduced functional levels in the early stages of CKD among older adults, suggesting that physical or mental maintenance is not seriously addressed, which may be a risk factor for poorer HRQoL outcomes in this population. In other words, poor physical function and mental health can be surrogate parameters indicating an increase in the multi-morbidity burden that older adults feel.

The guidelines for the management of individuals with multiple coexisting chronic diseases [42] suggest that clinicians should assess physical performance such as gait speed, balance, and self-reported health status. They should also be aware of mental health issues. This is compatible with the concept of healthy aging by the World Health Organization [43], which defines healthy aging as a "process of developing and maintaining the functional ability that enables well-being in older age". Our findings provide evidence that this approach is important in older adults even in the early stages of CKD, for which no clinical treatment is provided. Physical performance and mental state as potentially modifiable factors with an independent association with HRQoL are also important clinical considerations. When managing care for older adults, clinicians should provide care that will particularly treat physical function and mental health, since these issues affect the HRQoL of their patients. This could include planning a joint treatment with other healthcare professionals.

The strengths of our study are its meticulous protocol with a large and heterogeneous sample of respondents from different European countries and Israel. The combined use of subjective and classification-like scales reinforced analytical opportunities, as shown. It must be noted that the heterogeneous sample of older adults may also increase the variability of our outcome measures, specifically the objective measures of HRQoL. The prospective design allowed us to test the influence of physical and mental outcomes on change in HRQoL over time and to assess whether kidney function sub-stages affect HRQoL. The use of a physical performance examination such as the SPPB, which provides an objective measure of function, is also a strength of the study. However, the limitations of the current study must be noted. The main limitation of this study is the fact that our findings are based on a sample of older people who had a relatively high functional level and were in the early CKD stages, not allowing for a generalization of these conclusions to more frail older adults and ESRD patients. Second, the 713 participants who were excluded from the analysis due to incomplete information on the HRQoL may impact the results due to a selection bias. In a separate analysis, we found that the excluded older adults were older, more frequently widowed, had lower MMSE and lower SPPB at baseline, and had more frequently co-morbidities such as stroke, hypertension, diabetes, hip fractures, and depression than the 1748 individuals who were included in this study (see Supplementary Table S1). This might have affected our findings. However, it must be noted that the eGFR, depression, physical function, and handgrip strength over a two-year follow-up period, which were the main outcome parameters in the present study, were not different between groups. Finally, this observational study cannot resolve the difficulty of all hidden bias and confounding factors, despite the adjustments. Despite all these issues, longitudinal observational studies are useful for evaluating epidemiological associations and enable us to analyze the relationship between HRQoL and renal, physical, and mental outcomes through statistical techniques.

5. Conclusions

The findings of our study suggest that among older adults aged 75 years and older, HRQoL decline was not related to kidney function decline in the early stages of CKD. However, physical function and depressive symptoms, separately, have a low yet significant impact on HRQoL among older adults. This is an important message to clinicians and policymakers that a change in HRQoL should be taken into account to evaluate health interventions in this age group. Whether HRQoL change should be used for an evaluation depends strongly on the aims of the intervention and the characteristics of the participants. Due to the nature of this observational study, a careful interpretation of the findings as well as further research are needed. These studies are required to test whether the implementation of physical and psychological interventions in the early stages of CKD influences clinical outcomes, specifically HRQoL, among older adults.

Supplementary Materials: The following supporting information can be downloaded at: https://www.mdpi.com/article/10.3390/jcm12123959/s1, Supplementary Table S1.

Author Contributions: R.A.-M. and I.M.: participated in study protocol design, data collection, leading statistical analysis, manuscript drafting, and revision. F.L.: conceived the study, coordinated study protocol and data collection, and participated in statistical analysis and manuscript revision. M.D.R.: participated in statistical analysis and manuscript revision. R.K., A.C., I.Y., R.E.R.-W., G.H.W., F.U.S.M.-R., L.T., P.G.G., F.F., R.M.-G., T.K., A.G., J.Ä., A.C.C. and E.F.: participated in the study protocol and data collection and in manuscript revision. All authors have read and agreed to the published version of the manuscript.

Funding: The work reported in this publication was supported by the European Union Horizon 2020 program, under the Grant Agreement no. 634869, following a peer review process.

Institutional Review Board Statement: The study protocol was approved by ethics committees at all participating institutions and complies with the Declaration of Helsinki and Good Clinical Practice Guidelines. Only baseline data are used in the present study. Ethics approvals have been obtained by the ethics committees in participating institutions as follows:

- Italian National Research Center on Aging (INRCA), Italy, #2015 0522 IN, 17 January 2016.
- University of Lodz, Poland, #RNN/314/15/KE, 17 November 2015.
- Medizinische Universität Graz, Austria, #28–314 ex 15/16, 5 August 2016.
- Erasmus Medical Center Rotterdam, The Netherland, #MEC-2016-036—#NL56039.078.15, v.4, 7 March 2016.
- Hospital Clínico San Carlos, Madrid, Spain, # 15/532-E_BC, 16 September 2016.
- Bellvitge University Hospital Barcellona, Spain, #PR204/15, 29 January 2016.
- Friedrich-Alexander University Erlangen-Nürnberg, Germany, #340_15B, 21 January 2016.
- Helsinki committee in Maccabi Healthcare Services, Bait Ba-lev, Bat Yam, Israel, #45/2016, 24 July 2016.

Informed Consent Statement: Patients were asked to sign a written informed consent before entering the study.

Data Availability Statement: Data will be available for SCOPE researchers through the project website (www.scopeproject.eu) accessed on 25 February 2016.

Acknowledgments: The authors thank the volunteers who participated in this study. SCOPE study investigators, Coordinating Center: Fabrizia Lattanzio, Italian National Research Center on Aging (INRCA), Ancona, Italy–Principal Investigator. Andrea Corsonello, Silvia Bustacchini, Silvia Bolognini, Paola D'Ascoli, Raffaella Moresi, Giuseppina Di Stefano, Cinzia Giammarchi, Anna Rita Bonfigli, Roberta Galeazzi, Federica Lenci, Stefano Della Bella, Enrico Bordoni, Mauro Provinciali, Robertina Giacconi, Cinzia Giuli, Demetrio Postacchini, Sabrina Garasto, Annalisa Cozza–Italian National Research Center on Aging (INRCA), Ancona, Fermo and Cosenza, Italy—coordinating staff. Romano Firmani, Moreno Nacciariti, Mirko Di Rosa, Paolo Fabbietti—technical and statistical support; participating centers: Department of Internal Medicine, Medical University of Graz, Austria: Gerhard Hubert Wirnsberger, Regina Elisabeth Roller-Wirnsberger, Carolin Herzog, Sonja Lindner; Section of Geriatric Medicine, Department of Internal Medicine, Erasmus MC, University Medical Center Rotterdam, The Netherlands: Francesco Mattace-Raso, Lisanne Tap, Gijsbertus Ziere, Jeannette Goudzwaard, Harmke Polinder-Bos; Department of Geriatrics, Healthy Ageing Research Centre, Medical University of Lodz, Poland: Tomasz Kostka, Agnieszka Guligowska, Łukasz Kroc, Bartłomiej K Sołtysik, Małgorzata Pigłowska, Agnieszka Wójcik, Zuzanna Chrząstek, Natalia Sosowska, Anna Telążka, Joanna Kostka, Elizaveta Fife, Katarzyna Smyj, Kinga Zel; The Recanati School for Community Health Professions at the Faculty of Health Sciences at Ben-Gurion University of the Negev, Israel: Rada Artzi-Medvedik, Yehudit Melzer, Mark Clarfield, Itshak Melzer; Maccabi Healthcare Services southern region, Israel: Rada Artzi-Medvedik, Ilan Yehoshua, Yehudit Melzer; Geriatric Unit, Internal Medicine Department and Nephrology Department, Hospital Universitari de Bellvitge, Institut d'Investigació Biomèdica de Bellvitge-IDIBELL, L'Hospitalet de Llobregat, Barcelona, Spain: Francesc Formiga, Rafael Moreno-González, Xavier Corbella, Yurema Martínez, Carolina Polo, Josep Maria Cruzado; Department of Geriatric Medicine, Hospital Clínico San Carlos, Madrid: Pedro Gil Gregorio, Sara Laínez Martínez, Mónica González Alonso, Jose A. Herrero Calvo, Fernando Tornero Molina, Lara Guardado Fuentes, Pamela Carrillo García, María Mombiedro Pérez; Department of General Internal Medicine and Geriatrics, Krankenhaus Barmherzige Brüder Regensburg and Institute for Biomedicine of Aging, Friedrich-Alexander-Universität Erlangen-Nürnberg, Germany: Alexandra Renz, Susanne Muck, Stephan Theobaldy, Andreas Bekmann, Revekka Kaltsa, Sabine Britting, Robert Kob, Christian Weingart, Ellen Freiberger, Cornel Sieber; Department of Medical Sciences, Uppsala University, Sweden: Johan Ärnlöv, Axel Carlsson, Tobias Feldreich.

Conflicts of Interest: The authors declare no conflict of interest. The funders had no role in the design of the study; in the collection, analysis, or interpretation of data; in the writing of the manuscript, or in the decision to publish the results.

References

1. Kurella, M.; Chertow, G.M.; Fried, L.F.; Cummings, S.R.; Harris, T.; Simonsick, E.; Satterfield, S.; Ayonayon, H.; Yaffe, K. Chronic kidney disease and cognitive impairment in the elderly: The health, aging, and body composition study. *J. Am. Soc. Nephrol.* **2005**, *16*, 2127–2133. [CrossRef]
2. Lattanzio, F.; Corsonello, A.; Abbatecola, A.M.; Volpato, S.; Pedone, C.; Pranno, L.; Laino, I.; Garasto, S.; Corica, F.; Passarino, G.; et al. Relationship between renal function and physical performance in elderly hospitalized patients. *Rejuvenation Res.* **2012**, *15*, 545–552. [CrossRef]
3. Pedone, C.; Corsonello, A.; Bandinelli, S.; Pizzarelli, F.; Ferrucci, L.; Incalzi, R.A. Relationship between renal function and functional decline: Role of the estimating equation. *J. Am. Med. Dir. Assoc.* **2012**, *13*, e11–e14. [CrossRef] [PubMed]
4. Duenhas, M.R.; Draibe, S.A.; Avesani, C.M.; Sesso, R.; Cuppari, L. Influence of renal function on spontaneous dietary intake and on nutritional status of chronic renal insufficiency patients. *Eur. J. Clin. Nutr.* **2003**, *57*, 1473–1478. [CrossRef]
5. Foley, R.N.; Wang, C.; Ishani, A.; Collins, A.J.; Murray, A.M. Kidney function and sarcopenia in the United States general population: NHANES III. *Am. J. Nephrol.* **2007**, *27*, 279–286. [CrossRef]
6. Fried, L.F.; Lee, J.S.; Shlipak, M.; Chertow, G.M.; Green, C.; Ding, J.; Harris, T.; Newman, A.B. Chronic kidney disease and functional limitation in older people: Health, aging and body composition study. *J. Am. Geriatr. Soc.* **2006**, *54*, 750–756. [CrossRef]
7. Roshanravan, B.; Khatri, M.; Robinson-Cohen, C.; Levin, G.; Patel, K.V.; de Boer, I.H.; Seliger, S.; Ruzinski, J.; Himmelfarb, J.; Kestenbaum, B. A prospective study of frailty in nephrology-referred patients with CKD. *Am. J. Kidney Dis.* **2012**, *60*, 912–921. [CrossRef] [PubMed]
8. Arora, P.; Vasa, P.; Brenner, D.; Iglar, K.; McFarlane, P.; Morrison, H.; Badawi, A. Prevalence estimates of chronic kidney disease in Canada: Results of a nationally representative survey. *CMAJ* **2013**, *185*, E417–E423. [CrossRef] [PubMed]
9. Oh, T.R.; Choi, H.S.; Kim, C.S.; Bae, E.H.; Oh, Y.K.; Kim, Y.-S.; Choi, K.H.; Kim, S.W.; Ma, S.K. Association between health related quality of life and progression of chronic kidney disease. *Sci. Rep.* **2019**, *9*, 19595. [CrossRef]
10. Chadban, S.J.; Briganti, E.M.; Kerr, P.G.; Dunstan, D.W.; Welborn, T.A.; Zimmet, P.Z.; Atkins, R.C. Prevalence of kidney damage in Australian adults: The AusDiab kidney study. *J. Am. Soc. Nephrol.* **2003**, *7*, S131–S138. [CrossRef]

11. Hunsicker, L.G. The consequences and costs of chronic kidney disease before ESRD. *J. Am. Soc. Nephrol.* **2004**, *15*, 1363–1364. [CrossRef]
12. Kim, S.H.; Jo, M.W.; Go, D.S.; Ryu, D.R.; Park, J. Economic burden of chronic kidney disease in Korea using national sample cohort. *J. Nephrol.* **2017**, *30*, 787–793. [CrossRef]
13. Artzi-Medvedik, R.; Kob, R.; Fabbietti, P.; Lattanzio, F.; Corsonello, A.; Melzer, Y.; Roller-Wirnsberger, R.; Wirnsberger, G.; Mattace-Raso, F.; Tap, L.; et al. SCOPE investigators. Impaired kidney function is associated with lower quality of life among community-dwelling older adults: The screening for CKD among older people across Europe (SCOPE) study. *BMC Geriatr.* **2020**, *20*, 340. [CrossRef]
14. National Kidney Foundation. K/DOQI clinical practice guidelines for chronic kidney disease: Evaluation, classification, and stratification. *Am. J. Kidney Dis* **2002**, *39*, S1–S266.
15. Centers of Disease Control and Prevention. Health-Related Quality of Life (HRQoL). Available online: https://www.cdc.gov/hrqol/index.htm#:~:text=Related%20Pages,and%20mental%20health%20over%20time (accessed on 14 December 2022).
16. Kalantar-Zadeh, K.; Kopple, J.D.; Block, G.; Humphreys, M.H. Association among SF36 quality of life measures and nutrition, hospitalization, and mortality in hemodialysis. *J. Am. Soc. Nephrol.* **2001**, *12*, 2797–2806. [CrossRef] [PubMed]
17. Lopes, A.A.; Bragg-Gresham, J.L.; Satayathum, S.; McCullough, K.; Pifer, T.; Goodkin, D.A.; Mapes, D.L.; Young, E.W.; Wolfe, R.A.; Held, P.J.; et al. Worldwide Dialysis Outcomes and Practice Patterns Study Committee. Health-related quality of life and associated outcomes among hemodialysis patients of different ethnicities in the United States: The Dialysis Outcomes and Practice Patterns Study (DOPPS). *Am. J. Kidney Dis.* **2003**, *41*, 605–615. [CrossRef]
18. Perl, J.; Karaboyas, A.; Morgenstern, H.; Sen, A.; Rayner, H.C.; Vanholder, R.C.; Combe, C.; Hasegawa, T.; Finkelstein, F.O.; Lopes, A.A.; et al. Association between changes in quality of life and mortality in hemodialysis patients: Results from the DOPPS. *Nephrol. Dial. Transplant.* **2017**, *32*, 521–527. [CrossRef] [PubMed]
19. Picariello, F.; Moss-Morris, R.; Macdougall, I.C.; Chilcot, A.J. The role of psychological factors in fatigue among end-stage kidney disease patients: A critical review. *Clin. Kidney J.* **2017**, *10*, 79–88. [CrossRef]
20. Ju, A.; Unruh, M.L.; Davison, S.N.; Dapueto, J.; Dew, M.A.; Fluck, R.; Germain, M.; Jassal, S.V.; Obrador, G.; O'donoghue, D.; et al. Patient-reported outcome measures for fatigue in patients on hemodialysis: A systematic review. *Am. J. Kidney Dis.* **2018**, *71*, 327–343. [CrossRef]
21. Perlman, R.L.; Finkelstein, F.O.; Liu, L.; Roys, E.; Kiser, M.; Eisele, G.; Burrows-Hudson, S.; Messana, J.M.; Levin, N.; Rajagopalan, S.; et al. Quality of life in chronic kidney disease (CKD): A cross-sectional analysis in the Renal Research Institute-CKD study. *Am. J. Kidney Dis.* **2005**, *45*, 658–666. [CrossRef]
22. Kalender, B.; Ozdemir, A.C.; Dervisoglu, E.; Ozdemir, O. Quality of life in chronic kidney disease: Effects of treatment modality, depression, malnutrition and inflammation. *Int. J. Clin. Pract.* **2007**, *61*, 569–576. [CrossRef]
23. Rosansky, S.J. Renal function trajectory is more important than chronic kidney disease stage for managing patients with chronic kidney disease. *Am. J. Nephrol.* **2012**, *36*, 1–10. [CrossRef] [PubMed]
24. Yapa, H.E.; Purtell, L.; Chambers, S.; Bonner, A. The relationship between chronic kidney disease, symptoms and health-related quality of life: A systematic review. *J. Ren. Care* **2020**, *46*, 74–84. [CrossRef]
25. Fukuhara, S.; Yamazaki, S.; Marumo, F.; Akiba, T.; Akizawa, T.; Fujimi, S.; Haruki, S.; Kawaguchi, Y.; Nihei, H.; Shoji, T.; et al. Health-related quality of life of predialysis patients with chronic renal failure. *Nephron. Clin. Pract.* **2007**, *105*, c1–c8. [CrossRef]
26. Porter, A.; Fischer, M.J.; Wang, X.; Brooks, D.; Bruce, M.; Charleston, J.; Cleveland, W.H.; Dowie, D.; Faulkner, M.; Gassman, J.; et al. AASK Study Group. Quality of life and outcomes in African Americans with CKD. *J. Am. Soc. Nephrol.* **2014**, *25*, 1849–1855. [CrossRef]
27. Porter, A.C.; Lash, J.P.; Xie, D.; Pan, Q.; DeLuca, J.; Kanthety, R.; Kusek, J.W.; Lora, C.M.; Nessel, L.; Ricardo, A.C.; et al. CRIC Study Investigators. Predictors and outcomes of health-related quality of life in adults with CKD. *Clin. J. Am. Soc. Nephrol.* **2016**, *11*, 1154–1162. [CrossRef]
28. Tsai, Y.-C.; Hung, C.-C.; Hwang, S.-J.; Wang, S.-L.; Hsiao, S.-M.; Lin, M.-Y.; Kung, L.-F.; Hsiao, P.-N.; Chen, H.-C. Quality of life predicts risks of end-stage renal disease and mortality in patients with chronic kidney disease. *Nephrol. Dial. Transplant.* **2010**, *25*, 1621–1626. [CrossRef] [PubMed]
29. Corsonello, A.; on behalf of SCOPE investigators; Tap, L.; Roller-Wirnsberger, R.; Wirnsberger, G.; Zoccali, C.; Kostka, T.; Guligowska, A.; Mattace-Raso, F.; Gil, P.; et al. SCOPE investigators. Design and methodology of the screening for CKD among older patients across Europe (SCOPE) study: A multicenter cohort observational study. *BMC Nephrol.* **2018**, *19*, 260. [CrossRef]
30. Folstein, M.F.; Folstein, S.E.; McHugh, P.R. "Mini-mental state". A practical method for grading the cognitive state of patients for the clinician. *J. Psychiatr. Res.* **1975**, *12*, 189–198. [CrossRef] [PubMed]
31. Rosenberg, M.T.; Staskin, D.R.; Kaplan, S.A.; MacDiarmid, S.A.; Newman, D.K.; Ohl, D.A. A practical guide to the evaluation and treatment of male lower urinary tract symptoms in the primary care setting. *Int. J. Clin. Pract.* **2007**, *61*, 1535–1546. [CrossRef]
32. Conwell, Y.; Forbes, N.T.; Cox, C.; Caine, E.D. Validation of a measure of physical illness burden at autopsy: The Cumulative Illness Rating Scale. *J. Am. Geriatr. Soc.* **1993**, *41*, 38–41. [CrossRef] [PubMed]
33. Lesher, E.L.; Berryhill, J.S. Validation of the Geriatric Depression Scale--Short Form among inpatients. *J. Clin. Psychol.* **1994**, *50*, 256–260. [CrossRef]

34. Guralnik, J.M.; Simonsick, E.M.; Ferrucci, L.; Glynn, R.J.; Berkman, L.F.; Blazer, D.G.; Scherr, P.A.; Wallace, R.B. A short physical performance battery assessing lower extremity function: Association with self-reported disability and prediction of mortality and nursing home admission. *J. Gerontol.* **1994**, *49*, M85–M94. [CrossRef] [PubMed]
35. Roberts, H.C.; Denison, H.J.; Martin, H.J.; Patel, H.P.; Syddall, H.; Cooper, C.; Sayer, A.A. A review of the measurement of grip strength in clinical and epidemiological studies: Towards a standardised approach. *Age Ageing* **2011**, *40*, 423–429. [CrossRef]
36. EuroQol Research Foundation. EQ-5D-5L User Guide. 2019. Available online: https://euroqol.org/publications/user-guides (accessed on 14 December 2022).
37. Schaeffner, E.S.; Ebert, N.; Delanaye, P.; Frei, U.; Gaedeke, J.; Jakob, O.; Kuhlmann, M.K.; Schuchardt, M.; Tölle, M.; Ziebig, R.; et al. Two novel equations to estimate kidney function in persons aged 70 years or older. *Ann. Intern. Med.* **2012**, *157*, 471–481. [CrossRef]
38. Shardlow, A.; McIntyre, N.J.; Fluck, R.J.; McIntyre, C.W.; Taal, M.W. Chronic kidney disease in primary care: Outcomes after five years in a prospective cohort study. *PLoS Med.* **2016**, *13*, e1002128. [CrossRef]
39. Wyld, M.; Morton, R.L.; Hayen, A.; Howard, K.; Webster, A.C. A systematic review and meta-analysis of utility-based quality of life in chronic kidney disease treatments. *PLoS Med.* **2012**, *9*, e1001307. [CrossRef]
40. Krishnan, A.; Teixeira-Pinto, A.; Lim, W.H.; Howard, K.; Chapman, J.R.; Castells, A.; Roger, S.D.; Bourke, M.J.; Macaskill, P.; Williams, G.; et al. Health-related quality of life in people across the spectrum of CKD. *Kidney Int. Rep.* **2020**, *5*, 2264–2274. [CrossRef]
41. Fraser, S.D.; Barker, J.; Roderick, P.J.; Yuen, H.M.; Shardlow, A.; E Morris, J.; McIntyre, N.J.; Fluck, R.J.; McIntyre, C.W.; Taal, M.W. Health-related quality of life, functional impairment and comorbidity in people with mild-to-moderate chronic kidney disease: A cross-sectional study. *BMJ Open* **2020**, *10*, e040286. [CrossRef] [PubMed]
42. National Institute for Health and Care Excellence (NICE). Multimorbidity: Clinical Assessment and Management (NG56). 2016. Available online: https://www.nice.org.uk/guidance/ng56 (accessed on 16 December 2022).
43. World Health Organization. World Health Assembly, 69. Multisectoral Action for a Life Course Approach to Healthy Ageing: Draft Global Strategy and Plan of Action on Ageing and Health: Report by the Secretariat. 2016. Available online: https://apps.who.int/iris/handle/10665/252671 (accessed on 16 December 2022).

Disclaimer/Publisher's Note: The statements, opinions and data contained in all publications are solely those of the individual author(s) and contributor(s) and not of MDPI and/or the editor(s). MDPI and/or the editor(s) disclaim responsibility for any injury to people or property resulting from any ideas, methods, instructions or products referred to in the content.

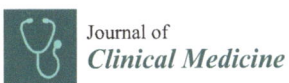 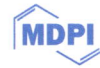

Article

Correlates of Restless Legs Syndrome in Older People

Magdalena Szklarek [1], Tomasz Kostka [1] and Joanna Kostka [2,*]

[1] Department of Geriatrics, Medical University of Lodz, 90-647 Lodz, Poland; magdalena.szklarek@gmail.com (M.S.); tomasz.kostka@umed.lodz.pl (T.K.)
[2] Department of Gerontology, Medical University of Lodz, 93-113 Lodz, Poland
* Correspondence: joanna.kostka@umed.lodz.pl

Abstract: Background: We examined the association between restless legs syndrome (RLS) and comprehensive geriatric assessment (CGA) data in two older European populations. The second goal was to evaluate correlates of their quality of life (QoL). **Methods**: Diagnostic criteria of the International RLS Study Group (IRLSSG) and elements of CGA were used in this study. **Results**: Among the examined 246 participants, 77 (31.3%) suffered from RLS, more often in the UK (39.4%) than in Poland (25.4%) ($p = 0.019$). In the multivariate logistic regression model, female sex [OR (CI) = 3.29 (1.51–7.21); $p = 0.0014$], the number of medications per day [OR (CI) = 1.11 (1.02–1.20); $p = 0.011$] and alcohol consumption [OR (CI) = 5.41 (2.67–10.95); $p < 0.001$] increased the probability of RLS. Residing in Poland [OR (CI) = 3.06 (1.36–6.88); $p = 0.005$], the presence of RLS [OR (CI) = 2.90 (1.36–6.17); $p = 0.004$], chronic heart failure, [OR (CI) = 3.60 (1.75–7.41); $p < 0.001$], osteoarthritis [OR (CI) = 2.85 (1.47–5.49); $p = 0.0016$], and urinary incontinence [OR (CI) = 4.74 (1.87–11.9); $p < 0.001$] were associated with a higher probability of mobility dimension problems in the QoL. Higher physical activity was related to a lower probability of mobility problems [OR (CI) = 0.85 (0.78–0.92); $p < 0.001$]. **Conclusions**: female sex, the number of medications and alcohol consumption are independent correlates of RLS in older adults. RLS together with several chronic medical conditions and a low physical activity level were independent correlates of the mobility dimension of the QoL.

Keywords: older adults; comprehensive geriatric assessment; alcohol consumption; number of medications; quality of life

Citation: Szklarek, M.; Kostka, T.; Kostka, J. Correlates of Restless Legs Syndrome in Older People. *J. Clin. Med.* **2024**, *13*, 1364. https://doi.org/10.3390/jcm13051364

Academic Editor: Edgar Ramos Vieira

Received: 17 January 2024
Revised: 14 February 2024
Accepted: 24 February 2024
Published: 28 February 2024

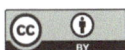

Copyright: © 2024 by the authors. Licensee MDPI, Basel, Switzerland. This article is an open access article distributed under the terms and conditions of the Creative Commons Attribution (CC BY) license (https://creativecommons.org/licenses/by/4.0/).

1. Introduction

Restless legs syndrome (RLS) is associated with unpleasant sensory experiences, with usual onsets in the evenings and nights. It occurs in the extremities and in extreme cases, it can also involve the torso, making rest difficult during a sleepless night. This sensory-motor neurologic disorder often dramatically affects sleep and QoL [1]. The lifetime prevalence of RLS is estimated to be within 2% to 3% of the adult population [2]. Since the very first description noted by Oxford physician Thomas Willis in the XVII century, RLS, also known as Willis–Ekbom disease, has been described in well over 5000 articles published on PubMed [3].

The pathophysiology of RLS is only partially understood [4,5]. The prevalence of RLS is higher in older people and females. RLS is most commonly related to iron deficiency and iron-deficiency anemia, pregnancy, uremia and polyneuropathies [6,7]. Brain iron deficiency, toxic metal exposure, concomitant diseases and postinfectious immunological mechanisms may influence the production of RLS symptoms [8–12]. Of individuals with conditions associated with iron-deficiency states, including pregnancy, renal failure, and anemia, 25–30% of them may develop RLS [13]. Patients with RLS could be deficient in vitamins D and B12 [14,15]. Various comorbidities such as kidney disease, cardiovascular diseases, diabetes mellitus, hypothyroidism, chronic liver disease, and neurological, rheumatological and respiratory disorders accompany RLS [2,16–19]. In our recent study, a significantly higher number of amalgam dental fillings were found in older adults with RLS as compared to the subjects without RLS symptoms [20].

As the prevalence of RLS increases with advancing age substantially decreasing the QoL of older adults, this population should be among the primary targets of research on RLS epidemiology and pathophysiology [21]. Several lifestyle factors have been linked to the occurrence of RLS in the general adult population [22]. Nevertheless, limited data exist on factors predisposing to RLS occurrence in older adults. Specfically, there are no studies relating RLS to comprehensive geriatric assessment (CGA) data and assessing the potential contribution of RLS to the quality of life (QoL) of older adults taking into account multiple covariates of CGA. Our study aimed to examine the association between RLS and an extensive set of CGA-potentially related factors such as smoking, alcohol consumption, concomitant diseases, physical and cognitive functioning, medications used, nutritional status and physical activity, in two older European populations. The second goal of the study was to evaluate correlates of the QoL of those subjects.

2. Materials and Methods

2.1. Subjects

The study population comprised 246 subjects (63 males and 183 females, median age 79 years) who volunteered to participate in the study, and was composed of two groups. The first was 104 subjects living in a Polish Housing Society in Penrhos, North Wales, founded in 1949, providing accommodation and support to Polish ex-service men and women who remained in the UK following World War II. The second group was 142 outpatients of the Geriatric Clinic of the Medical University of Lodz, Poland.

The exclusion criteria were having a known anemia, chronic kidney disease, known iron or vitamin deficiency, terminal illness, major disabilities or severe dementia. The criteria for inclusion in the study were being of an age > 60 years, having satisfactory verbal communication, the ability to perform functional tests and give written consent to participate in the study.

The study was approved by the Bioethics Committee of the Medical University of Lodz and complies with the Declaration of Helsinki and Good Clinical Practice Guidelines.

2.2. Methods

All subjects were interviewed to obtain a full medical history including regular medication taken. The medical history was supplemented based on the patient's medical records. In case of doubt, the interview was further supplemented by a conversation with a nurse or caregiver. Information about alcohol intake and smoking was gathered. Alcohol consumption was classified as "yes" if any amount of alcoholic beverages were consumed during the last 7 days. Current smoking was defined as smoking at least part or all of a cigarette during the past 30 days [23]. Arm blood pressure was measured once.

The diagnosis of RLS is purely clinical and is based on the information obtained during an interview with the patient. We applied the diagnostic criteria of the International Restless Legs Syndrome Study Group (IRLSSG) in the form of four questions from an internationally used questionnaire in order to determine the appearance of the problem of RLS [24].

The analysis of factors coexisting with RLS based on a comprehensive geriatric assessment (CGA) was conducted. A functional efficiency assessment was made using the ADL (Activities of Daily Living) scale [25] and the instrumental functioning scale—IADL (Instrumental Activities of Daily Living) [26]. The ADL scale is used to assess the basic activities of daily living, such as bathing, use of the toilet, continence, dressing, eating and mobility. One point (max 6 points in total) is awarded for the ability to perform a given activity. The IADL scale is a tool used to assess the ability to live independently in the community. It contains 8 questions (max 8 points in total) about complex daily activities regarding using the phone, shopping, food preparation, cleaning, washing, using means of transport, using medication and using money.

The TUG test is a popular test used to assess functional ability. It involves performing a series of activities over time (time is measured with a stopwatch): getting up from a chair, walking for a distance of 3 m, turning around, walking again for a distance of 3 m and sitting on the chair. A result above 14 s is considered to be at an increased risk of falling [27].

Physical activity assessments were conducted using two questionnaires: the seven-day recall PA questionnaire [28] and the Stanford questionnaire [29]. The seven-day recall PA questionnaire is designed to determine the average daily physical activity energy expenditure (PA-EE) over the past 7 days (kcal·kg^{-1} day^{-1}). Energy expenditure is calculated based on time spent sleeping and the light, moderate, vigorous and very hard activities over the past week. The Stanford Moderate Index was used to assess health behaviors related to physical activity (PA-HRB). This index is determined on the basis of 6 questions about habitual behaviors of light and moderate intensity. One point is awarded for each confirming answer (maximum 6 points in total).

The nutritional status of the study group was assessed using tools such as the MNA (Mini Nutritional Assessment) questionnaire [30], and anthropometric measures, including body mass and height (RADWAG personal weight scales, Radom, Poland) as well as waist and calf circumferences (SECA measuring tape, Hamburg, Germany). The body mass index (BMI) was calculated by dividing body weight by height in meters squared. The MNA is a questionnaire recommended for assessing the nutritional status of older people. It consists of parts such as a general assessment, anthropometric measures, dietary assessment and self-assessment. The full version was used in the study, consisting of 18 questions regarding various aspects of the risk of malnutrition. In the test, it is possible to obtain from 0 to 30 points, with a score of 24 points and above indicating a normal level of nutrition, 17–23.5 points indicating a risk of malnutrition, and a score below 17 points indicating malnutrition.

Mental state was assessed using the GDS (Geriatric Depression Scale) [31] and a short mental state assessment scale—the MMSE (mini-mental state examination) [32]. The short form of the GDS is a tool used to screen and assess symptoms of depression in older people. The scale consists of 15 questions related to mood disorders with possible answers of "yes" or "no". The GDS-15 is scored as follows: 0 to 5 points—normal, 6–10 points—a risk of depression and 11 points or more indicates depression. The MMSE is a clinical scale used to examine disorders in a patient's cognitive functioning. The scale assesses areas of mental abilities, including their orientation in time and place, attention/concentration, short-term memory, language skills, visuospatial abilities, and their ability to understand and follow instructions. During the test, it is possible to obtain a maximum of 30 points, where 27 to 30 points is normal, 24 to 26 points indicates mild cognitive impairment without dementia, 19 to 23 points—mild dementia, 11 to 18—moderate dementia and less than 11 suggests severe dementia.

The QoL was assessed by the international EQ-5D questionnaire [33]. The questionnaire consists of two parts. The first one assesses the existence of a problem in five domains of functioning (mobility, self-care, usual activities, pain/discomfort, and anxiety/depression). Each domain is assessed on a 3-point scale (1—no problem, 2—some problems, 3—severe problems). In the second part, using a 100-point visual analog scale (VAS), participants determine their perception of their overall health. Zero on this scale means the worst imaginable health status, while 100 means excellent health.

2.3. Statistical Analysis

The results were verified for their normality of distribution and equality of variance. The one-way analysis of variance (ANOVA), Mann–Whitney test or chi-square test were used to compare the groups. The EQ-5D dimension data were dichotomized (no problems vs. any problem) for statistical analyses. A multiple logistic regression was used to select independent correlates of RLS or QoL data with independent variables significant in bivariate associations entering the regression models. A multivariate logistic regression model was constructed by employing the forward–backward stepwise selection procedure.

Odds ratios (OR) and confidence intervals (CI) with 95% confidence limits were calculated. The quantitative variables are presented as the mean ± standard deviation or median and interquartile range [25–75%], qualitative variables as numbers and percentages. The statistical analysis was performed using Statistica (version 13.3) software (StatSoft, Kraków, Poland). The limit of significance was set at $p = 0.05$ for all analyses.

3. Results

3.1. Demographic and Clinical Data

Among the examined 246 participants, 183 (74.4%) were women. The proportion of men was smaller in Poland (19%) than in the UK (34.6%), $p < 0.001$. The English group was significantly older, $p < 0.001$ (the mean age in the UK was 83.5 ± 7.6 and in Poland was 75.8 ± 8.4 years). Seventy-seven (31.3%) subjects suffered from RLS, significantly more often in the UK (39.4%) than in Poland (25.4%) ($p = 0.019$). People from the Polish group smoked more cigarettes per day but consumed less alcohol (both $p < 0.001$).

Among the 246 participants, 71.1% were diagnosed with arterial hypertension, 37.4% had hypercholesterolemia, 22.8% suffered from diabetes mellitus, 39.4% had ischemic heart disease, 49.6% had chronic heart failure, 13.8% of the individuals had a myocardial infarction while 15.4% had a stroke in the past. The Polish group suffered more often from arterial hypertension ($p = 0.001$), ischemic heart disease and chronic heart failure (both $p < 0.001$), and stroke ($p = 0.030$). The English group suffered more often from hypercholesterolemia ($p = 0.003$) and ophthalmologic diseases ($p = 0.012$). The number of infections per year was higher in the Polish group and this group had fewer influenza vaccinations per year (both $p < 0.001$). The English group was taking more medications per day than the Polish ($p = 0.005$) and had higher systolic blood pressure ($p < 0.001$). English participants had higher ADL and IADL, MNA screening and EQ-5D VAS scores, but lower GDS and EQ5D dimensions scores ($p < 0.001$). The English group had a lower total energy expenditure (kcal/kg/day) ($p < 0.001$) but higher score for the Stanford Moderate Index ($p = 0.041$).

Table 1 shows the characteristics of the whole studied population divided into two groups, with and without RLS. Both groups had a similar age and smoking status. RLS was more frequent in women than in men. The consumption of alcohol was significantly higher in the group with symptoms of RLS (39.0%) than in those without RLS (16.0%), which was similar when analyzed separately in women and men ($p < 0.001$). The prevalence of alcohol consumption in relation to the presence of RLS according to sex and country is shown in Figure 1. The prevalence of concomitant diseases was not different between the RLS and non-RLS groups. The number of medications used per day and IADL scores (borderline significance) were higher in the RLS group. Other measures of the comprehensive geriatric assessment were not statistically different between the RLS and non-RLS groups.

Table 1. Characteristics for all subjects with and without restless legs syndrome (RLS).

	Subjects with RLS (n = 77)	Subjects without RLS (n = 169)	*p*-Value
Age (years)	80.0 ± 8.5 81 (74; 87)	78.6 ± 9.1 80 (72; 86)	0.26
Males (n; %)	13; 16.9	50; 29.6	**0.03**
Smoking (n; %)	3; 3.9	14; 8.3	0.21
Alcohol/7 days (n; %)	30; 39.0	27; 16.0	**<0.001**
Arterial hypertension (n; %)	56; 72.7	119; 70.4	0.71
Hypercholesterolemia (n; %)	29; 37.7	63; 37.3	0.95
Diabetes mellitus (n; %)	15; 19.5	41; 24.3	0.41

Table 1. *Cont.*

	Subjects with RLS (n = 77)	Subjects without RLS (n = 169)	*p*-Value
Myocardial infarction (n; %)	10; 13.0	24; 14.2	0.80
Ischemic heart disease (n; %)	27; 35.1	70; 41.4	0.34
Chronic heart failure (n; %)	36; 46.8	86; 50.9	0.55
Stroke (n; %)	8; 10.4	30; 17.8	0.14
Chronic obstructive pulmonary disease (n; %)	18; 23.4	30; 17.8	0.30
Osteoarthritis (n; %)	49; 63.6	88; 52.1	0.09
Osteoporosis (n; %)	27; 35.1	59; 34.9	0.98
Digestive tract diseases (n; %)	18; 23.4	33; 19.5	0.49
Past or present cancer (n; %)	8; 10.4	26; 15.4	0.29
Ophthalmologic diseases (n; %)	28; 36.4	54; 32.1	0.52
Depression (n; %)	17; 22.1	22; 13.1	0.07
Urinary incontinence (n; %)	27; 35.1	57; 33.9	0.86
Faecal incontinence (n; %)	12; 15.6	35; 20.8	0.33
Infections last year	1.0 ± 1.1 1 (0; 2)	1.1 ± 1.2 1 (0; 2)	0.49
Influenza vaccination last year (n; %)	41; 53.2	91; 54.5	0.86
Medications/day	7.0 ± 3.4 6 (5; 9)	5.9 ± 3.6 5 (3; 8)	**0.023**
RRs	143.0 ± 19.8 140 (130; 152)	143.2 ± 19.6 140 (130; 155)	0.94
RRd	80.1 ± 11.0 80 (75; 85)	81.6 ± 10.9 80 (75; 90)	0.33
BMI (kg/m^2)	26.4 ± 4.8 26 (23; 30)	26.3 ± 4.2 26 (23; 29)	0.77
Calf circumference (cm)	34.9 ± 4.8 35 (32; 38)	34.6 ± 4.5 35 (32; 37)	0.62
ADL	4.9 ± 1.7 5.5 (5; 6)	4.6 ± 1.9 5.5 (4; 6)	0.19
IADL	5.3 ± 2.9 6 (3; 8)	4.4 ± 3.2 5 (1; 8)	**0.050**
TUG test (sec)	16.7 ± 9.5 14 (10; 21)	17.2 ± 10.7 14 (10; 21)	0.73
MNA	22.5 ± 4.2 24 (20; 26)	23.5 ± 3.7 24 (22; 27)	0.063
MMSE	24.8 ± 4.6 25 (21; 29)	23.8 ± 5.6 25 (20; 29)	0.15
GDS	5.3 ± 3.7 5 (2; 8)	5.1 ± 3.7 5 (2; 8)	0.67
Energy expenditure kcal/kg/day	37.1 ± 4.3 35 (34; 39)	37.7 ± 5.0 36 (34; 40)	0.34
Stanford Moderate index	1.8 ± 1.5 2 (1; 3)	1.7 ± 1.6 1 (0; 3)	0.78

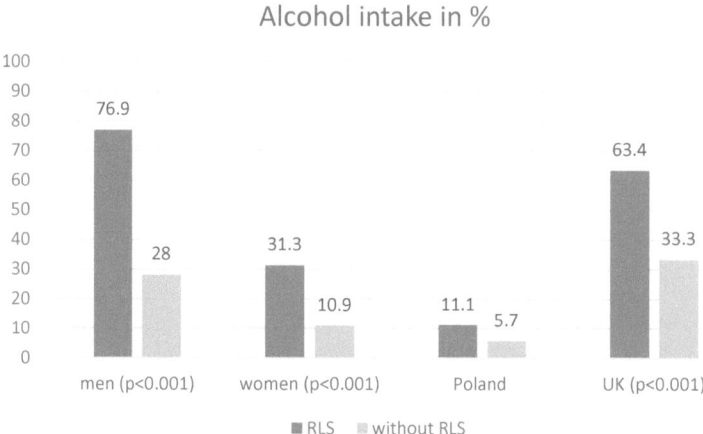

Figure 1. Prevalence of alcohol consumption in relation to the presence of RLS according to sex and country.

Table 2 shows the QoL indices in the groups with and without RLS. The prevalence of mobility problems was higher in the RLS group, other indices were not statistically different.

Table 2. QoL for all subjects with and without RLS examined using the EQ-5D questionnaire.

	Subjects with RLS (n = 77)	Subjects without RLS (n = 169)	p-Value
Mobility [%]			
no problems	20.8	36.3	
moderate	63.6	44.0	**0.01**
severe	15.6	19.6	
Self-care [%]			
no problems	61.0	57.1	
moderate	26.0	23.2	0.44
severe	13.0	19.6	
Usual activities [%]			
no problems	37.7	42.9	
moderate	39.0	29.2	0.31
severe	23.4	28.0	
Pain/discomfort [%]			
no problems	11.7	23.2	
moderate	79.2	70.2	0.10
severe	9.1	6.5	
Anxiety, depression [%]			
no problems	29.9	36.9	
moderate	62.3	59.5	0.25
severe	7.8	3.6	
Self-assessment of health (EQ-5D Visual Analogue Scale)	56.9 ± 18.9 50 (50; 70)	55.8 ± 20 50 (45; 70)	0.67

3.2. Multivariate Regression Models

The age, sex, country of participants and all variables significantly related to RLS in bivariate associations entered the multivariate logistic regression model. The results are presented in Table 3. In the stepwise selection procedure, sex, the number of medications per day and alcohol consumption were identified as independent correlates of RLS. Female sex [OR (CI) = 3.29 (1.51–7.21); p = 0.0014], the number of medications per day [OR (CI) = 1.11 (1.02–1.20); p = 0.011] and alcohol consumption [OR (CI) = 5.41 (2.67–10.95); p < 0.001] increased the probability of RLS. Forward and backward stepwise regression models gave the same results.

Table 3. Results of the multiple logistic regression with age, sex, country of participants, and all variables significantly related to RLS in bivariate associations.

Factor	Odds Ratios (95.0% Confidence Intervals)	p-Value
Age	1.008 (0.97–1.05)	0.69
Medications/day	1.11 (1.02–1.20)	0.018
IADL	1.04 (0.93–1.17)	0.51
Sex	3.22 (1.47–7.08)	0.0019
Country	1.07 (0.47–2.43)	0.87
Alcohol/7 days	5.04 (2.24–11.32)	<0.001

Age, physical activity (kcal/kg/day), RLS, and the presence of chronic heart failure, osteoarthritis and urinary incontinence were related to mobility dimension problems of the EQ-5D questionnaire. These variables were included in the multivariate regression models together with sex and country of residence. Although related to the mobility dimension, TUG and ADL results were not included in the multivariate models because of their obvious overlapping characteristics to mobility. Country of residence, RLS, the presence of chronic heart failure, osteoarthritis and urinary incontinence as well as physical activity level (kcal/kg/day) were selected as independent correlates of mobility dimension problems. Residing in Poland was related to a higher probability of mobility problems [OR (CI) = 3.06 (1.36–6.88); p = 0.005]. The presence of RLS [OR (CI) = 2.90 (1.36–6.17); p = 0.004], chronic heart failure, [OR (CI) = 3.60 (1.75–7.41); p < 0.001], osteoarthritis [OR (CI) = 2.85 (1.47–5.49); p = 0.0016], and urinary incontinence [OR (CI) = 4.74 (1.87–11.9); p < 0.001] were associated with a higher probability of mobility problems. Higher physical activity was related to a lower probability of mobility problems—a 15% lower probability for an increase of energy expenditure of 1 kcal/kg/day [OR (CI) = 0.85 (0.78–0.92); p < 0.001].

As the RLS relationship to the pain/anxiety dimension of the EQ-5D questionnaire was of borderline significance, this association was also checked in the multivariate design. Variables selected as independent correlates of the pain/anxiety dimension of the EQ-5D were RRs [OR (CI) = 1.03 (1.01–1.05); p = 0.014], the GDS [OR (CI) = 1.30 (1.15–1.48); p < 0.001], and osteoarthritis [OR (CI) = 4.08 (1.93–8.70); p < 0.001].

4. Discussion

In the present study, we have assessed the prevalence of RLS in relation to the comprehensive geriatric assessment in two populations of older subjects, living in Poland and the United Kingdom. The obtained data shed some light on the epidemiology and possible pathophysiology of RLS in an advanced-aged population. We found that female sex, the number of medications taken per day and alcohol consumption are independent correlates of RLS in older adults. RLS together with chronic heart failure, osteoarthritis and urinary incontinence as well as physical activity level were independent correlates of the mobility dimension of the QoL. These data only partially conform to the results obtained in younger populations.

RLS can present alone or with comorbidities that make proper diagnosis difficult [34]. The background literature review covered correlates from various areas such as environmental factors, including heavy metals, dietary factors, lifestyle factors, medical conditions and drug interactions [5,12]. RLS has been associated with obesity [35], an increased body mass index and diabetes [36,37]. People with a normal weight had a lower risk of developing RLS [22]. Obesity increased the risk of sleep disturbances in the long term, and both obesity and sleep disturbances had negative effects on health [38]. Smoking was related to an increased RLS risk in several studies [22,35,36,39]. In our study, when multiple other potential covariates were assessed, the BMI or smoking status did not emerge as independent correlates of RLS presence.

Various comorbidities such as kidney disease, cardiovascular diseases, obstructive lung disease, diabetes mellitus, hypothyroidism, chronic liver disease, and neurological, rheumatological and respiratory disorders may accompany RLS [2,16–19,40]. In a cross-sectional study including 5324 subjects, high cholesterol and hypertension were associated with RLS [41]. In a large population-based study, having RLS at baseline was not a significant predictor of any subsequent cardiovascular risk factors and/or vascular diseases, but cardiovascular risk factors and diseases predicted the subsequent development of RLS in the general population [42]. Similarly, we have not found a correlation between vascular diseases and restless legs syndrome in our groups. Other age-related medical conditions associated with sleep disturbances, including respiratory diseases such as asthma, infections, digestive tract diseases, physical disability, dementia, pain, depression, anxiety, and sleep itself, were taken into account. Except for some tendency for depressive symptoms, no strong correlation of accompanying diseases was found in relation to RLS in our study.

Of special interest is a statistically significant and independent-of-other-factors correlation between the prevalence of RLS and the consumption of alcohol in older men and women, assessed separately, as well as a whole group from Poland and the United Kingdom. In several studies, an association between RLS and alcohol consumption has been suggested [35,36,43]. In an Indian population study, chronic daily alcohol consumption was found to be associated with RLS [44]. Aldrich and Shipley found that in a significant proportion of alcohol users, periodic leg movements contributed to sleep disturbance. Additionally, women who consumed two or more drinks per day were more likely to report symptoms of restless legs and to be diagnosed with RLS [45]. In contrast, a non-significant trend between a higher alcohol consumption and a lower risk of RLS was observed in one study [22]. Likewise, in a sample of 317 psychiatric inpatients, RLS was associated with lower alcohol consumption [37]. Interestingly, not indifferent to this could also be alcohol detoxification therapy. The results of the study by Jiménez-Jiménez et al. show that a significant percentage of patients undergoing alcohol detoxification therapy develop RLS symptoms [43]. Mackie et al. show that alcohol withdrawal may involve generalized physical and psychological discomfort and insomnia, and patients with alcohol withdrawal experience symptoms that meet the criteria for RLS [46].

Alcohol consumption, regardless of the dose, affects the occurrence of sleep disorders, including sleep onset latency, consolidation in the first sleep period and disruptions in the second half of sleep [47]. Alcohol adds to aging-related sleep disturbances and cognitive impairment by affecting the brain. This occurs because the function of neurons, neuron survival, cell migration and glia, and glial cell (astrocytes and oligodendrocytes) differentiation are disrupted by alcohol [47]. However, despite extensive inquiry, we could not find one study that confirms a statistical significance between alcohol usage and RLS in an older population, taking into account possible covariates. Therefore, our data strongly suggest an important contribution of alcohol consumption to the prevalence of RLS, independent of other multiple possible co-determinants.

We also found that the RLS group used significantly more medication than the group without RLS alongside the higher alcohol intake. It is possible that alcohol correlates with RLS directly as well as indirectly, e.g., by altering the effects of simultaneously taken medications. Drug–food/alcohol interactions are known to reduce the therapeutic effects of medications, as well as to induce potent adverse drug reactions [48]. Medications, such as antidepressants, antihistamines, and antipsychotics have been associated with RLS [1]. Secondary forms of RLS and possible interactions of medications require particular consideration in older adults [49]. Both alcohol and many medications are metabolized by the same enzymes in the liver, where pharmacokinetic interactions generally occur. Alcohol can interact with numerous classes of prescription medications including antibiotics, antidepressants, antihistamines, barbiturates, benzodiazepines, histamine H2 receptor antagonists, muscle relaxants, nonnarcotic pain medications and anti-inflammatory agents, opioids, and warfarin. It can also interact with over-the-counter medicines and herbal products, often with negative effects [50].

We were not able to demonstrate any relationship between physical activity and RLS. In one study, physical activity reduced the risk of RLS and had a positive effect on its symptoms [22]. The mechanism by which this happens remains unknown, although several theories have been postulated. For instance, better blood flow in the lower limbs or the increased release of endorphins and dopamine. Additionally, symptoms, which are experienced at rest are likely to be reduced in those who exercise [22]. In another study, exercise therapy significantly affected the manifestations of the illness. Stretching, fitness training, and reflexology were beneficial with no side effects [51].

In several studies RLS was associated with a significantly lower HRQL and a higher prevalence of depression [39,52]. In a few studies, in older adults, this was assessed in relation to some aspects of the CGA [53–55]. In a Turkish study of 492 subjects aged on average 73 years, sleep disturbance, depressive mood, the fear of falling, reduced QoL, frailty and polypharmacy were more prevalent in the RLS group [56]. In a recent small study (54 RLS patients, 30 people in the control group), RLS patients were prone to sleep disorders, anxiety, and depression. Sleep disorders increased with the severity of the RLS and had some influence on the patient's cognitive function [53]. In a recent systematic review, a negative association between RLS and global cognition and attention was found. No significant differences in memory, executive function, or spatial cognition were observed between the RLS and control groups [54]. In a cross-sectional study of 1008 subjects aged $\geq$54 years, RLS did not predict incident disability for aggregate measures but was associated with an increased risk for specific limitations, including difficulty with climbing several stair flights, prolonged sitting, rising from a chair, stooping, moving heavy objects, carrying ten pounds, raising arms, or picking up a dime [57]. Interestingly, a large study on 90,337 Chinese adults showed that RLS was associated with increased incidents of perceived olfactory and taste dysfunction [58]. In a small study of 32 older patients, five with RLS, there was no association of RLS with clinical, laboratory or neurophysiological findings [55]. In the present study, we found a nonsignificant trend of greater depression in RLS sufferers. Additionally, we found that mobility difficulties were significantly more frequent in those with RLS which might suggest impairment related to the symptoms of RLS.

Several limitations of the present study should be acknowledged. Because the study was performed in selected populations, the results of this study may lack generalizability. The difference in alcohol consumption between the UK and Poland was high. Nevertheless, the participants both in Poland and the UK were questioned by the same investigator (MS). Therefore, this difference may be likely attributed to cultural dissimilarities between the two populations. To minimize potential biases, subjects without known anemia, chronic kidney disease, known iron or vitamin deficiency, terminal illness, major disabilities or cognitive impairment were included in the study. Nevertheless, the study lacks laboratory data on iron or vitamin deficiency. Although we have adjusted for the presence of major chronic diseases and CGA data, other factors might have influenced the occurrence of RLS. Possible biases in the interview (patients' forgetfulness in older age) should also be taken into consideration. Therefore, current findings should be corroborated in future studies assessing other potential confounders in more general populations.

5. Conclusions

Female sex, the number of medications taken per day and alcohol consumption are independent correlates of RLS in older adults. RLS together with several chronic medical conditions and a low physical activity level were independent correlates of the mobility dimension of the QoL. Therefore, controlling alcohol consumption seems the most important clinical implication put forward to alleviate the burden of RLS in older adults, probably contributing also to a better QoL.

Author Contributions: Conceptualization, M.S., T.K. and J.K.; methodology, T.K. and J.K.; formal analysis, J.K. and T.K.; investigation, M.S., T.K. and J.K.; resources, T.K.; data curation, M.S., J.K. and T.K.; writing—original draft preparation, M.S., J.K. and T.K.; writing—review and editing, M.S., T.K. and J.K.; visualization, M.S.; supervision, T.K. and J.K.; project administration, T.K.; funding acquisition, J.K. All authors have read and agreed to the published version of the manuscript.

Funding: The authors were supported by grants founded by the Medical University of Lodz, Poland (503/6-077-01/503-61-001-19-00 and 503/6-127-06/503-61-001).

Institutional Review Board Statement: The study was conducted in accordance with the Declaration of Helsinki, and approved by the Committee on the Ethics of Research of Human Experimentation at the Medical University of Lodz, Poland (RNN/312/08/KB, 24 June 2008).

Informed Consent Statement: Informed consent was obtained from all individual participants included in the study.

Data Availability Statement: Data will be available on reasonable request from the corresponding author.

Conflicts of Interest: The authors declare no conflicts of interest.

References

1. Winkelman, J.W. Treating Severe Refractory and Augmented Restless Legs Syndrome. *Chest* **2022**, *162*, 693–700. [CrossRef] [PubMed]
2. Budhiraja, P.; Budhiraja, R.; Goodwin, J.L.; Allen, R.P.; Newman, A.B.; Koo, B.B.; Quan, S.F. Incidence of restless legs syndrome and its correlates. *J. Clin. Sleep Med.* **2012**, *8*, 119–124. [CrossRef]
3. Gonzalez-Latapi, P.; Malkani, R. Update on Restless Legs Syndrome: From Mechanisms to Treatment. *Curr. Neurol. Neurosci. Rep.* **2019**, *19*, 54. [CrossRef] [PubMed]
4. Ferré, S.; García-Borreguero, D.; Allen, R.P.; Earley, C.J. New Insights into the Neurobiology of Restless Legs Syndrome. *Neuroscientist* **2019**, *25*, 113–125. [CrossRef] [PubMed]
5. Antelmi, E.; Rocchi, L.; Latorre, A.; Belvisi, D.; Magrinelli, F.; Bhatia, K.P.; Tinazzi, M. Restless Legs Syndrome: Known Knowns and Known Unknowns. *Brain Sci.* **2022**, *12*, 118. [CrossRef]
6. Guo, S.; Huang, J.; Jiang, H.; Han, C.; Li, J.; Xu, X.; Zhang, G.; Lin, Z.; Xiong, N.; Wang, T. Restless Legs Syndrome: From Pathophysiology to Clinical Diagnosis and Management. *Front. Aging Neurosci.* **2017**, *9*, 171. [CrossRef]
7. Milligan, S.A.; Chesson, A.L. Restless legs syndrome in the older adult: Diagnosis and management. *Drugs Aging* **2002**, *19*, 741–751. [CrossRef]
8. Chen, P.; Bornhorst, J.; Patton, S.; Bagai, K.; Nitin, R.; Miah, M.; Hare, D.J.; Kysenius, K.; Crouch, P.J.; Xiong, L.; et al. A potential role for zinc in restless legs syndrome. *Sleep* **2021**, *44*, zsaa236. [CrossRef]
9. Weinstock, L.B.; Brook, J.B.; Walters, A.S.; Goris, A.; Afrin, L.B.; Molderings, G.J. Restless legs syndrome is associated with long-COVID in women. *J. Clin. Sleep Med.* **2022**, *18*, 1413–1418. [CrossRef]
10. Trenkwalder, C.; Allen, R.; Högl, B.; Paulus, W.; Winkelmann, J. Restless legs syndrome associated with major diseases: A systematic review and new concept. *Neurology* **2016**, *86*, 1336–1343. [CrossRef] [PubMed]
11. Jiménez-Jiménez, F.J.; Ayuso, P.; Alonso-Navarro, H.; Calleja, M.; Díez-Fairén, M.; Álvarez, I.; Pastor, P.; Plaza-Nieto, J.F.; Navarro-Muñoz, S.; Turpín-Fenoll, L.; et al. Serum Trace Elements Concentrations in Patients with Restless Legs Syndrome. *Antioxidants* **2022**, *11*, 272. [CrossRef]
12. Tutan, D.; Ulfberg, J.; Aydemir, N.; Eser, B.; Doğan, İ. The Relationship between Serum Selenium Levels and Restless Leg Syndrome in Chronic Kidney Disease Patients. *Medicina* **2023**, *59*, 1795. [CrossRef]
13. Ryan, M.; Slevin, J.T. Restless legs syndrome. *Am. J. Health Syst. Pharm.* **2006**, *63*, 1599–1612. [CrossRef]
14. Cederberg, K.L.J.; Silvestri, R.; Walters, A.S. Vitamin D and Restless Legs Syndrome: A Review of Current Literature. *Tremor Other Hyperkinetic Mov.* **2023**, *13*, 12. [CrossRef]
15. Geng, C.; Yang, Z.; Xu, P.; Zhang, H. Possible association between vitamin B12 deficiency and restless legs syndrome. *Clin. Neurol. Neurosurg.* **2022**, *223*, 107477. [CrossRef]
16. Manconi, M.; Garcia-Borreguero, D.; Schormair, B.; Videnovic, A.; Berger, K.; Ferri, R.; Dauvilliers, Y. Restless legs syndrome. *Nat. Rev. Dis. Primers* **2021**, *7*, 80. [CrossRef]
17. Ahmed, N.; Kandil, M.; Elfil, M.; Jamal, A.; Koo, B.B. Hypothyroidism in restless legs syndrome. *J. Sleep. Res.* **2021**, *30*, e13091. [CrossRef] [PubMed]

18. Gupta, R.; Gupta, R.; Kumar, N.; Rawat, V.S.; Ulfberg, J.; Allen, R.P. Restless legs syndrome among subjects having chronic liver disease: A systematic review and meta-analysis. *Sleep Med. Rev.* **2021**, *58*, 101463. [CrossRef] [PubMed]
19. Diaconu, Ș.; Irincu, L.; Ungureanu, L.; Ciopleiaș, B.; Țînț, D.; Falup-Pecurariu, C. Restless Legs Syndrome in Parkinson's Disease. *J. Pers. Med.* **2023**, *13*, 915. [CrossRef] [PubMed]
20. Szklarek, M.; Kostka, T. The impact of the use of amalgam in dental treatment on the prevalence of restless legs syndrome in older people. *Med. Pr.* **2019**, *70*, 9–16. [CrossRef] [PubMed]
21. Gulia, K.K.; Kumar, V.M. Sleep disorders in the elderly: A growing challenge. *Psychogeriatrics* **2018**, *18*, 155–165. [CrossRef] [PubMed]
22. Batool-Anwar, S.; Li, Y.; De Vito, K.; Malhotra, A.; Winkelman, J.; Gao, X. Lifestyle Factors and Risk of Restless Legs Syndrome: Prospective Cohort Study. *J. Clin. Sleep Med.* **2016**, *12*, 187–194. [CrossRef] [PubMed]
23. Ryan, H.; Trosclair, A.; Gfroerer, J. Adult current smoking: Differences in definitions and prevalence estimates—NHIS and NSDUH, 2008. *J. Environ. Public Health* **2012**, *2012*, 918368. [CrossRef] [PubMed]
24. Walters, A.S.; LeBrocq, C.; Dhar, A.; Hening, W.; Rosen, R.; Allen, R.P.; Trenkwalder, C. Validation of the International Restless Legs Syndrome Study Group rating scale for restless legs syndrome. *Sleep Med.* **2003**, *4*, 121–132. [CrossRef] [PubMed]
25. Katz, S.; Ford, A.B.; Moskowitz, R.W.; Jackson, B.A.; Jaffe, M.W. Studies of illness in the aged: The index of ADL, a standardized measure of biogical and psychosocial function. *JAMA* **1963**, *185*, 914–919. [CrossRef]
26. Lawton, M.P.; Brody, E.M. Instrumental Activities of Daily Living (IADL) Scale: Original observer-rated version. *Psychopharmacol. Bull.* **1988**, *24*, 785–792.
27. Podsiadlo, D.; Richardson, S. The timed "up & go": A test of basic functional mobility for frail elderly persons. *J. Am. Geriatr. Soc.* **1991**, *39*, 142–148.
28. Blair, S.N.; Haskell, W.L.; Ho, P.; Paffenbarger, R.S.J.; Vranizan, K.M.; Farquhar, J.W.; Wood, P.D. Assessment of habitual physical activity by a seven-day recall in a community survey and controlled experiments. *Am. J. Epidemiol.* **1985**, *122*, 794–804. [CrossRef]
29. Sallis, J.F.; Haskell, W.L.; Wood, P.D.; Fortmann, S.P.; Rogers, T.; Blair, S.N.; Paffenbarger, R.S.J. Physical activity assessment methodology in the Five-City Project. *Am. J. Epidemiol.* **1985**, *121*, 91–106. [CrossRef]
30. Guigoz, Y.B.; Vellas, B.; Garry, P.J. Mini Nutritional Assessment: A practical assessment tool for grading the nutritional state of elderly patients. *Facts Res. Gerontol.* **1994**, *2*, 15–59.
31. Yesavage, J.A.; Brink, T.L.; Rose, T.L.; Lum, O.; Huang, V.; Adey, M.; Leirer, V.O. Development and validation of a geriatric depression screening scale: A preliminary report. *J. Psychiatr. Res.* **1982**, *17*, 37–49. [CrossRef]
32. Folstein, M.F.; Folstein, S.E.; McHugh, P.R. "Minimental state" a practical method for grading the cognitive state of patients for the clinician. *J. Psychiatr. Res.* **1975**, *12*, 189–198. [CrossRef]
33. Brooks, R. EuroQol: The current state of play. *Health Policy* **1996**, *37*, 53–72. [CrossRef]
34. Trenkwalder, C.; Allen, R.; Högl, B.; Clemens, S.; Patton, S.; Schormair, B.; Winkelmann, J. Comorbidities, treatment, and pathophysiology in restless legs syndrome. *Lancet Neurol.* **2018**, *17*, 994–1005. [CrossRef]
35. Didriksen, M.; Rigas, A.S.; Allen, R.P.; Burchell, B.J.; Di Angelantonio, E.; Nielsen, M.H.; Jennum, P.; Werge, T.; Erikstrup, C.; Pedersen, O.B.; et al. Prevalence of restless legs syndrome and associated factors in an otherwise healthy population: Results from the Danish Blood Donor Study. *Sleep Med.* **2017**, *36*, 55–61. [CrossRef] [PubMed]
36. Phillips, B.; Young, T.; Finn, L.; Asher, K.; Hening, W.A.; Purvis, C. Epidemiology of Restless Legs Symptoms in Adults. *Arch. Intern. Med.* **2000**, *160*, 2137–2141. [CrossRef] [PubMed]
37. Weber, F.C.; Danker-Hopfe, H.; Dogan-Sander, E.; Frase, L.; Hansel, A.; Mauche, N.; Mikutta, C.; Nemeth, D.; Richter, K.; Schilling, C.; et al. Restless Legs Syndrome Prevalence and Clinical Correlates Among Psychiatric Inpatients: A Multicenter Study. *Front. Psychiatry* **2022**, *13*, 846165. [CrossRef] [PubMed]
38. Amiri, S. Body mass index and sleep disturbances: A systematic review and meta-analysis. *Postep. Psychiatr. Neurol.* **2023**, *32*, 96–109. [CrossRef]
39. AlShareef, S.M. The prevalence of and risk factors for restless legs syndrome: A nationwide study. *Front. Psychiatry* **2022**, *13*, 987689. [CrossRef]
40. Suwała, S.; Rzeszuto, J.; Glonek, R.; Krintus, M.; Junik, R. Is Restless Legs Syndrome De Facto Thyroid Disease? *Biomedicines* **2022**, *10*, 2502. [CrossRef]
41. Liu, Y.; Liu, G.; Li, L.; Yang, J.; Ma, S. Evaluation of Cardiovascular Risk Factors and Restless Legs Syndrome in Women and Men: A Preliminary Population-Based Study in China. *J. Clin. Sleep Med.* **2018**, *14*, 445–450. [CrossRef] [PubMed]
42. Szentkirályi, A.; Völzke, H.; Hoffmann, W.; Happe, S.; Berger, K. A time sequence analysis of the relationship between cardiovascular risk factors, vascular diseases and restless legs syndrome in the general population. *J. Sleep Res.* **2013**, *22*, 434–442. [CrossRef]
43. Jiménez-Jiménez, F.J.; Gómez-Tabales, J.; Alonso-Navarro, H.; Zurdo, M.; Turpín-Fenoll, L.; Millán-Pascual, J.; Adeva-Bartolomé, T.; Cubo, E.; Navacerrada, F.; Rojo-Sebastián, A.; et al. Association between the rs1229984 Polymorphism in the Alcohol Dehydrogenase 1B Gene and Risk for Restless Legs Syndrome. *Sleep* **2017**, *40*, zsx174. [CrossRef]
44. Rangarajan, S.; Rangarajan, S.; D'Souza, G.A. Restless legs syndrome in an Indian urban population. *Sleep Med.* **2007**, *9*, 88–93. [CrossRef]
45. Aldrich, M.S.; Shipley, J.E. Alcohol use and periodic limb movements of sleep. *Alcohol. Clin. Exp. Res.* **1993**, *17*, 192–196. [CrossRef] [PubMed]

46. Mackie, S.E.; McHugh, R.K.; McDermott, K.; Griffin, M.L.; Winkelman, J.W.; Weiss, R.D. Prevalence of restless legs syndrome during detoxification from alcohol and opioids. *J. Subst. Abuse Treat.* **2017**, *73*, 35–39. [CrossRef]
47. Ebrahim, I.O.; Shapiro, C.M.; Williams, A.J.; Fenwick, P.B. Alcohol and sleep I: Effects on normal sleep. *Alcohol. Clin. Exp. Res.* **2013**, *37*, 539–549. [CrossRef] [PubMed]
48. Paśko, P.; Rodacki, T.; Domagała-Rodacka, R.; Palimonka, K.; Marcinkowska, M.; Owczarek, D. Second generation H1-Antihistamines interaction with food and alcohol—A systematic review. *Biomed. Pharmacother.* **2017**, *93*, 27–39. [CrossRef]
49. Spiegelhalder, K.; Hornyak, M. Restless legs syndrome in older adults. *Clin. Geriatr. Med.* **2008**, *24*, 167–180. [CrossRef]
50. Weathermon, R.; Crabb, D.W. Alcohol and medication interactions. *Alcohol. Res. Health* **1999**, *23*, 40–54.
51. Ratnani, G.; Harjpal, P. Advancements in Restless Leg Syndrome Management: A Review of Physiotherapeutic Modalities and Their Efficacy. *Cureus* **2023**, *15*, e46779. [CrossRef]
52. Didriksen, M.; Allen, R.P.; Burchell, B.J.; Thørner, L.W.; Rigas, A.S.; Di Angelantonio, E.; Nielsen, M.H.; Jennum, P.J.; Werge, T.; Erikstrup, C.; et al. Restless legs syndrome is associated with major comorbidities in a population of Danish blood donors. *Sleep. Med.* **2018**, *45*, 124–131. [CrossRef]
53. Xu, Y.; Wen, H.; Li, J.; Yang, J.; Luo, K.; Chang, L. The relationship between sleep disorders, anxiety, depression, and cognitive function with restless legs syndrome (RLS) in the elderly. *Sleep Breath.* **2022**, *26*, 1309–1318. [CrossRef]
54. Wang, S.; Zheng, X.; Huang, J.; Lin, J.; Yang, T.; Xiao, Y.; Jiang, Q.; Li, C.; Shang, H. Restless legs syndrome and cognitive function among adults: A systematic review and meta-analysis. *J. Neurol.* **2023**, *270*, 1361–1370. [CrossRef]
55. Dantas, F.; Medeiros, J.; Farias, K.; Ribeiro, C. Restless legs syndrome in institutionalized elderly. *Arq. Neuro-Psiquiatr.* **2008**, *66*, 328–330. [CrossRef]
56. Özkök, S.; Aydın, Ç.Ö.; Erbaş Saçar, D.; Çatıkkaş, N.M.; Erdoğan, T.; Kılıç, C.; Karan, M.A.; Bahat, G. Is There Any Association with Other Geriatric Syndromes? *Eur. J. Geriatric Gerontol.* **2022**, *4*, 182–189. [CrossRef]
57. Cirillo, D.J.; Wallace, R.B. Restless legs syndrome and functional limitations among American elders in the Health and Retirement Study. *BMC Geriatr.* **2012**, *12*, 39. [CrossRef]
58. Zhuang, S.; Yuan, X.; Ma, C.; Yang, N.; Liu, C.F.; Na, M.; Winkelman, J.W.; Wu, S.; Gao, X. Restless legs syndrome and perceived olfactory and taste dysfunction: A community-based study. *Eur. J. Neurol.* **2021**, *28*, 2688–2693. [CrossRef] [PubMed]

Disclaimer/Publisher's Note: The statements, opinions and data contained in all publications are solely those of the individual author(s) and contributor(s) and not of MDPI and/or the editor(s). MDPI and/or the editor(s) disclaim responsibility for any injury to people or property resulting from any ideas, methods, instructions or products referred to in the content.

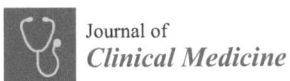

Review

Anemia and Its Connections to Inflammation in Older Adults: A Review

Eryk Wacka [1,*], Jan Nicikowski [1], Pawel Jarmuzek [2] and Agnieszka Zembron-Lacny [1]

1. Department of Applied and Clinical Physiology, Collegium Medicum University of Zielona Gora, 65-417 Zielona Gora, Poland; jan.nicikowski@gmail.com (J.N.); a.zembron-lacny@cm.uz.zgora.pl (A.Z.-L.)
2. Department of Neurosurgery and Neurology, Collegium Medicum University of Zielona Gora, 65-417 Zielona Gora, Poland; p.jarmuzek@cm.uz.zgora.pl
* Correspondence: e.wacka@cm.uz.zgora.pl

Abstract: Anemia is a common hematological disorder that affects 12% of the community-dwelling population, 40% of hospitalized patients, and 47% of nursing home residents. Our understanding of the impact of inflammation on iron metabolism and erythropoiesis is still lacking. In older adults, anemia can be divided into nutritional deficiency anemia, bleeding anemia, and unexplained anemia. The last type of anemia might be caused by reduced erythropoietin (EPO) activity, progressive EPO resistance of bone marrow erythroid progenitors, and the chronic subclinical pro-inflammatory state. Overall, one-third of older patients with anemia demonstrate a nutritional deficiency, one-third have a chronic subclinical pro-inflammatory state and chronic kidney disease, and one-third suffer from anemia of unknown etiology. Understanding anemia's pathophysiology in people aged 65 and over is crucial because it contributes to frailty, falls, cognitive decline, decreased functional ability, and higher mortality risk. Inflammation produces adverse effects on the cells of the hematological system. These effects include iron deficiency (hypoferremia), reduced EPO production, and the elevated phagocytosis of erythrocytes by hepatic and splenic macrophages. Additionally, inflammation causes enhanced eryptosis due to oxidative stress in the circulation. Identifying mechanisms behind age-related inflammation is essential for a better understanding and preventing anemia in older adults.

Keywords: aging; anemia diagnosis; erythropoiesis; geriatric diseases; inflammation; iro deficiency; hypoferremia; oxidative stress

1. Introduction

The world population is rapidly aging, and this demographic shift is expected to continue over the coming decades. This phenomenon is characterized by an increase in both the number and the percentage of older adults worldwide. Currently, 10% of the world population is aged 65 years or older, but this figure is expected to reach 16% by 2050. Developing countries are particularly affected by this trend due to the declining levels of mortality, as reflected in the increased levels of life expectancy at birth [1]. As individuals grow older, their organic functionality naturally declines over time (aging), ultimately resulting in death. Aging is also associated with an increased likelihood of common conditions such as cardiovascular diseases, cancer, diabetes, or neurodegenerative diseases, which, in turn, elevate the risk of mortality [2].

Anemia, a condition that frequently occurs in older patients, has no standard definition. The World Health Organization (WHO) established the diagnostic criteria for anemia, which was defined as a hemoglobin (Hb) level < 13.0 g/dL for men and <12.0 g/dL for women [3]. Since the WHO definition of anemia was established more than five decades ago on the basis of a limited population sample and without proper documentation of the methodology used, understandably, there are now certain restrictions related to these thresholds. Nevertheless, the WHO definition continues to be the standard for anemia classification in older adults, despite suggestions from various studies that the definition be revised. Higher Hb reference values to define anemia were suggested after the analyses of American databases including the National Health and Nutrition Examination Survey III [4] and the Scripps-Kaiser database [5]. The Cardiovascular Health Study [6] identified optimal Hb levels of ≥ 13.7 g/dL for men and ≥ 12.6 g/dL for women, which were recorded to be associated with improved survival. The population study by Culleton et al. [7] determined that optimal Hb values of 13.0 to 15.0 g/dL for women and 14.0 to 17.0 g/dL for men could help avoid hospitalization and reduce the risk of mortality in old age. Wouters et al. recommended modifying Hb values to <13.0 g/dL for women over 60 years of age to align with the definition used for men [8].

Age-related, chronic, low-grade inflammation is not only a consequence of increasing chronological age, but also a marker of biological aging, multimorbidity, and mortality risk [9]. Systemic inflammation can significantly exacerbate health status and lead to a decline in overall well-being [10]. As the immune system ages, its ability to effectively respond to and manage inflammation diminishes, which renders the elderly more susceptible to a range of diseases such as anemia [11,12]. Therefore, the objective of this review was to explore the pathophysiological causes of anemia in the elderly, particularly those associated with inflammation, and to elucidate the underlying mechanisms and contributing factors for anemia in this age group.

Prevalence of Anemia

The prevalence of anemia varies across age groups, genders, and races, and the condition is more common in older individuals, with higher rates observed in men compared to women and in black individuals compared to white ones. However, it is noteworthy that most individuals classified as anemic according to the WHO criteria demonstrated anemia of a mild degree [3].

A systematic review of 34 studies showed that in people aged >65 years, the prevalence of anemia was recorded in 12% of community-dwelling persons, 40% of hospitalized patients, and 47% of nursing home residents [13], with the overall mean prevalence of 17% [14]. The increased prevalence of anemia among nursing home residents was often attributed to poorer health status and the higher occurrence of comorbidities in the elderly residents of these facilities compared to the community-dwelling age-matched population [15]. Insights into the prevalence of anemia across different populations and its findings, based on selected studies, are summarized in Table 1.

Table 1. Selected studies examining the prevalence of anemia across various populations and its findings.

Study Name/Author	Country	Findings	Reference
EMPIRE study	Portugal	- higher prevalence of anemia in men than women (22.2% vs. 19.9%, respectively). - anemia prevalence increased with age, with the rates of 17.3% in the 65–79 age group and 31.4% in those aged 80 years and above.	[16]
Third US National Health and Nutrition Examination Survey (NHANES III)	USA	- a progressive increase in anemia prevalence with increasing age in the study participants aged ≥ 65 years, where the prevalence of 13% and 23% was recorded in subgroups aged 75–84 vs. ≥ 85, respectively. - data demonstrated that anemia was more prevalent in men than in women.	[1]

Table 1. Cont.

Study Name/Author	Country	Findings	Reference
Zaninetti et al.	Italy	- anemia was prevalent in 62% of males aged ≥65 years compared to 44.1% prevalence in the group aged below 65 years. - similar observations pertained to female gender where the proportion of women ≥65 years with anemia reached 60.1% vs. 53.5% recorded in females below 65 years of age.	[17]
Muñoz et al.	Spain	- prevalence of anemia varied depending on the surgical intervention, ranging from 14% in prostate surgery to 61% in colorectal cancer cases.	[18]

The severity of anemia was found to be higher in skilled nursing facilities compared to community-based settings, as revealed in a survey of five such facilities where a hemoglobin level ≤ 10 g/dL was detected in 11.4% of the residents [19]. In hospitalized patients aged ≥65 years, the prevalence of anemia reached up to 48%, with 65% of patients exhibiting mild (Hb > 10 g/dL) to moderate (Hb 8–10 g/dL) anemia [20]. Interestingly, it was observed that the recognition and investigation of anemia were rarely undertaken [21]. These findings highlight the increased severity of anemia in skilled nursing facilities and the need to raise the awareness of the staff and the management of this condition in both health care settings.

It is evident that the analyzed issue differs depending on the geographical location and the economic status of various countries.

The identification of the putative factors underlying anemia of inflammation in older adults poses a considerable challenge as this age group is affected by a tremendous extent of subclinical and clinical morbidities as well as an age-related increase in the levels of proinflammatory cytokines. It is therefore hardly surprising that nearly a fifth of anemia cases (19.7%) in older adults have been classified as anemia of inflammation, also known as anemia of chronic disease [1]. However, distinguishing anemia of chronic inflammation from iron deficiency anemia is particularly challenging in older adults due to the comorbid effects of gastrointestinal bleeding and the effects of medications [22]. Serum ferritin levels can still fall within the reference range when both types of anemia are present, which might potentially have led to an overestimation of anemia of chronic inflammation prevalence in the NHANES III study [1] at the expense of iron deficiency anemia. Furthermore, even distinguishing anemia of chronic inflammation from anemia of chronic kidney disease is somewhat tenuous, given the emerging evidence of increased inflammation associated with renal function in older adults without chronic kidney disease [23,24].

2. Causes of Anemia in Older Adults

The processes responsible for the maintenance of homeostasis diminish with increasing age, and one of these processes involves a decrease in hematopoietic potential. However, there are no adequate hemoglobin reference values below which anemia can be diagnosed in adults aged over 65 years, so the referential range for the general population is still applied [25]. Figure 1 provides a visual representation of the main factors contributing to the development of aging-related inflammation that can further contribute to the development of anemia in the elderly.

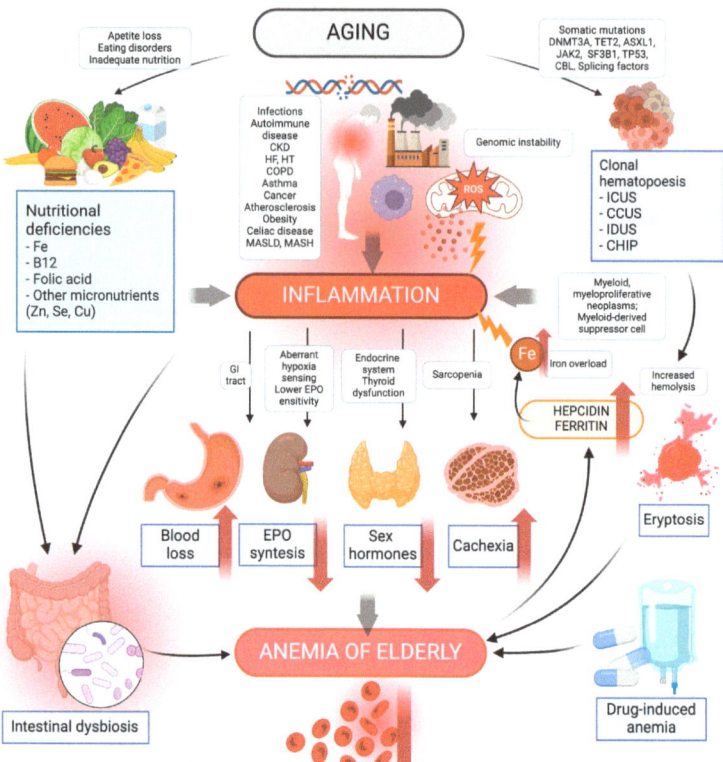

Figure 1. Causes of anemia in the elderly. The diagram shows the main causes of the development of aging-related inflammation that can contribute to anemia in the elderly. Aging processes such as genome instability, reactive oxygen species in the mitochondria, synthesis of pro-inflammatory cytokines, negative environmental factors, and chronic diseases lead to inflammation. Inadequate nutrition, eating disorders, and loss of appetite contribute to an increased risk of nutritional deficiencies—iron, vitamin B12, folic acid, zinc, selenium, and copper. Their deficiency leads to inflammation and modulation of the intestinal microbiota to its detriment, increasing the risk of intestinal dysbiosis. The number of somatic mutations increasing with age can lead to clonal hematopoiesis. This, in turn, increases the incidence of myeloid myeloproliferative neoplasms, myeloid-derived suppressor cells causing inflammation. Clonal hematopoiesis shortens the lifespan and durability of erythrocytes, increasing their risk of hemolysis, the process of eryptosis. Chronic inflammatory processes further contribute to gastrointestinal inflammatory disease and blood loss; a decrease in sensitivity to hypoxia and EPO, thereby causing a reduction in EPO synthesis; endocrine dysfunction causing a decrease in sex hormones; and a decrease in muscle mass to sarcopenia, leading to the risk of cachexia. Pharmacotherapy with drug–drug interactions can produce adverse effects potentially contributing to anemia in older adults. Lately, anemia in the elderly has been reported to cause an increase in hepcidin, a plasma ferritin causing pro-inflammatory iron overload. CCUS, clonal cytopenia of unknown significance; CHIP, clonal hematopoiesis of indeterminate potential; CKD, chronic kidney disease; COPD, chronic obstructive pulmonary disease; EPO, erythropoietin; GI, gastrointestinal; HF, heart failure; HT, hypertensive; ICUS, idiopathic cytopenia of undetermined significance; IDUS, idiopathic dysplasia of undetermined significance; MASLD, metabolic dysfunction-associated steatotic liver disease; MASH, metabolic dysfunction-associated steatohepatitis; ROS, reactive oxygen species. Created with BioRender.com (accessed on 9 March 2024).

Genomic instability is a fundamental cause of the progressive aging process [26]. The factors favoring genome instability include environmental factors [27], the influence of chemicals [28], oxidative stress [29], hypoxia progression with aging [30], and chronic inflammation [31]. An increase in DNA instability results in elevated numbers of somatic mutations in the resulting cells [32]. With age, somatic mutations also affect all cells involved in hematopoiesis, resulting in clonal hematopoiesis [33]. The incidence of progressive clonal hematopoiesis increases with age [34]. The number of clonal abnormalities is correlated with the risk of developing myeloid and myeloproliferative neoplasms including acute myeloid leukemia, myelodysplastic syndromes, myeloproliferative syndromes, and mixed (myelodysplastic-myeloproliferative) syndromes. The list of the above-mentioned diseases also includes anaplastic anemia.

Increased mitochondrial damage in stem cells [35] and impaired mitochondrial function observed in chronic diseases during hematopoiesis [36] are further elements of the hypothesis concerning the etiology of anemia in old age. Accumulating damage to telomeres leads to aging of the mitochondria and the increased production of reactive oxygen species (ROS), which results in generalized hypoxia as a consequence [37,38]. In the longer term, a persistent increase in hypoxia activates systemic compensatory and adaptive mechanisms [39].

3. Pathophysiology of Inflammation Causing Anemia in Older Adults

As individuals age, the phenomenon known as inflammaging becomes increasingly prevalent. Inflammaging is characterized by chronic low-grade inflammation, and it is considered a significant contributor to the aging process. The underlying mechanism involves the release of a multitude of inflammatory mediators that are produced in response to tissue damage and stress. The key players in chronic inflammation include a variety of interleukins such as IL-1, IL-1b IL-2, IL-6, IL-8, IL-12, IL-13, IL-15, IL-18, IL-22, and IL-23. The pro-inflammatory activity of these cytokines initiates and amplifies the inflammatory response. Additionally, tumor necrosis factor α (TNFα) and interferon-γ (IFN-γ) are also prominent pro-inflammatory cytokines. Variations in the genetic sequences within the promoter regions of proinflammatory and controlled cytokine genes can influence the processes of inflammaging and vulnerability to age-related diseases [40].

On the other hand, attempts are made by anti-inflammatory cytokines including IL-1Ra, IL-4, IL-10, and transforming growth factor (TGF-β1) to counterbalance the pro-inflammatory response. These cytokines, in turn, are engaged in the suppression of inflammation and they promote a more balanced immune response. Along with the cytokines, a range of other molecules contribute to the complex network of inflammaging. For instance, lipoxin A4 plays the role of a lipid mediator with potent anti-inflammatory properties. Heat shock proteins are also involved in the regulation of inflammation, acting like chaperones that help to protect cells from stress-induced damage [41–43]. According to Minciullo et al. [43], inflammaging is a key to our understanding of the aging process, and anti-inflammaging may be one of the secrets of longevity. Therefore, anemia caused by inflammation is an important issue to be tackled more quickly and multidimensionally.

3.1. Iron Restriction (Hypoferremia)

During infection or inflammatory events, hypoferremia occurs quickly with a decrease in plasma iron level and transferrin saturation, which prevents the formation of nontransferrin-bound iron, a powerful trigger for the pathogenicity of Gram-negative bacteria and potentially also other microorganisms [44,45]. Iron consumption by erythropoiesis and the turnover of senescent or damaged erythrocytes by macrophages are the primary factors affected by various inflammatory processes. Therefore, maintaining strict control over iron levels during inflammation is crucial for host defense.

Hepcidin, a 25-amino-acid peptide released by liver cells, circulates in the blood and is expelled in the urine. Hepcidin serves as the primary governing factor for both iron absorption and distribution across different tissues [46,47]. Elevated levels of circulating hepcidin, induced by IL-6, inhibit the release of cellular iron into plasma by binding to the cellular iron efflux channel ferroportin [48]. Ferroportin occurs on the cells that serve as specialized iron managers within the body, and these cells include duodenal enterocytes that are responsible for the absorption of dietary iron, hepatic and splenic macrophages that recycle senescent erythrocytes, hepatocytes that are engaged in iron storage, and placental trophoblasts that facilitate iron transfer to the developing fetus during pregnancy [49].

Macrophages play a crucial role in recycling iron from aging red blood cells and once recycled, the iron is released into the bloodstream through ferroportin. Inflammation triggers an increase in hepcidin levels, thereby leading to enhanced internalization and the breakdown of ferroportin [50]. As a result, the release of ferrous iron from key iron transport tissues such as duodenal enterocytes, iron-recycling macrophages, and iron-storing hepatocytes into the bloodstream is reduced. This leads to the accumulation of iron within their cellular ferritin. Subsequently, the continuous utilization of iron by erythropoiesis depletes the extracellular iron pool, which results in low levels of iron and restricted erythropoiesis.

Anemia of inflammation is characterized by hypoferremia accompanied by increased plasma ferritin and hepcidin levels, whereas iron-deficiency anemia manifests itself in hypoferremia accompanied by low levels of plasma ferritin and hepcidin. Inflammatory hypoferremia, similar to hypoferremia in systemic iron deficiency, inhibits erythropoiesis, however, the inhibitory effect is detected at a relatively high threshold (transferrin saturation of 15 to 20%), which may suggest a protective function of this mechanism to ensure an adequate iron supply for other tissues such as muscles, the central nervous system, and nonerythroid marrow, which are less affected by decreased plasma iron levels (Figure 2) [51].

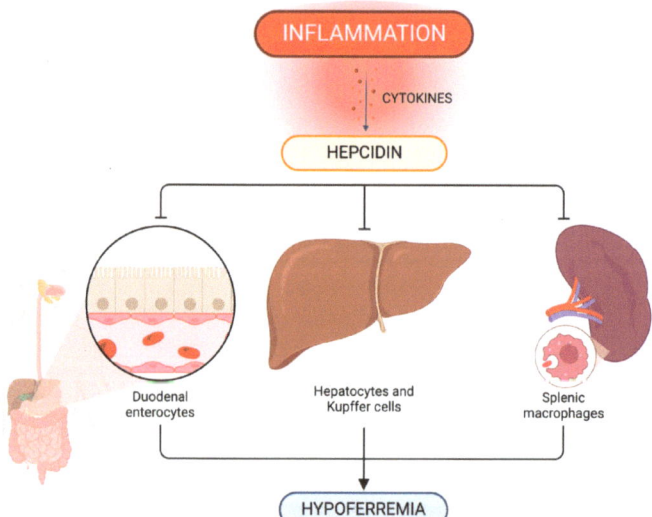

Figure 2. Inflammation impact on the regulation of systemic iron metabolism. Hepcidin plays a crucial role in systemic iron level control via ferroportin concentration in iron-exporting cells including duodenal enterocytes, hepatic and splenic iron-recycling macrophages and hepatocytes. Created with BioRender.com (accessed on 9 March 2024).

Our previous study demonstrated higher hepcidin levels in the group with anemia compared to non-anemic participants [52], which is consistent with other reports, for instance, the Leiden 85-plus Study, which also revealed elevated serum hepcidin levels in older adults with anemia of inflammation. However, the InCHIANTI study did not find an increase in urinary hepcidin levels [48,53]. The available studies also reported differences in hepcidin levels across the compared genders. On average, approximately 50% lower hepcidin levels were observed in premenopausal women than in the age-matched male groups. However, post-menopause hepcidin levels tend to become comparable in both gender groups, which was reported in the Val Borbera study [54] and the Nijmegen Biomedical Studies [55].

The impact of hepcidin–ferroportin interaction in iron homeostasis is shown in Figure 2.

3.2. Erythropoiesis Suppression

Pro-inflammatory cytokines, especially interferons and TNFα, appear to inhibit the proliferation and differentiation of erythroid progenitor cells, leading to ineffective erythropoiesis as a result [56].

Early inflammatory responses include leukocytosis and the increased production of leukocytes in the marrow, which is manifested by an increased number of myeloid precursors (>4:1 myeloid to erythroid precursors ratio). Inflammatory cytokines such as TNF-α [57] and interferon-γ [58] activate the transcription factor PU.1 and trigger bone marrow reprogramming, which promotes myelopoiesis and lymphopoiesis while suppressing erythropoiesis. Inflammatory cytokines also inhibit the ability of BFU-E to generate more differentiated erythroid cells [59,60].

Another bone marrow-reprogramming mechanism involves inflammation-induced suppression of erythropoietin production, the primary hormone responsible for erythropoiesis. In patients with systemic inflammation, serum erythropoietin levels are lower compared to the individuals with a similar degree of iron-deficiency anemia [61,62]. Inflammation also impairs the responsiveness of erythroid precursors to erythropoietin, as evidenced by increased exogenous erythropoietin requirements in end-stage kidney disease patients with inflammation [63,64]. Resistance to erythropoietin is partly mediated by a decrease in the number of erythropoietin receptors on erythroid progenitors, whose proliferative capacity is therefore reduced, which is a recently discovered effect of hypoferremia [65].

The Klotho enzyme, which is mainly expressed in humans in the kidney and brain by the KL gene, especially its alpha-Klotho variant activated by fibroblast growth factor 23 (FGF23), has been indicated as another potential cause of inflammatory anemia in old age [66,67]. Most of the early as well as current studies have focused on the role of alpha-Klotho in chronic kidney disease (CKD) in elderly populations, and reported an age-related Klotho reduction and association with increased likelihood of anemia [68]. Klotho is involved in hematopoiesis regulation through its impact on the hypoxia-inducible factor (HIF1α) pathway. Its deficiency interferes with hematopoietic stem cell development and erythropoiesis [69]. Klotho has the ability to modulate inflammation and oxidative stress through various mechanisms. As a suppressor gene of aging, Klotho protein expression, among other things, reduces phosphorus, ROS, and slows age-related renal fibrosis [70,71]. Increased Klotho levels could also potentially contribute to inflammation and anemia reduction in the elderly [70].

The production of erythropoietin, a major cytokine that affects the development of red blood cells, is triggered by a mechanism that detects low oxygen levels in anemia conditions. The relationship between the impaired response of hematopoietic stem cells to EPO and the development of anemia was observed in elderly patients [72]. The Baltimore Longitudinal Study on Aging [73] reported that EPO levels increased with age in healthy individuals without anemia, particularly in those without diabetes or hypertension. Conversely, individuals with anemia demonstrated a lower rate of EPO increase, suggesting that anemia is linked to a failure in the normal compensatory rise of EPO levels during aging. Although low EPO levels have specifically been associated with unexplained anemia in the elderly population, the exact cause of the inadequate EPO response is still unknown. Therefore, further studies on larger samples of elderly patients are necessary to confirm these findings [73]. A study by Chencheng et al. [68] suggested that low serum Klotho levels were associated with an increased likelihood of anemia in middle-aged and older adults regardless of kidney disease.

Overall, the age-dependent impairment of EPO response suggests a progressive resistance of hematopoietic stem cells to EPO as individuals age. The underlying reasons are yet to be determined, however, they could be attributed to impairments in normal EPO-dependent pathways caused by inflammatory cytokines, age-related comorbidities, declines in renal function, or a combination of these factors [74].

3.3. Shorter Erythrocyte Lifespan

The available studies on anemia of inflammation have consistently reported a moderate reduction (approximately 2–5%) in the lifespan of red blood cells with a decrease to approximately 90 days. However, a shortened erythrocyte lifespan was also observed in many cases of non-anemic inflammation, which indicates that anemia develops only when the compensatory response of red blood cell production is impaired [75].

The shortened lifespan of erythrocytes during inflammation has been ascribed to macrophage activation triggered by inflammatory cytokines, which results in premature phagocytosis and erythrocyte elimination. Macrocytic anemia and heightened erythrophagocytosis are prominent manifestations observed in macrophage activation syndromes, particularly those associated with systemic juvenile rheumatoid arthritis [76]. Multiple cytokines including interferon-γ and IL-4 have been implicated in macrophage activation for erythrophagocytosis in mouse models [57,77].

Except for rare cases of fulminant hemophagocytic states, erythrophagocytosis in anemia of inflammation exhibits only a mild increase, and the increase could easily be compensated if the production of erythrocytes is unimpaired [78,79].

Furthermore, the inflammatory cascade involves the generation of reactive oxygen and nitrogen species, shaping the intricate interrelationship between inflammation and the behavior of erythrocytes in the circulatory system. The oxidative stress within the vascular bed exerts multifaceted effects on the structural integrity of red blood cells, characterized by lipid peroxidation and the oxidation of membrane skeletal proteins. These biochemical alterations do not only compromise the molecular architecture of red blood cell membranes, but they also have profound implications for their functional properties [80–83].

The consequence of oxidative stress-induced modifications extends beyond mere structural compromise, significantly impacting the physiological characteristics of red blood cells. Notably, the reduction in osmotic resistance and deformability of red blood cells has emerged as a pivotal outcome of oxidative stress in the vascular microenvironment [84]. The compromised osmotic resistance renders erythrocytes more susceptible to premature removal from circulation as their resilience to environmental challenges diminishes [81,82,85,86].

The intricate relationship between oxidative stress and red blood cell dynamics underscores the accelerated elimination of these cells from the circulatory system. This phenomenon, although crucial in our understanding of broader implications of inflammation-induced alterations, unfortunately remains unexplored in the current discourse. An in-depth exploration of this aspect of oxidative stress is imperative for our thorough comprehension of the intricate mechanisms underpinning anemia in the context of inflammation.

Figure 3 provides a comprehensive overview of the interconnected processes contributing to inflammation-induced anemia. The schematic representation serves as a visual guide to illustrating the complex dynamics involving the key elements in the pathogenesis of inflammation-associated anemia.

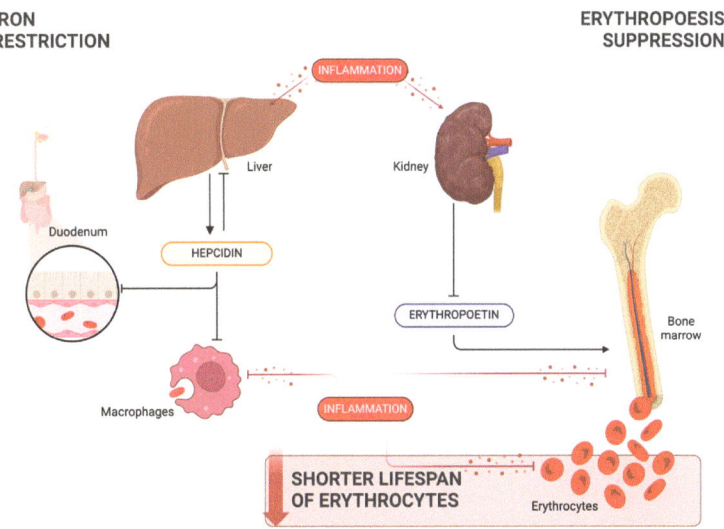

Figure 3. Overview of the processes linked to inflammation-induced anemia: iron restriction (yellow background), erythropoiesis suppression (blue background), and shortened erythrocyte lifespan (red background). Created with BioRender.com (accessed on 9 March 2024).

4. Diseases Associated with Anemia in Older Adults

Anemia in older adults has a multifactorial cause. Consequently, there are no and major and clear-cut contributors to anemia in the elderly. Overlapping diseases leading to multimorbidity and an increased risk of frailty syndrome make the identification of the causes of anemia even more challenging [87,88]. Nonetheless, the disease entities that are associated with reduced synthesis, disruption of normal hematopoiesis to achieve the desired volume and number of red blood cells and hemoglobin content, can be included in the list of potential anemia-inducing conditions. This section discusses the most common diseases associated with anemia in older adults. As depicted in Table 2, there are numerous common diseases prevalent among the elderly that have the potential to lead to anemia. Understanding these diseases is vital for health care professionals to accurately diagnose and manage anemia in this population.

The commonly reported reasons include the increased risk of nutritional disorders due to an excessive intake or negative balance in dietary supply of energy, nutrients, vitamins, and the inability to replenish the effects of catabolic processes [89]. Cachexia, defined as disease-related malnutrition (DRM) with inflammation in the ESPEN guidelines on definitions and terminology of clinical nutrition [90], has been reported in relevant analyses.

The process of aging is associated with epigenetic changes that lead to somatic mutations of cells beginning with pluripotent hematopoietic stem cells (PHSCs), which are further growth pathways in hematopoiesis. These alterations result in shorter erythrocyte lifespan and increased eryptosis rate. As a consequence, augmented oxidative stress increases inflammation and the risk of age-related chronic diseases as well as hematopoietic disorders [91,92]. The progressive deterioration of kidney and liver function in elderly populations is a key element in the development of anemia and it involves: firstly, macroscopic changes, mainly a lower mass of the organs and, secondly, microscopic pathological tissue and cells changes such as atherosclerosis of capillaries, atrophy, fibrosis, and collagen deposition. Functional and structural changes in the aging organs increase the probability of erythropoiesis suppression [93–95].

Table 2. Examples of common diseases potentially leading to anemia in older adults.

Chronic inflammatory diseases	Pulmonary infectious Infective endocarditis Chronic urinary tract infection Chronic liver diseases Arthritis Chronic fungal infections COPD Chronic kidney disease Chronic heart failure Atherosclerosis
Autoimmune disorders	Rheumatoid arthritis Rheumatic fever Vasculitis Sarcoidosis
Hematological diseases	ICUS, CCUS, IDUS, CHIP, MDS Aplastic anemia
Cancer disease	Hematological malignancy, lymphomas, solid tumors
Endocrinological and metabolic diseases	Metabolic syndrome Overweight Sarcopenia Cachexia Malnutrition
Gastrointestinal diseases	Esophagitis, gastroenteritis, peptic ulcers, ulcerative colitis—GI bleeding Intestinal malabsorption syndrome (lactose, gluten intolerance) Celiac disease *Helicobacter pylori, Clostridioides difficile* Dysbiosis
Nutritional deficiency	B12, folic acid, vitamin D Amino acids Iron, zinc, selenium, copper,
Drug-induced anemia	Antibiotics, NSAIDs Proton pump inhibitors (PPIs), Chemotherapy Radiotherapy Polypharmacy

Abbreviations: CCUS, clonal cytopenia of unknown significance; CHIP, clonal hematopoiesis of indeterminate potential; COPD, chronic obstructive pulmonary disease; GI, gastrointestinal; ICUS, idiopathic cytopenia of undetermined significance; IDUS, idiopathic dysplasia of undetermined significance; MDS, myelodysplastic syndromes; NSAIDs, non-steroidal anti-inflammatory drugs.

4.1. Hematopoietic Disorders

Hematopoiesis-regulating mechanisms that involve players such as cytokines, chemokines, hormones, adhesion molecules, and transcription factors occur at each stage of the cell lines, ranging from the process of renewal, through differentiation to maturation of blood cells. However, the process of aging is linked to the impairment to the processes of self-renewal, differentiation, proliferation, and maturation of cells involved in hematopoiesis.

Age-related progressive changes such as epigenetic alterations, genetic instability, telomere shortening, and accumulation of p53 damage have all been reported to affect cellular aging [96,97]. Progressive somatic mutations cause an increase in clonal hematopoiesis of indeterminate potential (CHIP) in an average of 25% of the human population aged over 65 years, with a further increase observed with aging. The most common mutations concern the following genes: DNMT3A, TET2, ASXL1, JAK2, SF3B1, and TP53 [33,98–100]. Clonal changes correlate with increased heterogeneity of the cell size indices such as the red cell distribution width (RDW) [100]. These findings have been supported by recent genome-wide association studies. Furthermore, studies have also demonstrated correlations with an increase in inflammatory markers such as CRP, IL-1b, and IL-18, but with a decrease in hemoglobin [98,99,101]. These somatic mutations result in an increased risk of chronic diseases typical of old age, myeloproliferative diseases, and mortality.

Changes associated with clonal hematopoiesis can also lead to aplastic anemias [102]. Along with changes in the cell population in the hematopoietic lineage, the bone marrow undergoes conversion from hematopoietically active red marrow to hematopoietically inactive yellow bone marrow [103]. A decrease in bone density and disturbances to homeostasis in osteoblast–osteoclast communication are also correlated with an increased risk of anemia in elderly people [104].

Consequently, the balance between new erythrocyte formation and their erythrophagocytosis and hemolysis is disrupted and can lead to a decrease in the number of erythrocytes in the bloodstream. Since oxidative stress is known to affect erythrocyte lifespan, one of the hypotheses for anemia involves the activity of reactive oxygen species on erythrocytes in the course of chronic inflammation in a progressive process of aging.

In the 1980s, Tozzi-Ciancarelli and Fedele showed that the structural properties of erythrocytes differed between older and young adults [105]. The age-related accumulation of defective proteins has further consequences for hematopoiesis, ultimately creating defects in the structure of reticulocytes and erythrocytes such as changes in the spectrin-4.1-actin complex, cytoskeleton structure, glycocalyx, and band protein III, which causes hemolysis [106–110].

4.2. Kidney Disease

Chronic kidney disease was defined by the KDIGO (Kidney Disease; Improving Global Outcomes) 2012 Clinical Practice Guideline for the Evaluation and Management of Chronic Kidney Disease as a progressive abnormality of kidney structure and function, a condition leading to end-stage renal disease requiring renal replacement therapy [111]. Uremia progression is accompanied by an increase in chronic inflammation and oxidative stress. The processes of hematopoiesis and eryptosis are therefore disrupted by the accumulation of pro-inflammatory molecules such as CRP, NOS, ROS, IL-1, IL-6, TNF-α, and other inflammatory mediators. Normal nephron functioning deteriorates with age, as shown by a decrease in the glomerular filtration rate (GFR) in the aging population. In a population study of 12,381 Germans, Waas and Schulz [112] recorded a decrease by 1 mL/min/m^2 estimated GFR (eGFR) per year from the third decade of life. The increased risk of developing progressive nephropathy includes age-related chronic diseases such as hypertension, diabetes, and glomerulonephritis [113]. An epidemiological study by Kovesda et al. [114] recorded 25.3% prevalence of anemia in people with stages 3–5 CKD (eGFR < 60 mL/min/1.73 m^2). With regard to age groups, anemia was more likely to develop in patients aged $\geq$75 years, who also demonstrated a significant correlation with lower mean hemoglobin concentrations. According to Stauffer et al. [115], anemia was twice as prevalent in people with CKD as in the general population (15.4% vs. 7.6%, respectively).

The phenomena of polypharmacy and polypragmasy, which belong to the risk factors for kidney disease, are frequently recorded in the elderly [116]. Increased use of drugs available without prescription, primarily, non-steroidal anti-inflammatory drugs (NSAIDs), herbal remedies, and dietary supplements can lead to drug-induced nephrotoxicity [117] with potential consequences being acute kidney injury (AKI), possibly leading to irreversible CKD [118].

Other risk factors of AKI and CKD progression include water–electrolyte disturbances. Older adults belong to the age group at increased risk of disruption of physiological homeostasis such as thirst control disturbances and water–electrolyte imbalance. Dysfunction of central nervous system mechanisms of thirst control results in reduced thirst in response to current water–electrolyte needs [119,120]. These tendencies toward dehydration are the risk factors for hemodynamic weakness, which significantly contributes to the increased risk of kidney damage [121,122].

Erythropoietin, the major regulator in erythropoiesis renewal, is prenatally synthesized in the liver, but hepatic EPO production is switched to the kidneys and taken over perinatally by peritubular interstitial fibroblasts (which belong to renal erythropoietin-producing cells (REPCs)) [123]. In chronic kidney disease, the number of REPCs is reduced due to their differentiation into myofibroblasts, which lose their ability to produce EPO. Therefore, an insufficient number of hypoxia-inducible factor (HIF)-sensitive REPCs in response to hypoxic stimuli causes an EPO decrease and erythropoiesis, leading to the development of anemia [124].

Vlasschaert et al. [125] observed more rapid development of progressive chronic kidney disease and greater severity of anemia in patients with previous CKD and current CHIP.

4.3. Hormonal Factors

Hormonal regulation is also affected by age-related changes, which pertains to both genders: menopausal and postmenopausal changes in women and andropausal transition in men have been widely investigated. In both genders, a reduction in circulating estrogen and testosterone plasma levels have been recorded. An age-related decrease in muscle mass due to lower testosterone levels also results in reduced sensitivity of erythropoietin forming [126,127]. Significant correlations between sarcopenia and anemia were detected in population-based studies [128–130]. A reduction in erythropoiesis may also result from decreased thyroid hormonal activity, which slows down the anabolic hormone level. Fatigue, weakness, and loss of appetite are among the significant effects of decreased numbers of blood erythrocytes [131].

With aging, the endocrine abnormalities decrease the production of hormones and consequently affect red blood cell homeostasis. A potential impact of anabolic hormones (IGF-1, testosterone, TSH, T3, T4) on hepcidin regulation and the expression of progenitor cells involved in hematopoiesis has been recorded [132] The late-onset hypogonadism in andropausal elderly males and hypoestrogenism in postmenopausal elderly females are the hormonal factors that potentially contribute to anemia development. Adequate plasma testosterone levels modulate pro-inflammatory cytokines, mainly IL-6, which ensure appropriate hepcidin levels and proper hematopoietic cell differentiation without clonal cells. These are the elements that favorably affect the hemoglobin and hematocrit levels in older men [133,134]. Reduced testosterone levels correlate with a negative response to erythropoiesis-stimulating factors [135].

It should be noted, however, that in elderly patients with prostate cancer treated with hormone replacement therapy (androgen deprivation), radiotherapy, and brachytherapy procedures, their hemoglobin levels were observed to fall by an average of 1–2.5 g/dL, which should not be directly linked to inflammatory processes and anemia [132,136].

Progenitor cells contain estrogen receptors (ER-α and ER-β) that are influenced by estrogen during differentiation [137]. Zhou and Tseng [138] showed that estrogen regulated erythropoiesis by ROS and NOS modulation on the progenitor erythroid cells, which affected proliferation and differentiation. The research conducted to date has also confirmed the protective cardiovascular effects of estrogens in women as their NOS and ROS-modulating activity produces anti-inflammatory effects [139]. Moreover, estrogen has an erythropoiesis-stimulating effect on bone marrow stem cells, which has been proven to support erythrocyte count and hemoglobin levels in pregnant women [140].

Estrogens participate in the estrogen–iron axis through their ability to inhibit hepcidin formation. A decrease in hepcidin results in an increase in iron storage, while an inflammation-induced increase of hepcidin levels, among other factors, negatively affects iron metabolism.

4.4. Gastrointestinal Diseases

Gastrointestinal (GI) changes are common in the elderly, with some GI disorders being more prevalent in this age group such as changes in the oral cavity, esophagitis, gastroesophageal reflux disease (GERD), chronic atrophic gastritis, Clostridioides difficile and Helicobacter pylori infection, peptic ulcer disease, celiac disease, small bowel bleeding, angiodysplasias, small bowel ulcers, inflammatory bowel disease (IBD), small intestinal bacterial overgrowth (SIBO), abdominal hernia, constipation, and diarrheal illnesses [141].

Decreased production of pepsin and hydrochloric acid limits the bioavailability of dietary and supplementary vitamin B12 [141,142]. Examples of bioavailability limitations include the use of acid suppressants to protect against medication side-effects (mainly NSAIDs), the presence of gastritis and/or duodenal inflammation, and esophageal disorders. Age-associated changes to intestinal epithelial cells and enterocyte function may result in insufficient nutrient absorption [143]. These limitations are also related to the higher prevalence of celiac disease in the elderly, reaching from 4 to about 25 percent [144]. In fact, this difference may be due to delayed diagnosis for celiac disease, mainly because of the atypical clinical manifestations of this enteropathy [141,143,145]. A higher incidence of hernias, adhesions, diverticulosis, and risk of obstruction may also contribute to bacterial overgrowth (SIBO) and chronic intestinal inflammation. Diverticular disease is rare in the general population, but it was found to affect 65% of people aged ≥65 years [141,146,147].

Abnormal hematological indicators such as inflammation-related normocytic anemia occur in approximately half of patients with hepatic cirrhosis [148]. Hepcidin plays a major role in hepatic disorders due to iron restriction. On the other hand, information regarding patients with cirrhosis is limited, and there is debate about the plasma erythropoietin (EPO) levels in these individuals. It is plausible that EPO elevation could be a result of renal hypoperfusion, hypoxia, anemia, or a hepato-protective and regenerative mechanism mediated by EPO. In contrast, inadequate EPO response in advanced cirrhosis might be attributed to poor hepatic synthesis capacity, decreasing co-factor levels, and inflammatory feedback mechanisms. Ultimately, the source of a potential increase in EPO production during certain stages of cirrhosis—whether from the kidney or liver—remains a lingering question [149].

While some changes associated with an aging GI system are physiologic, others are pathological and particularly more prevalent among those above 65 years of age [141]. Such GI diseases increase the risk of gastrointestinal bleeding.

Diseases of the gastrointestinal tract in old age are among the main causes of anemia due to the reduced absorption of micro- and macronutrients necessary for cell synthesis in erythropoiesis up to the erythrocytes themselves. It is challenging to unequivocally demonstrate anemia in the elderly as a result of chronic inflammation due to the overlapping causes of anemia such as disorders, impaired iron absorption, and the intake of other micronutrients.

4.5. Intestinal Dysbiosis

Our microbiota is subject to constant variation over our life course. The risk of intestinal dysbiosis (i.e., a significant reduction in beneficial microorganisms and an increase in opportunistic or pathobiont microbes in the gastrointestinal tract) is on the increase in old age depending on our health status, lifestyle, previous illnesses, and general inflammation [150,151]. Intestinal epithelial barrier dysfunction and increased permeability with aging, previously confirmed only in patients with inflammatory bowel diseases, have raised particular concerns. This is especially relevant for individuals with inflammatory bowel disease, nutritional deficiencies, overweight, metabolic syndrome, or those undergoing antibiotic therapy [152].

Josefsdottir et al. [153] demonstrated that the gut microbiota supports adequate hematopoiesis. Previous hypotheses suggested a signaling model involving the gut microbiome and the bone marrow.

The gut microbiome–macrophage–iron axis recently discovered by Zhang and Gao [154] shows that microbiota-derived metabolites increase iron availability in a manner dependent on bone marrow macrophage erythrophagocytosis, which affects hematopoietic differentiation and blood regeneration. These include STAT1 signaling, type I IFN signaling in hematopoietic cells [155]. The presence of a favorable gut microbiota population ensuring adequate synthesis of short-chain fatty acids (SCFAs) such as acetate, butyrate, and propionate may contribute to erythrophagocytosis and favorable hematopoietic regeneration [156–158]. Soriano-Lerma and García-Burgos [159] reported a potential mediatory function of SCFAs in iron absorption, and possibly in anemia status modulation. A gradual increase in unfavorable intestinal microbiota contributes to an increased risk of intestinal absorption disorders in the elderly [143,160].

4.6. Autoimmune Diseases

The risk of chronic inflammation including autoimmunization increases with age. Paradoxically, an increase in the incidence of new autoimmune pathologies in all autoimmune diseases has not been recorded in older adults [161]. A recent population-based study by Conrad et al. [162] confirmed that they occurred almost twice as often in women as in men, and the mean age of diagnosis was 54 years. Only in entities such as Graves' disease, pernicious anemia, and rheumatoid arthritis (RA) did the risk increase with age. For the other diseases (coeliac disease, inflammatory bowel disease and vasculitis), the incidence reached three different peaks: in childhood, early adulthood, and old age.

Even if we assume that the components of immunescence such as chronic inflammation, increased production of autoantibodies, and a decline in the immune response are most likely to be chronic autoimmunity rather than autoimmune diseases, they are still potential contributors to anemia in the elderly [163,164]. Some scientific reports support the link between anemia and autoimmune diseases, however, other causes of anemia should be considered such as anti-inflammatory drugs, glucocorticosteroids, biologic drugs that reduce iron-bioavailability and other essential micro- and macro-nutrients for erythropoiesis, or increased macrophage release [165]. This hypothesis may be supported by the decrease in Hb levels in RA, and the degree of clinical exacerbation of rheumatic disease. However, more research is needed into the relationships between anemia and autoimmunity and autoimmune diseases in older adults, taking into account confounding factors such as the use of medications that increase the risk of gastrointestinal diseases and limit bioavailability as well as other chronic diseases (e.g., CKD, hematological diseases, malnutrition, or hepatic diseases) [165–169].

Numerous research papers have reported that erythropoiesis-enhancing treatment reduced the severity of autoimmune diseases [170–174]. However, the conclusions should be treated with caution, as in some autoimmune diseases, EPO may produce pro-inflammatory or anti-inflammatory effects [175].

It is possible that the response of B and T lymphocytes in the autoimmunity process is potentially related to the increased risk of stress erythropoiesis, which does not allow older people to keep pace with the demand for erythrocytes [176,177].

5. Summary

Extensive studies on anemia in older adults have revealed significant outcomes including increased mortality, hospitalization rates, frailty, falls, mobility limitations, cognitive decline, dementia, functional dependence, and reduced quality of life. These findings are consistent across major cohort studies that excluded individuals with other conditions [6,178–181]. The multifactorial and highly prevalent nature of anemia in older adults is directly correlated with age. While the degree of anemia is mostly mild in the ambulatory setting, institutionalized patients exhibit higher rates of anemia of increased severity.

Aging-related changes are evident in the frequent occurrence of both anemia and indicators of inflammation in the elderly. It is crucial to recognize the interconnectedness of anemia and inflammaging, as they are, to some extent, manifestations of the same biological processes such as elevated levels of various proinflammatory mediators. Both conditions, anemia and inflammation, contribute to a heightened mortality risk, with the underlying causes of decreased survival likely stemming from a variety of factors. To enhance the clinical management of individual patients, a deeper understanding of the molecular mechanisms driving anemia and inflammation is essential. Our perspective emphasizes the need for personalized care based on the comprehensive clinical context when dealing with elderly patients.

A critical facet involves recalibrating reference values for older adults for key hematological parameters such as hemoglobin and hematocrit to align with the unique physiological changes associated with aging. This should make the diagnostic process more accurate and reflective of the health status of older individuals. Moreover, a diagnostic panel should be devised to encompass a spectrum of markers essential for comprehensive anemia assessment in older age. In addition to conventional indicators, special attention should be directed to hepcidin and inflammatory biomarkers such as CRP and cytokines such as IL-1β and TNF-α [52]. These indicators provide a more nuanced insight into the underlying causes of anemia, enabling tailored interventions that could address specific clinical conditions common in the elderly population.

Stratifying the elderly population into distinct age groups is another crucial modification proposal in the diagnostic approach. While anemia can affect individuals at various life stages, placing emphasis on those aged 65 and above recognizes the increased susceptibility to anemia-related issues in this demographic. Moreover, pinpointing high-risk groups such as individuals with specific chronic diseases ensures targeted and more frequent screenings for those who need it the most. Notably, persons aged 80 and above as well as institutionalized patients require even more vigilant monitoring, considering their advanced age and higher vulnerability to potential anemia-associated complications.

Moving beyond diagnostic measures, the multifaceted nature of combating anemia in the elderly necessitates the consideration of both non-pharmacological and pharmacological interventions. Non-pharmacological strategies, particularly dietary adjustments, have emerged as a cornerstone in anemia management.

However, when pharmacological interventions are warranted, a judicious approach is essential. Considering the likelihood of elderly individuals already being on a myriad of medications, potential interactions must be carefully evaluated.

In essence, addressing anemia in the elderly requires a meticulous balance between comprehensive diagnostic measures and tailored interventions. By embracing these modifications in diagnostic testing and intervention strategies, health care professionals can navigate the complexities of anemia management in older individuals with greater precision and efficacy.

We ought to incorporate every accessible data found in the Clinical Practice Guidelines, which shall support the comprehensive management of these patients through a multidisciplinary and multimodal approach.

This review provides valuable insights that can guide future endeavors in refining the approach to anemia in the elderly, ultimately contributing to improved health care outcomes for this demographic population.

Author Contributions: Conceptualization, E.W.; Writing—Original Draft Preparation, E.W. and J.N.; Visualization, E.W. and J.N.; Supervision, A.Z.-L. and P.J.; Funding Acquisition, A.Z.-L. and P.J. All authors have read and agreed to the published version of the manuscript.

Funding: This work was supported by funds from the University of Zielona Gora (No. 2023/2024 Ministry of Science and High Education, Poland).

Conflicts of Interest: The authors declare no conflicts of interest.

References

1. Guralnik, J.M.; Eisenstaedt, R.S.; Ferrucci, L.; Klein, H.G.; Woodman, R.C. Prevalence of Anemia in Persons 65 Years and Older in the United States: Evidence for a High Rate of Unexplained Anemia. *Blood* **2004**, *104*, 2263–2268. [CrossRef]
2. Aunan, J.R.; Watson, M.M.; Hagland, H.R.; Søreide, K. Molecular and Biological Hallmarks of Ageing. *Br. J. Surg.* **2016**, *103*, e29–e46. [CrossRef]
3. WHO Scientific Group on Nutritional Anaemias; World Health Organization. *Nutritional Anaemias: Report of a WHO Scientific Group [Meeting Held in Geneva from 13 to 17 March 1967]*; World Health Organization: Geneva, Switzerland, 1968.
4. Shavelle, R.M.; MacKenzie, R.; Paculdo, D.R. Anemia and Mortality in Older Persons: Does the Type of Anemia Affect Survival? *Int. J. Hematol.* **2012**, *95*, 248–256. [CrossRef]
5. Beutler, E.; Waalen, J. The Definition of Anemia: What Is the Lower Limit of Normal of the Blood Hemoglobin Concentration? *Blood* **2006**, *107*, 1747–1750. [CrossRef]
6. Zakai, N.A.; Katz, R.; Hirsch, C.; Shlipak, M.G.; Chaves, P.H.M.; Newman, A.B.; Cushman, M. A Prospective Study of Anemia Status, Hemoglobin Concentration, and Mortality in an Elderly Cohort: The Cardiovascular Health Study. *Arch. Intern. Med.* **2005**, *165*, 2214–2220. [CrossRef]
7. Culleton, B.F.; Manns, B.J.; Zhang, J.; Tonelli, M.; Klarenbach, S.; Hemmelgarn, B.R. Impact of Anemia on Hospitalization and Mortality in Older Adults. *Blood* **2006**, *107*, 3841–3846. [CrossRef]
8. Wouters, H.J.C.M.; van der Klauw, M.M.; de Witte, T.; Stauder, R.; Swinkels, D.W.; Wolffenbuttel, B.H.R.; Huls, G. Association of Anemia with Health-Related Quality of Life and Survival: A Large Population-Based Cohort Study. *Haematologica* **2019**, *104*, 468–476. [CrossRef]
9. Teissier, T.; Boulanger, E.; Cox, L.S. Interconnections between Inflammageing and Immunosenescence during Ageing. *Cells* **2022**, *11*, 359. [CrossRef]
10. Brognara, L.; Luna, O.C.; Traina, F.; Cauli, O. Inflammatory Biomarkers and Gait Impairment in Older Adults: A Systematic Review. *Int. J. Mol. Sci.* **2024**, *25*, 1368. [CrossRef] [PubMed]
11. Nemeth, E.; Ganz, T. Anemia of Inflammation. *Hematol./Oncol. Clin. N. Am.* **2014**, *28*, 671–681. [CrossRef] [PubMed]
12. Liberale, L.; Badimon, L.; Montecucco, F.; Lüscher, T.F.; Libby, P.; Camici, G.G. Inflammation, Aging, and Cardiovascular Disease. *J. Am. Coll. Cardiol.* **2022**, *79*, 837–847. [CrossRef] [PubMed]
13. Gaskell, H.; Derry, S.; Andrew Moore, R.; McQuay, H.J. Prevalence of Anaemia in Older Persons: Systematic Review. *BMC Geriatr.* **2008**, *8*, 1. [CrossRef] [PubMed]
14. Bach, V.; Schruckmayer, G.; Sam, I.; Kemmler, G.; Stauder, R. Prevalence and Possible Causes of Anemia in the Elderly: A Cross-Sectional Analysis of a Large European University Hospital Cohort. *Clin. Interv. Aging* **2014**, *9*, 1187–1196. [CrossRef] [PubMed]
15. Sahin, S.; Tasar, P.T.; Simsek, H.; Çiçek, Z.; Eskiizmirli, H.; Aykar, F.S.; Sahin, F.; Akcicek, F. Prevalence of Anemia and Malnutrition and Their Association in Elderly Nursing Home Residents. *Aging Clin. Exp. Res.* **2016**, *28*, 857–862. [CrossRef] [PubMed]
16. Robalo Nunes, A.; Fonseca, C.; Marques, F.; Belo, A.; Brilhante, D.; Cortez, J. Prevalence of Anemia and Iron Deficiency in Older Portuguese Adults: An EMPIRE Substudy. *Geriatr. Gerontol. Int.* **2017**, *17*, 1814–1822. [CrossRef] [PubMed]
17. Zaninetti, C.; Klersy, C.; Scavariello, C.; Bastia, R.; Balduini, C.L.; Invernizzi, R. Prevalence of Anemia in Hospitalized Internal Medicine Patients: Correlations with Comorbidities and Length of Hospital Stay. *Eur. J. Intern. Med.* **2018**, *51*, 11–17. [CrossRef] [PubMed]
18. Muñoz, M.; Laso-Morales, M.J.; Gómez-Ramírez, S.; Cadellas, M.; Núñez-Matas, M.J.; García-Erce, J.A. Pre-Operative Haemoglobin Levels and Iron Status in a Large Multicentre Cohort of Patients Undergoing Major Elective Surgery. *Anaesthesia* **2017**, *72*, 826–834. [CrossRef]
19. Artz, A.S.; Fergusson, D.; Drinka, P.J.; Gerald, M.; Gravenstein, S.; Lechich, A.; Silverstone, F.; Finnigan, S.; Janowski, M.C.; McCamish, M.A.; et al. Prevalence of Anemia in Skilled-Nursing Home Residents. *Arch. Gerontol. Geriatr.* **2004**, *39*, 201–206. [CrossRef]
20. Migone De Amicis, M.; Poggiali, E.; Motta, I.; Minonzio, F.; Fabio, G.; Hu, C.; Cappellini, M.D. Anemia in Elderly Hospitalized Patients: Prevalence and Clinical Impact. *Intern. Emerg. Med.* **2015**, *10*, 581–586. [CrossRef]
21. Nathavitharana, R.L.; Murray, J.A.; D'Sousa, N.; Sheehan, T.; Frampton, C.M.; Baker, B.W. Anaemia Is Highly Prevalent among Unselected Internal Medicine Inpatients and Is Associated with Increased Mortality, Earlier Readmission and More Prolonged Hospital Stay: An Observational Retrospective Cohort Study. *Intern. Med. J.* **2012**, *42*, 683–691. [CrossRef]
22. Weiss, G.; Goodnough, L.T. Anemia of Chronic Disease. *N. Engl. J. Med.* **2005**, *352*, 1011–1023. [CrossRef]
23. Keller, C.R.; Odden, M.C.; Fried, L.F.; Newman, A.B.; Angleman, S.; Green, C.A.; Cummings, S.R.; Harris, T.B.; Shlipak, M.G. Kidney Function and Markers of Inflammation in Elderly Persons without Chronic Kidney Disease: The Health, Aging, and Body Composition Study. *Kidney Int.* **2007**, *71*, 239–244. [CrossRef]
24. Patel, K.V. Epidemiology of Anemia in Older Adults. *Semin. Hematol.* **2008**, *45*, 210–217. [CrossRef]
25. Stauder, R.; Valent, P.; Theurl, I. Anemia at Older Age: Etiologies, Clinical Implications, and Management. *Blood* **2018**, *131*, 505–514. [CrossRef]
26. Melzer, D.; Pilling, L.C.; Ferrucci, L. The Genetics of Human Ageing. *Nat. Rev. Genet.* **2020**, *21*, 88–101. [CrossRef]
27. Wang, H.; Lou, D.; Wang, Z. Crosstalk of Genetic Variants, Allele-Specific DNA Methylation, and Environmental Factors for Complex Disease Risk. *Front. Genet.* **2018**, *9*, 695. [CrossRef]

28. Langie, S.A.S.; Koppen, G.; Desaulniers, D.; Al-Mulla, F.; Al-Temaimi, R.; Amedei, A.; Azqueta, A.; Bisson, W.H.; Brown, D.G.; Brunborg, G.; et al. Causes of Genome Instability: The Effect of Low Dose Chemical Exposures in Modern Society. *Carcinogenesis* **2015**, *36* (Suppl. S1), S61–S88. [CrossRef]
29. Cooke, M.S.; Evans, M.D.; Dizdaroglu, M.; Lunec, J. Oxidative DNA Damage: Mechanisms, Mutation, and Disease. *FASEB J.* **2003**, *17*, 1195–1214. [CrossRef]
30. Wei, Y.; Giunta, S.; Xia, S. Hypoxia in Aging and Aging-Related Diseases: Mechanism and Therapeutic Strategies. *Int. J. Mol. Sci.* **2022**, *23*, 8165. [CrossRef]
31. Kay, J.; Thadhani, E.; Samson, L.; Engelward, B. Inflammation-Induced DNA Damage, Mutations and Cancer. *DNA Repair* **2019**, *83*, 102673. [CrossRef]
32. Liu, W.; Deng, Y.; Li, Z.; Chen, Y.; Zhu, X.; Tan, X.; Cao, G. Cancer Evo-Dev: A Theory of Inflammation-Induced Oncogenesis. *Front. Immunol.* **2021**, *12*, 768098. [CrossRef]
33. Jaiswal, S.; Ebert, B.L. Clonal Hematopoiesis in Human Aging and Disease. *Science* **2019**, *366*, eaan4673. [CrossRef]
34. Mitchell, E.; Spencer Chapman, M.; Williams, N.; Dawson, K.J.; Mende, N.; Calderbank, E.F.; Jung, H.; Mitchell, T.; Coorens, T.H.H.; Spencer, D.H.; et al. Clonal Dynamics of Haematopoiesis across the Human Lifespan. *Nature* **2022**, *606*, 343–350. [CrossRef]
35. Morganti, C.; Ito, K. Mitochondrial Contributions to Hematopoietic Stem Cell Aging. *Int. J. Mol. Sci.* **2021**, *22*, 11117. [CrossRef]
36. Zampino, M.; Brennan, N.A.; Kuo, P.-L.; Spencer, R.G.; Fishbein, K.W.; Simonsick, E.M.; Ferrucci, L. Poor Mitochondrial Health and Systemic Inflammation? Test of a Classic Hypothesis in the Baltimore Longitudinal Study of Aging. *Geroscience* **2020**, *42*, 1175–1182. [CrossRef]
37. Yeo, E.-J. Hypoxia and Aging. *Exp. Mol. Med.* **2019**, *51*, 1–15. [CrossRef]
38. Lee, P.; Chandel, N.S.; Simon, M.C. Cellular Adaptation to Hypoxia through Hypoxia Inducible Factors and Beyond. *Nat. Rev. Mol. Cell Biol.* **2020**, *21*, 268–283. [CrossRef]
39. Tojo, Y.; Sekine, H.; Hirano, I.; Pan, X.; Souma, T.; Tsujita, T.; Kawaguchi, S.; Takeda, N.; Takeda, K.; Fong, G.-H.; et al. Hypoxia Signaling Cascade for Erythropoietin Production in Hepatocytes. *Mol. Cell. Biol.* **2015**, *35*, 2658–2672. [CrossRef]
40. Xia, S.; Zhang, X.; Zheng, S.; Khanabdali, R.; Kalionis, B.; Wu, J.; Wan, W.; Tai, X. An Update on Inflamm-Aging: Mechanisms, Prevention, and Treatment. *J. Immunol. Res.* **2016**, *2016*, 8426874. [CrossRef]
41. Franceschi, C.; Campisi, J. Chronic Inflammation (Inflammaging) and Its Potential Contribution to Age-Associated Diseases. *J. Gerontol. A Biol. Sci. Med. Sci.* **2014**, *69* (Suppl. S1), S4–S9. [CrossRef]
42. Wawrzyniak-Gramacka, E.; Hertmanowska, N.; Tylutka, A.; Morawin, B.; Wacka, E.; Gutowicz, M.; Zembron-Lacny, A. The Association of Anti-Inflammatory Diet Ingredients and Lifestyle Exercise with Inflammaging. *Nutrients* **2021**, *13*, 3696. [CrossRef] [PubMed]
43. Minciullo, P.L.; Catalano, A.; Mandraffino, G.; Casciaro, M.; Crucitti, A.; Maltese, G.; Morabito, N.; Lasco, A.; Gangemi, S.; Basile, G. Inflammaging and Anti-Inflammaging: The Role of Cytokines in Extreme Longevity. *Arch. Immunol. Ther. Exp.* **2016**, *64*, 111–126. [CrossRef] [PubMed]
44. Stefanova, D.; Raychev, A.; Deville, J.; Humphries, R.; Campeau, S.; Ruchala, P.; Nemeth, E.; Ganz, T.; Bulut, Y. Hepcidin Protects against Lethal Escherichia Coli Sepsis in Mice Inoculated with Isolates from Septic Patients. *Infect. Immun.* **2018**, *86*, e00253-18. [CrossRef]
45. Stefanova, D.; Raychev, A.; Arezes, J.; Ruchala, P.; Gabayan, V.; Skurnik, M.; Dillon, B.J.; Horwitz, M.A.; Ganz, T.; Bulut, Y.; et al. Endogenous Hepcidin and Its Agonist Mediate Resistance to Selected Infections by Clearing Non-Transferrin-Bound Iron. *Blood* **2017**, *130*, 245–257. [CrossRef] [PubMed]
46. Nemeth, E.; Ganz, T. The Role of Hepcidin in Iron Metabolism. *Acta Haematol.* **2009**, *122*, 78–86. [CrossRef] [PubMed]
47. Park, C.H.; Valore, E.V.; Waring, A.J.; Ganz, T. Hepcidin, a Urinary Antimicrobial Peptide Synthesized in the Liver. *J. Biol. Chem.* **2001**, *276*, 7806–7810. [CrossRef] [PubMed]
48. den Elzen, W.P.J.; de Craen, A.J.M.; Wiegerinck, E.T.; Westendorp, R.G.J.; Swinkels, D.W.; Gussekloo, J. Plasma Hepcidin Levels and Anemia in Old Age. The Leiden 85-Plus Study. *Haematologica* **2013**, *98*, 448–454. [CrossRef] [PubMed]
49. Donovan, A.; Lima, C.A.; Pinkus, J.L.; Pinkus, G.S.; Zon, L.I.; Robine, S.; Andrews, N.C. The Iron Exporter Ferroportin/Slc40a1 Is Essential for Iron Homeostasis. *Cell Metab.* **2005**, *1*, 191–200. [CrossRef] [PubMed]
50. Nemeth, E.; Tuttle, M.S.; Powelson, J.; Vaughn, M.B.; Donovan, A.; Ward, D.M.; Ganz, T.; Kaplan, J. Hepcidin Regulates Cellular Iron Efflux by Binding to Ferroportin and Inducing Its Internalization. *Science* **2004**, *306*, 2090–2093. [CrossRef]
51. Ganz, T. Anemia of Inflammation. *N. Engl. J. Med.* **2019**, *381*, 1148–1157. [CrossRef]
52. Wacka, E.; Wawrzyniak-Gramacka, E.; Tylutka, A.; Morawin, B.; Gutowicz, M.; Zembron-Lacny, A. The Role of Inflammation in Age-Associated Changes in Red Blood System. *Int. J. Mol. Sci.* **2023**, *24*, 8944. [CrossRef] [PubMed]
53. Ferrucci, L.; Semba, R.D.; Guralnik, J.M.; Ershler, W.B.; Bandinelli, S.; Patel, K.V.; Sun, K.; Woodman, R.C.; Andrews, N.C.; Cotter, R.J.; et al. Proinflammatory State, Hepcidin, and Anemia in Older Persons. *Blood* **2010**, *115*, 3810–3816. [CrossRef]
54. Campostrini, N.; Traglia, M.; Martinelli, N.; Corbella, M.; Cocca, M.; Manna, D.; Castagna, A.; Masciullo, C.; Silvestri, L.; Olivieri, O.; et al. Serum Levels of the Hepcidin-20 Isoform in a Large General Population: The Val Borbera Study. *J. Proteom.* **2012**, *76*, 28–35. [CrossRef] [PubMed]

55. Galesloot, T.E.; Vermeulen, S.H.; Geurts-Moespot, A.J.; Klaver, S.M.; Kroot, J.J.; van Tienoven, D.; Wetzels, J.F.M.; Kiemeney, L.A.L.M.; Sweep, F.C.; den Heijer, M.; et al. Serum Hepcidin: Reference Ranges and Biochemical Correlates in the General Population. *Blood* **2011**, *117*, e218–e225. [CrossRef] [PubMed]
56. Morceau, F.; Dicato, M.; Diederich, M. Pro-Inflammatory Cytokine-Mediated Anemia: Regarding Molecular Mechanisms of Erythropoiesis. *Mediat. Inflamm.* **2009**, *2009*, 405016. [CrossRef] [PubMed]
57. Orsini, M.; Chateauvieux, S.; Rhim, J.; Gaigneaux, A.; Cheillan, D.; Christov, C.; Dicato, M.; Morceau, F.; Diederich, M. Sphingolipid-Mediated Inflammatory Signaling Leading to Autophagy Inhibition Converts Erythropoiesis to Myelopoiesis in Human Hematopoietic Stem/Progenitor Cells. *Cell Death Differ.* **2019**, *26*, 1796–1812. [CrossRef]
58. Libregts, S.F.; Gutiérrez, L.; de Bruin, A.M.; Wensveen, F.M.; Papadopoulos, P.; van Ijcken, W.; Ozgür, Z.; Philipsen, S.; Nolte, M.A. Chronic IFN-γ Production in Mice Induces Anemia by Reducing Erythrocyte Life Span and Inhibiting Erythropoiesis through an IRF-1/PU.1 Axis. *Blood* **2011**, *118*, 2578–2588. [CrossRef] [PubMed]
59. Means, R.T.; Dessypris, E.N.; Krantz, S.B. Inhibition of Human Erythroid Colony-Forming Units by Interleukin-1 Is Mediated by Gamma Interferon. *J. Cell Physiol.* **1992**, *150*, 59–64. [CrossRef]
60. Means, R.T.; Krantz, S.B. Inhibition of Human Erythroid Colony-Forming Units by Gamma Interferon Can Be Corrected by Recombinant Human Erythropoietin. *Blood* **1991**, *78*, 2564–2567. [CrossRef]
61. Miller, C.B.; Jones, R.J.; Piantadosi, S.; Abeloff, M.D.; Spivak, J.L. Decreased Erythropoietin Response in Patients with the Anemia of Cancer. *N. Engl. J. Med.* **1990**, *322*, 1689–1692. [CrossRef]
62. Cazzola, M.; Ponchio, L.; de Benedetti, F.; Ravelli, A.; Rosti, V.; Beguin, Y.; Invernizzi, R.; Barosi, G.; Martini, A. Defective Iron Supply for Erythropoiesis and Adequate Endogenous Erythropoietin Production in the Anemia Associated with Systemic-Onset Juvenile Chronic Arthritis. *Blood* **1996**, *87*, 4824–4830. [CrossRef]
63. Macdougall, I.C.; Cooper, A.C. Erythropoietin Resistance: The Role of Inflammation and pro-Inflammatory Cytokines. *Nephrol. Dial. Transplant.* **2002**, *17* (Suppl. S11), 39–43. [CrossRef]
64. Kimachi, M.; Fukuma, S.; Yamazaki, S.; Yamamoto, Y.; Akizawa, T.; Akiba, T.; Saito, A.; Fukuhara, S. Minor Elevation in C-Reactive Protein Levels Predicts Incidence of Erythropoiesis-Stimulating Agent Hyporesponsiveness among Hemodialysis Patients. *Nephron* **2015**, *131*, 123–130. [CrossRef]
65. Khalil, S.; Delehanty, L.; Grado, S.; Holy, M.; White, Z.; Freeman, K.; Kurita, R.; Nakamura, Y.; Bullock, G.; Goldfarb, A. Iron Modulation of Erythropoiesis Is Associated with Scribble-Mediated Control of the Erythropoietin Receptor. *J. Exp. Med.* **2018**, *215*, 661–679. [CrossRef]
66. Buchanan, S.; Combet, E.; Stenvinkel, P.; Shiels, P.G. Klotho, Aging, and the Failing Kidney. *Front. Endocrinol.* **2020**, *11*, 560. [CrossRef]
67. Xu, Y.; Sun, Z. Molecular Basis of Klotho: From Gene to Function in Aging. *Endocr. Rev.* **2015**, *36*, 174–193. [CrossRef]
68. An, C.; Chen, X.; Zheng, D. Association between Anemia and Serum Klotho in Middle-Aged and Older Adults. *BMC Nephrol.* **2023**, *24*, 38. [CrossRef]
69. Vadakke Madathil, S.; Coe, L.M.; Casu, C.; Sitara, D. Klotho Deficiency Disrupts Hematopoietic Stem Cell Development and Erythropoiesis. *Am. J. Pathol.* **2014**, *184*, 827–841. [CrossRef]
70. Kanbay, M.; Copur, S.; Ozbek, L.; Mutlu, A.; Cejka, D.; Ciceri, P.; Cozzolino, M.; Haarhaus, M.L. Klotho: A Potential Therapeutic Target in Aging and Neurodegeneration beyond Chronic Kidney Disease—A Comprehensive Review from the ERA CKD-MBD Working Group. *Clin. Kidney J.* **2024**, *17*, sfad276. [CrossRef] [PubMed]
71. Yang, H.-C.; Fogo, A.B. Fibrosis and Renal Aging. *Kidney Int. Suppl.* **2014**, *4*, 75–78. [CrossRef] [PubMed]
72. Tsiftsoglou, A.S. Erythropoietin (EPO) as a Key Regulator of Erythropoiesis, Bone Remodeling and Endothelial Transdifferentiation of Multipotent Mesenchymal Stem Cells (MSCs): Implications in Regenerative Medicine. *Cells* **2021**, *10*, 2140. [CrossRef]
73. Ershler, W.B.; Sheng, S.; McKelvey, J.; Artz, A.S.; Denduluri, N.; Tecson, J.; Taub, D.D.; Brant, L.J.; Ferrucci, L.; Longo, D.L. Serum Erythropoietin and Aging: A Longitudinal Analysis. *J. Am. Geriatr. Soc.* **2005**, *53*, 1360–1365. [CrossRef]
74. Macciò, A.; Madeddu, C. Management of Anemia of Inflammation in the Elderly. *Anemia* **2012**, *2012*, 563251. [CrossRef]
75. Mitlyng, B.L.; Singh, J.A.; Furne, J.K.; Ruddy, J.; Levitt, M.D. Use of Breath Carbon Monoxide Measurements to Assess Erythrocyte Survival in Subjects with Chronic Diseases. *Am. J. Hematol.* **2006**, *81*, 432–438. [CrossRef]
76. Correll, C.K.; Binstadt, B.A. Advances in the Pathogenesis and Treatment of Systemic Juvenile Idiopathic Arthritis. *Pediatr. Res.* **2014**, *75*, 176–183. [CrossRef]
77. Milner, J.D.; Orekov, T.; Ward, J.M.; Cheng, L.; Torres-Velez, F.; Junttila, I.; Sun, G.; Buller, M.; Morris, S.C.; Finkelman, F.D.; et al. Sustained IL-4 Exposure Leads to a Novel Pathway for Hemophagocytosis, Inflammation, and Tissue Macrophage Accumulation. *Blood* **2010**, *116*, 2476–2483. [CrossRef]
78. Cartwright, G.E.; Lee, G.R. The Anaemia of Chronic Disorders. *Br. J. Haematol.* **1971**, *21*, 147–152. [CrossRef]
79. Freireich, E.J.; Ross, J.F.; Bayles, T.B.; Emerson, C.P.; Finch, S.C. Radioactive Iron Metabolism and Erythrocyte Survival Studies of the Mechanism of the Anemia Associated with Rheumatoid Arthritis. *J. Clin. Investig.* **1957**, *36*, 1043–1058. [CrossRef]
80. Kvietys, P.R.; Granger, D.N. Role of Reactive Oxygen and Nitrogen Species in the Vascular Responses to Inflammation. *Free Radic. Biol. Med.* **2012**, *52*, 556–592. [CrossRef]
81. Orrico, F.; Laurance, S.; Lopez, A.C.; Lefevre, S.D.; Thomson, L.; Möller, M.N.; Ostuni, M.A. Oxidative Stress in Healthy and Pathological Red Blood Cells. *Biomolecules* **2023**, *13*, 1262. [CrossRef]

137. Kim, H.-R.; Lee, J.-H.; Heo, H.-R.; Yang, S.-R.; Ha, K.-S.; Park, W.S.; Han, E.-T.; Song, H.; Hong, S.-H. Improved Hematopoietic Differentiation of Human Pluripotent Stem Cells via Estrogen Receptor Signaling Pathway. *Cell Biosci.* **2016**, *6*, 50. [CrossRef] [PubMed]
138. Tian, H.; Gao, Z.; Wang, G.; Li, H.; Zheng, J. Estrogen Potentiates Reactive Oxygen Species (ROS) Tolerance to Initiate Carcinogenesis and Promote Cancer Malignant Transformation. *Tumour Biol.* **2016**, *37*, 141–150. [CrossRef] [PubMed]
139. Guajardo-Correa, E.; Silva-Agüero, J.F.; Calle, X.; Chiong, M.; Henríquez, M.; García-Rivas, G.; Latorre, M.; Parra, V. Estrogen Signaling as a Bridge between the Nucleus and Mitochondria in Cardiovascular Diseases. *Front. Cell Dev. Biol.* **2022**, *10*, 968373. [CrossRef] [PubMed]
140. Nakada, D.; Oguro, H.; Levi, B.P.; Ryan, N.; Kitano, A.; Saitoh, Y.; Takeichi, M.; Wendt, G.R.; Morrison, S.J. Oestrogen Increases Haematopoietic Stem-Cell Self-Renewal in Females and during Pregnancy. *Nature* **2014**, *505*, 555–558. [CrossRef]
141. Dumic, I.; Nordin, T.; Jecmenica, M.; Stojkovic Lalosevic, M.; Milosavljevic, T.; Milovanovic, T. Gastrointestinal Tract Disorders in Older Age. *Can. J. Gastroenterol. Hepatol.* **2019**, *2019*, 6757524. [CrossRef]
142. Porter, K.M.; Hoey, L.; Hughes, C.F.; Ward, M.; Clements, M.; Strain, J.; Cunningham, C.; Casey, M.C.; Tracey, F.; O'Kane, M.; et al. Associations of Atrophic Gastritis and Proton-Pump Inhibitor Drug Use with Vitamin B-12 Status, and the Impact of Fortified Foods, in Older Adults. *Am. J. Clin. Nutr.* **2021**, *114*, 1286–1294. [CrossRef] [PubMed]
143. Hohman, L.S.; Osborne, L.C. A Gut-Centric View of Aging: Do Intestinal Epithelial Cells Contribute to Age-Associated Microbiota Changes, Inflammaging, and Immunosenescence? *Aging Cell* **2022**, *21*, e13700. [CrossRef]
144. Cappello, M.; Morreale, G.C.; Licata, A. Elderly Onset Celiac Disease: A Narrative Review. *Clin. Med. Insights Gastroenterol.* **2016**, *9*, CGast.S38454. [CrossRef]
145. Ching, C.K.; Lebwohl, B. Celiac Disease in the Elderly. *Curr. Treat. Options Gastro* **2022**, *20*, 238–249. [CrossRef] [PubMed]
146. Sopeña, F.; Lanas, A. Management of Colonic Diverticular Disease with Poorly Absorbed Antibiotics and Other Therapies. *Ther. Adv. Gastroenterol.* **2011**, *4*, 365–374. [CrossRef] [PubMed]
147. Efremova, I.; Maslennikov, R.; Poluektova, E.; Vasilieva, E.; Zharikov, Y.; Suslov, A.; Letyagina, Y.; Kozlov, E.; Levshina, A.; Ivashkin, V. Epidemiology of Small Intestinal Bacterial Overgrowth. *World J. Gastroenterol.* **2023**, *29*, 3400–3421. [CrossRef] [PubMed]
148. Manrai, M.; Dawra, S.; Kapoor, R.; Srivastava, S.; Singh, A. Anemia in Cirrhosis: An Underestimated Entity. *WJCC* **2022**, *10*, 777–789. [CrossRef]
149. Risør, L.M.; Fenger, M.; Olsen, N.V.; Møller, S. Hepatic Erythropoietin Response in Cirrhosis. A Contemporary Review. *Scand. J. Clin. Lab. Investig.* **2016**, *76*, 183–189. [CrossRef]
150. Ghosh, T.S.; Shanahan, F.; O'Toole, P.W. The Gut Microbiome as a Modulator of Healthy Ageing. *Nat. Rev. Gastroenterol. Hepatol.* **2022**, *19*, 565–584. [CrossRef]
151. Weiss, G.A.; Hennet, T. Mechanisms and Consequences of Intestinal Dysbiosis. *Cell Mol. Life Sci.* **2017**, *74*, 2959–2977. [CrossRef]
152. Wilms, E.; Troost, F.J.; Elizalde, M.; Winkens, B.; De Vos, P.; Mujagic, Z.; Jonkers, D.M.A.E.; Masclee, A.A.M. Intestinal Barrier Function Is Maintained with Aging—A Comprehensive Study in Healthy Subjects and Irritable Bowel Syndrome Patients. *Sci. Rep.* **2020**, *10*, 475. [CrossRef] [PubMed]
153. Josefsdottir, K.S.; Baldridge, M.T.; Kadmon, C.S.; King, K.Y. Antibiotics Impair Murine Hematopoiesis by Depleting the Intestinal Microbiota. *Blood* **2017**, *129*, 729–739. [CrossRef] [PubMed]
154. Tian, Y.; Tian, Y.; Yuan, Z.; Zeng, Y.; Wang, S.; Fan, X.; Yang, D.; Yang, M. Iron Metabolism in Aging and Age-Related Diseases. *Int. J. Mol. Sci.* **2022**, *23*, 3612. [CrossRef]
155. Yan, Y.; Walker, F.C.; Ali, A.; Han, H.; Tan, L.; Veillon, L.; Lorenzi, P.L.; Baldridge, M.T.; King, K.Y. The Bacterial Microbiota Regulates Normal Hematopoiesis via Metabolite-Induced Type 1 Interferon Signaling. *Blood Adv.* **2022**, *6*, 1754–1765. [CrossRef]
156. Manzo, V.E.; Bhatt, A.S. The Human Microbiome in Hematopoiesis and Hematologic Disorders. *Blood* **2015**, *126*, 311–318. [CrossRef] [PubMed]
157. Rackerby, B.; Kim, H.J.; Dallas, D.C.; Park, S.H. Understanding the Effects of Dietary Components on the Gut Microbiome and Human Health. *Food Sci. Biotechnol.* **2020**, *29*, 1463–1474. [CrossRef]
158. Caiado, F.; Manz, M.G. A Microbiome-Macrophage-Iron Axis Guides Stressed Hematopoietic Stem Cell Fate. *Cell Stem Cell* **2022**, *29*, 177–179. [CrossRef]
159. Soriano-Lerma, A.; García-Burgos, M.; Alférez, M.J.M.; Pérez-Carrasco, V.; Sanchez-Martin, V.; Linde-Rodríguez, Á.; Ortiz-González, M.; Soriano, M.; García-Salcedo, J.A.; López-Aliaga, I. Gut Microbiome-Short-Chain Fatty Acids Interplay in the Context of Iron Deficiency Anaemia. *Eur. J. Nutr.* **2022**, *61*, 399–412. [CrossRef]
160. Ragonnaud, E.; Biragyn, A. Gut Microbiota as the Key Controllers of "Healthy" Aging of Elderly People. *Immun. Ageing* **2021**, *18*, 2. [CrossRef]
161. Miller, F.W. The Increasing Prevalence of Autoimmunity and Autoimmune Diseases: An Urgent Call to Action for Improved Understanding, Diagnosis, Treatment, and Prevention. *Curr. Opin. Immunol.* **2023**, *80*, 102266. [CrossRef]
162. Conrad, N.; Misra, S.; Verbakel, J.Y.; Verbeke, G.; Molenberghs, G.; Taylor, P.N.; Mason, J.; Sattar, N.; McMurray, J.J.V.; McInnes, I.B.; et al. Incidence, Prevalence, and Co-Occurrence of Autoimmune Disorders over Time and by Age, Sex, and Socioeconomic Status: A Population-Based Cohort Study of 22 Million Individuals in the UK. *Lancet* **2023**, *401*, 1878–1890. [CrossRef] [PubMed]
163. Moskalec, O.V. Characteristics of immune response in elderly and autoimmunity. *Adv. Gerontol.* **2020**, *33*, 246–255. [PubMed]

164. Watad, A.; Bragazzi, N.L.; Adawi, M.; Amital, H.; Toubi, E.; Porat, B.-S.; Shoenfeld, Y. Autoimmunity in the Elderly: Insights from Basic Science and Clinics—A Mini-Review. *Gerontology* **2017**, *63*, 515–523. [CrossRef] [PubMed]
165. Chen, Y.-F.; Xu, S.-Q.; Xu, Y.-C.; Li, W.-J.; Chen, K.-M.; Cai, J.; Li, M. Inflammatory Anemia May Be an Indicator for Predicting Disease Activity and Structural Damage in Chinese Patients with Rheumatoid Arthritis. *Clin. Rheumatol.* **2020**, *39*, 1737–1745. [CrossRef] [PubMed]
166. Vadasz, Z.; Haj, T.; Kessel, A.; Toubi, E. Age-Related Autoimmunity. *BMC Med.* **2013**, *11*, 94. [CrossRef] [PubMed]
167. Imanuel, C.A.; Sivatheesan, S.; Koyanagi, A.; Smith, L.; Konrad, M.; Kostev, K. Associations between Rheumatoid Arthritis and Various Comorbid Conditions in Germany-A Retrospective Cohort Study. *J. Clin. Med.* **2023**, *12*, 7265. [CrossRef] [PubMed]
168. Shadick, N.; Hagino, O.; Praestgaard, A.; Fiore, S.; Weinblatt, M.; Burmester, G. Association of Hemoglobin Levels with Radiographic Progression in Patients with Rheumatoid Arthritis: An Analysis from the BRASS Registry. *Arthritis Res. Ther.* **2023**, *25*, 88. [CrossRef] [PubMed]
169. Günther, F.; Straub, R.H.; Hartung, W.; Fleck, M.; Ehrenstein, B.; Schminke, L. Usefulness of Soluble Transferrin Receptor in the Diagnosis of Iron Deficiency Anemia in Rheumatoid Arthritis Patients in Clinical Practice. *Int. J. Rheumatol.* **2022**, *2022*, 7067262. [CrossRef] [PubMed]
170. Peng, B.; Kong, G.; Yang, C.; Ming, Y. Erythropoietin and Its Derivatives: From Tissue Protection to Immune Regulation. *Cell Death Dis.* **2020**, *11*, 79. [CrossRef]
171. Nairz, M.; Schroll, A.; Moschen, A.R.; Sonnweber, T.; Theurl, M.; Theurl, I.; Taub, N.; Jamnig, C.; Neurauter, D.; Huber, L.A.; et al. Erythropoietin Contrastingly Affects Bacterial Infection and Experimental Colitis by Inhibiting Nuclear Factor-κB-Inducible Immune Pathways. *Immunity* **2011**, *34*, 61–74. [CrossRef]
172. Eswarappa, M.; Cantarelli, C.; Cravedi, P. Erythropoietin in Lupus: Unanticipated Immune Modulating Effects of a Kidney Hormone. *Front. Immunol.* **2021**, *12*, 639370. [CrossRef]
173. Moransard, M.; Bednar, M.; Frei, K.; Gassmann, M.; Ogunshola, O.O. Erythropoietin Reduces Experimental Autoimmune Encephalomyelitis Severity via Neuroprotective Mechanisms. *J. Neuroinflamm.* **2017**, *14*, 202. [CrossRef] [PubMed]
174. Fattizzo, B.; Pedone, G.L.; Brambilla, C.; Pettine, L.; Zaninoni, A.; Passamonti, F.; Barcellini, W. Recombinant Erythropoietin in Autoimmune Hemolytic Anemia with Inadequate Bone Marrow Response: A Prospective Analysis. *Blood Adv.* **2023**, *8*, 1322–1327. [CrossRef]
175. Wu, G.; Cao, B.; Zhai, H.; Liu, B.; Huang, Y.; Chen, X.; Ling, H.; Ling, S.; Jin, S.; Yang, X.; et al. EPO Promotes the Progression of Rheumatoid Arthritis by Inducing Desialylation via Increasing the Expression of Neuraminidase 3. *Ann. Rheum. Dis.* **2024**. [CrossRef] [PubMed]
176. Paulson, R.F.; Ruan, B.; Hao, S.; Chen, Y. Stress Erythropoiesis Is a Key Inflammatory Response. *Cells* **2020**, *9*, 634. [CrossRef] [PubMed]
177. Bennett, L.F.; Liao, C.; Quickel, M.D.; Yeoh, B.S.; Vijay-Kumar, M.; Hankey-Giblin, P.; Prabhu, K.S.; Paulson, R.F. Inflammation Induces Stress Erythropoiesis through Heme-Dependent Activation of SPI-C. *Sci. Signal.* **2019**, *12*, eaap7336. [CrossRef]
178. Denny, S.D.; Kuchibhatla, M.N.; Cohen, H.J. Impact of Anemia on Mortality, Cognition, and Function in Community-Dwelling Elderly. *Am. J. Med.* **2006**, *119*, 327–334. [CrossRef]
179. Izaks, G.J.; Westendorp, R.G.; Knook, D.L. The Definition of Anemia in Older Persons. *JAMA* **1999**, *281*, 1714–1717. [CrossRef]
180. Patel, K.V.; Harris, T.B.; Faulhaber, M.; Angleman, S.B.; Connelly, S.; Bauer, D.C.; Kuller, L.H.; Newman, A.B.; Guralnik, J.M. Racial Variation in the Relationship of Anemia with Mortality and Mobility Disability among Older Adults. *Blood* **2007**, *109*, 4663–4670. [CrossRef]
181. Penninx, B.W.J.H.; Pahor, M.; Woodman, R.C.; Guralnik, J.M. Anemia in Old Age Is Associated with Increased Mortality and Hospitalization. *J. Gerontol. A Biol. Sci. Med. Sci.* **2006**, *61*, 474–479. [CrossRef]

Disclaimer/Publisher's Note: The statements, opinions and data contained in all publications are solely those of the individual author(s) and contributor(s) and not of MDPI and/or the editor(s). MDPI and/or the editor(s) disclaim responsibility for any injury to people or property resulting from any ideas, methods, instructions or products referred to in the content.

28. Langie, S.A.S.; Koppen, G.; Desaulniers, D.; Al-Mulla, F.; Al-Temaimi, R.; Amedei, A.; Azqueta, A.; Bisson, W.H.; Brown, D.G.; Brunborg, G.; et al. Causes of Genome Instability: The Effect of Low Dose Chemical Exposures in Modern Society. *Carcinogenesis* **2015**, *36* (Suppl. S1), S61–S88. [CrossRef]
29. Cooke, M.S.; Evans, M.D.; Dizdaroglu, M.; Lunec, J. Oxidative DNA Damage: Mechanisms, Mutation, and Disease. *FASEB J.* **2003**, *17*, 1195–1214. [CrossRef]
30. Wei, Y.; Giunta, S.; Xia, S. Hypoxia in Aging and Aging-Related Diseases: Mechanism and Therapeutic Strategies. *Int. J. Mol. Sci.* **2022**, *23*, 8165. [CrossRef]
31. Kay, J.; Thadhani, E.; Samson, L.; Engelward, B. Inflammation-Induced DNA Damage, Mutations and Cancer. *DNA Repair* **2019**, *83*, 102673. [CrossRef]
32. Liu, W.; Deng, Y.; Li, Z.; Chen, Y.; Zhu, X.; Tan, X.; Cao, G. Cancer Evo-Dev: A Theory of Inflammation-Induced Oncogenesis. *Front. Immunol.* **2021**, *12*, 768098. [CrossRef]
33. Jaiswal, S.; Ebert, B.L. Clonal Hematopoiesis in Human Aging and Disease. *Science* **2019**, *366*, eaan4673. [CrossRef]
34. Mitchell, E.; Spencer Chapman, M.; Williams, N.; Dawson, K.J.; Mende, N.; Calderbank, E.F.; Jung, H.; Mitchell, T.; Coorens, T.H.H.; Spencer, D.H.; et al. Clonal Dynamics of Haematopoiesis across the Human Lifespan. *Nature* **2022**, *606*, 343–350. [CrossRef]
35. Morganti, C.; Ito, K. Mitochondrial Contributions to Hematopoietic Stem Cell Aging. *Int. J. Mol. Sci.* **2021**, *22*, 11117. [CrossRef]
36. Zampino, M.; Brennan, N.A.; Kuo, P.-L.; Spencer, R.G.; Fishbein, K.W.; Simonsick, E.M.; Ferrucci, L. Poor Mitochondrial Health and Systemic Inflammation? Test of a Classic Hypothesis in the Baltimore Longitudinal Study of Aging. *Geroscience* **2020**, *42*, 1175–1182. [CrossRef]
37. Yeo, E.-J. Hypoxia and Aging. *Exp. Mol. Med.* **2019**, *51*, 1–15. [CrossRef]
38. Lee, P.; Chandel, N.S.; Simon, M.C. Cellular Adaptation to Hypoxia through Hypoxia Inducible Factors and Beyond. *Nat. Rev. Mol. Cell Biol.* **2020**, *21*, 268–283. [CrossRef]
39. Tojo, Y.; Sekine, H.; Hirano, I.; Pan, X.; Souma, T.; Tsujita, T.; Kawaguchi, S.; Takeda, N.; Takeda, K.; Fong, G.-H.; et al. Hypoxia Signaling Cascade for Erythropoietin Production in Hepatocytes. *Mol. Cell. Biol.* **2015**, *35*, 2658–2672. [CrossRef]
40. Xia, S.; Zhang, X.; Zheng, S.; Khanabdali, R.; Kalionis, B.; Wu, J.; Wan, W.; Tai, X. An Update on Inflamm-Aging: Mechanisms, Prevention, and Treatment. *J. Immunol. Res.* **2016**, *2016*, 8426874. [CrossRef]
41. Franceschi, C.; Campisi, J. Chronic Inflammation (Inflammaging) and Its Potential Contribution to Age-Associated Diseases. *J. Gerontol. A Biol. Sci. Med. Sci.* **2014**, *69* (Suppl. S1), S4–S9. [CrossRef]
42. Wawrzyniak-Gramacka, E.; Hertmanowska, N.; Tylutka, A.; Morawin, B.; Wacka, E.; Gutowicz, M.; Zembron-Lacny, A. The Association of Anti-Inflammatory Diet Ingredients and Lifestyle Exercise with Inflammaging. *Nutrients* **2021**, *13*, 3696. [CrossRef] [PubMed]
43. Minciullo, P.L.; Catalano, A.; Mandraffino, G.; Casciaro, M.; Crucitti, A.; Maltese, G.; Morabito, N.; Lasco, A.; Gangemi, S.; Basile, G. Inflammaging and Anti-Inflammaging: The Role of Cytokines in Extreme Longevity. *Arch. Immunol. Ther. Exp.* **2016**, *64*, 111–126. [CrossRef] [PubMed]
44. Stefanova, D.; Raychev, A.; Deville, J.; Humphries, R.; Campeau, S.; Ruchala, P.; Nemeth, E.; Ganz, T.; Bulut, Y. Hepcidin Protects against Lethal Escherichia Coli Sepsis in Mice Inoculated with Isolates from Septic Patients. *Infect. Immun.* **2018**, *86*, e00253-18. [CrossRef]
45. Stefanova, D.; Raychev, A.; Arezes, J.; Ruchala, P.; Gabayan, V.; Skurnik, M.; Dillon, B.J.; Horwitz, M.A.; Ganz, T.; Bulut, Y.; et al. Endogenous Hepcidin and Its Agonist Mediate Resistance to Selected Infections by Clearing Non-Transferrin-Bound Iron. *Blood* **2017**, *130*, 245–257. [CrossRef] [PubMed]
46. Nemeth, E.; Ganz, T. The Role of Hepcidin in Iron Metabolism. *Acta Haematol.* **2009**, *122*, 78–86. [CrossRef] [PubMed]
47. Park, C.H.; Valore, E.V.; Waring, A.J.; Ganz, T. Hepcidin, a Urinary Antimicrobial Peptide Synthesized in the Liver. *J. Biol. Chem.* **2001**, *276*, 7806–7810. [CrossRef] [PubMed]
48. den Elzen, W.P.J.; de Craen, A.J.M.; Wiegerinck, E.T.; Westendorp, R.G.J.; Swinkels, D.W.; Gussekloo, J. Plasma Hepcidin Levels and Anemia in Old Age. The Leiden 85-Plus Study. *Haematologica* **2013**, *98*, 448–454. [CrossRef] [PubMed]
49. Donovan, A.; Lima, C.A.; Pinkus, J.L.; Pinkus, G.S.; Zon, L.I.; Robine, S.; Andrews, N.C. The Iron Exporter Ferroportin/Slc40a1 Is Essential for Iron Homeostasis. *Cell Metab.* **2005**, *1*, 191–200. [CrossRef] [PubMed]
50. Nemeth, E.; Tuttle, M.S.; Powelson, J.; Vaughn, M.B.; Donovan, A.; Ward, D.M.; Ganz, T.; Kaplan, J. Hepcidin Regulates Cellular Iron Efflux by Binding to Ferroportin and Inducing Its Internalization. *Science* **2004**, *306*, 2090–2093. [CrossRef]
51. Ganz, T. Anemia of Inflammation. *N. Engl. J. Med.* **2019**, *381*, 1148–1157. [CrossRef]
52. Wacka, E.; Wawrzyniak-Gramacka, E.; Tylutka, A.; Morawin, B.; Gutowicz, M.; Zembron-Lacny, A. The Role of Inflammation in Age-Associated Changes in Red Blood System. *Int. J. Mol. Sci.* **2023**, *24*, 8944. [CrossRef] [PubMed]
53. Ferrucci, L.; Semba, R.D.; Guralnik, J.M.; Ershler, W.B.; Bandinelli, S.; Patel, K.V.; Sun, K.; Woodman, R.C.; Andrews, N.C.; Cotter, R.J.; et al. Proinflammatory State, Hepcidin, and Anemia in Older Persons. *Blood* **2010**, *115*, 3810–3816. [CrossRef]
54. Campostrini, N.; Traglia, M.; Martinelli, N.; Corbella, M.; Cocca, M.; Manna, D.; Castagna, A.; Masciullo, C.; Silvestri, L.; Olivieri, O.; et al. Serum Levels of the Hepcidin-20 Isoform in a Large General Population: The Val Borbera Study. *J. Proteom.* **2012**, *76*, 28–35. [CrossRef] [PubMed]

55. Galesloot, T.E.; Vermeulen, S.H.; Geurts-Moespot, A.J.; Klaver, S.M.; Kroot, J.J.; van Tienoven, D.; Wetzels, J.F.M.; Kiemeney, L.A.L.M.; Sweep, F.C.; den Heijer, M.; et al. Serum Hepcidin: Reference Ranges and Biochemical Correlates in the General Population. *Blood* **2011**, *117*, e218–e225. [CrossRef] [PubMed]
56. Morceau, F.; Dicato, M.; Diederich, M. Pro-Inflammatory Cytokine-Mediated Anemia: Regarding Molecular Mechanisms of Erythropoiesis. *Mediat. Inflamm.* **2009**, *2009*, 405016. [CrossRef] [PubMed]
57. Orsini, M.; Chateauvieux, S.; Rhim, J.; Gaigneaux, A.; Cheillan, D.; Christov, C.; Dicato, M.; Morceau, F.; Diederich, M. Sphingolipid-Mediated Inflammatory Signaling Leading to Autophagy Inhibition Converts Erythropoiesis to Myelopoiesis in Human Hematopoietic Stem/Progenitor Cells. *Cell Death Differ.* **2019**, *26*, 1796–1812. [CrossRef]
58. Libregts, S.F.; Gutiérrez, L.; de Bruin, A.M.; Wensveen, F.M.; Papadopoulos, P.; van Ijcken, W.; Ozgür, Z.; Philipsen, S.; Nolte, M.A. Chronic IFN-γ Production in Mice Induces Anemia by Reducing Erythrocyte Life Span and Inhibiting Erythropoiesis through an IRF-1/PU.1 Axis. *Blood* **2011**, *118*, 2578–2588. [CrossRef] [PubMed]
59. Means, R.T.; Dessypris, E.N.; Krantz, S.B. Inhibition of Human Erythroid Colony-Forming Units by Interleukin-1 Is Mediated by Gamma Interferon. *J. Cell Physiol.* **1992**, *150*, 59–64. [CrossRef]
60. Means, R.T.; Krantz, S.B. Inhibition of Human Erythroid Colony-Forming Units by Gamma Interferon Can Be Corrected by Recombinant Human Erythropoietin. *Blood* **1991**, *78*, 2564–2567. [CrossRef]
61. Miller, C.B.; Jones, R.J.; Piantadosi, S.; Abeloff, M.D.; Spivak, J.L. Decreased Erythropoietin Response in Patients with the Anemia of Cancer. *N. Engl. J. Med.* **1990**, *322*, 1689–1692. [CrossRef]
62. Cazzola, M.; Ponchio, L.; de Benedetti, F.; Ravelli, A.; Rosti, V.; Beguin, Y.; Invernizzi, R.; Barosi, G.; Martini, A. Defective Iron Supply for Erythropoiesis and Adequate Endogenous Erythropoietin Production in the Anemia Associated with Systemic-Onset Juvenile Chronic Arthritis. *Blood* **1996**, *87*, 4824–4830. [CrossRef]
63. Macdougall, I.C.; Cooper, A.C. Erythropoietin Resistance: The Role of Inflammation and pro-Inflammatory Cytokines. *Nephrol. Dial. Transplant.* **2002**, *17* (Suppl. S11), 39–43. [CrossRef]
64. Kimachi, M.; Fukuma, S.; Yamazaki, S.; Yamamoto, Y.; Akizawa, T.; Akiba, T.; Saito, A.; Fukuhara, S. Minor Elevation in C-Reactive Protein Levels Predicts Incidence of Erythropoiesis-Stimulating Agent Hyporesponsiveness among Hemodialysis Patients. *Nephron* **2015**, *131*, 123–130. [CrossRef]
65. Khalil, S.; Delehanty, L.; Grado, S.; Holy, M.; White, Z.; Freeman, K.; Kurita, R.; Nakamura, Y.; Bullock, G.; Goldfarb, A. Iron Modulation of Erythropoiesis Is Associated with Scribble-Mediated Control of the Erythropoietin Receptor. *J. Exp. Med.* **2018**, *215*, 661–679. [CrossRef]
66. Buchanan, S.; Combet, E.; Stenvinkel, P.; Shiels, P.G. Klotho, Aging, and the Failing Kidney. *Front. Endocrinol.* **2020**, *11*, 560. [CrossRef]
67. Xu, Y.; Sun, Z. Molecular Basis of Klotho: From Gene to Function in Aging. *Endocr. Rev.* **2015**, *36*, 174–193. [CrossRef]
68. An, C.; Chen, X.; Zheng, D. Association between Anemia and Serum Klotho in Middle-Aged and Older Adults. *BMC Nephrol.* **2023**, *24*, 38. [CrossRef]
69. Vadakke Madathil, S.; Coe, L.M.; Casu, C.; Sitara, D. Klotho Deficiency Disrupts Hematopoietic Stem Cell Development and Erythropoiesis. *Am. J. Pathol.* **2014**, *184*, 827–841. [CrossRef]
70. Kanbay, M.; Copur, S.; Ozbek, L.; Mutlu, A.; Cejka, D.; Ciceri, P.; Cozzolino, M.; Haarhaus, M.L. Klotho: A Potential Therapeutic Target in Aging and Neurodegeneration beyond Chronic Kidney Disease—A Comprehensive Review from the ERA CKD-MBD Working Group. *Clin. Kidney J.* **2024**, *17*, sfad276. [CrossRef] [PubMed]
71. Yang, H.-C.; Fogo, A.B. Fibrosis and Renal Aging. *Kidney Int. Suppl.* **2014**, *4*, 75–78. [CrossRef] [PubMed]
72. Tsiftsoglou, A.S. Erythropoietin (EPO) as a Key Regulator of Erythropoiesis, Bone Remodeling and Endothelial Transdifferentiation of Multipotent Mesenchymal Stem Cells (MSCs): Implications in Regenerative Medicine. *Cells* **2021**, *10*, 2140. [CrossRef]
73. Ershler, W.B.; Sheng, S.; McKelvey, J.; Artz, A.S.; Denduluri, N.; Tecson, J.; Taub, D.D.; Brant, L.J.; Ferrucci, L.; Longo, D.L. Serum Erythropoietin and Aging: A Longitudinal Analysis. *J. Am. Geriatr. Soc.* **2005**, *53*, 1360–1365. [CrossRef]
74. Macciò, A.; Madeddu, C. Management of Anemia of Inflammation in the Elderly. *Anemia* **2012**, *2012*, 563251. [CrossRef]
75. Mitlyng, B.L.; Singh, J.A.; Furne, J.K.; Ruddy, J.; Levitt, M.D. Use of Breath Carbon Monoxide Measurements to Assess Erythrocyte Survival in Subjects with Chronic Diseases. *Am. J. Hematol.* **2006**, *81*, 432–438. [CrossRef]
76. Correll, C.K.; Binstadt, B.A. Advances in the Pathogenesis and Treatment of Systemic Juvenile Idiopathic Arthritis. *Pediatr. Res.* **2014**, *75*, 176–183. [CrossRef]
77. Milner, J.D.; Orekov, T.; Ward, J.M.; Cheng, L.; Torres-Velez, F.; Junttila, I.; Sun, G.; Buller, M.; Morris, S.C.; Finkelman, F.D.; et al. Sustained IL-4 Exposure Leads to a Novel Pathway for Hemophagocytosis, Inflammation, and Tissue Macrophage Accumulation. *Blood* **2010**, *116*, 2476–2483. [CrossRef]
78. Cartwright, G.E.; Lee, G.R. The Anaemia of Chronic Disorders. *Br. J. Haematol.* **1971**, *21*, 147–152. [CrossRef]
79. Freireich, E.J.; Ross, J.F.; Bayles, T.B.; Emerson, C.P.; Finch, S.C. Radioactive Iron Metabolism and Erythrocyte Survival Studies of the Mechanism of the Anemia Associated with Rheumatoid Arthritis. *J. Clin. Investig.* **1957**, *36*, 1043–1058. [CrossRef]
80. Kvietys, P.R.; Granger, D.N. Role of Reactive Oxygen and Nitrogen Species in the Vascular Responses to Inflammation. *Free Radic. Biol. Med.* **2012**, *52*, 556–592. [CrossRef]
81. Orrico, F.; Laurance, S.; Lopez, A.C.; Lefevre, S.D.; Thomson, L.; Möller, M.N.; Ostuni, M.A. Oxidative Stress in Healthy and Pathological Red Blood Cells. *Biomolecules* **2023**, *13*, 1262. [CrossRef]

82. Williams, A.; Bissinger, R.; Shamaa, H.; Patel, S.; Bourne, L.; Artunc, F.; Qadri, S. Pathophysiology of Red Blood Cell Dysfunction in Diabetes and Its Complications. *Pathophysiology* **2023**, *30*, 327–345. [CrossRef]
83. Barshtein, G. Biochemical and Biophysical Properties of Red Blood Cells in Disease. *Biomolecules* **2022**, *12*, 923. [CrossRef]
84. Chaudhary, R.; Katharia, R. Oxidative Injury as Contributory Factor for Red Cells Storage Lesion during Twenty Eight Days of Storage. *Blood Transfus.* **2012**, *10*, 59. [CrossRef]
85. Huisjes, R.; Bogdanova, A.; Van Solinge, W.W.; Schiffelers, R.M.; Kaestner, L.; Van Wijk, R. Squeezing for Life—Properties of Red Blood Cell Deformability. *Front. Physiol.* **2018**, *9*, 656. [CrossRef]
86. Ammendolia, D.A.; Bement, W.M.; Brumell, J.H. Plasma Membrane Integrity: Implications for Health and Disease. *BMC Biol.* **2021**, *19*, 71. [CrossRef]
87. Skou, S.T.; Mair, F.S.; Fortin, M.; Guthrie, B.; Nunes, B.P.; Miranda, J.J.; Boyd, C.M.; Pati, S.; Mtenga, S.; Smith, S.M. Multimorbidity. *Nat. Rev. Dis. Primers* **2022**, *8*, 48. [CrossRef]
88. Steinmeyer, Z.; Delpierre, C.; Soriano, G.; Steinmeyer, A.; Ysebaert, L.; Balardy, L.; Sourdet, S. Hemoglobin Concentration; a Pathway to Frailty. *BMC Geriatr.* **2020**, *20*, 202. [CrossRef]
89. Muscaritoli, M.; Imbimbo, G.; Jager-Wittenaar, H.; Cederholm, T.; Rothenberg, E.; Di Girolamo, F.G.; Amabile, M.I.; Sealy, M.; Schneider, S.; Barazzoni, R.; et al. Disease-Related Malnutrition with Inflammation and Cachexia. *Clin. Nutr.* **2023**, *42*, 1475–1479. [CrossRef]
90. Cederholm, T.; Barazzoni, R.; Austin, P.; Ballmer, P.; Biolo, G.; Bischoff, S.C.; Compher, C.; Correia, I.; Higashiguchi, T.; Holst, M.; et al. ESPEN Guidelines on Definitions and Terminology of Clinical Nutrition. *Clin. Nutr.* **2017**, *36*, 49–64. [CrossRef]
91. Alghareeb, S.A.; Alfhili, M.A.; Fatima, S. Molecular Mechanisms and Pathophysiological Significance of Eryptosis. *Int. J. Mol. Sci.* **2023**, *24*, 5079. [CrossRef]
92. Bissinger, R.; Bhuyan, A.A.M.; Qadri, S.M.; Lang, F. Oxidative Stress, Eryptosis and Anemia: A Pivotal Mechanistic Nexus in Systemic Diseases. *FEBS J.* **2019**, *286*, 826–854. [CrossRef]
93. O'Sullivan, E.D.; Hughes, J.; Ferenbach, D.A. Renal Aging: Causes and Consequences. *J. Am. Soc. Nephrol.* **2017**, *28*, 407–420. [CrossRef]
94. Zhao, Y.; Yang, Y.; Li, Q.; Li, J. Understanding the Unique Microenvironment in the Aging Liver. *Front. Med.* **2022**, *9*, 842024. [CrossRef]
95. Bolignano, D.; Mattace-Raso, F.; Sijbrands, E.J.G.; Zoccali, C. The Aging Kidney Revisited: A Systematic Review. *Ageing Res. Rev.* **2014**, *14*, 65–80. [CrossRef]
96. Ou, H.-L.; Schumacher, B. DNA Damage Responses and P53 in the Aging Process. *Blood* **2018**, *131*, 488–495. [CrossRef]
97. Walsh, K.; Raghavachari, N.; Kerr, C.; Bick, A.G.; Cummings, S.R.; Druley, T.; Dunbar, C.E.; Genovese, G.; Goodell, M.A.; Jaiswal, S.; et al. Clonal Hematopoiesis Analyses in Clinical, Epidemiologic, and Genetic Aging Studies to Unravel Underlying Mechanisms of Age-Related Dysfunction in Humans. *Front. Aging* **2022**, *3*, 841796. [CrossRef]
98. Bick, A.G.; Weinstock, J.S.; Nandakumar, S.K.; Fulco, C.P.; Bao, E.L.; Zekavat, S.M.; Szeto, M.D.; Liao, X.; Leventhal, M.J.; Nasser, J.; et al. Inherited Causes of Clonal Haematopoiesis in 97,691 Whole Genomes. *Nature* **2020**, *586*, 763–768. [CrossRef]
99. Kar, S.P.; Quiros, P.M.; Gu, M.; Jiang, T.; Mitchell, J.; Langdon, R.; Iyer, V.; Barcena, C.; Vijayabaskar, M.S.; Fabre, M.A.; et al. Genome-Wide Analyses of 200,453 Individuals Yield New Insights into the Causes and Consequences of Clonal Hematopoiesis. *Nat. Genet.* **2022**, *54*, 1155–1166. [CrossRef]
100. Hoermann, G. Clinical Significance of Clonal Hematopoiesis of Indeterminate Potential in Hematology and Cardiovascular Disease. *Diagnostics* **2022**, *12*, 1613. [CrossRef]
101. Jaiswal, S.; Natarajan, P.; Silver, A.J.; Gibson, C.J.; Bick, A.G.; Shvartz, E.; McConkey, M.; Gupta, N.; Gabriel, S.; Ardissino, D.; et al. Clonal Hematopoiesis and Risk of Atherosclerotic Cardiovascular Disease. *N. Engl. J. Med.* **2017**, *377*, 111–121. [CrossRef]
102. Mangaonkar, A.A.; Patnaik, M.M. Clonal Hematopoiesis of Indeterminate Potential and Clonal Cytopenias of Undetermined Significance: 2023 Update on Clinical Associations and Management Recommendations. *Am. J. Hematol.* **2023**, *98*, 951–964. [CrossRef]
103. Kovtonyuk, L.V.; Fritsch, K.; Feng, X.; Manz, M.G.; Takizawa, H. Inflamm-Aging of Hematopoiesis, Hematopoietic Stem Cells, and the Bone Marrow Microenvironment. *Front. Immunol.* **2016**, *7*, 502. [CrossRef]
104. Kim, S.-Y.; Yoo, D.-M.; Min, C.; Choi, H.-G. Association between Osteoporosis and Low Hemoglobin Levels: A Nested Case–Control Study Using a National Health Screening Cohort. *Int. J. Environ. Res. Public Health* **2021**, *18*, 8598. [CrossRef]
105. Tozzi-Ciancarelli, M.G.; Fedele, F.; Tozzi, E.; Di Massimo, C.; Oratore, A.; De Matteis, G.; D'Alfonso, A.; Troiani-Sevi, E.; Gallo, P.; Prencipe, M. Age-Dependent Changes in Human Erythrocyte Properties. *CH* **2016**, *9*, 999–1007. [CrossRef]
106. Higuchi-Sanabria, R.; Paul, J.W.; Durieux, J.; Benitez, C.; Frankino, P.A.; Tronnes, S.U.; Garcia, G.; Daniele, J.R.; Monshietehadi, S.; Dillin, A. Spatial Regulation of the Actin Cytoskeleton by HSF-1 during Aging. *MBoC* **2018**, *29*, 2522–2527. [CrossRef]
107. Li, H.; Yang, J.; Chu, T.T.; Naidu, R.; Lu, L.; Chandramohanadas, R.; Dao, M.; Karniadakis, G.E. Cytoskeleton Remodeling Induces Membrane Stiffness and Stability Changes of Maturing Reticulocytes. *Biophys. J.* **2018**, *114*, 2014–2023. [CrossRef]
108. Ciana, A.; Achilli, C.; Minetti, G. Spectrin and Other Membrane-Skeletal Components in Human Red Blood Cells of Different Age. *Cell Physiol. Biochem.* **2017**, *42*, 1139–1152. [CrossRef]
109. Kim, Y.J.; Cho, M.J.; Yu, W.D.; Kim, M.J.; Kim, S.Y.; Lee, J.H. Links of Cytoskeletal Integrity with Disease and Aging. *Cells* **2022**, *11*, 2896. [CrossRef]

110. Remigante, A.; Morabito, R.; Marino, A. Band 3 Protein Function and Oxidative Stress in Erythrocytes. *J. Cell. Physiol.* **2021**, *236*, 6225–6234. [CrossRef]
111. Levin, A.S.; Bilous, R.W.; Coresh, J. Chapter 1: Definition and Classification of CKD. *Kidney Int. Suppl.* **2013**, *3*, 19–62. [CrossRef]
112. Waas, T.; Schulz, A.; Lotz, J.; Rossmann, H.; Pfeiffer, N.; Beutel, M.E.; Schmidtmann, I.; Münzel, T.; Wild, P.S.; Lackner, K.J. Distribution of Estimated Glomerular Filtration Rate and Determinants of Its Age Dependent Loss in a German Population-Based Study. *Sci. Rep.* **2021**, *11*, 10165. [CrossRef] [PubMed]
113. Bikbov, B.; Purcell, C.A.; Levey, A.S.; Smith, M.; Abdoli, A.; Abebe, M.; Adebayo, O.M.; Afarideh, M.; Agarwal, S.K.; Agudelo-Botero, M.; et al. Global, Regional, and National Burden of Chronic Kidney Disease, 1990–2017: A Systematic Analysis for the Global Burden of Disease Study 2017. *Lancet* **2020**, *395*, 709–733. [CrossRef] [PubMed]
114. Kovesdy, C.P.; Davis, J.R.; Duling, I.; Little, D.J. Prevalence of Anaemia in Adults with Chronic Kidney Disease in a Representative Sample of the United States Population: Analysis of the 1999–2018 National Health and Nutrition Examination Survey. *Clin. Kidney J.* **2023**, *16*, 303–311. [CrossRef]
115. Stauffer, M.E.; Fan, T. Prevalence of Anemia in Chronic Kidney Disease in the United States. *PLoS ONE* **2014**, *9*, e84943. [CrossRef] [PubMed]
116. Sutaria, A.; Liu, L.; Ahmed, Z. Multiple Medication (Polypharmacy) and Chronic Kidney Disease in Patients Aged 60 and Older: A Pharmacoepidemiologic Perspective. *Ther. Adv. Cardiovasc. Dis.* **2016**, *10*, 242–250. [CrossRef] [PubMed]
117. Fusco, S.; Garasto, S.; Corsonello, A.; Vena, S.; Mari, V.; Gareri, P.; Ruotolo, G.; Luciani, F.; Roncone, A.; Maggio, M.; et al. Medication-Induced Nephrotoxicity in Older Patients. *CDM* **2016**, *17*, 608–625. [CrossRef]
118. Khan, S.; Loi, V.; Rosner, M.H. Drug-Induced Kidney Injury in the Elderly. *Drugs Aging* **2017**, *34*, 729–741. [CrossRef]
119. Luckey, A.E.; Parsa, C.J. Fluid and Electrolytes in the Aged. *Arch. Surg.* **2003**, *138*, 1055–1060. [CrossRef]
120. Begg, D.P. Disturbances of Thirst and Fluid Balance Associated with Aging. *Physiol. Behav.* **2017**, *178*, 28–34. [CrossRef]
121. Docherty, N.G.; Delles, C.; D'Haese, P.; Layton, A.T.; Martínez-Salgado, C.; Vervaet, B.A.; López-Hernández, F.J. Haemodynamic Frailty—A Risk Factor for Acute Kidney Injury in the Elderly. *Ageing Res. Rev.* **2021**, *70*, 101408. [CrossRef]
122. El-Sharkawy, A.M.; Devonald, M.A.J.; Humes, D.J.; Sahota, O.; Lobo, D.N. Hyperosmolar Dehydration: A Predictor of Kidney Injury and Outcome in Hospitalised Older Adults. *Clin. Nutr.* **2020**, *39*, 2593–2599. [CrossRef] [PubMed]
123. Fandrey, J. Why Not the Liver Instead of the Kidney? *Blood* **2012**, *120*, 1760–1761. [CrossRef]
124. Haase, V.H. Regulation of Erythropoiesis by Hypoxia-Inducible Factors. *Blood Rev.* **2013**, *27*, 41–53. [CrossRef]
125. Vlasschaert, C.; McNaughton, A.J.M.; Chong, M.; Cook, E.K.; Hopman, W.; Kestenbaum, B.; Robinson-Cohen, C.; Garland, J.; Moran, S.M.; Paré, G.; et al. Association of Clonal Hematopoiesis of Indeterminate Potential with Worse Kidney Function and Anemia in Two Cohorts of Patients with Advanced Chronic Kidney Disease. *JASN* **2022**, *33*, 985–995. [CrossRef]
126. Takata, T.; Mae, Y.; Yamada, K.; Taniguchi, S.; Hamada, S.; Yamamoto, M.; Iyama, T.; Isomoto, H. Skeletal Muscle Mass Is Associated with Erythropoietin Response in Hemodialysis Patients. *BMC Nephrol.* **2021**, *22*, 134. [CrossRef] [PubMed]
127. Rundqvist, H.; Rullman, E.; Sundberg, C.J.; Fischer, H.; Eisleitner, K.; Ståhlberg, M.; Sundblad, P.; Jansson, E.; Gustafsson, T. Activation of the Erythropoietin Receptor in Human Skeletal Muscle. *Eur. J. Endocrinol.* **2009**, *161*, 427–434. [CrossRef]
128. Zeng, F.; Huang, L.; Zhang, Y.; Hong, X.; Weng, S.; Shen, X.; Zhao, F.; Yan, S. Additive Effect of Sarcopenia and Anemia on the 10-Year Risk of Cardiovascular Disease in Patients with Type 2 Diabetes. *J. Diabetes Res.* **2022**, *2022*, 2202511. [CrossRef] [PubMed]
129. Tseng, S.-H.; Lee, W.-J.; Peng, L.-N.; Lin, M.-H.; Chen, L.-K. Associations between Hemoglobin Levels and Sarcopenia and Its Components: Results from the I-Lan Longitudinal Study. *Exp. Gerontol.* **2021**, *150*, 111379. [CrossRef] [PubMed]
130. Hirani, V.; Naganathan, V.; Blyth, F.; Le Couteur, D.G.; Seibel, M.J.; Waite, L.M.; Handelsman, D.J.; Hsu, B.; Cumming, R.G. Low Hemoglobin Concentrations Are Associated with Sarcopenia, Physical Performance, and Disability in Older Australian Men in Cross-Sectional and Longitudinal Analysis: The Concord Health and Ageing in Men Project. *Gerona* **2016**, *71*, 1667–1675. [CrossRef]
131. Boelaert, K. Thyroid Dysfunction in the Elderly. *Nat. Rev. Endocrinol.* **2013**, *9*, 194–204. [CrossRef]
132. Maggio, M.; De Vita, F.; Fisichella, A.; Lauretani, F.; Ticinesi, A.; Ceresini, G.; Cappola, A.; Ferrucci, L.; Ceda, G.P. The Role of the Multiple Hormonal Dysregulation in the Onset of "Anemia of Aging": Focus on Testosterone, IGF-1, and Thyroid Hormones. *Int. J. Endocrinol.* **2015**, *2015*, 292574. [CrossRef] [PubMed]
133. Bhasin, S.; Brito, J.P.; Cunningham, G.R.; Hayes, F.J.; Hodis, H.N.; Matsumoto, A.M.; Snyder, P.J.; Swerdloff, R.S.; Wu, F.C.; Yialamas, M.A. Testosterone Therapy in Men with Hypogonadism: An Endocrine Society Clinical Practice Guideline. *J. Clin. Endocrinol. Metab.* **2018**, *103*, 1715–1744. [CrossRef] [PubMed]
134. Al-Sharefi, A.; Mohammed, A.; Abdalaziz, A.; Jayasena, C.N. Androgens and Anemia: Current Trends and Future Prospects. *Front. Endocrinol.* **2019**, *10*, 754. [CrossRef] [PubMed]
135. Carrero, J.J.; Bárány, P.; Yilmaz, M.I.; Qureshi, A.R.; Sonmez, A.; Heimbürger, O.; Ozgurtas, T.; Yenicesu, M.; Lindholm, B.; Stenvinkel, P. Testosterone Deficiency Is a Cause of Anaemia and Reduced Responsiveness to Erythropoiesis-Stimulating Agents in Men with Chronic Kidney Disease. *Nephrol. Dial. Transplant.* **2012**, *27*, 709–715. [CrossRef]
136. Magné, N.; Daguenet, E.; Bouletour, W.; Conraux, L.; Tinquaut, F.; Grangeon, K.; Moreno-Acosta, P.; Suchaud, J.-P.; Rancoule, C.; Guy, J.-B. Impact of Radiation Therapy on Biological Parameters in Cancer Patients: Sub-Analysis from the RIT Prospective Epidemiological Study. *Cancer Investig.* **2023**, *41*, 109–118. [CrossRef] [PubMed]

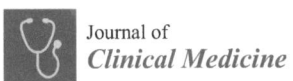

Systematic Review

Effects of Exercise on Frailty in Older People Based on ACSM Recommendations: A Systematic Review and Meta-Analysis of Randomized Controlled Trials

Neng Pan [1,*], Zbigniew Ossowski [1], Jun Tong [2], Dan Li [3] and Shan Gao [3]

1. Faculty of Physical Culture, Akademia Wychowania Fizycznego I Sportu, 80-336 Gdansk, Poland; zbigniew.ossowski@awf.gda.pl
2. Department of Sport, Kunming Medical University, Kunming 650000, China; tongjun080511@163.com
3. Academy of Sport, Yunnan Normal University, Kunming 650000, China; 17279123996@163.com (D.L.); gaoshan199608@163.com (S.G.)
* Correspondence: neng.pan@awf.gda.pl; Tel.: +48-734-908-103

Abstract: Objectives: The objective of the study was to carry out an analysis of the methodological quality of clinical trials (effects of exercise on frailty in older people) based on ACSM recommendations. **Methods**: The search scope included PubMed, Embase, Web of Science, Cochrane, and literature that cannot be retrieved from the database. The topic was the impact of exercise on frailty in elderly people. Changes in five outcome measures (FP, BI, SPPB, GS, and BMI) were assessed using mean differences (MD) and 95% confidence intervals (95% CI). A random effects model (RE) was used to conduct a meta-analysis and compare the results between subgroups. **Results:** The intervention effects of exercise on the five outcome indicators of frailty in elderly people were all significant ($p < 0.05$). The effect of a high-consistency subgroup on outcome indicators FP and GS was more significant than that of the low- or uncertain-consistency subgroup (MD: −1.09 < −0.11, MD: 2.39 >1.1). There was no significant difference in the intervention effect as reflected in the outcome measures SPPB and BMI in the high-consistency subgroup ($p = 0.07$, $p = 0.34$). There was no significant difference in the impact of the intervention on the outcome measure BI between the two subgroups ($p = 0.06$, $p = 0.14$). **Conclusions:** Exercise prescriptions with high consistency with ACSM recommendations may be more effective in both FP and GS interventions than those with uncertain or low consistency. However, it is essential to note that the data derived from the meta-analysis is still subject to the small number of studies, the unknown degree of consistency of participants in individual studies, and the different mix of cases in the studies.

Keywords: frailty; elderly; ACSM recommendations; exercise intervention; exercise dose

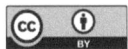

1. Introduction

The clinical syndrome that meets three or more of the following criteria is referred to as frailty: unexpected weight loss (10 pounds in the last year), poor physical activity, self-reported tiredness, grip strength weakening, and sluggish walking [1]. The clinical condition known as frailty is defined by an individual's extreme susceptibility to both internal and external stimuli [2]. The world's aging population is one of the demographic groups seeing the most drastic changes. Current estimates indicate that between 2015 and 2030, there will be 1.4 billion persons worldwide who are 60 years of age or older, up from 901 million in 2015. By 2050, that number is expected to approach 2.1 billion [3]. Frailty in elderly people is a multi-dimensional syndrome that involves the interaction of biological, psychological, and social factors. It is associated with a higher risk of adverse outcomes, such as a decline in functional ability, falls, delirium, institutionalization, hospitalization, and death [4,5]. Exercises, dietary intervention, multi-component treatments, and individually customized geriatric care models are the four main kinds of interventions that have been tried to enhance the health outcomes of weak patients or, more recently, to battle frailty [6]. Many macronutrients and micronutrients have been shown to either directly cause or interact with frailty, indicating that diet plays a crucial role in both avoiding and exacerbating frailty syndrome [7]. However, more longitudinal studies on this topic are required to further understand the potential role of nutrition in preventing, postponing, or reversing frailty syndrome [8]. In elderly patients, frailty and polypharmacy are prevalent and well-researched conditions, but little is known about how they could affect one another [9]. Reducing polypharmacy could be a cautious strategy to prevent and manage frailty. Further research is needed to confirm the possible benefits of reducing polypharmacy in frailty development, reversion, or delay [10]. Low-level care could be promoted as a primary intervention [11]. Exercise reduces age-related oxidative damage and chronic inflammation, increases autophagy, and improves mitochondrial function, the myokine profile, the insulin-like growth factor-1 (IGF-1) signaling pathway, and insulin sensitivity [12]. Consequently, physical activity and exercise are regarded as one of the primary methods for preventing the physical deterioration associated with frailty in elderly people.

Lifestyle behaviors like physical activity can help manage frailty levels [13]. Frailty is not a reason to avoid physical activity; in fact, it can be one of the most significant reasons to recommend it [14]. Although the optimal level of exercise intervention intensity (duration and frequency) is yet unknown, consistency is consistently high across different programs [4]. Physical performance tests have been used as alternative measures of frailty since they are associated with, or predictive of, frailty [15–17]. Although the Short Physical Performance Battery (SPPB) was originally designed to assess lower limb function, it has also been used to gauge physical frailty in earlier research [18,19]. Grip strength is a viable test to administer in a clinical context and has been utilized as a single item measure for frailty in several investigations [16,20]. One of the most used frailty assessments, the Fried Frailty Phenotype (FP), operationalizes frailty as a biological phenotype into five quantifiable criteria [1]. The Barthel Index is a valid measure of disability [21]. These are important predictors of health outcomes and are therefore useful outcome measures to assess the effectiveness of exercise. A person's height and weight are used to calculate their body mass index (BMI), which enables them to be categorized as overweight or obese [22]. Body fat contributes to the association between BMI and frailty, and a larger proportion of body fat is linked to frailty [23]. All of the indicators mentioned above can be affected by exercise. For older persons who are at risk of frailty, exercise is the medication that may reverse or alleviate frailty, maintain quality of life, and restore independent functioning [24].The best approach for enhancing gait, balance, and strength in older adults while also lowering their fall risk and preserving their functional ability as they age appears to be a multi-component exercise intervention program that includes strength, endurance, and balance training [25]. Nonetheless, some academics have suggested that in order to choose the most beneficial exercise regimen, additional research on this subject that also includes fragile populations is required [26].

The American College of Sports Medicine (ACSM) has created exercise regimens that are advised for older folks. These regimens include specific recommendations for the dosage of cardiorespiratory exercise, resistance training, and balancing exercise for frail people [27,28]. However, it is currently unclear whether exercise interventions based on the ACSM recommendations will significantly impact frailty in elderly people more than exercise interventions with low or uncertain consistency. This systematic review aims to analyze the methodological quality of clinical randomized controlled trials (effects of exercise on frailty in older adults) based on ACSM recommendations.

2. Materials and Methods

The Preferred Reporting Items for Systematic Reviews and Meta-Analyses (PRISMA) statement have been followed in reporting the systematic review and meta-analyses, and will be registered in PROSPERO (CRD42024517899).

2.1. Search Strategy

Our search strategy was based on the PICOS principle. We searched the PubMed, Embase, Web of Science, and Cochrane databases from their inception to 20 January 2024. It was last searched on 25 January 2024. It focused on disease type, study population, intervention, and research methodology. The search terms included the following: ("Asthenia" or "Frailty" or "Fatigue" or "Neurasthenia" or "Muscle Weakness" or "Frailties" or "Frailness" or "Frailty Syndrome" or "Debility" or "Debilities") AND ("Exercise" or "walking" or "Nordic Walking" or "Exercises" or "Physical Activity" or "Activities, Physical" or "Activity, Physical" or "Physical Activities" or "Exercise, Physical" or "Exercises, Physical" or "Physical Exercise" or "Physical Exercises" or "Exercise, Aerobic" or "Aerobic Exercise" or "Aerobic Exercises" or "Exercises, Aerobic" or "Exercise Training" or "Exercise Trainings" or "Training, Exercise" or "Trainings, Exercise" or "Training, Resistance" or "Strength Training" or "Training, Strength" or "Balance" or "Ambulation" or "Stair Climbing" or "Walking, Nordic" or "Pole Walking" or "Walking, Pole") AND ("Randomized controlled trial" or "controlled clinical trial" or "randomized" or "placebo" or "randomly") AND ("aged" or "elderly"). The detailed search strategy is shown in Supplementary Materials. We manually searched for the literature that could not be retrieved from the database. When necessary, we contacted the authors by email for further information.

2.2. Criteria for Selection of Studies

First of all, we need to state that there are no restrictions on the publication time and language of the included articles. The study inclusion criteria were as follows: (a) published studies using randomized controls (RCTs); (b) the participants consisted of older adults who had previously received a diagnosis of pre-frailty or frailty, as well as those exhibiting suspected symptoms of frailty (either during hospitalization or shortly after discharge). Different clinical trials have used different criteria to identify frailty in patients. Some trials have used a Barthel Index score of 50 or higher and the MEC-35, which is a modified and validated version of the mini-mental state test in Spanish. Other trials have used a walking pace test and a chair standing test to identify frailness. Some trials have even used patients' self-reports and the number of falls they have experienced as criteria for determining frailty. These methods are able to derive participants in a state that approximates, but is not exactly equivalent to, pre-frailty or frailty; (c) any kind of exercise program, such as resistance, flexibility, or aerobic training, might be used as an intervention; (d) the control group only received routine care that did not include exercise or carried out daily life; (e) outcome measures included at least one of five outcomes related to frailty in elderly people: grip strength, BI, SPPB, the Fried scale, and BMI.

The research exclusion criteria included the following: (a) reports, meeting minutes, comments, etc., were not considered; (b) in the intervention group, interventions that combined exercise, nutrition, drug treatment, etc.; (c) in the control group, in addition to routine care and daily life, all interventions; (d) redundant experimental data that appeared in many papers related to the same research were excluded.

The titles and abstracts of the literature that satisfied the inclusion requirements were separately examined by two writers (N.P. and J.T.). The whole text of the paper was retrieved if one of the writers determined that a research paper satisfied the criteria. Subsequently, two writers separately evaluated whether the whole text satisfied the requirements. In the event that an agreement could not be reached, debate led to the decision being taken by the fourth author (D.L.). Subjects were defined as older individuals without regard to language, body mass index, gender, or publication date constraints.

2.3. Data Synthesis and Analyses

Two authors (N.P. and J.T.) independently extracted data for the included studies. Grip strength and Fried scale were the primary outcomes; SPPB, BI, and BMI were the secondary outcomes. An Excel spreadsheet was designed in advance to extract the relevant data, including publication characteristics (author name, country, publication year), methodological characteristics (interventions, sample size), participant characteristics (age, gender), campaign characteristics (intervention period, intervention frequency, duration), risk assessment, and outcome characteristics.

When extracting the result data, Engauge Digitizer 4.1 software was used to extract the research data presented in the form of pictures. We extracted data only immediately after the intervention for studies with multiple follow-up assessments.

After the data extraction, the exercise intervention was evaluated for dose and consistency. The exercise intervention doses in this study were assessed against ACSM recommendations for developing and maintaining cardiorespiratory, muscle, skeletal, and neurological function in healthy adults [29]. According to ACSM recommendations, two authors (NP and JT) independently evaluated each study's exercise intervention based on different criteria defined for exercise dose (frequency, intensity, duration, etc.) to assess consistency to exercise dose (Table 1).

Table 1. The ACSM guidelines for muscular strength, flexibility, and cardiorespiratory fitness in individuals who seem to be in good health.

Exercise Dose	Cardiorespiratory Exercise	Resistance Exercise	Flexibility Exercise
Frequency	4–5 days/week	On non-consecutive days, 1–2 days each week, progressively rising to 2–3 days per week.	5–7 days/week
Intensity/workload	Moderate intensity, 40–59%VO^2R/HRR, CR-10 scale rating of 3–4	The last two sets should be difficult; adjust the resistance accordingly. If it's manageable, high-intensity exercise may be done.	Stretch until you feel your muscles being pulled tight or a slight discomfort.
Duration	Gradually increase from 20 min to at least 30 min (up to 45–60 min)	After approximately two weeks, work your way up to two sets of eight to twelve repetitions. Don't exceed 8–10 exercises in a single session.	Repeated 2–4 times, static stretching is sustained for 10–30 s.

HRR: heart rate reserve. VO^2R: oxygen uptake reserve.

The scoring criteria for each indicator in this meta-analysis was 0 points for not completely meeting the standards; 1 point for not being sure whether it meets or may meet the standards; 2 points for completely meeting the standards. If two authors had different opinions during the review process, a third author was invited to discuss this until a consensus was reached. This scoring rubric was used to calculate the proportion of each metric that meets the ACSM recommended exercise measures. When the proportion was $\geq 70\%$, this meant a high-consistency relationship with ACSM recommendations; when <70%, this meant a low- or uncertain-consistency relationship with ACSM recommendations.

2.4. Biased Risk Assessment

Two pairs of authors completed quality assessments (NP and JT and ZO, DL, and SG). The evaluation tool used was the Cochrane risk of bias tool (Rob). The evaluation reference standard was Cochrane Collaboration's tool for assessing the risk of bias [30]. This study's investigations were all randomized controlled trials. Evaluation indicators include incomplete outcome data (attrition bias), biased reporting (reporting bias), blinding of personnel and participants (performance bias), allocation concealment (selection bias), random sequence generation (selection bias), and other bias [30]. Three categories were used to categorize bias risk: "low risk," "unclear risk", and "high risk".

2.5. Statistical Analyses

This meta-analysis used REVIEW MANAGER 5.4.1 to perform statistics and analysis on the data, divided into two groups: high consistency with ACSM guidelines and low or uncertain consistency with ACSM guidelines. In the heterogeneity test within the subgroup, if $I^2 > 50\%$, the random effects model was used, and if $I^2 < 50\%$, the random effects model or the fixed effect model was used [31]. When the included literature used scales to evaluate outcome indicators, if the scales used were different, standard mean difference for analysis was used; if the scales used were the same, mean difference for analysis was used.

3. Results

3.1. Study Selection

The retrieved literature included PubMed (2027), Embase (45), Web of Science (3712), and Cochrane (8401), totaling 14,185 articles. A total of seven articles were found through other search methods. After removing duplicates (2027), 12,165 articles remained. After a preliminary review of titles and abstracts, 743 articles remained; after a final evaluation of whole texts, 20 remained [32–51] (Figure 1).

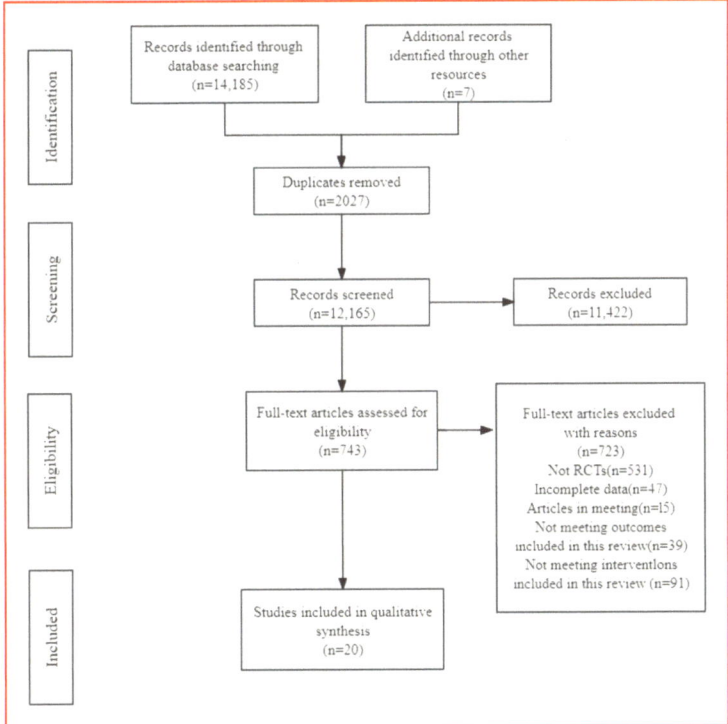

Figure 1. PRISMA study flow diagram.

3.2. Study Characteristics

In total, 2016 persons over 60 were enrolled in the 20 investigations (1004 in the intervention group and 1012 in the control group). The studies that were considered include the following outcome indicators: "BMI," "grip strength," "SPPB," "Fried," and "BI." There are thirteen articles on "grip strength" result indicators, six on "Fried" outcome indicators, eight on "BI" outcome indicators, eleven on "SPPB" outcome indicators, and three on "BMI" outcome indicators [32–51]. The included articles are from France, Turkey, Spain, Denmark, Japan, Taiwan, Singapore, Ireland, Canada, Thailand, and China (Table 2).

Table 2. Included article characteristics.

Author	Country	Year	Population	Age (Mean + SD)	Total/Male/Female	Intervention	Control	Outcome
Juan Luis Sánchez-Sánchez [39]	France	2022	Frailty Pre-frailty	T:84.15(4.76) C:83.99(4.8)	T:88/28/60 C:100/40/60	Vivifrail training Length of Intervention: 12 weeks Freq: 3–5 times a week Duration: 30–60 min	CON	SPPB Grip strength
Ulku K. Sahin [34]	Turkey	2018	Frailty	T:84.18(6.85) C:85.37(4.7)	T:16/NA/NA C:16/NA/NA	Resistance training Length of Intervention: 8 weeks Freq: 3 times a week Duration: 40 min	CON	Grip strength BI
Haritz Arrieta [42]	Spain	2019	Frailty	T:85.1(7.6) C:84.7(6.1)	T:57/15/42 C:55/18/37	MEP Length of Intervention: 24 weeks Freq: 2 times a week Duration: 60 min	CON	SPPB BI
Maria Giné-Garriga [33]	Spain	2010	Frailty	T:83.9(2.8) C:84.1(3)	T:22/9/13 C:19/7/12	FCT Length of Intervention: 12 weeks Freq: 2 times a week Duration: 45 min	CON	BI
Sonja Vestergaard [45]	Denmark	2008	Frailty	T:81(3.3) C:82.7(3.8)	T:25/0/25 C:28/0/28	Vivifrail training Length of Intervention: 12 weeks Freq: 3–5 times a week Duration: 30–60 min	CON	Grip strength
Yoshiji Kato [38]	Japan	2018	Frailty	T:77.6(7.2) C:79.6(7.7)	T:18/11/7 C:13/7/6	NHK&MP&CR Length of Intervention: 12 weeks Freq: 7 times a week Duration: 25 min	CON	BMI BI
Francisco José Tarazona-Santabalbina [48]	Spain	2016	Frailty	T:79.7(3.6) C:80.3(3.7)	T:51/22/29 C:49/24/25	MEP Length of Intervention: 24 weeks Freq: 5 times a week Duration: 65 min	CON	SPPB BI Fried
Tsung-Jen Hsieh [47]	Taiwan	2019	Frailty Pre-frailty	T:72.0(6.0) C:72.5(5.5)	T:79/28/60 C:80/40/60	Exercise training Length of Intervention: 24 weeks Freq: 3–7 times a week Duration: 5–60 min	CON	Fried Grip strength
Tze Pin Ng [50]	Singapore	2015	Frailty Pre-frailty	T:70.3(5.25) C:70.1(5.02)	T:48/21/27 C:50/22/28	Physical training Length of Intervention: 12 weeks Freq: 2 times a week Duration: 90 min	CON	BMI Fried

Table 2. Cont.

Author	Country	Year	Population	Age (Mean + SD)	Total/Male/Female	Intervention	Control	Outcome
Álvaro Casas-Herrero [43]	Spain	2022	Frailty	T:84.2(4.8) C:84.0(4.8)	T:88/25/63 C:100/31/69	Vivifrail training Length of Intervention: 12 weeks Freq: 5 times a week Duration: 30 min	CON	SPPB BI Grip strength
John Travers [32]	Ireland	2023	Frailty	T:77.6(5.2) C:76.5(5.2)	T:79/25/54 C:77/26/51	Home-based exercise Length of Intervention: 12 weeks Freq: 4 times a week Duration: 45–60 min	CON	Grip strength
Mario Ulises Pérez-Zepeda [46]	Canada	2022	Frailty	T:87.1(4.8) C:87.9(4.5)	T:163/72/91 C:160/69/91	Vivifrail training Length of Intervention: 12 weeks Freq: 3–5 times a week Duration: 30–60 min	CON	BI SPPB Grip strength
Rujie Chen [41]	China	2020	Pre-frailty	T:76.97(5.19) C:75.27(5.98)	T:33/12/21 C:33/11/22	Elastic band training Length of Intervention: 8 weeks Freq: 3 times a week Duration: 45–60 min	CON	Grip strength
T. Liu [40]	China	2022	Frailty	T:80.75(2.99) C:80.74(2.82)	T:67/16/51 C:68/24/44	Integrated exercise Length of Intervention: 12 weeks Freq: 5 times a week Duration: 40 min	CON	Fried
Zhang Xiaohong [44]	China	2023	Frailty	T:64.75(4.35) C:64.94(4.29)	T:36/13/23 C:36/20/16	Dance training Length of Intervention: 16 weeks Freq: 5 times a week Duration: 60 min	CON	SPPB Grip strength
Joaquín Barrachina-Igual [37]	Spain	2021		T:74.83(5.78) C:75.25(8.20)	T:23/7/16 C:20/5/15	MEP Length of Intervention: 12 weeks Freq: 2 times a week Duration: 65 min	CON	BI SPPB Grip strength
Nien Xiang Tou [36]	Singapore	2021	Frailty	T:79.5(4.2) C:74.6(6.5)	T:23/NA/NA C:27/NA/NA	FPT Length of Intervention: 12 weeks Freq: 2 times a week Duration: 60 min	CON	Fried SPPB Grip strength
Pedro Otones [51]	Spain	2020	Frailty	T:79.5(4.2) C:74.6(6.5)	T:17/5/12 C:15/2/13	Physical training Length of Intervention: 32 weeks Freq: 1 time a week Duration: 60 min	CON	SPPB Grip strength

Table 2. *Cont.*

Author	Country	Year	Population	Age (Mean + SD)	Total/Male/Female	Intervention	Control	Outcome
Uratcha Sadjapong [49]	Thailand	2020	Frailty	T:76.68(1.14) C:78.87(1.32)	T:32/16/16 C:32/23/9	MEP Length of Intervention: 12 weeks Freq: 3 times a week Duration: 60 min	CON	Fried Grip strength
Fermín García-Gollarte [35]	Spain	2023	Frailty	T:86(5.9) C:84.9(6)	T:39/9/30 C:34/13/21	OEP training Length of Intervention: 24 weeks Freq: 3 times a week Duration: 40–60 min	CON	SPPB Grip strength

Note: SD: standard deviation, CON: control group with routine care (no exercise), T: experimental group, C: control group; MEP: multi-component exercise program, FCT: functional circuit training, NHK: NHK radio calisthenics, MP: marching in place, CR: chair rising, FPT: functional power training, OEP: Otago Exercise Program. SPPB: Short Physical Performance Battery, BI: Barthel Index, BMI: body mass index, Fried: Fried scale.

The intervention periods in the included literature ranged from 8 to 32 weeks, ranging from 1 to 7 days per week, and the duration of a single intervention ranged from 5 to 90 min. Interventions included regular exercise training, individualized physical activity programs, multi-component physical exercise, dance, and Tai Chi. The intervention measures in the control group were daily life without participating in any physical exercise (Table 2).

Among the included literature, 14 studies were about cardiopulmonary exercise, 18 were about resistance exercise, and 11 were about flexibility exercise. Among them, a total of 10 articles have high consistency to ACSM recommendations (consistency ≥70%), and the remaining ten articles have low or uncertain consistency (consistency <70%) (Table 3).

3.3. Risk of Bias

Low risk of bias >50%, include three indicators: bias in reporting (selective reporting), bias in random sequence generation (selection bias), and additional biases. Three signs indicate an unclear risk of bias ≥50%: allocation concealment (selection bias), staff and participant blinding (performance bias), and outcome assessment blinding (detection bias). Incomplete outcome data (attrition bias) present an unclear risk of bias and a high risk of bias ≥75%, as well as a high risk of bias ≈25% (Figure 2).

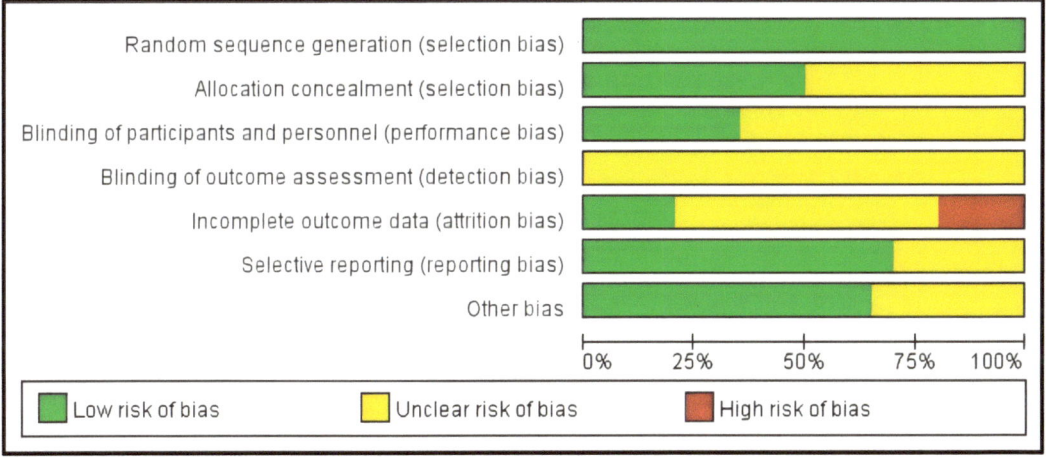

Figure 2. The risk of bias graph displays the percentages representing the review authors' assessments of each risk of bias item for all the included research.

All 20 included articles were randomized controlled trials. Ten articles did not report their allocation methods. Only 13 articles used one blinding method because exercise intervention is difficult to implement under double-masked conditions. None of the 20 articles reported whether blinding was used when processing the results. Experimental samples were lost in 16 articles (12 articles lost samples <10 people, and 4 articles lost samples >10 people). Six articles have the possibility of selective reporting. It was unclear whether there were other risks of bias in seven articles (Figure 3).

Table 3. Exercise interventions evaluated according to the American College of Sports Medicine's (ACSM) recommendations.

Author, Year	Cardiorespiratory Exercise				Resistance Exercise					Flexibility Exercise			ACSM Consistency
	Frequency	Intensity/Workload	Duration	Frequency	Intensity/Workload	Repetitions	Sets	Frequency	Intensity/Workload	Duration			Points (Percent)
	4–5 d/wk	40–59% VO2R/HRR, Moderate Exertion, with a CR-10 Scale Grade of 3–4.	Increase by 20 Minutes Gradually to at Least 30 Min (or Up to 45–60 Min).	1–2 Days per Week, Rising to 2–3 Days per Week over Time	Change the Resistance from Medium to High.	8–12	1–2	5–7 d/wk	Stretch until You Start to Feel a Mild Soreness or a Tugging Sensation in Your Muscles.	Repeated 2–4 Times, Static Stretching Is Sustained for 10–30 s.			
Juan Luis Sánchez-Sánchez, 2022 [39]	5 ☺	Walk at the usual pace.	50–105 (s) ☺	3 ☺	30 RM ☺	12–15 ☺	2 ☺	3 ☺	NR	20–30 (s)	☺		11/20 (55%)
Ulku K. Sahin, 2018 [34]				3 ☺	40–70% 1 RM ☺	6–10 ☺	NR ☺						7/8 (88%)
Haritz Arrieta, 2019 [42]	7 ☺	NR ☺	20 min ☺	2 ☺	40–70% 1 RM ☺	NR ☺	NR ☺	2 ☺	NR	5 (min)	☺		10/20 (50%)
Maria Giné-Garriga, 2010 [33]	2 ☺	Walk at the usual pace.	10 min ☺	2 ☺	12–14 RM ☺	6–15 ☺	1–2 ☺	2 ☺	NR	5 (min)	☺		11/20 (55%)
Sonja Vestergaard, 2008 [45]	3 ☺	Walking on the spot	5 min ☺	3 ☺	NR ☺	NR ☺	NR ☺	3 ☺	NR	15 (min)	☺		6/20 (30%)
Yoshiji Kato, 2018 [38]	7 ☺	Walking on the spot	15 min ☺	7 ☺	NR ☺	NR ☺	NR ☺	7 ☺	NR	5 (min)	☺		6/20 (30%)
Francisco José Tarazona-Santabalbina, 2016 [48]	3 ☺	Moderate intensity	40 min ☺	2 ☺	75%1 RM ☺	8 ☺	3 ☺	5 ☺	NR	20 (s)	☺		15/20 (75%)
Tsung-Jen Hsieh, 2019 [47]				3–7 ☺	ACSM intensity ☺	8–12 ☺	1–2 ☺	3–7 ☺	ACSM intensity	10–30 s	☺		12/14 (86%)
Tze Pin Ng, 2015 [50]				2 ☺	ACSM intensity ☺	8–15 ☺	NR ☺						7/8 (88%)
Álvaro Casas-Herrero, 2022 [43]	5 ☺	Walk at the usual pace.	24 min ☺	3 ☺	NR ☺	12 ☺	3 ☺	3 ☺	NR	10 s	☺		14/20 (70%)
John Travers, 2023 [32]	3–4 ☺	Walking	35–45 min ☺	4–7 ☺	NR ☺	10–15 ☺	≥4 ☺						8/14 (57%)
Mario Ulises Pérez-Zepeda, 2022 [46]	NR ☺	Walk at the usual pace.	24 min ☺	NR ☺	30–60% 1 RM ☺	8–10 ☺	2–3 ☺						10/14 (71%)
Rujie Chen, 2020 [41]				3 ☺	NR ☺	10–15 ☺	2 ☺						7/8 (88%)
T. Liu, 2022 [40]	5 ☺	Tai Chi	40 min ☺					5 ☺	NR	NR	☺		10/12 (83%)

316

Table 3. Cont.

Author, Year	Cardiorespiratory Exercise				Resistance Exercise					Flexibility Exercise			ACSM Consistency
	Frequency	Intensity/Workload	Duration	Frequency	Intensity/Workload	Repetitions	Sets	Frequency	Intensity/Workload	Duration			Points (Percent)
	4–5 d/wk	40–59% VO2R/HRR, Moderate Exertion, with a CR-10 Scale Grade of 3–4.	Increase by 20 Minutes Gradually to at Least 30 Min (or Up to 45–60 Min).	1–2 Days per Week, Rising to 2–3 Days per Week over Time	Change the Resistance from Medium to High.	8–12	1–2	5–7 d/wk	Stretch until You Start to Feel a Mild Soreness or a Tugging Sensation in Your Muscles.	Repeated 2–4 Times, Static Stretching Is Sustained for 10–30 s.			
Sonja Vestergaard, 2008 [45]	5 ☺	Dance ☺	40 min ☺					5 ☺	NR	NR ☺			10/12 (83%)
Yoshiji Kato, 2018 [38]	2 ☺	Walking ☺	10 min ☺	2 ☺	≥70%1 RM ☺	10–15 ☺	3 ☺	2 ☺	NR	NR ☺			10/20 (50%)
Francisco José Tarazona-Santabalbina, 2016 [48]				2 ☺	NR ☺	10–20 ☺	3 ☺						5/8 (63%)
Tsung-Jen Hsieh, 2019 [47]				NR ☺	NR ☺	NR ☺	NR ☺						4/8 (50%)
Tze Pin Ng, 2015 [50]	≥3 ☺	40–65% HRR ☺	10–20 min ☺	≥3 ☺	65–100%1 RM ☺	8–12 ☺	2–3 ☺						10/14 (71%)
Álvaro Casas-Herrero, 2022 [43]	NR ☺	NR ☺	NR ☺	NR ☺	NR ☺	NR ☺	NR ☺						7/14 (50%)

ACSM: American College of Sports Medicine. NR: not reported. Happy/green face: meets the recommendations (2 points), neutral/yellow face: not sure if the recommendations are met (1 point), unhappy/red face: does not meet the recommendations (0 points).

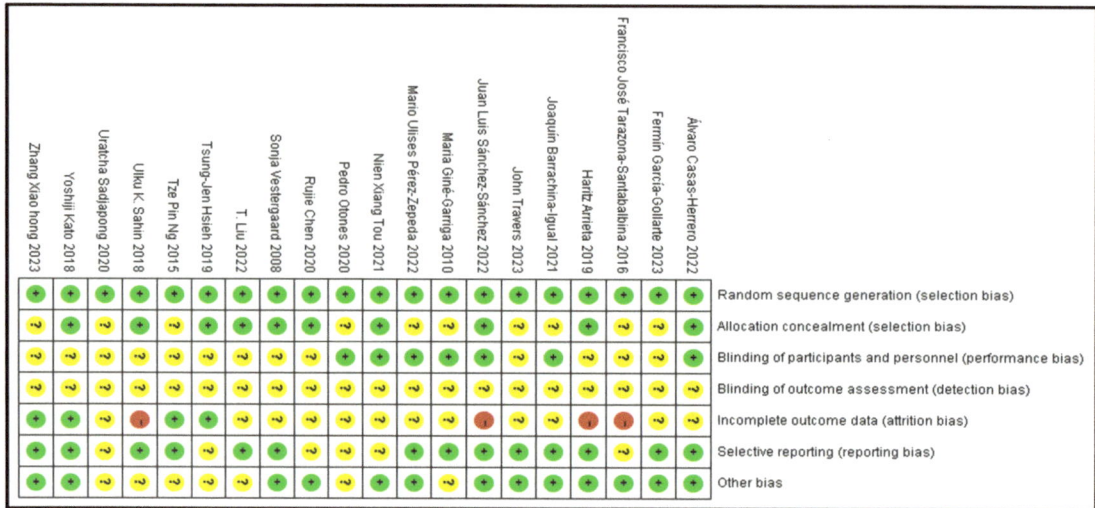

Figure 3. Review the authors' assessments of each risk of bias item for every research article that is included in the risk of bias summary [32–51]. Red: there is a risk. Yellow: it is uncertain whether the risk exists. Green: there is no risk.

3.4. The Impact of Consistency with ACSM Recommendations on the Fried Frailty Phenotype

Outcome indicator 1 (Fried Frailty Phenotype) contains a total of six articles, with 300 people in the intervention group and 306 people in the control group; there was high consistency with ACSM guidelines in five articles, and low or uncertain consistency with ACSM guidelines in one article. After the heterogeneity test ($I^2 = 97\%$), the random effects model was used for statistical analysis. All articles used the same scale for this outcome indicator, so mean difference (MD) was used for statistics and analysis.

Data analysis showed that the overall impact of exercise on the Fried Frailty Phenotype (FP) was −0.93 (95% CI: −1.75, −0.1), which was significantly different ($p = 0.03$). This shows that exercise has a significant intervention effect on FP.

The results of the subgroup analysis showed that in the high-consistency group, the MD was −1.09 (95% CI: −2.01, −0.16) and $I^2 = 98\%$, which was significantly different ($p = 0.02$). This indicates that exercise prescription with high consistency to ACSM guidelines significantly affects the FP intervention.

The results of the subgroup analysis showed that in the low- or uncertain-consistency group, the MD was −0.11 (95% CI: −0.53, 0.31), which was not significantly different ($p = 0.61$). It is unclear whether exercise prescription with low or uncertain consistency to ACSM guidelines significantly influences FP.

In summary, exercise has a significant intervention effect on FP indicators; the MD was −0.93 (95% CI: −1.75, −0.1) and ($p = 0.03$). Exercise prescription with high consistency to ACSM guidelines has a more significant impact on FP than exercise prescription with low or uncertain consistency to ACSM guidelines (−1.09 < −0.11), and the intervention effect is better. Because the FP score is more significant, it indicates a higher degree of frailty [1] (Figure 4). However, the higher heterogeneity in the high-consistency subgroup may be due to the intervention period, intervention measures, and study sample characteristics (Table 2).

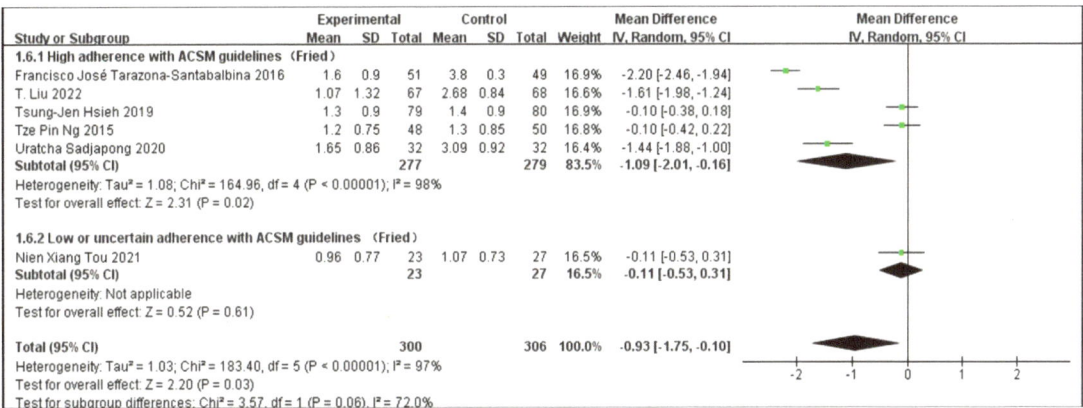

Figure 4. Forest plot for meta-analysis of the impact of exercise on FP indicators in frail elderly people [36,40,47–50]

Subsequently, we conducted publication bias testing through REVIEW MANAGER 5.4.1. We observed the funnel plot and found that both sides were approximately symmetrical, indicating no obvious publication bias (Figure 5).

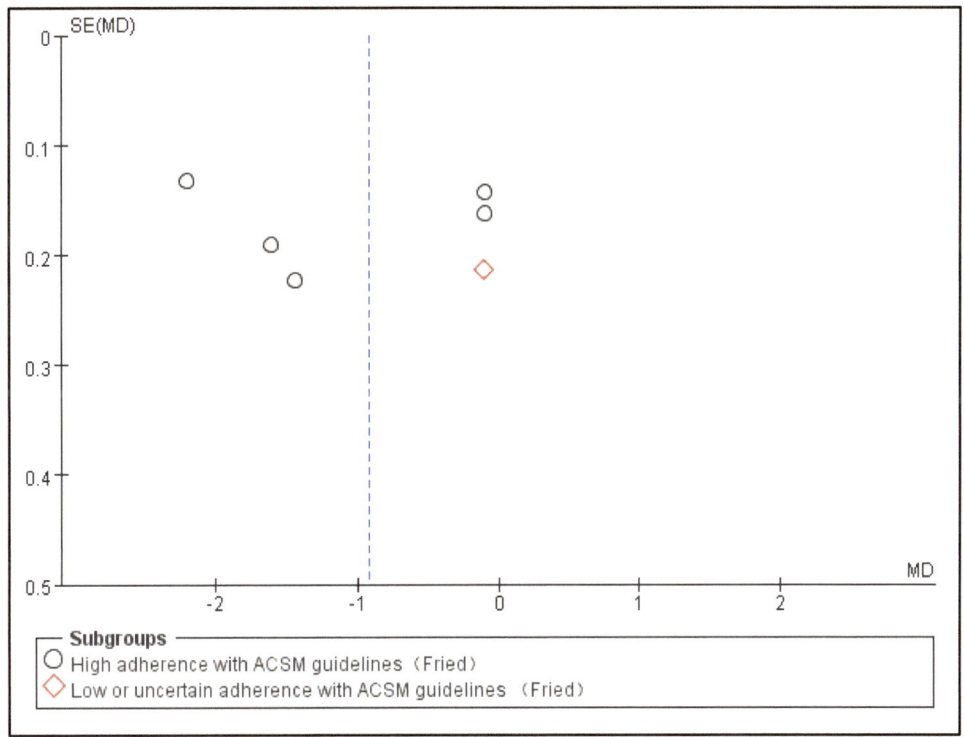

Figure 5. Funnel plot for FP indicator.

3.5. The Impact of Consistency with ACSM Recommendations on the Barthel Index

Outcome indicator 2 (Barthel Index) contains a total of eight articles, with 438 people in the intervention group and 432 people in the control group; there was high consistency with

ACSM guidelines (four articles), and low or uncertain consistency with ACSM guidelines (four articles). After the heterogeneity test ($I^2 = 94\%$), the random effects model was used for statistical analysis. All articles used the same scale for this outcome indicator, so mean difference (MD) was used for statistics and analysis.

Data analysis showed that the overall impact of exercise on the Barthel Index (BI) was 5.79 (95% CI: 1.11, 10.46), which was significantly different ($p = 0.02$). This shows that exercise has a significant intervention effect on BI.

The results of the subgroup analysis showed that in the high-consistency group, the MD was 5.72 (95% CI: −0.16, 11.6) and $I^2 = 87\%$, which was not significantly different ($p = 0.06$). This indicates that it is unclear whether exercise prescription with high consistency to ACSM guidelines has a significant intervention effect on BI.

The results of the subgroup analysis showed that in the low- or uncertain-consistency group, the MD was 5.85 (95% CI: −1.95, 13.65), which was not significantly different ($p = 0.14$). It is unclear whether exercise prescription with low or uncertain consistency to ACSM guidelines has a significant intervention effect on BI.

In summary, exercise has a significant intervention effect on BI indicators; the MD was 5.79 (95% CI: 1.11, 10.46) and ($p = 0.02$). However, it is unclear whether exercise prescriptions with high consistency to ACSM guidelines or with low or uncertain consistency to ACSM guidelines have a significant intervention effect on BI indicators (Figure 6). The higher heterogeneity in the two subgroups may be due to the intervention period, intervention measures, and study sample characteristics (Table 2). It should be noted here that the higher the BI score, the stronger the independence and the lower the dependence.

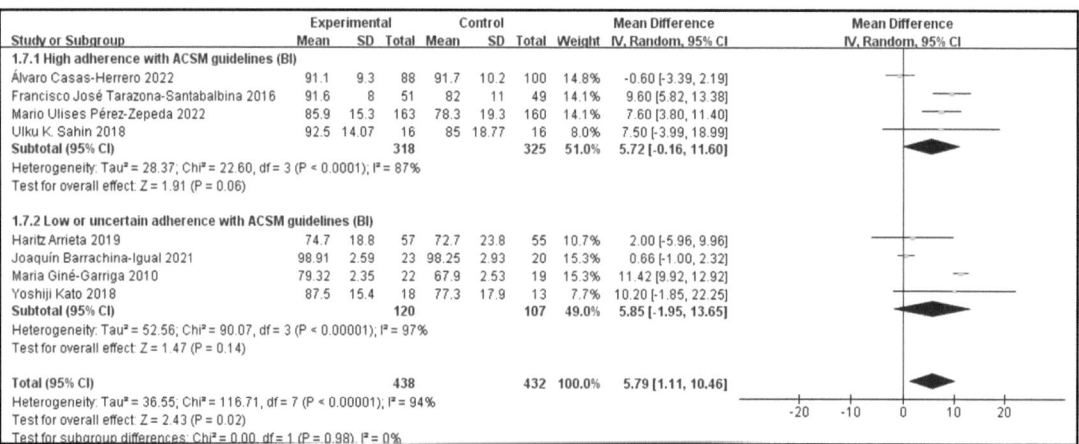

Figure 6. Forest plot for meta-analysis of the impact of exercise on BI indicators in frail elderly people [33,34,37,38,42,43,46,48].

Subsequently, we conducted publication bias testing through REVIEW MANAGER 5.4.1. We observed the funnel plot and found that both sides were approximately symmetrical, indicating no obvious publication bias (Figure 7).

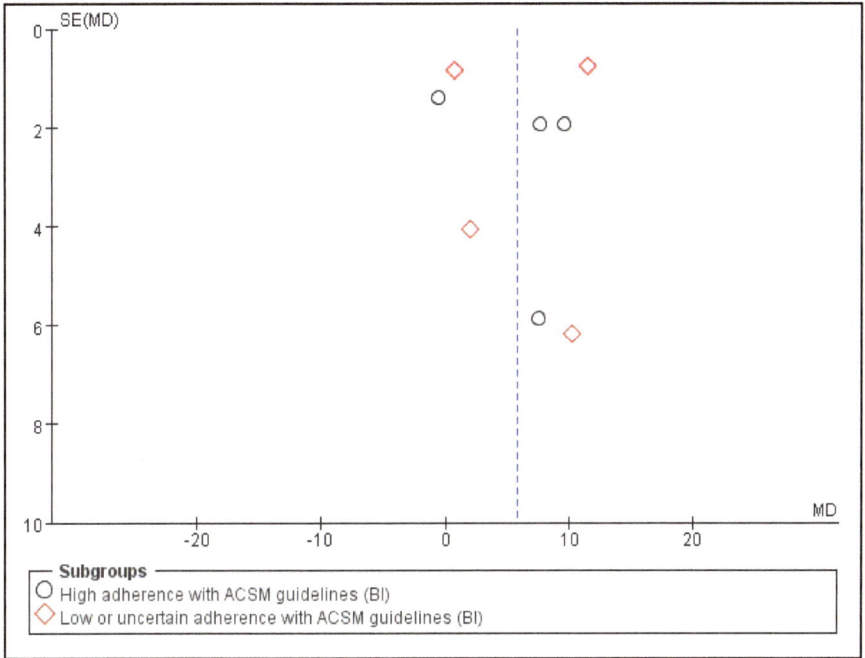

Figure 7. Funnel plot for BI indicator.

3.6. The Impact of Consistency with ACSM Recommendations on the Short Physical Performance Battery

Outcome indicator 3 (Short Physical Performance Battery) contains a total of 10 articles, with 585 people in the intervention group and 596 people in the control group; there was high consistency with ACSM guidelines in 4 articles, and low or uncertain consistency with ACSM guidelines in 6 articles. After the heterogeneity test (I^2 = 93%), the random effects model was used for statistical analysis. All articles used the same scale for this outcome indicator, so mean difference (MD) was used for statistics and analysis.

Data analysis showed that the overall impact of exercise on Short Physical Performance Battery (SPPB) was 1.03 (95% CI: 0.28, 1.78), which was significantly different (p = 0.007). This shows that exercise has a significant intervention effect on SPPB.

The results of the subgroup analysis showed that in the high-consistency group, the MD was 1.42 (95% CI: −0.12, 2.96) and I^2 = 95%, which was not significantly different (p = 0.07). This indicates that it is unclear whether exercise prescription with high consistency to ACSM guidelines has a significant intervention effect on SPPB.

The subgroup analysis findings revealed that the MD was 0.73 (95% CI: 0.01, 1.46) in the low- or unclear-consistency group, which was different (p = 0.05). This suggests that the SPPB intervention is impacted by exercise prescription that is inconsistent or poor in relation to ACSM standards.

In summary, exercise has a significant intervention effect on SPPB indicators, with an MD of 1.03 (95% CI: 0.28, 1.78) and (p = 0.007). Exercise prescriptions with low or uncertain ACSM guideline consistency had a more statistically significant impact on SPPB than those with high ACSM guideline consistency (p = 0.05 > p = 0.07). However, looking only at the mean of the intervention effect, the former is smaller than the latter (0.73 < 1.42). This suggests that exercise prescriptions with high consistency to ACSM guidelines may be more effective for SPPB intervention than those with low or uncertain consistency to ACSM guidelines (Figure 8). The higher heterogeneity in the two subgroups may be due to the intervention period, intervention measures, and study sample characteristics (Table 2). It should be noted that the higher the SPPB score, the better the physical function performance.

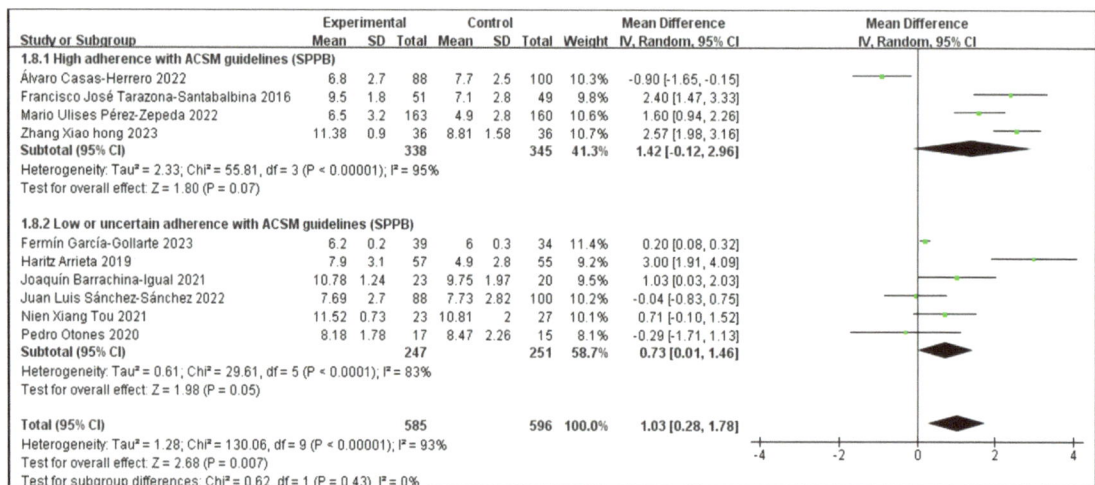

Figure 8. Forest plot for meta-analysis of the impact of exercise on SPPB indicators in frail elderly people [35–37,39,42–44,46,48,51].

Subsequently, we conducted publication bias testing through REVIEW MANAGER 5.4.1. We observed the funnel plot and found that both sides were approximately symmetrical, indicating no obvious publication bias (Figure 9).

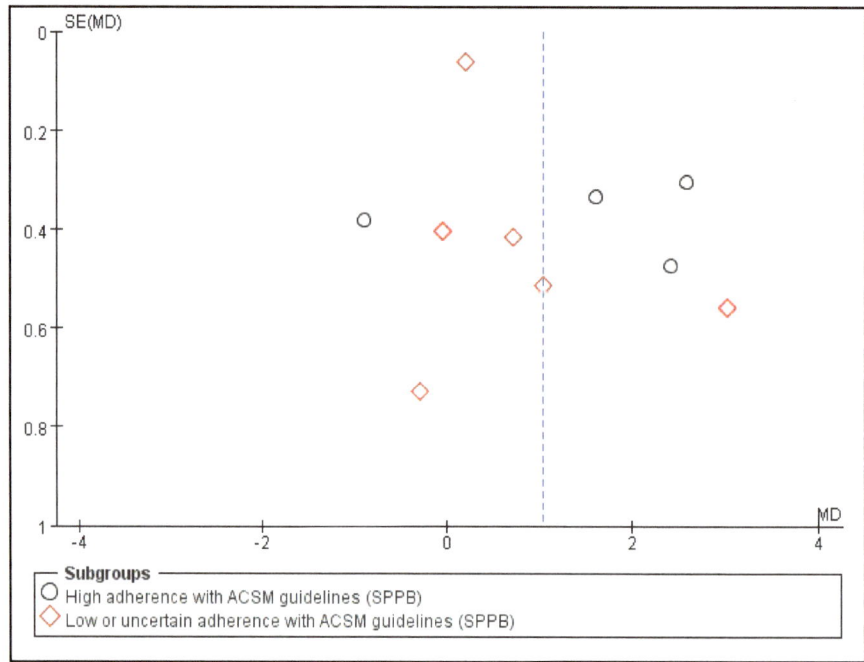

Figure 9. Funnel plot for SPPB indicator.

3.7. The Impact of Consistency with ACSM Recommendations on the Grip Strength

Outcome indicator 4 (grip strength) contains a total of 13 articles, with 712 people in the intervention group and 732 people in the control group; there was high consistency with ACSM guidelines in 7 articles, and low or uncertain consistency with ACSM guidelines in 6 articles. After the heterogeneity test ($I^2 = 78\%$), the random effects model was used for statistical analysis. All articles used the same scale for this outcome indicator, so mean difference (MD) was used for statistics and analysis.

Data analysis showed that the overall impact of exercise on the grip strength (GS) was 1.86 (95% CI: 0.75, 2.97), which was significantly different ($p = 0.001$). This shows that exercise has a significant intervention effect on GS.

The results of the subgroup analysis showed that in the high-consistency group, the MD was 2.39 (95% CI: 0.69, 4.09) and $I^2 = 74\%$, which was significantly different ($p = 0.006$). This indicates that exercise prescription with high consistency to ACSM guidelines significantly affects GS intervention.

The results of the subgroup analysis showed that in the low- or uncertain-consistency group, the MD was 1.1 (95% CI: −0.89, 3.09) and $I^2 = 84\%$, which was not significantly different ($p = 0.28$). It is unclear whether exercise prescription with low or uncertain consistency to ACSM guidelines has a significant intervention effect on GS.

In summary, exercise has a significant intervention effect on GS indicators; the MD was 1.86 (95% CI: 0.75, 2.97) and ($p = 0.001$). Exercise prescription with high consistency to ACSM guidelines has a more significant impact on GS than exercise prescription with low or uncertain consistency to ACSM guidelines (2.39 > 1.1), and the intervention effect is better. Because the GS score number is more significant, It indicates a lower degree of frailty [16] (Figure 10). The higher heterogeneity in the two subgroups may be due to the intervention period, intervention measures, and study sample characteristics (Table 2).

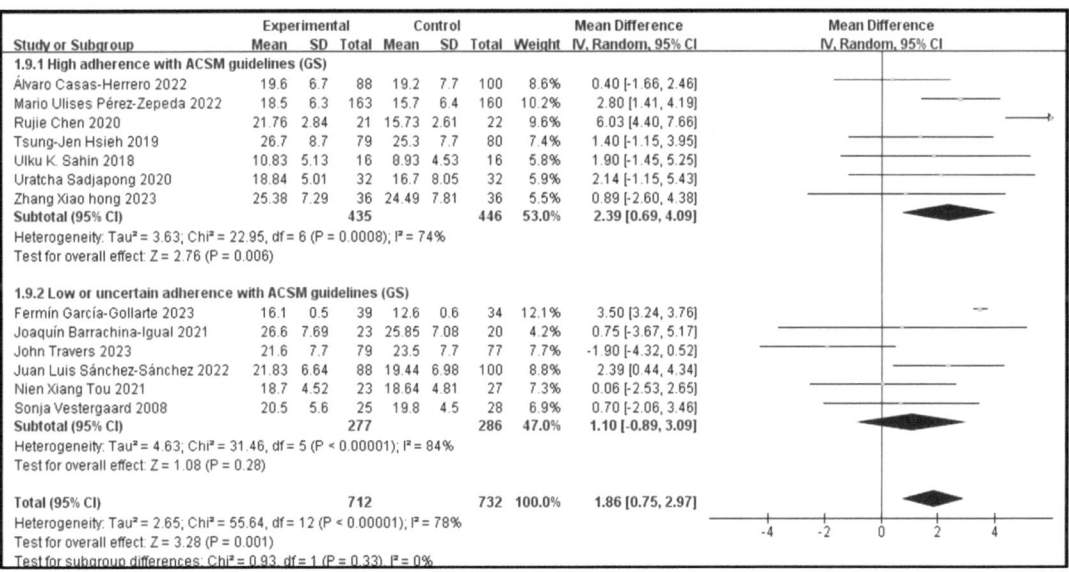

Figure 10. Forest plot for meta-analysis of the impact of exercise on GS indicators in frail elderly people [32,34–37,39,41,43–47,49].

Subsequently, we conducted publication bias testing through REVIEW MANAGER 5.4.1. We observed the funnel plot and found that both sides were approximately symmetrical, indicating no obvious publication bias (Figure 11).

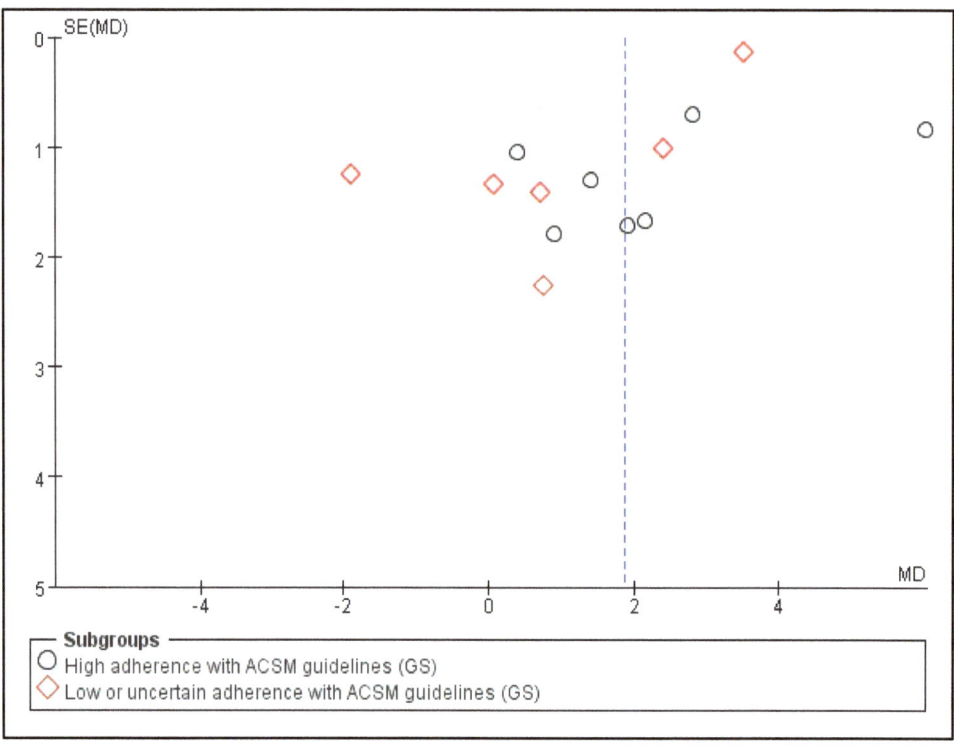

Figure 11. Funnel plot for GS indicator.

3.8. The Impact of Consistency with ACSM Recommendations on the Body Mass Index

There are three publications for outcome indicator 5 (BMI), with 89 participants in the intervention group and 83 participants in the control group. One study showed excellent consistency with ACSM standards, while the other two showed poor or questionable consistency (two articles). For statistical analysis, the fixed effects model was used after the heterogeneity test ($I^2 = 31\%$). Since this outcome variable was used on the same scale across all publications, statistics and analysis were performed using mean difference (MD).

Data analysis showed that the overall impact of exercise on body mass index (BMI) was −1.14 (95% CI: −2.17, −0.11), which was significantly different ($p = 0.03$). This shows that exercise has a significant intervention effect on BMI.

The results of the subgroup analysis showed that in the high-consistency group, the MD was −0.6 (95% CI: −1.84, 0.64), which was not significantly different ($p = 0.34$). This indicates that it is unclear whether exercise prescription with high consistency to ACSM guidelines significantly influences BMI.

The results of the subgroup analysis showed that in the low- or uncertain-consistency group, the MD was −2.37 (95% CI: −4.24, −0.5) and $I^2 = 0\%$, which was significantly different ($p = 0.01$). This indicates that exercise prescription with low or uncertain consistency to ACSM guidelines significantly affects BMI intervention.

In summary, exercise significantly influences BMI indicators; the MD was −1.14 (95% CI: −2.17, −0.11) and ($p = 0.03$). Exercise prescription with low or uncertain consistency to ACSM guidelines has a more significant impact on BMI than exercise prescription with high consistency to ACSM guidelines (−2.37 > −0.6) (Figure 12). It is worth mentioning that BMI is a range index, and a noticeable intervention effect does not mean the actual impact is better.

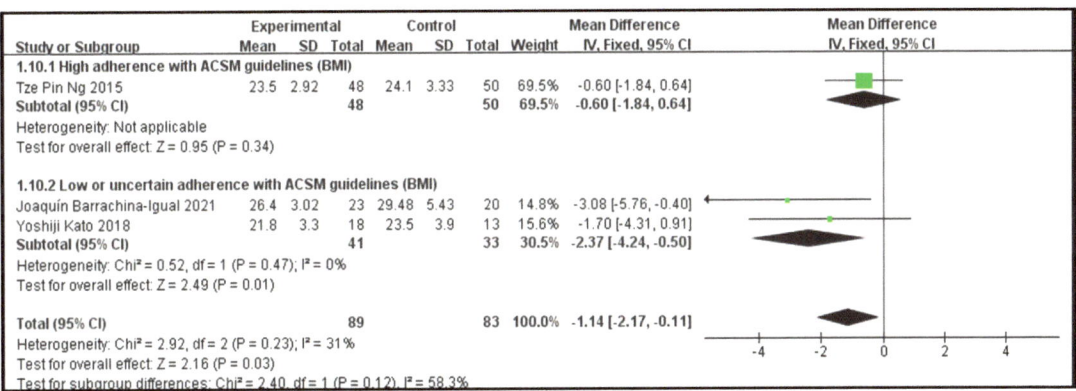

Figure 12. Forest plot for meta-analysis of the impact of exercise on BMI indicators in frail elderly people [37,38,50].

Subsequently, we conducted publication bias testing through REVIEW MANAGER 5.4.1. We observed the funnel plot and found that both sides were approximately symmetrical, indicating no obvious publication bias (Figure 13).

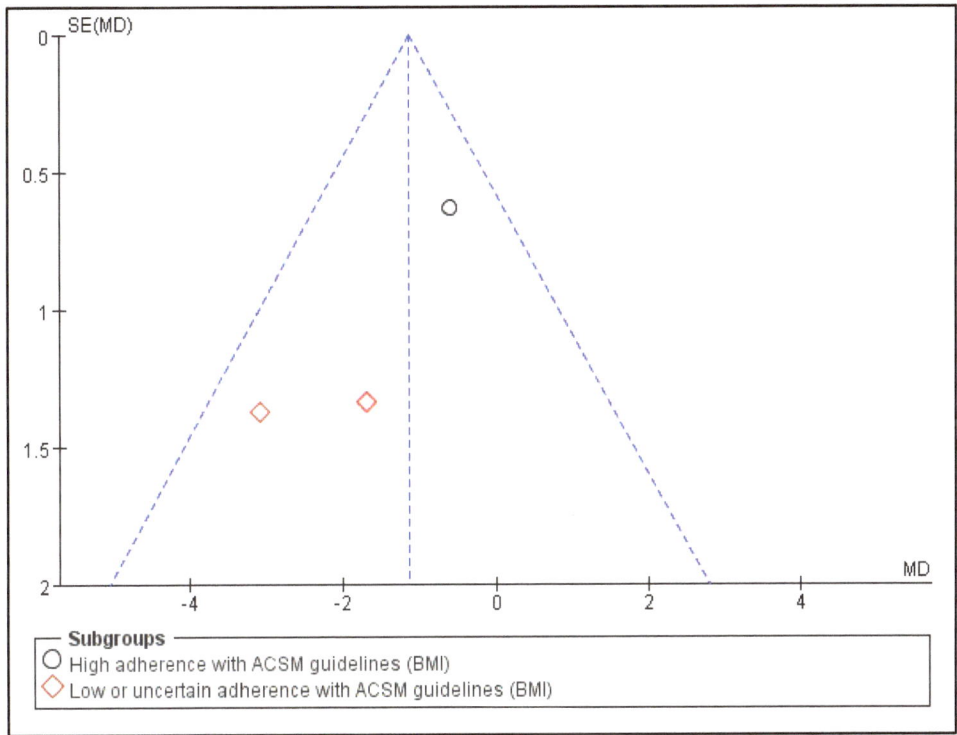

Figure 13. Funnel plot for BMI indicator.

4. Discussion

This study is based on the exercise prescriptions recommended by ACSM. It compares the effects of exercise prescriptions with high consistency and low or uncertain consistency recommended by ACSM on frailty in elderly people. A total of 20 studies were included, including 11 different exercise interventions and 2016 frail older adults. Exercise has once again proven to be a very effective intervention in improving frailty in elderly people [12]. It is worth mentioning that through meta-analysis, we found that exercise prescriptions with high consistency to ACSM recommendations have a significant intervention effect on two outcome indicators related to frailty in elderly people (Fried Frailty Phenotype and grip strength) and are better than exercise prescriptions with low or uncertain consistency to ACSM recommendations. However, exercise prescriptions with low or uncertain consistency to ACSM recommendations have a significant intervention effect on BMI, but this does not mean that there is an excellent actual effect. Finally, we found that exercise prescriptions with different consistency had no significant intervention effect on the two outcome indicators (Barthel Index, Short Physical Performance Battery). None of the 20 studies we included explicitly showed blinding of data analysts, so there is a risk of selection bias. It is important to note here that we did not assess the methodological quality and certainty of the included studies, so these viewpoints need to be viewed critically.

Exercise has a significant intervention effect on FP indicators. The requirements include five components: unintentional weight loss, fatigue, poor muscle strength, sluggishness, and physical inactivity [1]. First of all, it is well known that exercise has a direct intervention effect on these components, which is why both high consistency and low or uncertain consistency with the exercise prescription recommended by the ACSM can have a significant intervention effect on this indicator. Secondly, we found that the intervention effects differ depending on the frequency, intensity, and exercise duration. An ineffectively low dose will not impart full benefits, whereas the adverse effects stemming from an excessively high dose may overshadow potential benefits and introduce detriments [52]. This is also why high consistency to the exercise prescription recommended by the ACSM can improve this indicator's intervention.

Through meta-analysis, we found that only exercise prescriptions with high consistency to ACSM recommendations have a significant intervention effect on this indicator (MD: 2.39, $p = 0.006$). It is worth mentioning that an increase in grip strength of more than 1.6 kg can be called a fundamental change [53]. Resistance training is considered an efficient treatment for age-related sarcopenia and can improve muscle strength and quality in patients [54], but it must also include grip strength. Therefore, a suitable resistance exercise program is essential. We believe that the resistance training program recommended by the ACSM is trustworthy because its training frequency, intensity, number of repetitions, and number of sets are similar to other resistance exercise programs for elderly people. These exercise prescriptions have been proven to be effective in improving the grip strength of elderly people [55–57] (Table 4).

Table 4. Comparison of ACSM recommended exercise prescriptions and other exercise prescriptions in resistance exercise.

	Frequency	Intensity/Workload	Repetitions	Sets
ACSM exercise prescriptions	1–2 d/wk, 2–3 d/wk	Change the resistance from medium to high	8–12	1–2
Other exercise prescriptions (1)	2–3 d/wk	1 RM 50–80%	5–8	1–2
Other exercise prescriptions (2)	2 d/wk	1 RM 51–69%	7–9	2–3
Other exercise prescriptions (3)	2 d/wk	relatively high degree of effort	6–12	1–3

Subsequently, we found that exercise prescriptions with low or uncertain consistency to ACSM recommendations were not detailed enough when designing resistance exercise programs (Table 3), which resulted in insignificant intervention effects for patients (MD: 1.1, $p = 0.28$).

Exercise has been shown to improve ADL, which is consistent with the results of our meta-analysis (MD: 5.79, $p = 0.02$). However, whether it is high or low or uncertain consistency with the exercise prescription recommended by the ACSM, the intervention effect on BI indicator is insignificant ($p = 0.06$, $p = 0.14$). The intervention effect of exercise on SPPB indicator is also significant (MD: 1.03, $p = 0.007$). However, whether it is high or low or uncertain consistency with the exercise prescription recommended by the ACSM, the intervention effect on this indicator is insignificant ($p = 0.07$, $p = 0.05$). We speculate that this may be because the BI and SPPB indicators do not lead to apparent differences in intervention effects due to specific exercise doses. This is why they are widely used as secondary outcome indicators in some exercise dosage experiments. Exercise has a significant intervention effect on BMI (MD: -1.14, $p = 0.03$). However, only the intervention effect of high consistency to ASCM recommended exercise prescription is not substantial ($p = 0.34$). This may be because only one article in the high-consistency group includes this indicator. In addition, BMI is only a statistical index used to estimate body fat; the impact of obesity on health outcomes in elderly people is complex; this has been described as the obesity paradox [58]. This is also why most experiments use BMI as a baseline measurement or secondary outcome indicator.

In summary, although exercise has a significant intervention effect on five outcome indicators related to frailty in elderly people, exercise prescriptions with high consistency to ACSM recommendations have a more substantial impact on two frequently used primary outcome indicators (Fried Frailty Phenotype, grip strength). Different exercise doses did not affect the differences in the intervention effects of the remaining three outcome indicators.

5. Strengths and Limitations

Firstly, the topic of our meta-analysis is novel and has high clinical significance. Currently, many studies focus on the intervention effects of different exercise prescriptions on frailty in elderly people. The most critical part of the intervention in these studies was the dose of exercise [59]. However, many studies or scholars have disagreed on how much exercise should be given to pre-frail or frail older adults. Of course, this is also because people consider the clinical value of personalized exercise prescription [60]. Nonetheless, the standardized application of exercise dose is still a topic worthy of discussion.

Secondly, our meta-analysis has the following limitations: 1: The number of articles included in the final study is small, although we tried to obtain as many articles as possible through various methods. We did not search the databases SCOPUS, CINAHL, PEDro, LILACS, and some gray literature; 2: The research results are interfered with by some confounding factors (age, gender, weight, physical condition, etc.), so it is difficult for us to avoid heterogeneity between studies; 3: We did not assess the quality and certainty of the included studies; 4: We did not test for MICD (minimum significant clinical difference).

Finally, readers need to be cautious when interpreting our findings, especially among those outcomes with small sample sizes.

6. Conclusions

This review again supports and demonstrates that exercise can improve frailty in older adults. In exploring the optimal exercise dose for older adults with pre-frailty and frailty, we found that exercise prescriptions with high consistency with ACSM recommendations may be more effective as reflected in the outcome measures of FP and GS than for those with uncertain or low consistency. However, it is essential to note that the data derived from the meta-analysis is still subject to the small number of studies, the unknown degree of adherence to the exercise of the participants in individual studies, and the different mix of cases in the studies. There is, therefore, a need to expand the sample size in this field to verify the impact of interventions on the five outcomes related to frailty in elderly people. In addition, there are many methodological biases in the evidence based on the included interventions, so the above conclusions can only be preliminary.

Supplementary Materials: The following supporting information can be downloaded at: https://www.mdpi.com/article/10.3390/jcm13113037/s1, Table S1: Search Strategy.

Author Contributions: N.P. conceived and designed the study, and the screening of titles and abstracts was completed by N.P. and J.T., with disputes resolved by D.L., Z.O. and S.G. completed the data inclusion; Z.O. and S.G. independently scored the consistency of each exercise intervention with the ACSM recommended dose. All authors participated in the quality assessment of the included literature. N.P. and J.T. completed the initial draft of the manuscript. All authors have read and agreed to the published version of the manuscript.

Funding: This research was supported by a grant from Akademia Wychowania Fizycznego I Sportu. The funders were not involved in the conception and implementation of the study, the analysis of the data, or the reporting of the results.

Institutional Review Board Statement: Not applicable.

Informed Consent Statement: Not applicable.

Data Availability Statement: The original contributions presented in the study are included in the article/Supplementary Materials; further inquiries can be directed to the corresponding author.

Conflicts of Interest: The authors declare that the research was conducted without any commercial or financial relationships that could be construed as a potential conflict of interest.

References

1. Fried, L.P.; Tangen, C.M.; Walston, J.; Newman, A.B.; Hirsch, C.; Gottdiener, J.; Seeman, T.; Tracy, R.; Kop, W.J.; Burke, G.; et al. Frailty in older adults: Evidence for a phenotype. *J. Gerontol. Ser. A Biol. Sci. Med. Sci.* **2001**, *56*, M146–M156. [CrossRef]
2. Proietti, M.; Cesari, M. Frailty: What Is It? *Adv. Exp. Med. Biol.* **2020**, *1216*, 1–7. [CrossRef]
3. United Nations Department of Economic and Social Affairs. *World Population Ageing 2020: Highlights: Living Arrangements of Older Persons*; UN: New York, NY, USA, 2021.
4. Clegg, A.; Young, J.; Iliffe, S.; Rikkert, M.O.; Rockwood, K. Frailty in elderly people. *Lancet* **2013**, *381*, 752–762. [CrossRef]
5. Carneiro, J.A.; Ramos, G.C.F.; Barbosa, A.T.F.; Mendonça, J.M.G.d.; Costa, F.M.d.; Caldeira, A.P. Prevalência e fatores associados à fragilidade em idosos não institucionalizados. *Rev. Bras. Enferm.* **2016**, *69*, 408–415. [CrossRef] [PubMed]
6. Walston, J.; Buta, B.; Xue, Q.L. Frailty Screening and Interventions: Considerations for Clinical Practice. *Clin. Geriatr. Med.* **2018**, *34*, 25–38. [CrossRef] [PubMed]
7. Woolford, S.J.; Sohan, O.; Dennison, E.M.; Cooper, C.; Patel, H.P. Approaches to the diagnosis and prevention of frailty. *Aging Clin. Exp. Res.* **2020**, *32*, 1629–1637. [CrossRef]
8. Lorenzo-López, L.; Maseda, A.; de Labra, C.; Regueiro-Folgueira, L.; Rodríguez-Villamil, J.L.; Millán-Calenti, J.C. Nutritional determinants of frailty in older adults: A systematic review. *BMC Geriatr.* **2017**, *17*, 108. [CrossRef]
9. Palmer, K.; Marengoni, A.; Russo, P.; Mammarella, F.; Onder, G. Frailty and Drug Use. *J. Frailty Aging* **2016**, *5*, 100–103. [CrossRef]
10. Gutiérrez-Valencia, M.; Izquierdo, M.; Cesari, M.; Casas-Herrero, Á.; Inzitari, M.; Martínez-Velilla, N. The relationship between frailty and polypharmacy in older people: A systematic review. *Br. J. Clin. Pharmacol.* **2018**, *84*, 1432–1444. [CrossRef]
11. Chan, D.D.; Tsou, H.H.; Chang, C.B.; Yang, R.S.; Tsauo, J.Y.; Chen, C.Y.; Hsiao, C.F.; Hsu, Y.T.; Chen, C.H.; Chang, S.F.; et al. Integrated care for geriatric frailty and sarcopenia: A randomized control trial. *J. Cachexia Sarcopenia Muscle* **2017**, *8*, 78–88. [CrossRef]
12. Angulo, J.; El Assar, M.; Álvarez-Bustos, A.; Rodríguez-Mañas, L. Physical activity and exercise: Strategies to manage frailty. *Redox Biol.* **2020**, *35*, 101513. [CrossRef] [PubMed]
13. Kehler, D.S.; Theou, O. The impact of physical activity and sedentary behaviors on frailty levels. *Mech. Ageing Dev.* **2019**, *180*, 29–41. [CrossRef] [PubMed]
14. Aguirre, L.E.; Villareal, D.T. Physical Exercise as Therapy for Frailty. *Nestle Nutr. Inst. Workshop Ser.* **2015**, *83*, 83–92. [CrossRef] [PubMed]
15. Abizanda, P.; Romero, L.; Sánchez-Jurado, P.M.; Atienzar-Núñez, P.; Esquinas-Requena, J.L.; García-Nogueras, I. Association between Functional Assessment Instruments and Frailty in Older Adults: The FRADEA Study. *J. Frailty Aging* **2012**, *1*, 162–168. [CrossRef] [PubMed]
16. Clegg, A.; Rogers, L.; Young, J. Diagnostic test accuracy of simple instruments for identifying frailty in community-dwelling older people: A systematic review. *Age Ageing* **2015**, *44*, 148–152. [CrossRef]
17. Dent, E.; Kowal, P.; Hoogendijk, E.O. Frailty measurement in research and clinical practice: A review. *Eur. J. Intern. Med.* **2016**, *31*, 3–10. [CrossRef]
18. Pritchard, J.M.; Kennedy, C.C.; Karampatos, S.; Ioannidis, G.; Misiaszek, B.; Marr, S.; Patterson, C.; Woo, T.; Papaioannou, A. Measuring frailty in clinical practice: A comparison of physical frailty assessment methods in a geriatric out-patient clinic. *BMC Geriatr.* **2017**, *17*, 264. [CrossRef] [PubMed]

19. Guralnik, J.M.; Simonsick, E.M.; Ferrucci, L.; Glynn, R.J.; Berkman, L.F.; Blazer, D.G.; Scherr, P.A.; Wallace, R.B. A short physical performance battery assessing lower extremity function: Association with self-reported disability and prediction of mortality and nursing home admission. *J. Gerontol.* **1994**, *49*, M85–M94. [CrossRef]
20. Sousa-Santos, A.R.; Amaral, T.F. Differences in handgrip strength protocols to identify sarcopenia and frailty—A systematic review. *BMC Geriatr.* **2017**, *17*, 238. [CrossRef]
21. Collin, C.; Wade, D.T.; Davies, S.; Horne, V. The Barthel ADL Index: A reliability study. *Int. Disabil. Stud.* **1988**, *10*, 61–63. [CrossRef]
22. Khanna, D.; Peltzer, C.; Kahar, P.; Parmar, M.S. Body Mass Index (BMI): A Screening Tool Analysis. *Cureus* **2022**, *14*, e22119. [CrossRef] [PubMed]
23. Jayanama, K.; Theou, O.; Godin, J.; Mayo, A.; Cahill, L.; Rockwood, K. Relationship of body mass index with frailty and all-cause mortality among middle-aged and older adults. *BMC Med.* **2022**, *20*, 404. [CrossRef] [PubMed]
24. Bray, N.W.; Smart, R.R.; Jakobi, J.M.; Jones, G.R. Exercise prescription to reverse frailty. *Appl. Physiol. Nutr. Metab. Physiol. Appl. Nutr. Et Metab.* **2016**, *41*, 1112–1116. [CrossRef] [PubMed]
25. Cadore, E.L.; Rodríguez-Mañas, L.; Sinclair, A.; Izquierdo, M. Effects of different exercise interventions on risk of falls, gait ability, and balance in physically frail older adults: A systematic review. *Rejuvenation Res.* **2013**, *16*, 105–114. [CrossRef] [PubMed]
26. de Labra, C.; Guimaraes-Pinheiro, C.; Maseda, A.; Lorenzo, T.; Millán-Calenti, J.C. Effects of physical exercise interventions in frail older adults: A systematic review of randomized controlled trials. *BMC Geriatr.* **2015**, *15*, 154. [CrossRef] [PubMed]
27. Leslie, E.; Luna, V.; Gibson, A.L. Older Adult Aerobic Capacity, Muscular Strength, Fitness and Body Composition After 20+ Years of Exercise Training: A Systematic Review and Meta-Analysis. *Int. J. Exerc. Sci.* **2023**, *16*, 620–637. [PubMed]
28. Gennuso, K.P.; Zalewski, K.; Cashin, S.E.; Strath, S.J. Resistance training congruent with minimal guidelines improves function in older adults: A pilot study. *J. Phys. Act. Health* **2013**, *10*, 769–776. [CrossRef] [PubMed]
29. Garber, C.E.; Blissmer, B.; Deschenes, M.R.; Franklin, B.A.; Lamonte, M.J.; Lee, I.M.; Nieman, D.C.; Swain, D.P. American College of Sports Medicine position stand. Quantity and quality of exercise for developing and maintaining cardiorespiratory, musculoskeletal, and neuromotor fitness in apparently healthy adults: Guidance for prescribing exercise. *Med. Sci. Sports Exerc.* **2011**, *43*, 1334–1359. [CrossRef] [PubMed]
30. Higgins, J.P.; Altman, D.G.; Gøtzsche, P.C.; Jüni, P.; Moher, D.; Oxman, A.D.; Savovic, J.; Schulz, K.F.; Weeks, L.; Sterne, J.A. The Cochrane Collaboration's tool for assessing risk of bias in randomised trials. *BMJ (Clin. Res. Ed.)* **2011**, *343*, d5928. [CrossRef]
31. Higgins, J.P.; Green, S. *Cochrane Handbook for Systematic Reviews of Interventions*; Wiley: Hoboken, NJ, USA, 2008.
32. Travers, J.; Romero-Ortuno, R.; Langan, J.; MacNamara, F.; McCormack, D.; McDermott, R.; McEntire, J.; McKiernan, J.; Lacey, S.; Doran, P.; et al. Building resilience and reversing frailty: A randomised controlled trial of a primary care intervention for older adults. *Age Ageing* **2023**, *52*, afad012. [CrossRef]
33. Giné-Garriga, M.; Guerra, M.; Pagès, E.; Manini, T.M.; Jiménez, R.; Unnithan, V.B. The effect of functional circuit training on physical frailty in frail older adults: A randomized controlled trial. *J. Aging Phys. Act.* **2010**, *18*, 401–424. [CrossRef]
34. Sahin, U.K.; Kirdi, N.; Bozoglu, E.; Meric, A.; Buyukturan, G.; Ozturk, A.; Doruk, H. Effect of low-intensity versus high-intensity resistance training on the functioning of the institutionalized frail elderly. *Int. J. Rehabil. Res.* **2018**, *41*, 211–217. [CrossRef]
35. García-Gollarte, F.; Mora-Concepción, A.; Pinazo-Hernandis, S.; Segura-Ortí, E.; Amer-Cuenca, J.J.; Arguisuelas-Martínez, M.D.; Lisón, J.F.; Benavent-Caballer, V. Effectiveness of a Supervised Group-Based Otago Exercise Program on Functional Performance in Frail Institutionalized Older Adults: A Multicenter Randomized Controlled Trial. *J. Geriatr. Phys. Ther.* **2023**, *46*, 15–25. [CrossRef] [PubMed]
36. Tou, N.X.; Wee, S.L.; Seah, W.T.; Ng, D.H.M.; Pang, B.W.J.; Lau, L.K.; Ng, T.P. Effectiveness of Community-Delivered Functional Power Training Program for Frail and Pre-frail Community-Dwelling Older Adults: A Randomized Controlled Study. *Prev. Sci. Off. J. Soc. Prev. Res.* **2021**, *22*, 1048–1059. [CrossRef] [PubMed]
37. Barrachina-Igual, J.; Martínez-Arnau, F.M.; Pérez-Ros, P.; Flor-Rufino, C.; Sanz-Requena, R.; Pablos, A. Effectiveness of the PROMUFRA program in pre-frail, community-dwelling older people: A randomized controlled trial. *Geriatr. Nurs.* **2021**, *42*, 582–591. [CrossRef]
38. Kato, Y.; Islam, M.M.; Koizumi, D.; Rogers, M.E.; Takeshima, N. Effects of a 12-week marching in place and chair rise daily exercise intervention on ADL and functional mobility in frail older adults. *J. Phys. Ther. Sci.* **2018**, *30*, 549–554. [CrossRef]
39. Sánchez-Sánchez, J.L.; de Souto Barreto, P.; Antón-Rodrigo, I.; Ramón-Espinoza, F.; Marín-Epelde, I.; Sánchez-Latorre, M.; Moral-Cuesta, D.; Casas-Herrero, Á. Effects of a 12-week Vivifrail exercise program on intrinsic capacity among frail cognitively impaired community-dwelling older adults: Secondary analysis of a multicentre randomised clinical trial. *Age Ageing* **2022**, *51*, afac303. [CrossRef] [PubMed]
40. Liu, T.; Wang, C.; Sun, J.; Chen, W.; Meng, L.; Li, J.; Cao, M.; Liu, Q.; Chen, C. The Effects of an Integrated Exercise Intervention on the Attenuation of Frailty in Elderly Nursing Homes: A Cluster Randomized Controlled Trial. *J. Nutr. Health Aging* **2022**, *26*, 222–229. [CrossRef]
41. Chen, R.; Wu, Q.; Wang, D.; Li, Z.; Liu, H.; Liu, G.; Cui, Y.; Song, L. Effects of elastic band exercise on the frailty states in pre-frail elderly people. *Physiother. Theory Pract.* **2020**, *36*, 1000–1008. [CrossRef]
42. Arrieta, H.; Rezola-Pardo, C.; Gil, S.M.; Virgala, J.; Iturburu, M.; Antón, I.; González-Templado, V.; Irazusta, J.; Rodriguez-Larrad, A. Effects of Multicomponent Exercise on Frailty in Long-Term Nursing Homes: A Randomized Controlled Trial. *J. Am. Geriatr. Soc.* **2019**, *67*, 1145–1151. [CrossRef]

43. Casas-Herrero, Á.; Sáez de Asteasu, M.L.; Antón-Rodrigo, I.; Sánchez-Sánchez, J.L.; Montero-Odasso, M.; Marín-Epelde, I.; Ramón-Espinoza, F.; Zambom-Ferraresi, F.; Petidier-Torregrosa, R.; Elexpuru-Estomba, J.; et al. Effects of Vivifrail multicomponent intervention on functional capacity: A multicentre, randomized controlled trial. *J. Cachexia Sarcopenia Muscle* **2022**, *13*, 884–893. [CrossRef]
44. Zhang, X.; van der Schans, C.P.; Liu, Y.; Krijnen, W.P.; Hobbelen, J.S.M. Efficacy of Dance Intervention for Improving Frailty Among Chinese Older Adults Living in the Community: A Randomized Controlled Trial. *J. Aging Phys. Act.* **2023**, *31*, 806–814. [CrossRef]
45. Vestergaard, S.; Kronborg, C.; Puggaard, L. Home-based video exercise intervention for community-dwelling frail older women: A randomized controlled trial. *Aging Clin. Exp. Res.* **2008**, *20*, 479–486. [CrossRef]
46. Pérez-Zepeda, M.U.; Martínez-Velilla, N.; Kehler, D.S.; Izquierdo, M.; Rockwood, K.; Theou, O. The impact of an exercise intervention on frailty levels in hospitalised older adults: Secondary analysis of a randomised controlled trial. *Age Ageing* **2022**, *51*, afac028. [CrossRef] [PubMed]
47. Hsieh, T.J.; Su, S.C.; Chen, C.W.; Kang, Y.W.; Hu, M.H.; Hsu, L.L.; Wu, S.Y.; Chen, L.; Chang, H.Y.; Chuang, S.Y.; et al. Individualized home-based exercise and nutrition interventions improve frailty in older adults: A randomized controlled trial. *Int. J. Behav. Nutr. Phys. Act.* **2019**, *16*, 119. [CrossRef]
48. Tarazona-Santabalbina, F.J.; Gómez-Cabrera, M.C.; Pérez-Ros, P.; Martínez-Arnau, F.M.; Cabo, H.; Tsaparas, K.; Salvador-Pascual, A.; Rodriguez-Mañas, L.; Viña, J. A Multicomponent Exercise Intervention that Reverses Frailty and Improves Cognition, Emotion, and Social Networking in the Community-Dwelling Frail Elderly: A Randomized Clinical Trial. *J. Am. Med. Dir. Assoc.* **2016**, *17*, 426–433. [CrossRef]
49. Sadjapong, U.; Yodkeeree, S.; Sungkarat, S.; Siviroj, P. Multicomponent Exercise Program Reduces Frailty and Inflammatory Biomarkers and Improves Physical Performance in Community-Dwelling Older Adults: A Randomized Controlled Trial. *Int. J. Environ. Res. Public Health* **2020**, *17*, 3760. [CrossRef] [PubMed]
50. Ng, T.P.; Feng, L.; Nyunt, M.S.; Feng, L.; Niti, M.; Tan, B.Y.; Chan, G.; Khoo, S.A.; Chan, S.M.; Yap, P.; et al. Nutritional, Physical, Cognitive, and Combination Interventions and Frailty Reversal Among Older Adults: A Randomized Controlled Trial. *Am. J. Med.* **2015**, *128*, 1225–1236. [CrossRef]
51. Otones, P.; García, E.; Sanz, T.; Pedraz, A. A physical activity program versus usual care in the management of quality of life for pre-frail older adults with chronic pain: Randomized controlled trial. *BMC Geriatr.* **2020**, *20*, 396. [CrossRef]
52. O'Keefe, J.H.; O'Keefe, E.L.; Lavie, C.J. The Goldilocks Zone for Exercise: Not Too Little, Not Too Much. *Mo. Med.* **2018**, *115*, 98–105.
53. Labott, B.K.; Bucht, H.; Morat, M.; Morat, T.; Donath, L. Effects of Exercise Training on Handgrip Strength in Older Adults: A Meta-Analytical Review. *Gerontology* **2019**, *65*, 686–698. [CrossRef] [PubMed]
54. Zhao, H.; Cheng, R.; Song, G.; Teng, J.; Shen, S.; Fu, X.; Yan, Y.; Liu, C. The Effect of Resistance Training on the Rehabilitation of Elderly Patients with Sarcopenia: A Meta-Analysis. *Int. J. Environ. Res. Public Health* **2022**, *19*, 15491. [CrossRef] [PubMed]
55. Borde, R.; Hortobágyi, T.; Granacher, U. Dose-Response Relationships of Resistance Training in Healthy Old Adults: A Systematic Review and Meta-Analysis. *Sports Med. (Auckl. N.Z.)* **2015**, *45*, 1693–1720. [CrossRef] [PubMed]
56. Hurst, C.; Robinson, S.M.; Witham, M.D.; Dodds, R.M.; Granic, A.; Buckland, C.; De Biase, S.; Finnegan, S.; Rochester, L.; Skelton, D.A.; et al. Resistance exercise as a treatment for sarcopenia: Prescription and delivery. *Age Ageing* **2022**, *51*, afac003. [CrossRef] [PubMed]
57. Rodrigues, F.; Domingos, C.; Monteiro, D.; Morouço, P. A Review on Aging, Sarcopenia, Falls, and Resistance Training in Community-Dwelling Older Adults. *Int. J. Environ. Res. Public Health* **2022**, *19*, 874. [CrossRef] [PubMed]
58. Bosello, O.; Vanzo, A. Obesity paradox and aging. *Eat. Weight Disord. EWD* **2021**, *26*, 27–35. [CrossRef] [PubMed]
59. Wasfy, M.M.; Baggish, A.L. Exercise Dose in Clinical Practice. *Circulation* **2016**, *133*, 2297–2313. [CrossRef]
60. Hawley, J.A. Commentary on viewpoint: Perspective on the future use of genomics in exercise prescription. *J. Appl. Physiol.* **2008**, *104*, 1253. [CrossRef]

Disclaimer/Publisher's Note: The statements, opinions and data contained in all publications are solely those of the individual author(s) and contributor(s) and not of MDPI and/or the editor(s). MDPI and/or the editor(s) disclaim responsibility for any injury to people or property resulting from any ideas, methods, instructions or products referred to in the content.

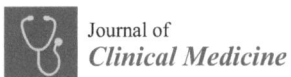

Article

Causal Roles of Ventral and Dorsal Neural Systems for Automatic and Control Self-Reference Processing: A Function Lesion Mapping Study

Jie Sui [1,*], Pia Rotshtein [2], Zhuoen Lu [1] and Magdalena Chechlacz [3,4]

1 School of Psychology, University of Aberdeen, Aberdeen AB24 3FX, UK
2 Neuroimaging Research Unit, University of Haifa, Haifa 3498838, Israel
3 Centre for Human Brain Health, University of Birmingham, Birmingham B15 2TT, UK
4 School of Psychology, University of Birmingham, Birmingham B15 2TT, UK
* Correspondence: jie.sui@abdn.ac.uk

Abstract: Background: Humans perceive and interpret the world through the lens of self-reference processes, typically facilitating enhanced performance for the task at hand. However, this research has predominantly emphasized the automatic facet of self-reference processing, overlooking how it interacts with control processes affecting everyday situations. **Methods**: We investigated this relationship between automatic and control self-reference processing in neuropsychological patients performing self-face perception tasks and the Birmingham frontal task measuring executive functions. **Results**: Principal component analysis across tasks revealed two components: one loaded on familiarity/orientation judgments reflecting automatic self-reference processing, and the other linked to the cross task and executive function indicating control processing requirements. Voxel-based morphometry and track-wise lesion-mapping analyses showed that impairments in automatic self-reference were associated with reduced grey matter in the ventromedial prefrontal cortex and right inferior temporal gyrus, and white matter damage in the right inferior fronto-occipital fasciculus. Deficits in executive control were linked to reduced grey matter in the bilateral inferior parietal lobule and left anterior insula, and white matter disconnections in the left superior longitudinal fasciculus and arcuate fasciculus. **Conclusions**: The causal evidence suggests that automatic and control facets of self-reference processes are subserved by distinct yet integrated ventral prefrontal–temporal and dorsal frontal–parietal networks, respectively.

Keywords: principal component analysis; voxel-based morphometry; white matter pathway; ventral neural network; dorsal control network

Citation: Sui, J.; Rotshtein, P.; Lu, Z.; Chechlacz, M. Causal Roles of Ventral and Dorsal Neural Systems for Automatic and Control Self-Reference Processing: A Function Lesion Mapping Study. J. Clin. Med. **2024**, 13, 4170. https://doi.org/10.3390/jcm13144170

Academic Editors: Francesco Mattace-Raso and Petra Klinge

Received: 29 May 2024
Revised: 10 July 2024
Accepted: 15 July 2024
Published: 16 July 2024

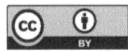

Copyright: © 2024 by the authors. Licensee MDPI, Basel, Switzerland. This article is an open access article distributed under the terms and conditions of the Creative Commons Attribution (CC BY) license (https://creativecommons.org/licenses/by/4.0/).

1. Introduction

Humans perceive and interpret the external world through the lens of their own sense of self [1–5]. This self-reference ability typically manifests as a self-prioritization effect (SPE) or self-bias, a processing advantage for self-related versus non-self information [6–10]. The effect occurs across cognitive domains spanning from perception, attention, and memory to decision-making [11–32]. However, due to its emphasis on automatic self-reference processing [33–37], this research has overlooked potential interactions with control processes that affect everyday situations. Recent theoretical frameworks propose distinct yet interactive mechanisms and neural networks for self-reference processing and cognitive control [38–50]. Specifically, ventral temporal–prefrontal networks support automatic self-referencing, while dorsal prefrontal–parietal networks mediate attentional and executive control processes that can regulate self-biases. Although the neural manifestation of each of these core cognitive processes is well characterized, the precise relationship between them in supporting adaptive self-prioritization remains elusive. Here, we aimed to address this question by examining the roles of automatic and executive control functions in the

SPE using previously reported patient data [51,52], combined with new neuropsychological assessments of control processing, to uncover latent cognitive factors underpinning the SPE. This new approach enabled the investigation of causal neural mechanisms underlying distinct components of self-prioritization processes, transcending traditional task-based analysis.

The Self Attentional Network model (SAN [38]) hypothesizes that social stimuli, such as self-related information, automatically attract attention, facilitating the SPE. It has been suggested to be mediated through the activation of ventral prefrontal–temporal networks. When self-related stimuli are task irrelevant, however, dorsal fronto-parietal networks are engaged for top-down control over this self-bias to maintain task goals. The SAN proposes that self-prioritization emerges from dynamic interactions between these ventral and dorsal control networks through key processing nodes [53,54]—the ventromedial prefrontal cortex (vmPFC) and left posterior superior temporal sulcus (LpSTS) within the ventral network, and the bilateral prefrontal cortex (DLPFC) and intraparietal sulcus (IPS) within the dorsal network. Notably, the vmPFC plays a prominent role in self-referencing, considered crucial for facilitating automatic self-prioritization as the central self-network node [55–60]. While there is some indirect evidence supporting contributions of each core network to the SAN model, direct evidence elucidating the precise relationship between them as a whole remains lacking [61,62].

The SAN model has been supported by functional neuroimaging studies in healthy participants. During a self-matching task [16], researchers reported increased activation in the vmPFC and the LpSTS in response to self-related stimuli compared to other-related stimuli [63]. These results suggest these regions as crucial nodes within the ventral self network. Specifically, the vmPFC functions as a central node for self-representation [64–67], while the LpSTS is implicated in social attention processes [68,69]. In the reverse comparison, processing other-related stimuli elicited greater activity in the DLPFC, a key region in the dorsal fronto-parietal network. This enhanced activation in the DLPFC indicates recruitment of cognitive control processes during the processing of other-related stimuli. Moreover, participants exhibited an inverse vmPFC–DLPFC relationship when matching self-related stimuli, with the SPE on behaviors (self vs. other) positively relating to activation of the vmPFC but negatively to DLPFC activation [70–72]. Dynamic causal modelling analysis revealed that the strength of neural couplings from the vmPFC to the LpSTS predicted the size of the SPE, suggesting dynamic interaction between the ventral (e.g., vmPFC and LpSTS) and dorsal frontoparietal (e.g., DLPFC) networks in the control of behaviors in the presence of self-related stimuli [63]. Further evidence for the regulatory role of DLPFC in self-reference processing comes from a paradigm that directly manipulates the task relevance of self-related stimuli [73]. When self-related distractors had to be ignored, left intra-parietal sulcus (a region part of the fronto-parietal network) activity increased, suggesting front-parietal control mechanisms in averting attention from social salient self-stimuli. Furthermore, focusing on self-face stimuli, an fMRI meta-analysis revealed increased responses to self- versus an other-face in ventral regions, including medial temporal, fusiform gyrus, superior temporal, inferior parietal, anterior cingulate, and inferior frontal cortices. The correlational nature of fMRI research precludes causal inferences, necessitating converging evidence from lesions.

Supporting the SAN model, a virtual-lesion study with transcranial direct current stimulation (tDCS) [74] reported diminished self-prioritization–hypos self-bias following vmPFC suppression stimulation (cathodal) (but see [70,75]). Disrupting the processes of LpSTS with a transcranial magnetic stimulation (TMS) caused reduced performances on self-related stimuli [76]. Similarly, TMS to the right posterior temporal parietal junction led to reduced egocentric self-biases [77]. These findings are further supported by neuropsychological studies in patients with acquired lesion, manifesting hypo or hyper self-biases. In a neuropsychological study, two left neuropsychological patients showed a double dissociation of the SPE. The patients performed the self-matching task and demonstrated opposing self-prioritization impairments [78]. Relative to controls, patient SC with lesions to the prefrontal cortex expanding from the vmPFC to insula and subcortical tracts showed a diminish self-prioritization effect–hypo self-bias. In contrast, patient BR with lesions to the temporal and parietal cortices, including the LpSTS, exhibited an enhanced self-prioritization–hyper self-bias. It is important to note that although the studies above demonstrated that distribution to the normal functionality of nodes within the SAN led to alteration in SPE, the direction of reported alteration was not consistent. Specifically, a virtual lesion to the left pSTS led to hypo self-bias [76], while an acquired lesion led to hyper self-bias [78]. We suggest that the left temporal–parietal region consists of multiple sub-nodes that contribute to the SAN, as revealed by the fine-tuned voxel-based analysis.

The neural substrates associated with hypo and hyper self-biases were further examined using voxel-based morphometry (VBM) in a heterogenic cohort of chronic neuropsychological patients performing a familiarity categorization task with faces [52]. Patients made familiarity judgments on their own face, a personally familiar face, and a stranger's face presented with different head orientations. Self-prioritization was computed by contrasting responses to self versus familiar other faces. Lesions to the inferior temporal extending to the hippocampus and disconnection of the right inferior occipito-frontal (IFOF) and inferior lateral frontal (ILF) fasciculi were associated with hypo self-bias, a diminished self-prioritization relative to matched healthy controls. In contrast, lesions to the LpSTS and superior prefrontal cortex yielded hyper self-bias. Notably, the extent of self-bias correlated with patients' executive function ability [52]. In a complementary study with the same cohort [51], researchers assessed the SPE using two different tasks with the same set of face images. In the orientation judgment task with faces as targets, participants judged the orientation of faces (left versus right). In the cross task with faces as distracters, participants judged the length of the horizontal or vertical feature of a cross. Hypo self-bias on the orientation task was predicted by lesions to the left anterior temporal pole, insula, superior parietal, and right superior frontal gyrus and disconnection of the left IFOF and ILF. For the cross task, hyper self-bias was predicted by lesions to the inferior parietal, superior temporal, and cingulate and disconnection of the cingulum. Critically, lesions to left supramarginal predicted SPE deficits irrespective of the task [51,52]. In summary, acquired lesion to ventral frontal and temporal regions is associated with hypo self-bias, while acquired lesion of the LpSTS is associated with hyper self-bias and lesion to a nearby area of the left supramarginal is associated with hypo-self.

Although the neuropsychological findings yield causal insights into the neural mechanisms of the SPE, a key challenge when making inferences from specific tasks is that the mapping of tasks to the underlying cognitive process of interest is not one-to-one. For example, the familiarity categorization task relies not only on self-reference processing but also face and picture recognition, episodic memory, and generic executive functions. Similarly, the face orientation task recruits spatial mapping, action perception, and generic executive function beyond self-reference per se. In addition, previous research only indirectly inferred involvement of executive functions and control processing. In other words, the extent to which executive function contributed to task performance and self-prioritization is unclear. Principal component analysis (PCA) [79] across tasks is one method that can overcome idiosyncratic effects of a specific self-task while directly quantifying the contribution of executive function to self-reference.

In the present study, to search for causal neural mechanisms underpinning automatic and control self-reference processing for the SPE, we combined PCA across multiple tasks with function lesion-mapping techniques. Specifically, we re-analyzed data from two previous studies assessing the SPE in different manners [51,52], combined with new neuropsychological assessments of executive functions using the Birmingham frontal task [80], to uncover latent cognitive factors underpinning the SPE. This combined approach enabled investigation of the causal neural mechanisms that underscore distinct manifestations of self-prioritization processes. Most tasks assessing self-related processing require cognitive flexibility to switch between self-related and non-self-related information. That is, processing non-self-related stimuli requires switching away from the self-prioritization rule to enable processing of other stimuli. Thus, we were particularly interested in examining the flexibility of executive functions, as measured by the Birmingham frontal task. We computed the SPE (self vs. familiar other) separately from each of the self-face processing tasks across the two studies for (i) the face familiarity categorization, (ii) a face orientation task, and (iii) the cross judgment task, where participants were instructed to disregard face stimuli while assessing the relative length of elements (horizontal versus vertical) of a cross superimposed on the faces. The Birmingham frontal task assessed patient's flexibility in learning and switching rules to predict a dot movement on a grid. The PCA was performed on the three face SPEs and the Birmingham frontal task. We computed function lesion mapping of grey matter using VBM analysis [81], and track-wise lesion deficits [82] for white matter disconnection associated with cognitive deficits.

2. Materials and Methods

2.1. Participants

2.1.1. Patients

We recruited 30 patients (age range from 36 to 78 years; mean 64.97 ± 10.91 years, 3 women, 27 men) from the panel of neuropsychological volunteers at the School of Psychology, University of Birmingham (Supplementary Table S1 shows demographic and clinical data for individual patients). All patients had chronic acquired brain lesions (i.e., were recruited at least 6 months post-injury). A total of 25 of 30 patients suffered stroke, 3 with carbon monoxide poisoning, 1 with herpes simplex encephalitis, and 1 with cortico-basal degeneration. All patients who participated in the study had no prosopagnosia and no contraindications to MRI. Prior to neuropsychological testing, each patient was presented with central images and required to discriminate their own faces, the faces of familiar others, and those of unfamiliar people. Participation was contingent on 100% discrimination accuracy. No other exclusion criteria were used. All patients provided written informed consent, in agreement with ethics protocols at the School of Psychology and Birmingham University Imaging Centre (BUIC). Lesion overlap across all patients is illustrated in Figure 1.

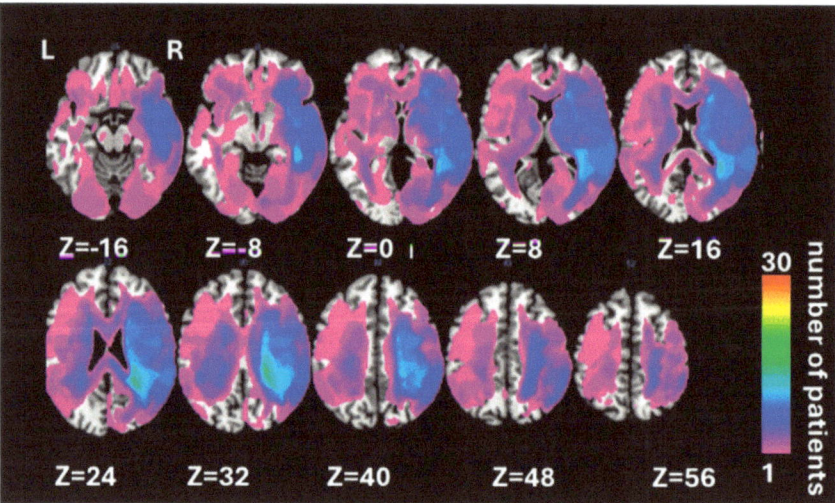

Figure 1. Lesion overlap map representing the spatial distribution of lesions among all 30 patients included in the current study. Lesion maps from individual patients were reconstructed based on [83]; see the Section 2—Materials and Methods for details. The lesion overlap map is shown for ten axial slices in standard MNI space with given MNI Z-coordinates of the presented axial sections. The color bar shows the number of patients with a lesion within a particular voxel (range 1–30).

2.1.2. Healthy Controls

For the lesion identification protocol (see below), we acquired T1-weighted images from 100 healthy controls (55 males and 45 females, mean age 54.5 years, range 20–87) with no history of stroke, brain damage, or neurological disorders. All the controls provided written informed consent in agreement with ethics protocols at the School of Psychology and the Birmingham University Imaging Centre (BUIC).

2.2. Neuropsychological Assessments

The study employed four tasks, as illustrated in Figure 2, including a face orientation task, a cross task, a categorization task, and a rule-finding and -switching task.

In the face orientation task, participants were presented with images of their own face (self), the face of a familiar other (friend), and the face of an unfamiliar person (stranger), and they had to judge the orientation of the face but not the identity. In the cross task, there was a cross simultaneously presented with the face image and participants had to judge which horizontal or vertical element of the cross was longer while ignoring the face in the background. In the categorization task, they were asked to classify the identity of the face stimuli into one of two groups, familiar (self and familiar other/friend) or unfamiliar (unfamiliar other/stranger). We took six photographs of each participant's face and six images of a gender-matched other person who was highly personally familiar to the participant. All images were taken with a neutral facial expression, comprising 3 left profiles and 3 right profiles of each individual. Each image was depicted at angles ranging from 15° to 45° in both directions. A gender-matched, unfamiliar other was randomly selected from the image dataset for inclusion in the current study.

In each task, the images subtended about 5° × 5° of the visual angle at a viewing distance of 60 cm. Each patient completed two blocks of seventy-two trials, with equal numbers of images in the self, familiar, and unfamiliar face conditions. Within each block, thirty-six trials were facial images oriented to the left and thirty-six oriented to the right. Therefore, there were forty-eight trials per face condition (self, familiar, or unfamiliar) for data analysis. Each trial began with the presentation of a white fixation cross at the center of screen for 500 ms. A face image was then displayed at the center of the screen until the patients made a response. The maximum duration of a face was 3000 ms, and this was followed by feedback for 1000 ms. In all three of the tasks described above, the SPE in the tasks was estimated by the differential scores in reaction times between the familiar other and the self conditions dividing by the sum of the two conditions in order to reduce individual difference. Higher or lower scores indicate the severity of the deficits—hyper or hypo self-prioritization. The data were published in two previous studies [51,52].

In the rule-finding and -switching task in the Birmingham frontal tasks from the BCoS assessment battery [80], each stimulus consists of a grid made of six columns and six lines. Most cells are grey, but two are red and two are green. Participants were asked to lean to predict the movement of a black marker across the grid. The marker moves in a lawful manner but then switches the rule by which it is operating. The switch either operates along a single dimension (e.g., moving in one direction then another) or it operates across dimensions (switch from a position rule to a color rule, where the marker jumps between squares of the same color). The rule-finding score gives measures of control function [84]. The BCoS assessment battery includes healthy control norms.

Overall, in the orientation task and categorization task, self-related information was task-relevant. In contrast, self-related stimuli were task-irrelevant in the cross task, where control processing was required to inhibit self-related distractors to keep efficient responses to targets. Likewise, in the rule-finding and -switching task, patients had to keep findings the rules while switching between the rules in order to complete the task, where again executive control processing was required. Supplementary Table S1 presents patients' performance across the tasks. These SPE and rule-finding scores were entered into the principal component analysis (PCA).

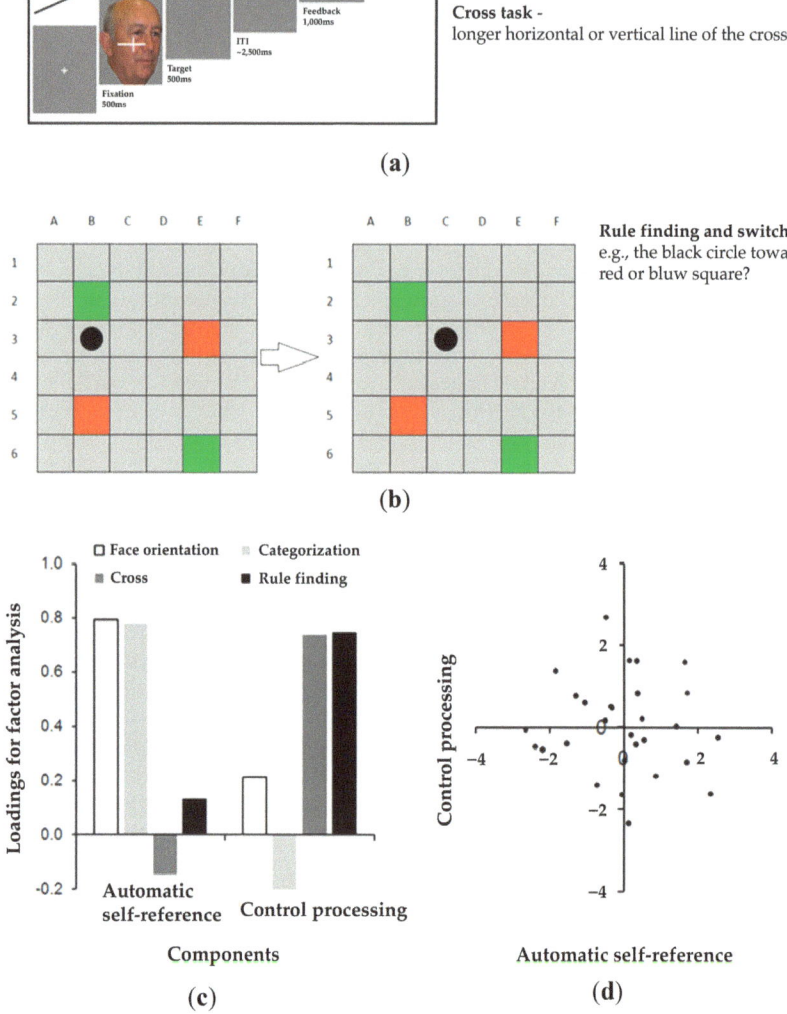

Figure 2. Neuropsychological assessments. (**a**) Experimental stimuli and protocols in the face tasks. Participants display their own face, the face of a friend, or the face of a stranger. They have to judge the orientation of the face in the face orientation task and categorize faces into the familiar (self and friend) or unfamiliar category in the categorization task. In the cross task, a cross appears on the top of the face, where participants are required to judge which horizontal or vertical element of the cross is longer while ignoring the face in the background. (**b**) In the rule-finding and -switching task in the Birmingham frontal task, participants are asked to predict the next movement of the black dot. (**c**) Principal component analysis identifies two components among the four assessments and the loadings of the four assessments for the automatic self-reference and control processing components. (**d**) No significant correlation between the two components demonstrates their separate functions of the four assessments (the distribution of participants' loading scores in the two components).

2.3. Principal Component Analysis (PCA)

The PCA was performed to isolate cognitive functions underlying various symptoms associated with lesion location across the whole group of patients. This aimed at identifying independent factors across the four assessments, as well as the loading of each assessment on common factors [85,86]. The individual SPEs or rule-finding score were normalized by subtracting the averaged group mean and divided by one standard deviation. Normalized data were entered into factor analyses using a principal component approach with an orthogonal rotational (Varimax) procedure. Factors were chosen based on eigen values greater than 1. The adequacy of the correlation matrix for the factor analysis was assessed with Bartlett's test and the Kaiser–Meyer–Olkin measure [87,88].

As predicted, there were two components—one reflecting automatic self-reference processing associated with the orientation task and the categorization task, and the other reflecting control processing based on the cross task and the Birmingham frontal task. The neuropsychological assessments were then re-calculated based on the components instead of single tasks for all individual patients. Principal component scores were measured by the sum of the associated task scores multiplying the relevant loadings. The scores were then used for the VBM analysis and tract-wise lesion deficit analysis.

2.4. Neuroimaging Assessment

2.4.1. Image Acquirement

All patients and healthy controls were scanned at the Birmingham University Imaging Centre (BUIC) on a 3T Philips Achieva MRI system with an 8-channel phased array SENSE head coil. Patients' scans were obtained in close proximity to the time of neuropsychological assessments. The anatomical scans were acquired using a sagittal T1-weighted sequence (sagittal orientation, TE/TR = 3.8/8.4 ms, voxel size $1 \times 1 \times 1$ mm^3).

2.4.2. Image Pre-Processing

All T1 scans (both from 30 patients and 100 controls) were first converted and reoriented using MRICro (Chris Rorden, Georgia Tech, Atlanta, GA, USA). The pre-processing of all T1 scans was completed using SPM5 (Statistical Parametric Mapping, Welcome Department of Cognitive Neurology, London, UK). All brain scans were transformed into the standard MNI space using the unified segmentation procedure [81]. The unified segmentation procedure involves tissue classification based on the signal intensity in each voxel and on a priori knowledge of the expected location of grey matter (GM), white matter (WM), and cerebrospinal fluid (CSF) in the brain. The unified segment procedure as implemented in SPM5 has been shown to be optimal for spatial normalization of lesioned brains [89]. Furthermore, to improve tissue classification and spatial normalization of lesioned brains, a modified segmentation procedure was used (see [83] for details). The modified approach was to resolve misclassification of damaged tissue by including an additional prior for an atypical tissue class (an added "extra" class) to account for the "abnormal" voxels within lesions and thus allowing for classification of the outlier voxels. The segmented images (GM and WM maps) were smoothed with an 8 mm FWHM Gaussian filter to accommodate the assumption of random field theory used in statistical analysis [90]. The choice of intermediate smoothing of an 8 mm FWHM was previously shown to be optimal for lesion detection and further analysis of segmented images [83,91]. The pre-processed GM and WM images were used for the automated lesion reconstruction, and in the analyses to determine voxel-by-voxel relationships between grey matter damage and the self and attentional control factors.

2.4.3. Lesion Reconstruction

Lesion maps from individual patients were reconstructed by using a modified segmentation procedure and an outlier detection algorithm based on fuzzy clustering [83,92,93]. This procedure identifies voxels that are different in the lesioned brain compared with a set of 100 healthy controls. The GM and WM outlier voxels are then combined into a single outlier image and thresholded to generate to a binary map of the lesion [83]. The results of lesion reconstruction were verified against the patient's T1 scans. We used the lesion maps for all patients in the track-wise lesion-deficit analysis and to calculate lesion volumes. The lesion volumes for patients were computed using Matlab 7.14/R2012a [94].

2.4.4. Voxel-Based Morphometry (VBM)

To delineate anatomical structures involved in the automatic self-reference and control components and examine contributions of grey matter changes, VBM was chosen as the analysis approach [95] since it does not require patient classification with respect to anatomical symptoms and so the analysis can include patients with a wide range of damage, including left, right, and bilateral lesions. Since our patients were not pre-selected based on clinical, anatomical, or neuropsychological criteria, VBM analysis allowed us to look for common anatomical function relationships across the whole brain, irrespective of etiology (stroke, degenerative changes) [95].

We assessed the relationship between grey matter damage and the deficits in the automatic self-reference and control functions derived from the PCA, respectively, using VBM carried out with SPM8 (Statistical Parametric Mapping, Wellcome Department of Cognitive Neurology, London, UK). We used parametric statics within the framework of the general linear model [96] and performed the analyses with the segmented GM images, with deficits associated with the two components as the main covariate of interest, while including covariates, age, gender, time since lesion, and lesion volume. We report results only showing a significant effect at the $p < 0.05$ cluster level, corrected for multiple comparisons, with the amplitude of voxels surviving at $p < 0.005$ uncorrected across the whole brain and an extent threshold of 100 mm^3 (>50 voxels). The brain coordinates are presented in the MNI space. The anatomical location of the brain regions identified in VBM analyses is based on [97], Automated Anatomical Labeling of Activations [98], and the Woolsey Brain Atlas [99].

2.4.5. Track-Wise Lesion-Deficit Analysis

To assess the relationship between white matter damage and the deficits in the automatic self-reference and control components, we conducted tract-wise lesion-deficit analyses based on an approach [82] utilizing DTI tractography atlases of all major human white matter tracts (association, projection, and commissural) for a total of 8 pathways in each hemisphere, including the inferior frontal occipital fasciculus (IFOF), inferior longitudinal fasciculus (ILF), and uncinate, arcuate, cingulum, and 3 branches of the superior longitudinal fasciculus (SLF I, SLF II, SLFIII [100,101]). By using the patients' reconstructed lesion maps (in MNI space), and the maps of white matter tracts from the above atlases (also in MNI space), we first evaluated the pattern of disconnection within these white matter tracts for each individual patient. All maps of white matter tracts represent a probability of a given voxel belonging to that tract, and these maps were overlapped with patients' lesion maps. We then considered a given white matter tract to be disconnected (binary measure) if the individual patient lesion overlapped on a voxel within the white matter pathway map with a probability of at least 50% (above the chance level). Finally, we calculated the percentage of patients with the disconnection within specific white matter tracts within the left and right hemispheres, i.e., patients with versus patients without automatic self-reference processing deficits and patients with versus patients without control processing deficits (see Figure 3).

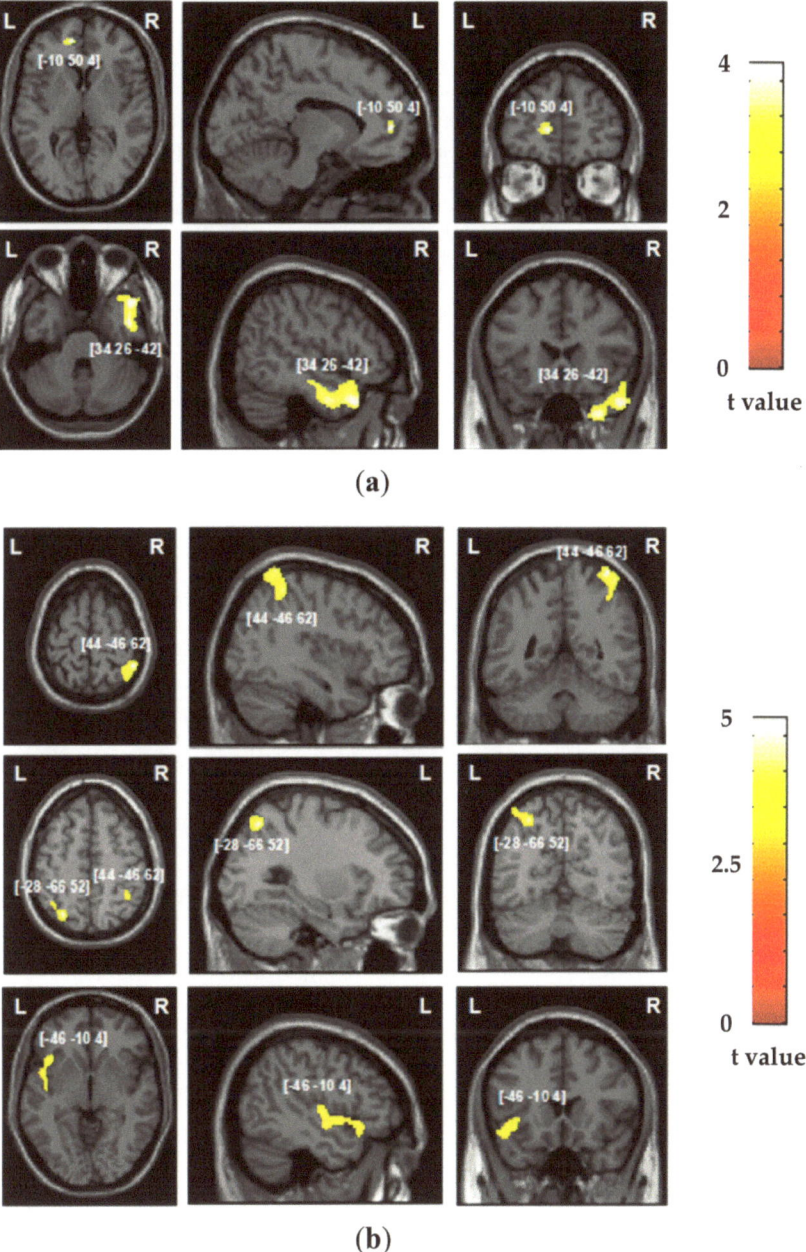

Figure 3. Voxel-based morphometry analysis: grey matter substrates of the two components identified in the principal component analysis for (**a**) automatic self-reference processing and (**b**) control processing. The areas of damage associated with both components of deficits are colored according to the level of significance in the VBM analysis, where brighter colors represent higher t-values. The numbers in brackets indicate peak MNI coordinates.

We also calculated the continuous measure of the pathway disconnection by calculating the size of the overlap (in cubic centimeters) between each patient's lesion map and each thresholded (50%) pathway map using Matlab7.14/R2012a [94]. We used these continuous measures of white matter disconnections in the statistical track-wise lesion-deficit analyses based on linear regression. In the linear regression, we entered the lesion volume, age, and each individual pathway disconnection measure as independent variables to test whether the disconnection within specific pathways (controlling for age, injury type, and lesion location: left, right, or bilateral) predicts automatic self-reference deficits and/or control deficits (measures corresponding to the two components identified in the PCA analysis) as the dependent variable. The regression analyses were carried out separately for the left and right hemispheres. Each tract-wise lesion-deficit analysis was subjected to FDR correction. These significant effects survived FDR correction across all comparisons.

3. Results

3.1. Neuropsychological Profiles and the Self and Attentional Control Factors

The PCA yielded two components that accounted for 62% of the variance. The first component emerged from the orientation task and categorization task (automatic self-reference). The second component was associated with the cross task and rule-finding and -switching task (control processing). The two components showed a dissociation in functions between automatic self-reference and control processing. This was loaded on all variables and accounted for 62% of the variance. Factor loadings for principal component analysis using varimax rotation for the four tasks are shown in Figure 2.

3.2. Neuroimaging Findings: Grey Matter Damage

In the studied group of patients, the overall lesion distribution was within both hemispheres, encompassing both grey and white matter substrates and with maximum overlap within the right hemisphere, as presented in Figure 1. We subsequently assessed the neural correlates of deficits in the components of automatic self-reference and control processing identified in the PCA analysis, first employing VBM to explore the grey matter correlates of the two components. Grey matter lesions in the left ventral medial prefrontal cortex and inferior temporal gyrus were associated with the automatic self-reference component (corresponding to hypo self-bias deficits; Table 1 and Figure 3a), while grey matter lesions in the bilateral inferior parietal lobule and the left anterior insular cortex were associated with the deficits in the control component (Table 1 and Figure 3b).

Table 1. Grey matter substrates of automatic self-reference and control processing components as identified in the VBM analysis.

Factor	Size (Voxels)	Z-Score	Coordinates (X, Y, Z)	Brain Structure
Automatic self-reference				
	1384	3.44	34 26 −42	Right ITG [1]
	50	3.41	−10 50 4	Left vmPFC [2]
Control processing				
	405	3.93	44 −46 62	Right IPL [3]
	275	3.74	−28 −66 52	Left IPL [3]
	343	3.39	−46 −10 4	Left AIC [4]

[1] ITG = inferior frontal gyrus. [2] vmPFC = ventral medial prefrontal cortex. [3] IPL = inferior parietal lobule. [4] AIC = anterior insular cortex.

3.3. Neuroimaging Findings: White Matter Disconnections

The patterns of white matter disconnections in the studied group of patients are depicted in Figure 4. To identify the contribution of white matter disconnections to deficits of automatic self-reference or control processing deficits, linear regression analysis was performed for each whiter matter pathway. The analyses revealed that disconnection in the right IFOF predicted deficits in the automatic self-reference component, $F(5, 24) = 4.018$, $p = 0.009$, with an R^2 of 0.456 (right IFOF: $b = 0.452$; $p = 0.036$; lesion location: $b = 0.399$; $p = 0.031$; Figure 4b, upper panel, and Figure 5a), while the left hemispheric white matter disconnections contributed specifically to the control processing deficit, $F (5, 24) = 3.062$, $p = 0.028$, with an R^2 of 0.389 (left SLFII, SLFIII, and arcuate: $b = 0.443$; $p = 0.037$; lesion location: $b = 0.413$; $p = 0.034$; Figure 4b, bottom panel, and Figure 5b). The effects for other white matter pathways failed to show any reliable results after FDR correction. These regression analyses indicate that asymmetrical white matter disconnections predicted impairment in automatic self-reference and control processing (see Figures 4b and 5).

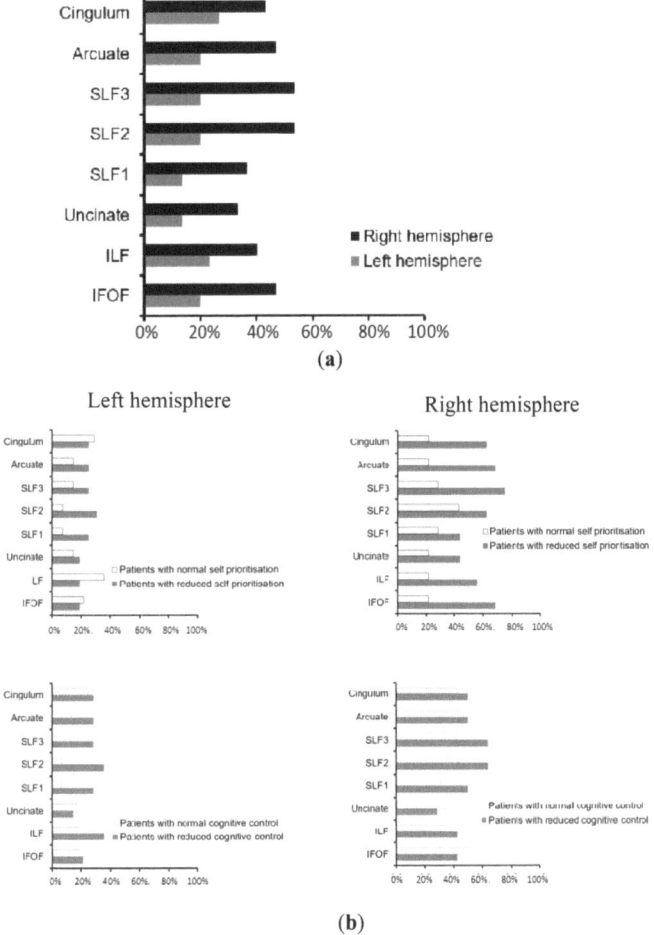

Figure 4. Tract-wise lesion deficits: (a). Percentage of patients with disconnection in the eight examined association, commissural, and projection white matter pathways within the left versus right hemisphere, plotted across the entire group of patients. (b). Percentage of patients with disconnection in the eight examined association, commissural, and projection white matter pathways within the left versus right hemisphere, calculated for groups with and without deficits in automatic self-reference and control processing (classified based on norms from healthy control participants. Note: We cannot directly classify patients with or without deficits based on the scores for the two components derived from PCA analysis). As indicated in the Methods section, the tract-wise lesion deficits include eight pathways within both the left and the right hemisphere (cingulum; arcuate; SLFI, II, III, 3 branches of the superior longitudinal fasciculus; uncinate; ILF, inferior longitudinal fasciculus; IFOF, inferior frontal occipital fasciculus).

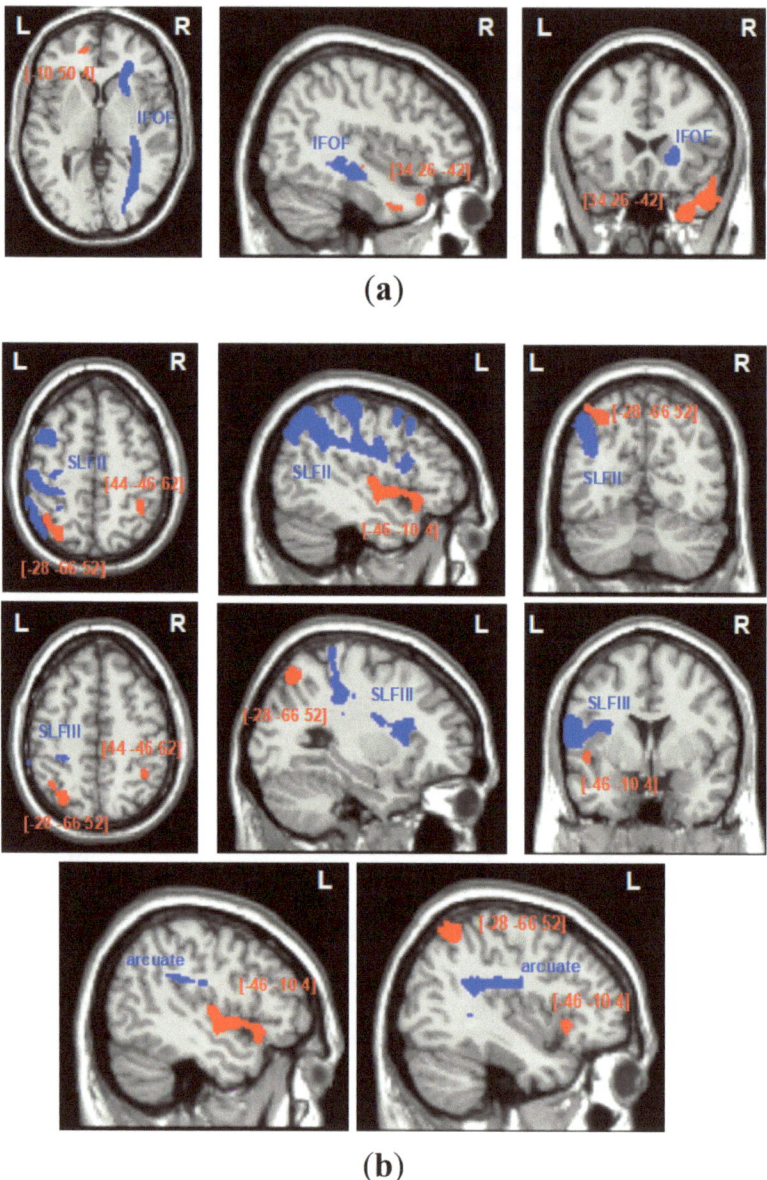

Figure 5. Tract-wise lesion deficits: the trajectories of white matter pathways (blue) presented in relation to cortical substrates for automatic self-reference (**a**) and control components (**b**), as identified in VBM analysis (red). The white matter pathways (IFOF, inferior frontal occipital fasciculus; SLF II, III, second and third branch of the superior longitudinal fasciculus; arcuate) are plotted as thresholded (50%) binary maps from the DTI tractography atlas of human white matter tracts [101,102], and the VBM results are presented as binary statistical maps thresholded at the significance level of $p < 0.005$.

4. Discussion

The PCA across four cognitive tasks revealed two distinct components accounting for the dynamics of the SPE, relating to automatic and control processing. This dichotomy, explaining approximately 2/3 of the variance in self-bias, elucidates the pivotal roles of automatic and controlled processes for the SPE. Neuroimaging analyses revealed the causal neural mechanisms underlying these functions—reduced grey matter in the vmPFC and right inferior temporal gyrus was associated with automatic self-reference processing deficits. This was compounded by disconnection of the right IFOF. In contrast, lesions in the bilateral dorsal parietal cortex and left inferior frontal cortex, alongside white matter damage in the left arcuate, SLF II, and SLF III fasciculus, were linked to decreased control functions. Such a dissociation between the ventral prefrontal–temporal network and the dorsal fronto-parietal control network is consistent with their roles in mediating automatic versus controlled self-reference processing.

We identified fundamental but distinct roles of the ventral prefrontal–temporal and dorsal bilatirial fronto-parietal networks in the SPE, supporting the SAN model. Our causal evaluation showed the critical functions of the vmPFC, right inferior temporal gyrus (ITG), and right IFOF in automatic self-reference processing for self-bias. These results were partially consistent with previous evidence that damage to the right inferior temporal and right IFOF disconnection reduced the SPE [52]. However, the role of vmPFC was newly revealed. These results likely stem from our cross task approach capturing this region's broader self-reference functions. Indeed, capturing robust latent variables across multiple task contexts, enabled by our PAC approach, may be critical for fully understanding the contributions of key nodes like vmPFC and connectivity to self-reference in stroke patients typically with bilateral hemisphere lesions (Figure 1). Specifically, the vmPFC constitutes a core "ventral self" network prominently engaged in many self-reference tasks [56,57]. The function of this region in self-processing is well documented, spanning from basic matching tasks to trait evaluation [63–65]. Our causal lesion evidence extends these findings, suggesting that the vmPFC may serve as a fundamental driver of automatic self-reference processing, operating independently of specific task demands [103–107].

The role of the vmPFC and the right ITG in automatic self-reference processing may have implications for understanding alterations in self-concept in various neuropsychiatric conditions. Disfunction of the prefrontal cortex, including the vmPFC, has been identified in major depressive disorder [108–110]. Recent research also reported that the right ITG might serve as a potential biomarker for major depressive disorder in individuals with childhood sexual abuse [111]. The evidence underlies the potential link between disrupted self-processing and the manifestation of depressive symptoms. Liu and colleagues provided evidence for this relationship, demonstrating that alterations in the SPE, as measured by matching tasks related to self- and emotion-processing, can predict the onset of depressive episodes in pre-clinical participants [112]. Critically, these tasks recruit the vmPFC and pSTS as central nodes in modulating the SPE [63]. This predictive ability of altered SPE indicates that subtle changes in automatic self-processing may serve as early indicators for the development of depressive symptoms. On the other hand, patients with brain disorders who retained vmPFC and SPE functionality can harness these aspects of maintained automatic self-processing to enhance cognitive performance, such as attention in patients with neglect [113].

Moreover, it has been shown that the dorsal fronto-parietal network plays a key role in regulating the SPE [63,73,78,114,115]. The current study indicated that control processing is mediated by the bilateral dorsal parietal context and left inferior frontal areas, aligning with our previous findings in specific tasks where patients with lesions to the left hemisphere, including the superior parietal lobe, cingulate gyrus, and prefrontal cortex, produced a hyper self-bias [51,52]. Critically, we found that this control function among these cortical regions may be mediated through white matter pathways, including the arcuate and superior longitudinal fasciculus. The current finding provides new evidence that the dynamic integration of automatic and control self-reference processes relies on the intricate white matter architecture linking the frontal and parietal regions, extending recent functional connectivity insights into the white matter pathways [116–119].

Our findings have several implications for theoretical models of social cognition and clinical practice. First, they provide empirical validation for the SAN account for self-prioritization, which posits a dynamic interaction between ventral self and dorsal control networks [38,40]. This interaction is crucial for understanding the relationship between the neural basis of adaptive self-reference processing and control functions in everyday situations. Second, the elucidation of the roles of specific white matter pathways in modulating self-bias opens new avenues for research into the structural and functional connectivity of the brain and how disconnections of white matter pathways produce social cognitive deficits. Importantly, understanding how disruptions in white matter pathways contribute to social cognitive deficits invites further exploration to reveal the underlying mechanisms. Third, the identification of causal neural substrates associated with deficits in self-reference and control processing post-stroke or brain injury could inform targeted therapeutic interventions to rehabilitate these cognitive and social cognitive impairments, given the potential compensatory role of these functions. It has been reported that self-association approaches can be used to enhance neuropsychological patients' memory and attention performance [113,120]. Techniques such as TMS and tDCS could be invaluable for revealing the complex neural dynamics that govern automatic and control facets of self-reference processing for neural rehabilitation [74,121].

In conclusion, our multiple-task, function lesion-mapping approach delineated the complementary ventral self and dorsal control networks mediating automatic versus regulated components of self-prioritization via their distributed grey and white matter substrates. These causal evaluations shed lights on neurobiological models of self-reference and inform therapeutic efforts for social cognitive impairments.

Supplementary Materials: The following supporting information can be downloaded at: https://www.mdpi.com/article/10.3390/jcm13144170/s1, Table S1: Self-prioritisation scores in the face tasks and the rule finding scores in the Birmingham frontal task in patients.

Author Contributions: Conceptualization, J.S.; Methodology, P.R. and Z.L.; Formal analysis, J.S. and M.C.; Investigation, J.S.; Writing—original draft, J.S.; Writing—review & editing, J.S., P.R., Z.L. and M.C.; Funding acquisition, J.S. All authors have read and agreed to the published version of the manuscript.

Funding: This research was funded by a Royal Society Newton Fellowship and an ESRC research grant (ES/J001597/1).

Institutional Review Board Statement: The study was conducted in accordance with the Declaration of Helsinki and approved by the Institutional Review Board of the University of Birmingham (protocol code ERN_11_0429 and approved in 2011).

Informed Consent Statement: Informed consent was obtained from all subjects involved in the study.

Data Availability Statement: The data presented in this study are available on request from the corresponding author. The data are not publicly available due to ongoing analyses for further investigation.

Conflicts of Interest: The authors declare no conflict of interest.

References

1. McGuire, W.J.; McGuire, C.V.; Cheever, J. The Self in Society: Effects of Social Contexts on the Sense of Self. *Br. J. Soc. Psychol.* **1986**, *25*, 259–270. [CrossRef] [PubMed]
2. Churchland, P.S. Self-Representation in Nervous Systems. *Science* **2002**, *296*, 308–310. [CrossRef] [PubMed]
3. Gallagher, S. Philosophical Conceptions of the Self: Implications for Cognitive Science. *Trends Cogn. Sci.* **2000**, *4*, 14–21. [CrossRef] [PubMed]
4. Zhu, Y.; Zhang, L. An Experimental Study on the Self-Reference Effect. *Sci. China C Life Sci.* **2002**, *45*, 120–128. [CrossRef] [PubMed]
5. Lichtenberg, J.D. The Development of the Sense of Self. *J. Am. Psychoanal. Assoc.* **1975**, *23*, 453–484. [CrossRef] [PubMed]
6. Conway, M.A.; Pleydell-Pearce, C.W. The Construction of Autobiographical Memories in the Self-Memory System. *Psychol. Rev.* **2000**, *107*, 261. [CrossRef]
7. Sui, J.; Humphreys, G.W. The Ubiquitous Self: What the Properties of Self-bias Tell Us about the Self. *Ann. N. Y. Acad. Sci.* **2017**, *1396*, 222–235. [CrossRef]

8. Desebrock, C.; Spence, C. The Self-Prioritization Effect: Self-Referential Processing in Movement Highlights Modulation at Multiple Stages. *Atten. Percept. Psychophys.* **2021**, *83*, 2656–2674. [CrossRef]
9. Singh, D.; Karnick, H. Self-Prioritization Effect in Children and Adults. *Front. Psychol.* **2022**, *13*, 726230. [CrossRef]
10. Palmero, L.B.; Martínez-Pérez, V.; Tortajada, M.; Campoy, G.; Fuentes, L.J. Testing the Modulation of Self-Related Automatic and Others-Related Controlled Processing by Chronotype and Time-of-Day. *Conscious. Cogn.* **2024**, *118*, 103633. [CrossRef]
11. Apps, M.A.J.; Tsakiris, M. The Free-Energy Self: A Predictive Coding Account of Self-Recognition. *Neurosci. Biobehav. Rev.* **2014**, *41*, 85–97. [CrossRef] [PubMed]
12. Cunningham, S.J.; Turk, D.J.; Macdonald, L.M.; Macrae, C.N. Yours or Mine? Ownership and Memory. *Conscious. Cogn.* **2008**, *17*, 312–318. [CrossRef]
13. Golubickis, M.; Macrae, C.N. That's Me in the Spotlight: Self-Relevance Modulates Attentional Breadth. *Psychon. Bull. Rev.* **2021**, *28*, 1915–1922. [CrossRef] [PubMed]
14. Woźniak, M.; Knoblich, G. Self-Prioritization of Fully Unfamiliar Stimuli. *Q. J. Exp. Psychol.* **2019**, *72*, 2110–2120. [CrossRef]
15. Woźniak, M.; Knoblich, G. Self-Prioritization Depends on Assumed Task-Relevance of Self-Association. *Psychol. Res.* **2022**, *86*, 1599–1614. [CrossRef] [PubMed]
16. Sui, J.; He, X.; Humphreys, G.W. Perceptual Effects of Social Salience: Evidence from Self-Prioritization Effects on Perceptual Matching. *J. Exp. Psychol. Hum. Percept. Perform.* **2012**, *38*, 1105. [CrossRef] [PubMed]
17. Sui, J.; Humphreys, G.W. Aging Enhances Cognitive Biases to Friends but Not the Self. *Psychon. Bull. Rev.* **2017**, *24*, 2021–2030. [CrossRef]
18. Sun, Y.; Fuentes, L.J.; Humphreys, G.W.; Sui, J. Try to See It My Way: Embodied Perspective Enhances Self and Friend-Biases in Perceptual Matching. *Cognition* **2016**, *153*, 108–117. [CrossRef]
19. Sui, J.; Cao, B.; Song, Y.; Greenshaw, A.J. Individual Differences in Self-and Value-Based Reward Processing. *Curr. Res. Behav. Sci.* **2023**, *4*, 100095. [CrossRef]
20. Żochowska, A.; Jakuszyk, P.; Nowicka, M.M.; Nowicka, A. The Self and a Close-Other: Differences between Processing of Faces and Newly Acquired Information. *Cereb. Cortex* **2023**, *33*, 2183–2199. [CrossRef]
21. Schäfer, S.; Frings, C. Understanding Self-Prioritisation: The Prioritisation of Self-Relevant Stimuli and Its Relation to the Individual Self-Esteem. *J. Cogn. Psychol.* **2019**, *31*, 813–824. [CrossRef]
22. Golubickis, M.; Persson, L.M.; Falbén, J.K.; Macrae, C.N. On Stopping Yourself: Self-Relevance Facilitates Response Inhibition. *Atten. Percept. Psychophys.* **2021**, *83*, 1416–1423. [CrossRef] [PubMed]
23. Martínez-Pérez, V.; Sandoval-Lentisco, A.; Tortajada, M.; Palmero, L.B.; Campoy, G.; Fuentes, L.J. Self-Prioritization Effect in the Attentional Blink Paradigm: Attention-Based or Familiarity-Based Effect? *Conscious. Cogn.* **2024**, *117*, 103607. [CrossRef] [PubMed]
24. Conty, L.; George, N.; Hietanen, J.K. Watching Eyes Effects: When Others Meet the Self. *Conscious. Cogn.* **2016**, *45*, 184–197. [CrossRef] [PubMed]
25. Renninger, K.A.; Hidi, S.E. Interest Development, Self-Related Information Processing, and Practice. *Theory Pract.* **2022**, *61*, 23–34. [CrossRef]
26. Tacikowski, P.; Weijs, M.L.; Ehrsson, H.H. Perception of Our Own Body Influences Self-Concept and Self-Incoherence Impairs Episodic Memory. *Iscience* **2020**, *23*, 101429. [CrossRef]
27. Keil, J.; Barutchu, A.; Desebrock, C.; Spence, C. More of Me: Self-Prioritization of Numeric Stimuli. *J. Exp. Psychol. Hum. Percept. Perform.* **2023**, *49*, 1518–1533. [CrossRef]
28. Roy, N.; Karnick, H.; Verma, A. Towards the Self and Away from the Others: Evidence for Self-Prioritization Observed in an Approach Avoidance Task. *Front. Psychol.* **2023**, *14*, 1041157. [CrossRef]
29. Bogdanova, O.V.; Bogdanov, V.B.; Dureux, A.; Farne, A.; Hadj-Bouziane, F. The Peripersonal Space in a Social World. *Cortex* **2021**, *142*, 28–46. [CrossRef]
30. Blanke, O.; Slater, M.; Serino, A. Behavioral, Neural, and Computational Principles of Bodily Self-Consciousness. *Neuron* **2015**, *88*, 145–166. [CrossRef]
31. Serino, A.; Alsmith, A.; Costantini, M.; Mandrigin, A.; Tajadura-Jimenez, A.; Lopez, C. Bodily Ownership and Self-Location: Components of Bodily Self-Consciousness. *Conscious. Cogn.* **2013**, *22*, 1239–1252. [CrossRef] [PubMed]
32. Symons, C.S.; Johnson, B.T. The Self-Reference Effect in Memory: A Meta-Analysis. *Psychol. Bull.* **1997**, *121*, 371. [CrossRef] [PubMed]
33. Liu, M.; He, X.; Rotshtein, P.; Sui, J. Dynamically Orienting Your Own Face Facilitates the Automatic Attraction of Attention. *Cogn. Neurosci.* **2016**, *7*, 37–44. [CrossRef] [PubMed]
34. Sui, J.; Sun, Y.; Peng, K.; Humphreys, G.W. The Automatic and the Expected Self: Separating Self- and Familiarity Biases Effects by Manipulating Stimulus Probability. *Atten. Percept. Psychophys.* **2014**, *76*, 1176–1184. [CrossRef] [PubMed]
35. Northoff, G. How Does the 'Rest-Self Overlap' Mediate the Qualitative and Automatic Features of Self-Reference? *Cogn. Neurosci.* **2016**, *7*, 18–20. [CrossRef] [PubMed]
36. Herbert, C.; Pauli, P.; Herbert, B.M. Self-Reference Modulates the Processing of Emotional Stimuli in the Absence of Explicit Self-Referential Appraisal Instructions. *Soc. Cogn. Affect. Neurosci.* **2011**, *6*, 653–661. [CrossRef] [PubMed]

37. Soares, A.P.; Macedo, J.; Oliveira, H.M.; Lages, A.; Hernández-Cabrera, J.; Pinheiro, A.P. Self-Reference Is a Fast-Acting Automatic Mechanism on Emotional Word Processing: Evidence from a Masked Priming Affective Categorisation Task. *J. Cogn. Psychol.* **2019**, *31*, 317–325. [CrossRef]
38. Humphreys, G.W.; Sui, J. Attentional Control and the Self: The Self-Attention Network (SAN). *Cogn. Neurosci.* **2016**, *7*, 5–17. [CrossRef]
39. Sui, J.; Gu, X. Self as Object: Emerging Trends in Self Research. *Trends Neurosci.* **2017**, *40*, 643–653. [CrossRef]
40. Sui, J.; Rotshtein, P. Self-Prioritization and the Attentional Systems. *Curr. Opin. Psychol.* **2019**, *29*, 148–152. [CrossRef]
41. Scalabrini, A.; Mucci, C.; Northoff, G. Is Our Self Related to Personality? A Neuropsychodynamic Model. *Front. Hum. Neurosci.* **2018**, *12*, 346. [CrossRef] [PubMed]
42. Lockwood, P.L.; Wittmann, M.K.; Apps, M.A.; Klein-Flügge, M.C.; Crockett, M.J.; Humphreys, G.W.; Rushworth, M.F. Neural Mechanisms for Learning Self and Other Ownership. *Nat. Commun.* **2018**, *9*, 4747. [CrossRef] [PubMed]
43. Qin, P.; Wang, M.; Northoff, G. Linking Bodily, Environmental and Mental States in the Self—A Three-Level Model Based on a Meta-Analysis. *Neurosci. Biobehav. Rev.* **2020**, *115*, 77–95. [CrossRef] [PubMed]
44. Soch, J.; Deserno, L.; Assmann, A.; Barman, A.; Walter, H.; Richardson-Klavehn, A.; Schott, B.H. Inhibition of Information Flow to the Default Mode Network during Self-Reference versus Reference to Others. *Cereb. Cortex* **2017**, *27*, 3930–3942. [CrossRef] [PubMed]
45. Schmitz, T.W.; Johnson, S.C. Self-Appraisal Decisions Evoke Dissociated Dorsal—Ventral aMPFC Networks. *Neuroimage* **2006**, *30*, 1050–1058. [CrossRef] [PubMed]
46. Yaoi, K.; Osaka, M.; Osaka, N. Neural Correlates of the Self-Reference Effect: Evidence from Evaluation and Recognition Processes. *Front. Hum. Neurosci.* **2015**, *9*, 383. [CrossRef] [PubMed]
47. Haciahmet, C.C.; Golubickis, M.; Schäfer, S.; Frings, C.; Pastötter, B. The Oscillatory Fingerprints of Self-prioritization: Novel Markers in Spectral EEG for Self-relevant Processing. *Psychophysiology* **2023**, *60*, e14396. [CrossRef] [PubMed]
48. Davey, C.G.; Pujol, J.; Harrison, B.J. Mapping the Self in the Brain's Default Mode Network. *NeuroImage* **2016**, *132*, 390–397. [CrossRef] [PubMed]
49. Damme, K.S.; Pelletier-Baldelli, A.; Cowan, H.R.; Orr, J.M.; Mittal, V.A. Distinct and Opposite Profiles of Connectivity during Self-Reference Task and Rest in Youth at Clinical High Risk for Psychosis. *Hum. Brain Mapp.* **2019**, *40*, 3254–3264. [CrossRef]
50. Gaubert, M.; Villain, N.; Landeau, B.; Mezenge, F.; Egret, S.; Perrotin, A.; Belliard, S.; de La Sayette, V.; Eustache, F.; Desgranges, B. Neural Correlates of Self-Reference Effect in Early Alzheimer's Disease. *J. Alzheimers Dis.* **2017**, *56*, 717–731. [CrossRef]
51. Sui, J.; Chechlacz, M.; Humphreys, G.W. Dividing the Self: Distinct Neural Substrates of Task-Based and Automatic Self-Prioritization after Brain Damage. *Cognition* **2012**, *122*, 150–162. [CrossRef] [PubMed]
52. Sui, J.; Chechlacz, M.; Rotshtein, P.; Humphreys, G.W. Lesion-Symptom Mapping of Self-Prioritization in Explicit Face Categorization: Distinguishing Hypo-and Hyper-Self-Biases. *Cereb. Cortex* **2015**, *25*, 374–383. [CrossRef] [PubMed]
53. Lu, Z.; He, X.; Yi, D.; Sui, J. Temporal Properties of Self-Prioritization. *Entropy* **2024**, *26*, 242. [CrossRef]
54. Sui, J.; He, X.; Golubickis, M.; Svensson, S.L.; Macrae, C.N. Electrophysiological Correlates of Self-Prioritization. *Conscious. Cogn.* **2023**, *108*, 103475. [CrossRef]
55. Frewen, P.; Schroeter, M.L.; Riva, G.; Cipresso, P.; Fairfield, B.; Padulo, C.; Kemp, A.H.; Palaniyappan, L.; Owolabi, M.; Kusi-Mensah, K. Neuroimaging the Consciousness of Self: Review, and Conceptual-Methodological Framework. *Neurosci. Biobehav. Rev.* **2020**, *112*, 164–212. [CrossRef]
56. Northoff, G.; Heinzel, A.; De Greck, M.; Bermpohl, F.; Dobrowolny, H.; Panksepp, J. Self-Referential Processing in Our Brain—A Meta-Analysis of Imaging Studies on the Self. *Neuroimage* **2006**, *31*, 440–457. [CrossRef]
57. Murray, R.J.; Schaer, M.; Debbané, M. Degrees of Separation: A Quantitative Neuroimaging Meta-Analysis Investigating Self-Specificity and Shared Neural Activation between Self- and Other-Reflection. *Neurosci. Biobehav. Rev.* **2012**, *36*, 1043–1059. [CrossRef]
58. D'Argembeau, A.; Collette, F.; Van der Linden, M.; Laureys, S.; Del Fiore, G.; Degueldre, C.; Luxen, A.; Salmon, E. Self-Referential Reflective Activity and Its Relationship with Rest: A PET Study. *Neuroimage* **2005**, *25*, 616–624. [CrossRef] [PubMed]
59. Qin, P.; Northoff, G. How Is Our Self Related to Midline Regions and the Default-Mode Network? *NeuroImage* **2011**, *57*, 1221–1233. [CrossRef]
60. Whitfield-Gabrieli, S.; Moran, J.M.; Nieto-Castañón, A.; Triantafyllou, C.; Saxe, R.; Gabrieli, J.D. Associations and Dissociations between Default and Self-Reference Networks in the Human Brain. *Neuroimage* **2011**, *55*, 225–232. [CrossRef]
61. Kolvoort, I.R.; Wainio-Theberge, S.; Wolff, A.; Northoff, G. Temporal Integration as "Common Currency" of Brain and Self-Scale-free Activity in Resting-state EEG Correlates with Temporal Delay Effects on Self-relatedness. *Hum. Brain Mapp.* **2020**, *41*, 4355–4374. [CrossRef] [PubMed]
62. Wolff, A.; Di Giovanni, D.A.; Gómez-Pilar, J.; Nakao, T.; Huang, Z.; Longtin, A.; Northoff, G. The Temporal Signature of Self: Temporal Measures of Resting-state EEG Predict Self-consciousness. *Hum. Brain Mapp.* **2019**, *40*, 789–803. [CrossRef] [PubMed]
63. Sui, J.; Rotshtein, P.; Humphreys, G.W. Coupling Social Attention to the Self Forms a Network for Personal Significance. *Proc. Natl. Acad. Sci. USA* **2013**, *110*, 7607–7612. [CrossRef] [PubMed]
64. Northoff, G.; Bermpohl, F. Cortical Midline Structures and the Self. *Trends Cogn. Sci.* **2004**, *8*, 102–107. [CrossRef] [PubMed]
65. Chavez, R.S.; Heatherton, T.F.; Wagner, D.D. Neural Population Decoding Reveals the Intrinsic Positivity of the Self. *Cereb. Cortex* **2017**, *27*, 5222–5229. [CrossRef] [PubMed]

66. Heleven, E.; Van Overwalle, F. The Neural Representation of the Self in Relation to Close Others Using fMRI Repetition Suppression. *Soc. Neurosci.* **2019**, *14*, 717–728. [CrossRef] [PubMed]
67. D'Argembeau, A. On the Role of the Ventromedial Prefrontal Cortex in Self-Processing: The Valuation Hypothesis. *Front. Hum. Neurosci.* **2013**, *7*, 372. [CrossRef]
68. Samson, D.; Apperly, I.A.; Chiavarino, C.; Humphreys, G.W. Left Temporoparietal Junction Is Necessary for Representing Someone Else's Belief. *Nat. Neurosci.* **2004**, *7*, 499–500. [CrossRef] [PubMed]
69. Smith, E.; Xiao, Y.; Xie, H.; Manwaring, S.S.; Farmer, C.; Thompson, L.; D'Souza, P.; Thurm, A.; Redcay, E. Posterior Superior Temporal Cortex Connectivity Is Related to Social Communication in Toddlers. *Infant Behav. Dev.* **2023**, *71*, 101831. [CrossRef]
70. Martínez-Pérez, V.; Campoy, G.; Palmero, L.B.; Fuentes, L.J. Examining the Dorsolateral and Ventromedial Prefrontal Cortex Involvement in the Self-Attention Network: A Randomized, Sham-Controlled, Parallel Group, Double-Blind, and Multichannel HD-tDCS Study. *Front. Neurosci.* **2020**, *14*, 683. [CrossRef]
71. Leszkowicz, E.; Maio, G.R.; Linden, D.E.J.; Ihssen, N. Neural Coding of Human Values Is Underpinned by Brain Areas Representing the Core Self in the Cortical Midline Region. *Soc. Neurosci.* **2021**, *16*, 486–499. [CrossRef] [PubMed]
72. Isoda, M. The Role of the Medial Prefrontal Cortex in Moderating Neural Representations of Self and Other in Primates. *Annu. Rev. Neurosci.* **2021**, *44*, 295–313. [CrossRef] [PubMed]
73. Sui, J.; Liu, M.; Mevorach, C.; Humphreys, G.W. The Salient Self: The Left Intraparietal Sulcus Responds to Social as Well as Perceptual-Salience after Self-Association. *Cereb. Cortex* **2015**, *25*, 1060–1068. [CrossRef] [PubMed]
74. Yin, S.; Bi, T.; Chen, A.; Egner, T. Ventromedial Prefrontal Cortex Drives the Prioritization of Self-Associated Stimuli in Working Memory. *J. Neurosci.* **2021**, *41*, 2012–2023. [CrossRef] [PubMed]
75. Schäfer, S.; Frings, C. Searching for the Inner Self: Evidence against a Direct Dependence of the Self-Prioritization Effect on the Ventro-Medial Prefrontal Cortex. *Exp. Brain Res.* **2019**, *237*, 247–256. [CrossRef]
76. Liang, Q.; Zhang, B.; Fu, S.; Sui, J.; Wang, F. The Roles of the LpSTS and DLPFC in Self-prioritization: A Transcranial Magnetic Stimulation Study. *Hum. Brain Mapp.* **2022**, *43*, 1381–1393. [CrossRef] [PubMed]
77. Soutschek, A.; Ruff, C.C.; Strombach, T.; Kalenscher, T.; Tobler, P.N. Brain Stimulation Reveals Crucial Role of Overcoming Self-Centeredness in Self-Control. *Sci. Adv.* **2016**, *2*, e1600992. [CrossRef] [PubMed]
78. Sui, J.; Enock, F.; Ralph, J.; Humphreys, G.W. Dissociating Hyper and Hypoself Biases to a Core Self-Representation. *Cortex* **2015**, *70*, 202–212. [CrossRef] [PubMed]
79. Abdi, H.; Williams, L.J. Principal Component Analysis. *WIREs Comput. Stat.* **2010**, *2*, 433–459. [CrossRef]
80. Bickerton, W.-L.; Riddoch, M.J.; Samson, D.; Balani, A.B.; Mistry, B.; Humphreys, G.W. Systematic Assessment of Apraxia and Functional Predictions from the Birmingham Cognitive Screen. *J. Neurol. Neurosurg. Psychiatry* **2012**, *83*, 513–521. [CrossRef]
81. Ashburner, J.; Friston, K.J. Unified Segmentation. *NeuroImage* **2005**, *26*, 839–851. [CrossRef] [PubMed]
82. Thiebaut de Schotten, M.; Tomaiuolo, F.; Aiello, M.; Merola, S.; Silvetti, M.; Lecce, F.; Bartolomeo, P.; Doricchi, F. Damage to White Matter Pathways in Subacute and Chronic Spatial Neglect: A Group Study and 2 Single-Case Studies with Complete Virtual "in Vivo" Tractography Dissection. *Cereb. Cortex* **2014**, *24*, 691–706. [CrossRef] [PubMed]
83. Seghier, M.L.; Ramlackhansingh, A.; Crinion, J.; Leff, A.P.; Price, C.J. Lesion Identification Using Unified Segmentation-Normalisation Models and Fuzzy Clustering. *NeuroImage* **2008**, *41*, 1253–1266. [CrossRef]
84. Humphreys, G.W. *BCoS Brain Behaviour Analysis*; Psychology Press: Hove, UK, 2012.
85. Fabrigar, L.R.; Wegener, D.T.; MacCallum, R.C.; Strahan, E.J. Evaluating the Use of Exploratory Factor Analysis in Psychological Research. *Psychol. Methods* **1999**, *4*, 272–299. [CrossRef]
86. Kim, J.-O.; Mueller, C.W. *Factor Analysis: Statistical Methods and Practical Issues*; SAGE: Beverly Hills, CA, USA, 1978; ISBN 978-0-8039-1166-6.
87. Bartlett, M.S.; Fowler, R.H. Properties of Sufficiency and Statistical Tests. *Proc. R. Soc. Lond. Ser.-Math. Phys. Sci.* **1997**, *160*, 268–282. [CrossRef]
88. Kaiser, H.F.; Rice, J. Little Jiffy, Mark Iv. *Educ. Psychol. Meas.* **1974**, *34*, 111–117. [CrossRef]
89. Crinion, J.; Ashburner, J.; Leff, A.; Brett, M.; Price, C.; Friston, K. Spatial Normalization of Lesioned Brains: Performance Evaluation and Impact on fMRI Analyses. *NeuroImage* **2007**, *37*, 866–875. [CrossRef]
90. Worsley, K.J. Developments in Random Field Theory. *Hum. Brain Funct.* **2003**, *2*, 881–886.
91. Leff, A.P.; Schofield, T.M.; Crinion, J.T.; Seghier, M.L.; Grogan, A.; Green, D.W.; Price, C.J. The Left Superior Temporal Gyrus Is a Shared Substrate for Auditory Short-Term Memory and Speech Comprehension: Evidence from 210 Patients with Stroke. *Brain* **2009**, *132*, 3401–3410. [CrossRef]
92. Chechlacz, M.; Terry, A.; Demeyere, N.; Douis, H.; Bickerton, W.-L.; Rotshtein, P.; Humphreys, G.W. Common and Distinct Neural Mechanisms of Visual and Tactile Extinction: A Large Scale VBM Study in Sub-Acute Stroke. *NeuroImage Clin.* **2013**, *2*, 291–302. [CrossRef]
93. Chechlacz, M.; Rotshtein, P.; Bickerton, W.-L.; Hansen, P.C.; Deb, S.; Humphreys, G.W. Separating Neural Correlates of Allocentric and Egocentric Neglect: Distinct Cortical Sites and Common White Matter Disconnections. *Cogn. Neuropsychol.* **2010**, *27*, 277–303. [CrossRef]
94. The MathWorks Inc. *MATLAB*, Version: 7.14.0 (R2012a); The MathWorks Inc.: Natick, MA, USA, 2012. Available online: https://www.mathworks.com (accessed on 28 May 2024).
95. Ashburner, J.; Friston, K.J. Voxel-Based Morphometry—The Methods. *Neuroimage* **2000**, *11*, 805–821. [CrossRef]

96. Kiebel, S.; Holmes, A. *The General Linear Model*; Elsevier: Amsterdam, The Netherlands, 2007; Chapter 8.
97. Duvernoy, H.M. *The Human Brain: Surface, Three-Dimensional Sectional Anatomy with MRI, and Blood Supply*; Springer Science & Business Media: Vienna, Austria, 1999.
98. Tzourio-Mazoyer, N.; Landeau, B.; Papathanassiou, D.; Crivello, F.; Etard, O.; Delcroix, N.; Mazoyer, B.; Joliot, M. Automated Anatomical Labeling of Activations in SPM Using a Macroscopic Anatomical Parcellation of the MNI MRI Single-Subject Brain. *NeuroImage* **2002**, *15*, 273–289. [CrossRef]
99. Woolsey, T.A.; Hanaway, J.; Gado, M.H. *The Brain Atlas: A Visual Guide to the Human Central Nervous System*; John Wiley & Sons: Hoboken, NJ, USA, 2017.
100. Thiebaut de Schotten, M.; Ffytche, D.H.; Bizzi, A.; Dell'Acqua, F.; Allin, M.; Walshe, M.; Murray, R.; Williams, S.C.; Murphy, D.G.; Catani, M. Atlasing Location, Asymmetry and Inter-Subject Variability of White Matter Tracts in the Human Brain with MR Diffusion Tractography. *Neuroimage* **2010**, *54*, 49–59. [CrossRef] [PubMed]
101. de Schotten, M.T.; Dell'Acqua, F.; Forkel, S.J.; Simmons, A.; Vergani, F.; Murphy, D.G.M.; Catani, M. A Lateralized Brain Network for Visuospatial Attention. *Nat. Neurosci.* **2011**, *14*, 1245–1246. [CrossRef] [PubMed]
102. Rojkova, K.; Volle, E.; Urbanski, M.; Humbert, F.; Dell'Acqua, F.; de Schotten, M.T. Atlasing the frontal lobe connections and their variability due to age and education: A spherical deconvolution tractography study. *Brain Struct. Funct.* **2016**, *221*, 1751–1766. [CrossRef]
103. Sui, J. Self-Reference Acts as a Golden Thread in Binding. *Trends Cogn. Sci.* **2016**, *20*, 482–483. [CrossRef]
104. Sui, J.; Humphreys, G.W. The Integrative Self: How Self-Reference Integrates Perception and Memory. *Trends Cogn. Sci.* **2015**, *19*, 719–728. [CrossRef]
105. Stendardi, D.; Biscotto, F.; Bertossi, E.; Ciaramelli, E. Present and Future Self in Memory: The Role of vmPFC in the Self-Reference Effect. *Soc. Cogn. Affect. Neurosci.* **2021**, *16*, 1205–1213. [CrossRef]
106. Philippi, C.L.; Duff, M.C.; Denburg, N.L.; Tranel, D.; Rudrauf, D. Medial PFC Damage Abolishes the Self-Reference Effect. *J. Cogn. Neurosci.* **2012**, *24*, 475–481. [CrossRef]
107. Wagner, D.D.; Haxby, J.V.; Heatherton, T.F. The Representation of Self and Person Knowledge in the Medial Prefrontal Cortex. *WIREs Cogn. Sci.* **2012**, *3*, 451–470. [CrossRef]
108. Pizzagalli, D.A.; Roberts, A.C. Prefrontal Cortex and Depression. *Neuropsychopharmacology* **2022**, *47*, 225–246. [CrossRef]
109. George, M.S.; Ketter, T.A.; Post, R.M. Prefrontal Cortex Dysfunction in Clinical Depression. *Depression* **1994**, *2*, 59–72. [CrossRef]
110. Murray, E.A.; Wise, S.P.; Drevets, W.C. Localization of Dysfunction in Major Depressive Disorder: Prefrontal Cortex and Amygdala. *Biol. Psychiatry* **2011**, *69*, e43–e54. [CrossRef]
111. Liu, Y.; Gao, Y.; Li, M.; Qin, W.; Xie, Y.; Zhao, G.; Wang, Y.; Yang, C.; Zhang, B.; Jing, Y. Childhood Sexual Abuse Related to Brain Activity Abnormalities in Right Inferior Temporal Gyrus among Major Depressive Disorder. *Neurosci. Lett.* **2023**, *806*, 137196. [CrossRef]
112. Liu, Y.S.; Song, Y.; Lee, N.A.; Bennett, D.M.; Button, K.S.; Greenshaw, A.; Cao, B.; Sui, J. Depression Screening Using a Non-Verbal Self-Association Task: A Machine-Learning Based Pilot Study. *J. Affect. Disord.* **2022**, *310*, 87–95. [CrossRef]
113. Sui, J.; Humphreys, G.W. The Self Survives Extinction: Self-Association Biases Attention in Patients with Visual Extinction. *Cortex* **2017**, *95*, 248–256. [CrossRef]
114. Molnar-Szakacs, I.; Uddin, L.Q. Self-Processing and the Default Mode Network: Interactions with the Mirror Neuron System. *Front. Hum. Neurosci.* **2013**, *7*, 571. [CrossRef]
115. Knyazev, G. EEG Correlates of Self-Referential Processing. *Front. Hum. Neurosci.* **2013**, *7*, 264. [CrossRef]
116. Tian, Y.; Margulies, D.S.; Breakspear, M.; Zalesky, A. Topographic Organization of the Human Subcortex Unveiled with Functional Connectivity Gradients. *Nat. Neurosci.* **2020**, *23*, 1421–1432. [CrossRef]
117. Caverzasi, E.; Papinutto, N.; Amirbekian, B.; Berger, M.S.; Henry, R.G. Q-Ball of Inferior Fronto-Occipital Fasciculus and Beyond. *PLoS ONE* **2014**, *9*, e100274. [CrossRef]
118. Martino, J.; Brogna, C.; Robles, S.G.; Vergani, F.; Duffau, H. Anatomic Dissection of the Inferior Fronto-Occipital Fasciculus Revisited in the Lights of Brain Stimulation Data. *Cortex* **2010**, *46*, 691–699. [CrossRef]
119. Zhang, F.; Daducci, A.; He, Y.; Schiavi, S.; Seguin, C.; Smith, R.E.; Yeh, C.-H.; Zhao, T.; O'Donnell, L.J. Quantitative Mapping of the Brain's Structural Connectivity Using Diffusion MRI Tractography: A Review. *Neuroimage* **2022**, *249*, 118870. [CrossRef]
120. Sui, J.; Humphreys, G.W. Self-Referential Processing Is Distinct from Semantic Elaboration: Evidence from Long-Term Memory Effects in a Patient with Amnesia and Semantic Impairments. *Neuropsychologia* **2013**, *51*, 2663–2673. [CrossRef]
121. Zhang, Y.; Wang, F.; Sui, J. Decoding Individual Differences in Self-Prioritization from the Resting-State Functional Connectome. *NeuroImage* **2023**, *276*, 120205. [CrossRef]

Disclaimer/Publisher's Note: The statements, opinions and data contained in all publications are solely those of the individual author(s) and contributor(s) and not of MDPI and/or the editor(s). MDPI and/or the editor(s) disclaim responsibility for any injury to people or property resulting from any ideas, methods, instructions or products referred to in the content.

MDPI AG
Grosspeteranlage 5
4052 Basel
Switzerland
Tel.: +41 61 683 77 34

Journal of Clinical Medicine Editorial Office
E-mail: jcm@mdpi.com
www.mdpi.com/journal/jcm

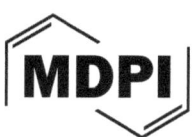

Disclaimer/Publisher's Note: The statements, opinions and data contained in all publications are solely those of the individual author(s) and contributor(s) and not of MDPI and/or the editor(s). MDPI and/or the editor(s) disclaim responsibility for any injury to people or property resulting from any ideas, methods, instructions or products referred to in the content.

www.ingramcontent.com/pod-product-compliance
Lightning Source LLC
LaVergne TN
LVHW072314090526
838202LV00019B/2284